Bone Biology, Harvesting, and Grafting for Dental Implants:
Rationale and Clinical Applications

BONE

Biology, Harvesting, & Grafting for Dental Implants

Rationale and Clinical Applications

Arun K. Garg, DMD

Professor of Surgery

Division of Oral and Maxillofacial Surgery

University of Miami School of Medicine

Miami, Florida

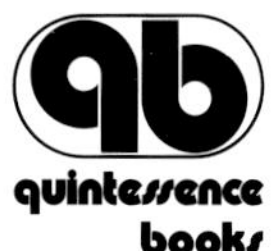

Quintessence Publishing Co, Inc

Chicago, Berlin, Tokyo, Copenhagen, London, Paris, Milan, Barcelona, Istanbul, São Paulo, New Delhi, Moscow, Prague, and Warsaw

Library of Congress Cataloging-in-Publication Data

Garg, Arun K., D.M.D.
Bone biology, harvesting, and grafting for dental implants : rationale and clinical applications / Arun K. Garg.
p. ; cm.
Includes bibliographical references and index.
ISBN 0-86715-441-1 (hardcover)
1. Dental implants. 2. Bone-grafting. 3. Bones--Physiology. I. Title.
[DNLM: 1. Dental Implantation--methods. 2. Bone Transplantation--methods. 3. Bone and Bones--physiology. WU 640 G231b 2004]
RK667.I45G375 2004
617.6'93--dc22

2004014770

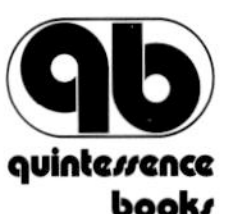

Quintessence Publishing Co, Inc
4350 Chandler Drive
Hanover Park, IL 60133
www.quintpub.com

Editors: Lisa C. Bywaters and Lindsay Harmon
Cover and internal design: Dawn Hartman
Production: Susan Robinson

Printed in China

Table of Contents

Part III: Bone Grafting

Part IV: Future Directions

Preface

For the past 10 years, many of the questions raised during my hands-on cadaver, live-surgery, and lecture programs have pertained to bone biology, graft materials, membranes, bone harvesting, or bone grafting. While it seems that most practitioners today have been adequately trained in the technical aspects of placing implants, I find that many lack knowledge of the basic biologic processes that allow us to harvest bone from one area of the mouth and graft it in another. Since the format of a short lecture or even a one-day course does not allow me to delve very far beyond the step-by-step procedures associated with harvesting and grafting bone, I conceived the idea of writing a book that would explain not only *how* to perform these and other procedures, but also *why* we do them one way and not another and what makes the procedures work. Above all, my aim in writing this book was to arm the clinician with a sufficient understanding of bone and bone grafting to be able to make decisions that will benefit individual patients, without overwhelming him or her with information that is not directly relevant to that purpose.

It is truly remarkable to consider how much implant dentistry has evolved over the past two decades. Today we are able to restore function in patients with as little as 1 mm of crestal bone height, providing they have adequate ridge width to accommodate the intended implant. This has significantly expanded the number of patients who qualify as candidates for implant therapy, but the clinician must be knowledgeable about the needs of these patients and how to meet them successfully. This book is designed to bridge that gap in knowledge. It begins with a broad overview of bone biology to refresh the reader's understanding of how bone develops at the microscopic level. This section also reviews graft materials and membrane barriers and recommends the situations and types of defects for which these materials are best suited. A section on bone harvesting describes surgical techniques and potential complications of harvesting bone grafts from the ramus, the anterior mandible, and the tibia. This is followed by a section on bone grafting for the maxillary sinus, anterior maxilla, and the subnasal area, including methods, materials, techniques, and postoperative considerations, all of them accompanied by numerous clinical photographs. Each procedure is described in the context of the biologic processes that it initiates so that the reader will understand not only how but also why it works. The book concludes with a look at the growth factors that are currently available and those being investigated for possible future applications in bone grafting for dental implants. It is my hope that this book will provide the profession with a comprehensive yet concise resource for understanding and providing care to patients who can benefit from bone harvesting and grafting.

This book is intended primarily for the advanced clinician in periodontics and oral and maxillofacial surgery who desires a comprehensive and clinically relevant review of both the background science and clinical applications of bone for dental implants. The book will also be useful for graduate students in oral and maxillofacial surgery, periodontics, and hospital dentistry residency training programs and for the academic surgeon with an interest in this important subject.

As I complete the writing of this book, I must acknowledge my division chief, Dr Robert E. Marx—colleague, teacher, mentor, and (I humbly add) friend. Internationally recognized as a pioneer in the development of major maxillofacial reconstruction, Dr Marx is the consummate academic surgeon, providing the highest quality of medical care, empathizing with patients, accomplishing significant research, and most importantly, teaching brilliantly. Words alone can never express the gratitude I feel for the privilege of sharing my ideas with him, listening to him, witnessing his work ethic, hearing his brilliant and innovative ideas, and applying all of this mentoring experience to the study of bone science generally and the practice of bone harvesting and grafting for dental implants specifically.

I am also deeply indebted to all of the researchers and clinicians whose published results helped me form the scientific basis of my work and of this book. In addition, I would like to gratefully acknowledge the enormous contributions of the students, residents, and colleagues with whom I have had the privilege of collaborating during the past 18 years at the University of Miami School of Medicine.

Thanks go especially to my editors at Quintessence, who constantly pushed me to do my personal best. The book has benefited significantly from their excellent editing and great guidance and ideas on additions and deletions. I also want to thank the entire team at Quintessence Publishing for their excellence in all that they do.

I have been exceptionally lucky to have so many truly talented and creative individuals on my team. I would like to thank my postdoctoral fellow, Dr Aura Picon, for her assistance in patient care and her organizational abilities, diligence, and work ethic. I would like to thank my clinical staff—Cathie Ellyn, RN, Gina Lewis, CDA, and Amy Guerra, CDA—for assisting with the patient care depicted in the book. The care and love they provide their patients is incomparable, and the teamwork and support they provide is appreciated.

I would like to thank Dr Morton Perel for his manuscript review, probing questions, guidance, and encouragement. My heartfelt gratitude goes to the friends and assistants who always stand by me: Rick, Kuy, Lillibeth, Leo, Michael, Karen, Robert, Katrina, Vivian, and Frank.

Finally, thanks to my family—Mom, Dad, Heather, Nathan, Jeremy, Kyle, Lovey, Ravi, Angela, and Anil—for their support and understanding and for providing an oasis of tranquility where I can retreat from my frequently chaotic schedule. Without their help, both directly and indirectly, this book would not have been possible.

PART

I

Bone Biology

CHAPTER

1 Bone Physiology for Dental Implantology

The entire adult skeleton exists in a dynamic state, constantly broken down and re-formed by the coordinated actions of osteoclasts and osteoblasts (Fig 1-1). Bone is a living tissue that serves two primary functions: structural support and calcium metabolism.[1] The bone matrix is composed of an extremely complex network of collagen protein fibers impregnated with mineral salts that include calcium phosphate (85%), calcium carbonate (10%), and small amounts of calcium fluoride and magnesium fluoride (5%).[2] The minerals in bone are present primarily in the form of hydroxyapatites. Bone also contains small quantities of noncollagen proteins embedded in its mineral matrix, including the all-important family of bone morphogenetic proteins (BMPs). Coursing through the bone is a rich vascular network that provides perfusion to the viable cells, as well as the network of nerves (Fig 1-2). To maintain normal bone structure, sufficient amounts of proteins and minerals must be present.

Because of its unique architecture, bone is a mass-efficient structure in which maximal strength is achieved with absolutely minimal mass (Fig 1-3). In humans, bone mass reaches its maximum level approximately 10 years after the end of linear growth. This level normally remains fairly constant as bone is continually deposited and absorbed throughout the skeleton until sometime in the fourth decade of life, when bone mass begins to gradually decrease. Although the reasons are not clearly understood, this decline is a result of an ongoing net loss effect that begins to occur in the bone remodeling process. By

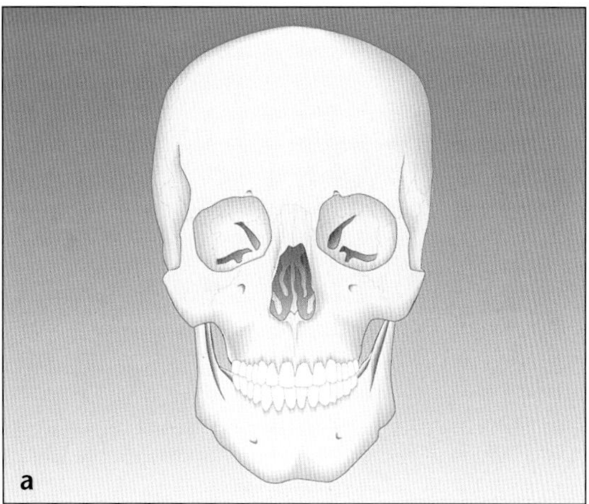

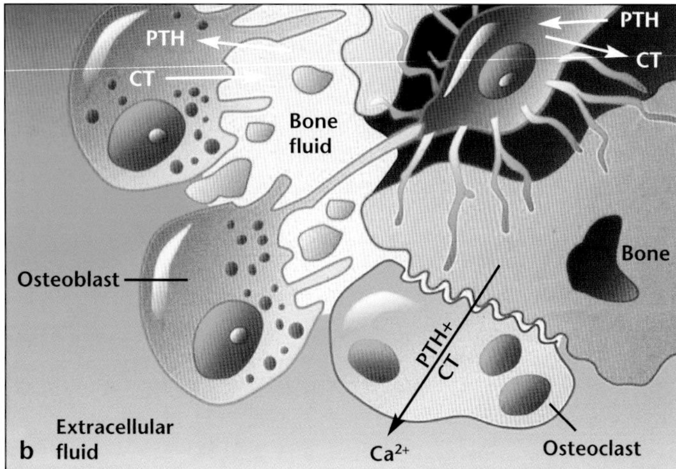

Fig 1-1
(a) A thorough knowledge of bone physiology is essential for understanding bone behavior during oral bone grafting, implant placement, osseointegration, and long-term bone maintenance.

(b) Osteoblasts and osteoclasts maintain metabolic equilibrium in all human bones, including the mandible and maxilla. When osteoblasts have successfully formed bone matrix and then become embedded in it, they transform into osteocytes. Osteocytes communicate with each other and with cells on the bone surface via dendritic processes encased in canaliculi. (PTH = parathyroid hormone; CT = calcitonin.)

age 80, both men and women typically have lost about half of their maximum bone mass value. Humans reach peak bone mineral density in their 30s, although it is lower in women than in men and in whites than in blacks. Women lose an estimated 35% of their cortical bone and 50% of cancellous bone as they age, while men lose only two-thirds of these amounts.[3] Bone deemed unnecessary by the body (eg, atrophy and bone loss in paraplegic patients) is also lost during a shift in the absorption-deposition balance in bone remodeling; in addition, turnover may be a response to metabolic reactions.

The skull and jaws are unquestionably affected in all of these scenarios; therefore, it is important for the clinician working with dental implants to have a good understanding of bone structure and metabolism as well as knowledge of the process of osseointegration when bone grafts and implants are placed.

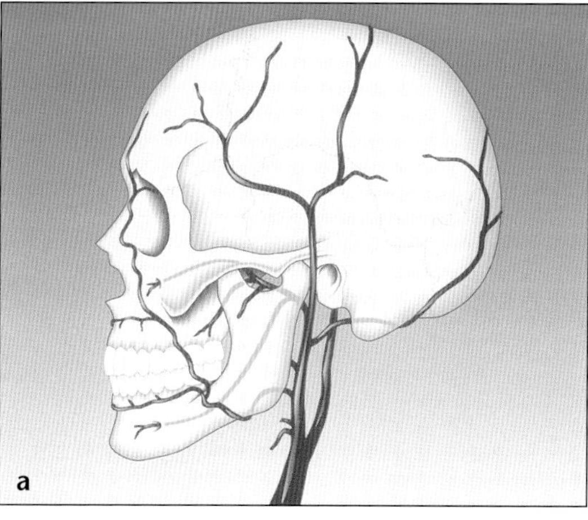

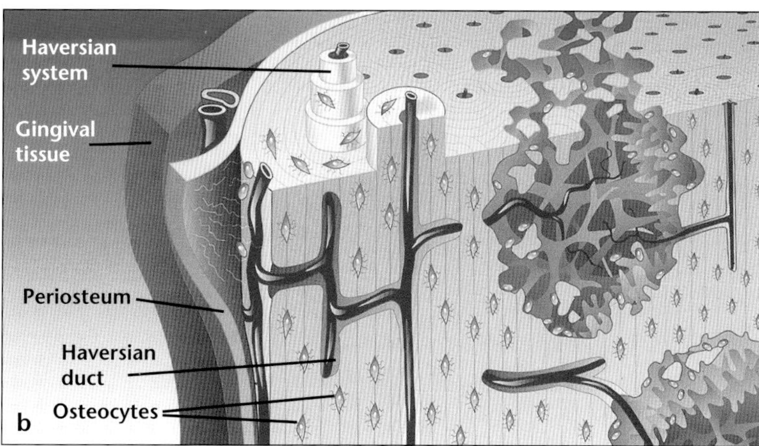

Fig 1-2
(a) Bone cells maintain viability as a result of the rich arterial supply, with smaller vessels reaching the cells embedded within the bone matrix.

(b) The vascular system within the lamellar bone emerges from the medullary spaces; the interconnected design irrigates the entire structure.

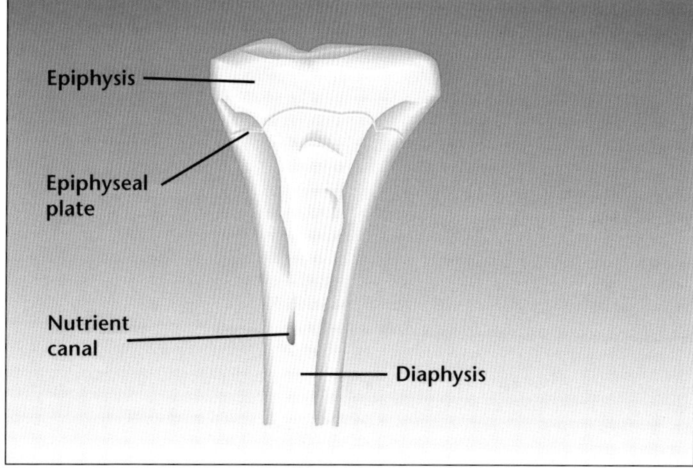

Fig 1-3
Bone, a mass-efficient tissue, has a trabecular configuration that provides resilience under functional load.

Bone Cells

Three main types of cells are involved in bone metabolism and physiology: osteoblasts, osteocytes, and osteoclasts.

Osteoblasts, which are involved in building bone, are located in two general areas. These cells deposit bone matrix (Fig 1-4) and are frequently referred to as either *endosteal osteoblasts* or *periosteal osteoblasts*. Periosteal osteoblasts are present on the outer surfaces of the bones beneath the periosteum, while endosteal osteoblasts line the vascular canals within bone. Mature osteoblasts are responsible for producing the proteins of bone matrix. Indeed, the cytoplasm of osteoblasts is intensely basophilic, suggesting the presence of ribonucleoproteins that are related to the synthesis of these protein components. Bone deposition continues in an active growth area for several months, with osteoblasts laying down new bone in successive layers of concentric circles on the inner surfaces of the cavity in which they are working. This activity continues until the tunnel is filled with new bone to the point that the new growth begins to encroach on the blood vessels running through it. In addition to mineralizing newly formed bone matrix, osteoblasts also produce other matrix constituents, such as phospholipids and proteoglycans, that may also be important in the mineralization process. During osteogenesis, the osteoblasts secrete growth factors, including transforming growth factor-beta (TGF-β), BMPs, platelet-derived growth factor (PDGF), and insulin-like growth factors (IGFs), which are stored in bone matrix.[4] Recent research suggests that osteoblasts may even act as helper cells for osteoclasts during normal bone resorption, possibly by preparing the bone surface for their attack.[4] However, further study is needed to clarify this possible role.

When osteoblasts have successfully formed bone matrix and then become embedded in it, they transform into osteocytes (see Fig 1-1b). Osteocytes are the most abundant bone cells, and they communicate with each other and with cells on the bone surface via dendritic processes encased in canaliculi. Osteocytes have a slightly basophilic cytoplasm, the prolongations of which extend from the osteocyte through a network of fine canaliculi that emerge from the lacunae. During bone formation, these prolongations extend beyond their normal limit, creating direct continuity with adjacent osteocyte lacunae and with the tissue spaces. Fluid in these spaces mixes with fluid from the canaliculi; this appears to allow an exchange of metabolic and biochemical messages between the bloodstream and osteocytes. In mature bone, there is almost no extension of these prolongations, but the canaliculi continue to function as a means of messenger exchange. This mechanism allows the osteocytes to remain alive, regardless of the calcified intercellular substance surrounding them. This duct system does not function, however, if it is located more than 0.5 mm from a capillary, which may explain the abundant blood supply in bone through capillaries that run through the Haversian systems and Volkmann canals (see below). Osteocytes have also been shown to express TGF-β and possibly other growth factors. Some researchers have also suggested that weight-bearing loads may influence the behavior of bone remodeling cells located on bone surfaces by their effects on the osteocytes buried within the bone, which subsequently release TGF-β into the canalicular system.[4] Other research suggests that osteocytes may play a role in transporting calcium through the bones.[5]

Osteoclasts are the cells responsible for bone resorption, and their activity is controlled by parathyroid hormone.[4] Osteo-

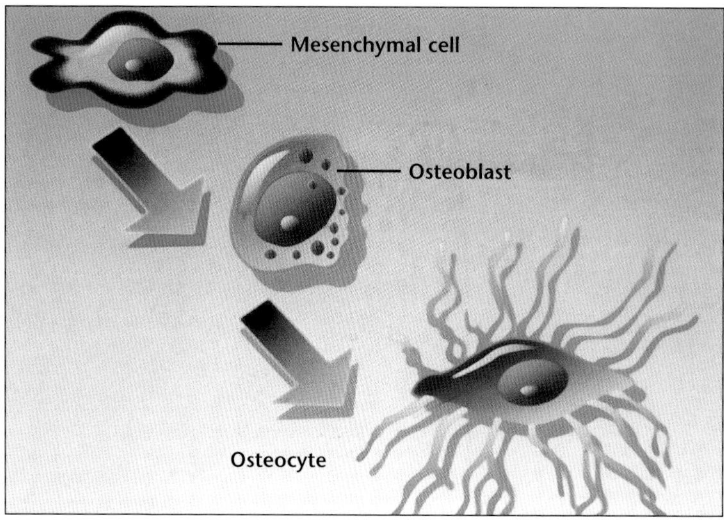

Fig 1-4
When influenced by the transforming growth factors secreted by platelets and osteoblasts, undifferentiated stem cells can transform into pre-osteoblasts, then osteoblasts, and eventually osteocytes, thus maturing into the tissues essential to the body.

clasts are fused monocytes that histologically appear as large, multinucleated giant cells (containing as many as 50 nuclei). They are located in shallow excavations (Howship lacunae) along the mineralized bone surfaces.[6] A specific area of their cell membrane forms adjacent to the bone surface to be resorbed. This area, known as the ruffled border, is formed by villus-like projections that the osteoclasts send out toward the bone. It consists of folds and invaginations that allow intimate contact between the cell membrane and the bone surface (see Fig 1-1b). Bone resorption occurs in the ruffled border as the villi secrete proteolytic enzymes that digest or dissolve the organic bone matrix and acids that cause dissolution of the bone cells. Via phagocytosis, osteoclasts also absorb minute particles of bone matrix and crystals, eventually dissolving them and releasing the products into the bloodstream. In adults, osteoclasts are usually active on fewer than 1% of bone surfaces at any one time.[7] They typically exist in small but concentrated masses. Once a mass has developed, it usually eats away at the bone for about 3 weeks, creating a tunnel that ranges from 0.2 to 1.0 mm in diameter and is several millimeters long. After local bone resorption is complete, the osteoclasts disappear, probably by degeneration. Subsequently, the tunnel is invaded by osteoblasts, and the bone formation segment of the continuous remodeling cycle begins again.

In addition to the three main types of bone cells, there is a fourth type, the bone-lining cell. These cells are similar to osteocytes in that they are "retired" osteoblasts—in other words, osteoblasts that do not become embedded in newly formed bone, but instead adhere to the outer bone surfaces when formation halts. Bone-lining cells become quiescent and flattened against the bone surface, but they do not form a contiguous gap-free barrier. They maintain communication with osteocytes and with each other via gap-junctioned processes, and they also appear to maintain their receptors for hormones such as parathyroid hormone and estrogens. As with osteocytes, bone-lining cells are thought to play a role in transferring mineral into and out of bone and in sensing mechanical strain.[8] They may also initiate bone remodeling in response to various chemicals or mechanical stimuli.[9]

Bone Metabolism

Bone is the body's primary reservoir of calcium. Its tremendous turnover capability allows it to respond to the body's metabolic needs and to maintain a stable serum calcium level.[1,2] Calcium has an essential life-support function. It works in conjunction with the lungs and kidneys to help maintain the body's pH balance by producing additional phosphates and carbonates. It also assists in the conduction of nerve and muscle electrical charges, including those involving the heart (see Fig 1-1b).

Bone structure and mass—including that of the skull and jaw—are directly affected by the body's metabolic state. Faced with unmet calcium requirements or certain diseases, the structural integrity of bone may be altered and even compromised. Consider the bone structure of postmenopausal women. In response to decreased estrogen hormone in the system, bone mass begins to dwindle, and the interconnections between bone trabeculae are lost. Because normal interconnections are crucial for making bone biomechanically rigid, the decrease in bone leads to an increase in fragility. This is an important phenomenon in dental implantology and related bone grafting because declining estrogen levels appear to significantly increase the risk of implant failure.[10] The effects of a disrupted balance in bone remodeling are also illustrated by Albers-Schoenberg, or "marble bone," disease, which involves defective osteoclasts. Because these osteoclasts do not resorb the existing bone matrix and liberate BMP, new bone is not formed, resulting in avascular and acellular bone (essentially, old bone) that is brittle and thus fractures easily and frequently becomes infected. Other diseases associated with bone remodeling abnormalities include cancer, primary hyperparathyroidism, and Paget disease. Although these disorders are common, in most cases little is known about what mechanisms are responsible for controlling normal bone remodeling or how it is coordinated and balanced.

Metabolic-hormonal interactions play a crucial role in maintaining bone structure. Most importantly, they help to maintain the coupled cycle of bone resorption and bone apposition through BMP. As previously mentioned, when osteoblasts form bone, they also secrete BMP into the mineral matrix. This acid-insoluble protein resides in the matrix until it is released during osteoclastic resorption. The acid insolubility is an evolutionary mechanism by which the pH of 1 created by osteoclasts is able to dissolve bone mineral without affecting BMP.[11] Once released, BMP binds to the cell surface of undifferentiated mesenchymal stem cells, where it causes a membrane signal protein to become activated with high-energy phosphate bonds. This, in turn, affects the gene sequence in the nucleus, causing expression of osteoblast differentiation and stimulation of new bone production. A disturbance in this process may be at the root of osteoporosis. Of current research interest is the therapeutic potential of applying BMPs directly to a healing site to induce bone formation. Some researchers suggest that in the future, this biologic material may replace or assist bone grafts in restorative therapy,[12] an issue discussed in more detail in chapter 11.

Normally, about 0.7% of the human skeleton is resorbed and replaced by new healthy bone each day (see Figs 1-1b and

1-2b). Therefore, normal turnover of the entire skeleton occurs approximately every 142 days. With aging and metabolic disease states, there may be a reduction in the normal turnover process and thus an increase in the average age of functional bone. This raises the risk for fatigue damage of old bone, compromised bone healing, failed implant integration, and loss of implant osseointegration.[13] Thus, it is important for dental clinicians to recognize that a compromised status must be considered before treatment planning because its effects may not be revealed until the clinician attempts to place implants or until the implants have been in place for some time.

Macroscopic Structure of Bone

The human skeleton is composed of two distinct kinds of bone based on porosity: dense cortical tissue and spongy cancellous tissue (Fig 1-5). In principle, the porosity of bone could vary continuously from 0% to 100%; however, most sites are either of very low or very high porosity. In most cases, both cortical and cancellous tissue is found at every bone site, but their quantity and distribution vary. The nonmineralized spaces within bone contain marrow, a tissue consisting of blood vessels, nerves, and various cell types. Marrow's chief function is to generate the principal cells present in blood; it is also a highly osteogenic material that can stimulate bone formation if placed in an extracellular skeletal location, as with bone grafting in the dental area.

Cortical or compact bone, which comprises about 85% of total bone in the body,[4] is found in the shafts of long bones and forms a shell around vertebral bodies and other spongy bones (Fig 1-6). This tissue is organized in bony cylinders consolidated around a central blood vessel, called a *Haversian system*. Haversian canals, which contain capillaries and nerves, are connected to each other and to the outside surfaces of the bone by short, transverse Volkmann canals.

Trabecular, or cancellous, bone, which comprises about 15% of the body's total bone, is found in cuboidal and flat bones and in the ends of long bones. Its pores are interconnected and filled with marrow. The bone matrix is in the form of plates (called *trabeculae*) arranged in a varied fashion; sometimes, they appear to be organized into orthogonal arrays, but often they are randomly arranged.[14] The medullary cavities are filled with marrow, which is red when there is active production of blood cells or a reserve population of mesenchymal stem cells and yellow when aging causes the cavity to be converted into a site for fat storage.

Except for the articular surfaces, the outer surface of bone is covered with periosteum, which forms a boundary between the hard tissue and its soft tissue covering. It is also the site of considerable metabolic, cellular, and biomechanical activities that modulate bone growth and shape (Fig 1-7). The periosteum is composed of two layers of specialized connective tissue. The outer fibrous layer, mainly formed from dense collagenous fibers and fibroblasts, provides toughness, while the inner cellular, or cambium, layer, which is in direct contact with bone, contains functional osteoblasts. The medullary cavities and spaces are covered by endosteum, a very thin and delicate membrane consisting of a single layer of osteoblasts. The endosteum is architecturally similar to the cambium layer of the periosteum because of the presence of osteoprogenitor cells, osteoblasts, and osteoclasts.

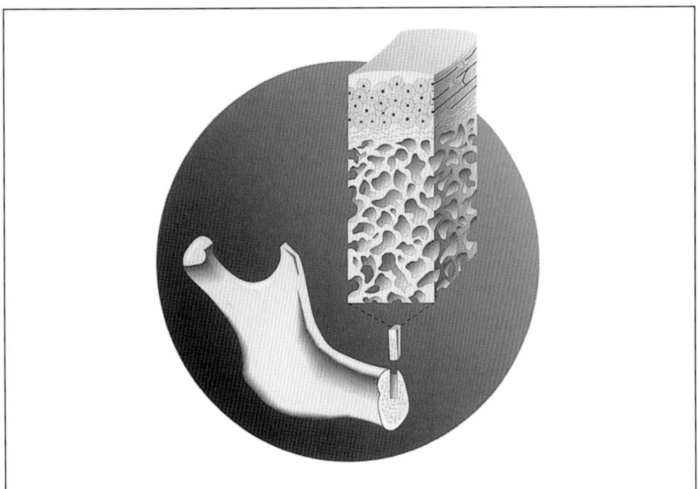

Fig 1-5
For successful bone harvesting, bone grafting, and osseointegration, bone density and the ratio of cortical to cancellous bone in the mandible and maxilla must be thoroughly evaluated.

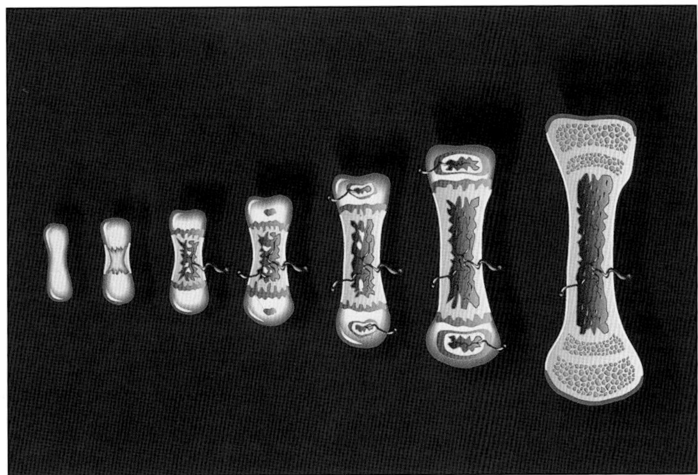

Fig 1-6
Formation and maturation of the long bones. Bone density and the ratio of cortical to cancellous bone in long bones used as harvest sites are essential factors in achieving clinical success with bone harvesting, bone grafting, and osseointegration.

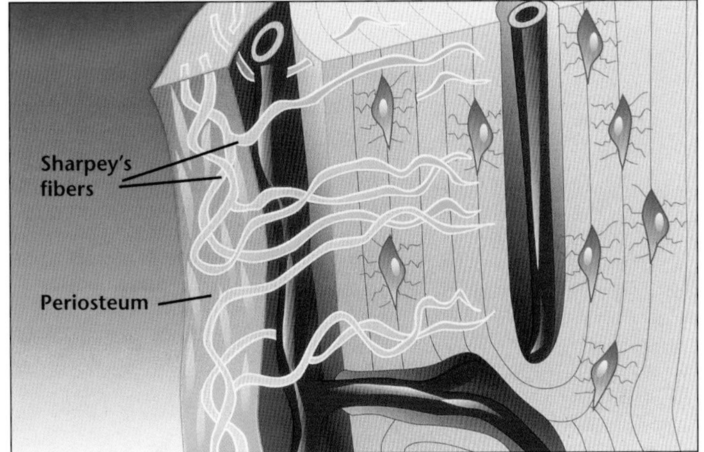

Fig 1-7
The periosteum, a connective tissue membrane surrounding cortical bone, should be carefully repositioned so that its osteogenic potential after surgery can nurture the graft and/or underlying bone.

Microstructure of Bone

At the microscopic level, there are four types of bone: woven, composite, lamellar, and bundle.

Woven bone plays a principal role in healing because it forms very quickly (approximately 30 to 60 mm/day). As a result, it develops in a very disorganized fashion, without lamellar architecture or Haversian systems. Thus, it is quite soft, has little biomechanical strength, and does not last long. On the plus side, however, woven bone can become more highly mineralized than lamellar bone, a fact that, mechanically speaking, may help to compensate for its lack of organization.[14] During healing, woven bone is often referred to as *phase I bone*. It is fairly quickly resorbed and replaced with more mature lamellar bone, referred to as *phase II bone*.

Composite bone refers to the transitional state between woven (phase I) bone and lamellar (phase II) bone, in which a woven bone lattice filled with lamellar bone can be seen.

Lamellar bone is the most abundant, mature, load-bearing bone in the body, and it is extremely strong. This type of bone forms slowly (approximately 0.6 to 1 mm/day) and thus has a well-organized collagen protein and mineralized structure. Lamellar bone consists of multiple oriented layers.

Bundle bone is the principal bone found around ligaments and joints and consists of striated interconnections with ligaments.

Molecular Structure of Bone

At the molecular level, bone is composed of collagen (primarily type I), water, hydroxyapatite material, and small amounts of proteoglycans and noncollagenous proteins. It is a cross-linked collagen matrix with a three-dimensional multiple arrangement of matrix fibers. The orientation of the collagen fibers determines the mineralization pattern. In this way, bone adapts to its biomechanical environment and projects maximal strength in the direction receiving compressive loads. Collagen gives bone tensile strength and flexibility and provides a place for the nucleation of bone mineral crystals, which give bone its rigidity and compressive strength.

The intercellular bone substance has an organized structure. The organic portion occupies 35% of the matrix and is primarily formed by osteocollagenous fibers, similar to collagen fibers in connective tissue. These are joined together by a cement-like substance that consists primarily of glucoaminoglycan (protein-polysaccharide).

The inorganic component comprises 65% of bone weight and is localized only in the interfibrinous cement. The minerals in bone consist mainly of hydroxyapatite crystals, which form dense deposits along the osteocollagenous fibers. It also contains other substances, such as carbonate, fluoride, other proteins, and peptides. Some of these materials are governed by the body fluid composition and affect the solubility of bone mineral.[14]

Other components, such as BMP, regulate how bone is laid down and maintained. Bone matrix has sequential layers that vary in thickness from 300 to 700 μm. These layers are the result of rhythmic and uniform matrix deposition. Also characteristic is the pattern of fibers within each layer, which are parallel with a spiral orientation that changes between layers so that the fibers in one layer run perpendicular to those in the adjacent layer. This pattern is what creates the distinguishable bone layers.

Bone Modeling and Remodeling

As previously mentioned, bone is continually being deposited by osteoblasts and absorbed by osteoclasts at active sites in the body. In adults, a small amount of new bone is continually being formed by osteoblasts, which work on about 4% of all surfaces at any given time.[7]

Although many orthopedists and bone scientists refer to both processes as *remodeling*, it is important to note that bone modeling and bone remodeling are two different processes in osseous repair. *Bone modeling* typically refers to the sculpting and shaping of bones after they have grown in length. This process involves the independent, uncoupled actions of osteoclasts and osteoblasts, so bone is resorbed in some areas and added in others. Bone modeling can also be controlled by mechanical factors, for example, during orthodontic tooth movement, in which the application of force causes the bone to resorb on the tooth surface, new bone to form on the opposite surface, and the tooth to move with the surrounding bone rather than through the alveolus. Bone modeling can change both the size and shape of the bones.

Bone remodeling, on the other hand, refers to the sequential, coupled actions by these two types of cells. It is a cyclical process that usually maintains the status quo and does not change the size or shape of bones. Bone remodeling removes a portion of old bone and replaces it with new bone.

Unlike bone modeling, which slows substantially after growth stops, bone remodeling occurs throughout life (although its rate also slows somewhat after growth). Bone remodeling also occurs throughout the skeleton in focal, discrete packets that are distinct in location and chronology. This suggests that the activation of the cellular sequence responsible for bone remodeling is controlled locally, possibly by an autoregulatory mechanism such as autocrine or paracrine factors generated in the bone microenvironment.

Bone modeling also occurs during wound healing (eg, during the stabilization of endosseous implants) and in response to bone loading. Unlike bone remodeling, it does not have to be preceded by resorption. The activation of cells that resorb and those that form bone can occur on different surfaces within the same bone. In addition, bone modeling may also be controlled by growth factors, as with bone healing, grafting, and osseointegration.

Whether bone is being modeled or remodeled, it is deposited in proportion to the compressional load it must carry. For instance, the bones of athletes become considerably heavier than those of nonathletes. Likewise, a person with one leg in a cast who continues to walk using only the opposite leg will experience a thinning of the unused leg bone.

Continuous physical stress stimulates osteoblastic activity and calcification of bone.[7] Bone stress also determines the shape of bones in some circumstances. To explain this, it has been theorized that bone compression causes a negative electrical potential in the compressed area and a positive electrical potential elsewhere in the bone. Minute amounts of electric current flowing in bone have been shown to cause osteoblastic activity at the negative end of the current flow, which may explain increased bone deposition in compression sites.[7] This is the basis of studies on the use of electrical stimulation to promote bone formation and osseointegration,[15–17] although further research is needed to support claims of benefit.

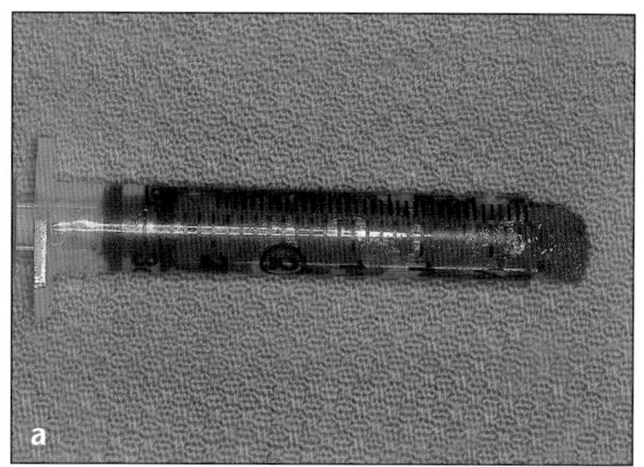

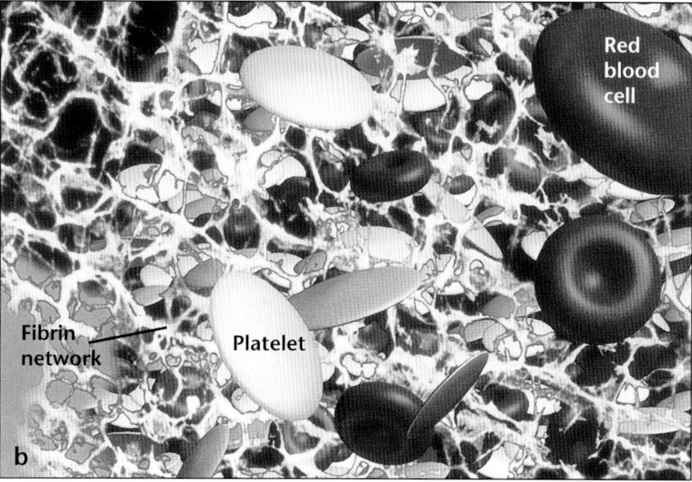

Fig 1-8
(a) Autogenous cancellous bone grafts have large quantities of osteocytes, osteoblasts, and osteoclasts, while the recipient site provides vascularity and cells.

(b) An autogenous bone graft contains fibrin, platelets, leukocytes, and red blood cells. The platelets release growth factors that trigger bone regeneration.

Bone Formation and Modeling with Bone Graft Materials

In most cases, the goal of placing a bone graft is to regenerate lost tissue as well as simply to repair or fill the defect. Thus, graft materials ideally should transfer an optimal quantity of viable osteocompetent cells—including osteoblasts and cancellous marrow stem cells—to the host site. For the osseointegration of the graft to proceed successfully, the host tissue must have sufficient vascularity to diffuse nutrients to the cells before revascularization occurs and to bud new capillaries into the graft to create a more permanent vascular network. Thus, depending on the amount of new bone that must be formed, donor sites are selected based on their osteocompetent cell density. The graft also consists of islands of mineralized cancellous bone, fibrin from blood clotting, and platelets within the clot (Fig 1-8). In descending order of available cancellous bone, autogenous donor sites include the posterior and anterior ilium, tibial plateau, femoral head, mandibular symphysis, calvaria, rib, and fibula.[18] Other intraoral sites may also be good choices for autogenous bone harvest, and nonautogenous materials may be used in some cases. (Specifics on material selection are discussed in more detail in chapter 2.) Placement of a graft that consists of endosteal osteoblasts and marrow stem cells and is surrounded by a vascular and cellular tissue bed creates a recipient site with a biochemistry that is hypoxic (O_2 tensions of 3 to 10 mm Hg), acidotic (pH of 4.0 to 6.0), and rich in lactate.[19] The osteoblasts and stem cells survive the first 3 to 5 days after transplant to the host site largely because of their surface position and ability to absorb nutrients from the recipient tissues. The osteocytes within the mineralized cancellous bone die as a result of their encasement in mineral, which acts as a nutritional barrier. Because the graft is inherently hypoxic and the surrounding tissue is normoxic (50 to 55 mm Hg), an oxygen gradient greater than the 20 mm Hg (usually 35 to 55 mm Hg) is set up and, in turn, the macrophages are stimulated to secrete macrophage-derived angiogenesis factor (MDAF) and macrophage-derived growth factor (MDGF).

Within the graft, the platelets trapped in the clot degranulate within hours of graft placement, releasing PDGF. Therefore, the inherent properties of the wound, particularly the oxygen gradient phenomenon and PDGF, initiate early angiogenesis from the surrounding capillaries and mitogenesis of the transferred osteocompetent cells.[13] By day 3, buds from existing capillaries outside the graft can be seen. These buds penetrate the graft and proliferate between the graft and the cancellous bone network to form a complete network by days 10 to 14. As these capillaries respond to the oxygen gradient, MDAF messengers effectively reduce the oxygen gradient as they perfuse the graft, thus creating a shut-off mechanism that prevents overangiogenesis.

Although PDGF seems to be the earliest messenger to stimulate early osteoid formation, it is probably replaced by MDGF and other mesenchymal tissue stimulators from the TGF-β family. During the first 3 to 7 days after graft placement, the stem cells and endosteal osteoblasts produce only a small amount of osteoid. Over the next few days, osteoid production accelerates after the vascular network is established, presumably because of the availability of oxygen and nutrients. The new osteoid initially forms on the surface of the mineralized cancellous trabeculae from the endosteal osteoblasts. Shortly thereafter, individual osteoid islands develop between the cancellous bone trabeculae, presumably from the stem cells transferred with the graft material. A third source of osteoid production is circulating stem cells, which are attracted to the wound and are believed to seed into the graft and proliferate.[20]

During the first 3 to 4 weeks, this biochemical and cellular phase of bone regeneration coalesces individual osteoid islands, surface osteoid on the cancellous trabeculae, and host bone to clinically consolidate the graft. This process uses the graft's fibrin network as a framework to build upon—a process referred to as *osteoconduction*. Normally nonmotile cells, such as osteoblasts, may be somewhat motile via the process of endocytosis along the scaffold-like fibrin. During endocytosis, the cell membrane is transferred from the retreating edge of the cell, through the cytoplasm, to the advancing edge to re-form a cell membrane. During this process, the cell slowly advances and secretes its product along the way—in this case, osteoid onto the fibrin network. This cellular regeneration phase is often referred to as *phase I bone regeneration*. It produces disorganized woven bone, similar to fracture callus, that is structurally sound but not as strong as mature bone.

The amount of bone formed during phase I depends on the osteocompetent cell density in the graft material. The bone yield can also be enhanced by compacting the graft material using a bone mill, followed by syringe compaction and then by further condensing it into the graft site with bone-packing instruments.

Current research and clinical experience also suggest that adding certain growth factors to the material may also increase the amount of phase I bone that forms. In laboratory studies and some early human trials involving graft enhancement, BMPs (particularly recombinant DNA–produced BMP), TGF-β, PDGF, and IGF have shown promise in their ability to increase the speed and quantity of bone regeneration.[21,22] Clinical studies on adding platelet-rich plasma (PRP) to graft material have demonstrated its ability to induce early consolidation and graft mineralization in half the time with a 15% to 30% improvement in trabecular bone density.[15,23-25] This material, an enhanced fibrin clot rich in platelets that in turn release PDGF, is discussed in greater detail in chapter 11. It has been theorized that the enhanced presence of PDGF initiates osteocompetent cell activity more completely than that which inherently occurs in the graft and clot milieu alone. The enhanced fibrin network created by PRP may also enhance osteoconduction throughout the graft, supporting consolidation.

Phase I bone undergoes resorption and remodeling, until it is eventually replaced by phase II bone, which is less cellular, more mineralized, and more structurally organized.

Phase II is initiated by osteoclasts that arrive at the graft site through the newly developed vascular network.[6,26] BMP is released during resorption of both the newly formed phase I bone and the nonviable cancellous trabecular graft. As with normal bone remodeling, BMP acts as the link or couple between bone resorption and new bone apposition. Stem cells in the graft and from the local tissues and the circulatory system respond by osteoblast differentiation and new bone formation. New bone forms while the jaw and graft are in function, developing in response to the demands placed on it. This bone develops into mature Haversian systems and lamellar bone that can withstand normal shear forces from the jaw and impact compressive forces that are typical of dentures and implant-supported prostheses. Histologically, grafts undergo long-term remodeling that is consistent with normal skeletal turnover. A periosteum and endosteum develop as part of this cycle. Although the graft cortex never grows as thick as a normal jaw cortex, the graft itself retains a dense cancellous trabecular pattern that is beneficial for placing dental implants because its density promotes osseointegration of the implant. It can also be beneficial for placing conventional dentures because the dense trabecular bone can easily adapt to a variety of functional stresses. Radiographically, the graft takes on the morphology and cortical outlines of the mandible or maxilla over several years. Preprosthetic procedures, such as soft tissue grafts, can be performed at 4 months when a functional periosteum has formed. Osseointegrated dental implants can also be placed at this point.

Osseointegration of Dental Implants

The healing and remodeling of tissues around an implant involves a complex array of events. In this case, *osseointegration* refers to direct bone anchorage to the implant body, which can provide a foundation to support a prosthesis and can transmit occlusal forces directly to the bone (Fig 1-9). This concept was developed and the term coined by Per-Ingvar Brånemark, a professor at the Institute for Applied Biotechnology at the University of Göteborg

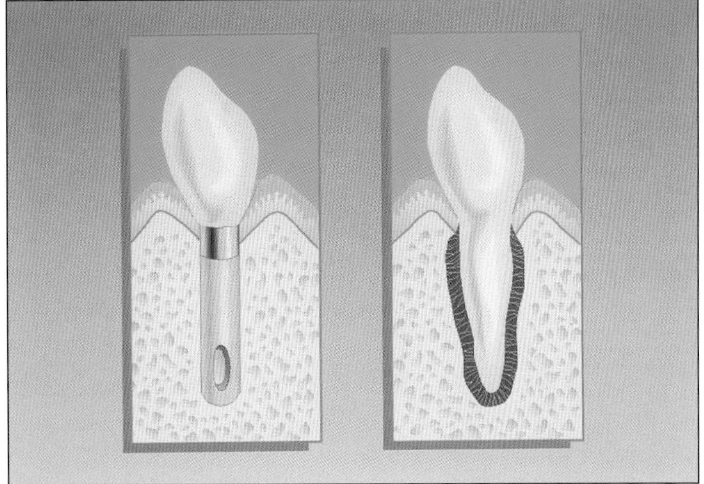

Fig 1-9
Unlike a natural tooth, which (unless ankylosed) is separated from the bone by periodontal ligament space and Sharpey's fibers, the implant surface directly contacts the bone, with only a small interpositional layer (similar to a cement line on newly laid down or existing remodeled bone).

in Sweden and the inventor of the well-known Brånemark implant system. During animal studies of microcirculation in bone repair during the 1950s, Brånemark discovered a strong bond between bone and titanium. Today, we know that a fully anchored prosthesis can provide patients with restored masticatory functions that are similar to the natural dentition.

Several key factors influence successful implant osseointegration.[27,28] These include the following:

- The characteristics of the implant material (some appear to chemically bond to bone better than others)[29] and maintenance of implant sterility prior to placement
- Implant design, shape, and macro- and microsurface topography
- Prevention of excessive heat generation during bone drilling

The long-term osseointegration of dental implants also relies on placement within bone that has adequate trabecular density, ridge height and width, and systemic health (particularly good vascularity).[13] When the recipient bone or graft is deficient in height, the portion of the implant prosthesis that is above the bone is greater than the length of the implant within it, possibly creating a destructive lever arm that will loosen the implant over time. A ridge that is too narrow (ie, less than 5 mm to accommodate standard 3.75-mm-diameter implants) will leave some of the implant placed outside the bone or will force the clinician to use less desirable small-diameter implants to gain the necessary osseointegrated surface area. Likewise, trabecular bone that is not sufficiently dense either will fail to osseointegrate or will lose its osseointegration over time. Ideally, the marginal and apical parts of the implant should be fully engaged in cortical bone or in cancellous bone that has a high proportion of bony trabeculae to support it. The ingrowth of fibrous tissue between the bone and implant also decreases the chances for long-term success and the ability to withstand mechanical and microbial insults. In some cases this can be prevented by protecting against micromobility and by using protective barrier membranes during healing. This is discussed in

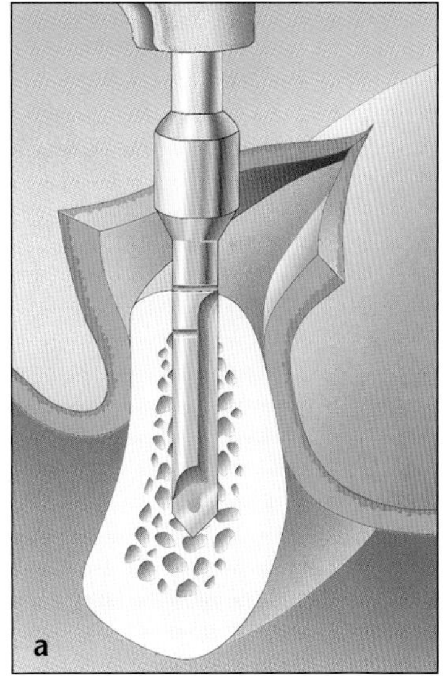

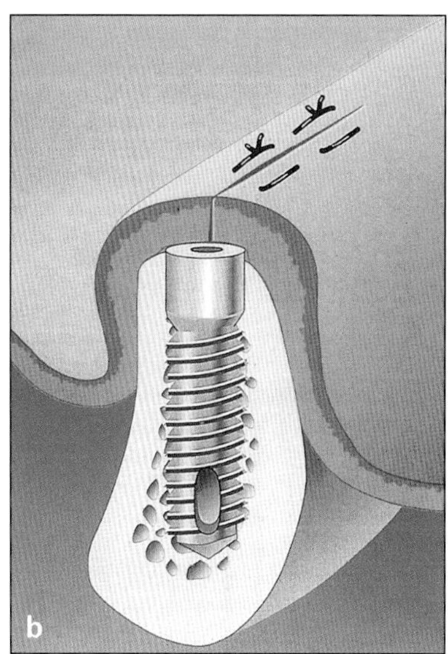

Fig 1-10
(a) Placing an implant traumatizes bone, stimulating a response to repair and remodel. Using sharp burs and good saline irrigation minimizes trauma to both bone and soft tissues, helping to maintain tissue viability.

(b) The rough surface of the dental implant allows for fibrin attachment and subsequent adhesion molecule production and cellular proliferation to enhance collagen synthesis and to regulate bone metabolism.

chapter 3. It is crucial to achieve initial stability and osseointegration because a clinically mobile implant has never been observed to become reosseointegrated.[28] Once stability is lost, the implant can only be removed.

Biologic Process of Implant Osseointegration

The healing process around an implant is the same as that which occurs in normal primary bone. Research with titanium dental implants suggests the following three-stage process.[13]

Osteophyllic Phase

When a rough-surface implant is placed into the cancellous marrow space of the mandible or maxilla, blood is initially present between the implant and bone, and a clot subsequently forms. Only a small amount of bone is in contact with the implant surface; the rest is exposed to extracellular fluid and cells. During the initial implant-host interaction, numerous cytokines are released that have a variety of functions, from regulating adhesion molecule production and altering cellular proliferation to enhancing collagen synthesis and regulating bone metabolism. These events also correspond to the beginning of the generalized inflammatory response to the surgical insult (Fig 1-10). By the end of the first week, inflammatory cells are responding to foreign antigens introduced by the surgical procedure.

While the inflammatory phase is still active, vascular ingrowth from the surrounding vital tissues begins by about day 3, developing into a more mature vascular network during the first 3 weeks following implant placement.[29] In addition, cellular differentiation, proliferation, and activation begin. Ossification also begins during the first week, and the initial response observed is the migration of osteoblasts from the endosteal surface of the trabecular bone and the inner surface of the buccal and lingual cortex to the implant surface. This migration is likely a response to the release of BMP during implant placement and the initial resorption of bone crushed against the metal surface. The osteophyllic phase lasts about 1 month.

Osteoconductive Phase

Once they reach the implant, the bone cells spread along the metal surface (osteoconduction), laying down osteoid. Initially, this is an immature connective tissue matrix, and the bone deposited is a thin layer of woven bone called a *foot plate* (basis stapedis). The fibrocartilaginous callus is eventually remodeled into bone callus (woven and, later, lamellar) in a process similar to endochondral ossification. This process occurs during the next 3 months (peaking between the third and fourth week) as more bone is added to the total surface area of the implant. Four months after implant placement, the maximum surface area is covered by bone. By this point, a relatively steady state has been reached and no further bone is deposited on the implant surface.[29]

Osteoadaptive Phase

The final, or osteoadaptive, phase begins approximately 4 months after implant placement. A balanced remodeling sequence has begun and continues even after the implants are exposed and loaded. Once loaded, the implants generally do not gain or lose bone contact, but the foot plates thicken in response to the load transmitted through the implant to the surrounding bone, and some reorientation of the vascular pattern may be seen.

Because grafted bone integrates with implants to a higher degree than does natural host bone,[13] bone grafting is recommended around implants placed in sites where bone volume or density is deficient or where there is a history of implant failure. When rehabilitating reconstructed jaws, it is even preferable to place implants in grafted bone rather than in normal bone, although each type of bone is acceptable. To achieve optimal results, an osseointegration period of 4 months prior to loading is recommended for implants placed in grafted bone, and 4 to 8 months prior to loading for implants placed in normal bone, depending on its density.

Summary

A thorough knowledge of bone physiology, biology, and mass is essential for understanding bone behavior during oral bone grafting, implant placement, osseointegration, and long-term bone maintenance. Osteoblasts, which are involved in building bone, deposit bone matrix in two general areas and are therefore referred to as periosteal and endosteal osteoblasts. Both types of osteoblasts are important in bone grafting and in bone modeling and remodeling. Bone modeling may be controlled by growth factors, as with bone healing, grafting, and osseointegration, or by mechanical factors; bone remodeling is locally controlled, possibly by an autoregulatory mechanism. Continuous physical stress stimulates osteoblastic activity and calcification of bone. Bone stress also determines the shape of bones in some circumstancs. In bone grafting, as in natural bone remodeling, growth factors act as the link or couple between bone resorption and new bone apposition. Because grafted bone integrates with implants to a higher degree than does natural host bone, bone grafting is recommended around implants placed in sites where bone volume or density is deficient or where there is a history of implant failure. When rehabilitating jaws that have been reconstructed, it is even preferable to place implants in grafted bone rather than in normal bone, although each type of bone is acceptable.

References

1. Roberts WE, Turley PK, Breznick N, Fielder PJ. Implants: Bone physiology and metabolism. CDA J 1987;15:54–61.
2. Dalen N, Olsson KE. Bone mineral content and physical activity. Acta Orthop Scand 1974;45:170–176.
3. Mazess RB. On aging bone loss. Clin Orthop 1982;165:239–252.
4. Mundy GR. Bone remodeling. In: Mundy GR (ed). Bone Remodeling and Its Disorders, ed 2. London: Martin Dunitz, 1999;1–11.
5. De Barnard C. Calcium metabolism and bone minerals. In: Hall BK (ed). Bone, vol 4. Boca Raton: CRC, 1990;73–98.
6. Bonucci E. New knowledge on the origin, function and fate of osteoclasts. Clin Orthop 1981; 158:252–269.
7. Guyton AC, Hall JE. Bone and its relations to extracellular calcium and phosphates. In: Guyton AC, Hall JE (eds). Textbook of Medical Physiology, ed 9. Philadelphia: Saunders, 1996;989–992.
8. Parfitt AM. Bone and plasma calcium homeostasis. Bone 1987;8(suppl 1):S1–S8.
9. Miller SC, Jee WSS. Bone lining cells. In: Hall BK (ed). Bone, vol 4. Boca Raton: CRC, 1990; 1–19.
10. August M, Chung K, Chang Y, Glowacki J. Influence of estrogen status on endosseous implant osseointegration. J Oral Maxillofac Surg 2001;59:1285–1291.
11. Urist MR. Bone morphogenetic protein. In: Habal MB, Reddi AR (eds). Bone Graft and Bone Substitute. Philadelphia: Saunders, 1992; 70–82.
12. Wang EA, Gerhart TN, Toriumi DM. BMPs and development. In: Slavkin HC, Price PA (eds). Chemistry and Biology of Mineralized Tissues. [Proceedings of the Fourth International Conference on Chemistry and Biology of Mineralized Tissues, 5-19 Feb 1992, Coronado, CA]. Amsterdam: Excerpta Medica, 1992: 352–360.
13. Marx RE, Ehler WJ, Peleg M. Mandibular and facial reconstruction: Rehabilitation of the head and neck cancer patient. Bone 1996;19(1 suppl):59S–82S.
14. Martin RB, Burr DB, Sharkey NA. Skeletal biology. In: Martin RB, Burr DB, Sharkey NA (eds). Skeletal Tissue Mechanics. New York: Springer-Verlag, 1998;29–78.
15. Kassolis JD, Rosen PS, Reynolds MA. Alveolar ridge and sinus augmentation utilizing platelet-rich plasma in combination with freeze-dried bone allograft: Case series. J Periodontol 2000;71:1654–1661.
16. Shigino T, Ochi M, Hirose Y, Hirayama H, Sakaguchi K. Enhancing osseointegration by capacitively coupled electrical field: A pilot study on early occlusal loading in the dog mandible. Int J Oral Maxillofac Implants 2001; 16:841–850.
17. Shigino T, Ochi M, Kagami H, Sakaguchi K, Nakade O. Application of capacitively coupled electrical field enhances periimplant osteogenesis in the dog mandible. Int J Prosthodont 2000;13:365–372.
18. Marx RE. Philosophy and particulars of autogenous bone grafting. Oral Maxillofac Surg Clin North Am 1993;5:599–612.
19. Knighton DR, Oredsson S, Banda M. Regulation of repair hypoxic control of macrophage-mediated angiogenesis. In: Hunt TK, Happenstall RB, Pennes E (eds). Soft and Hard Tissue Repair. New York: Prager, 1984;41–49.
20. Caplan AI. The mesengenic process. Clin Plast Surg 1995;21:429–435.
21. Lind M. Growth factors: Possible new clinical tools. Acta Orthop Scand 1996;67:407–417.
22. Garg AK. The future role of growth factors in bone grafting. Dent Implantol Update 1999; 10:5–7.
23. Marx RE, Carlson ER, Eichstaedt RM, Schimmele SR, Strauss JE, Georgeff KR. Platelet-rich plasma: Growth factor enhancement for bone grafts. Oral Surg Oral Med Oral Pathol Oral Radiol Endod 1998;85:638–646.

24. Kim SG, Chung CH, Kim YK, Park JC, Lim SC. Use of particulate dentin-plaster of Paris combination with/without platelet-rich plasma in the treatment of bone defects around implants. Int J Oral Maxillofac Implants 2002;17: 86–94.
25. Shanaman R, Filstein MR, Danesh-Meyer MJ. Localized ridge augmentation using GBR and platelet-rich plasma: Case reports. Int J Periodontics Restorative Dent 2001;21:345–355.
26. Marx RE. Clinical application of bone biology to mandibular and maxillary reconstruction. Clin Plast Surg 1994;21:377–392.
27. Hobo S, Ichida E, Garcia LT. Introduction. In: Osseointegration and Occlusal Rehabilitation. Tokyo: Quintessence, 1989:3–18.
28. Adell R. Surgical principles of osseointegration. In: Worthington P, Brånemark PI (eds). Advanced Osseointegration Surgery: Applications in the Maxillofacial Region. Chicago: Quintessence, 1992:94–119.
29. Zoldos J, Kent JN. Healing of endosseous implants. In: Block MS, Kent JN (eds). Endosseous Implants for Maxillofacial Reconstruction. Philadelphia: Saunders, 1995:40–70.

CHAPTER

2

Review of Bone-Grafting Materials

Although alveolar bone can be a contraindication for dental implants, bone grafting can provide the structural or functional support necessary in such cases. Grafts can provide scaffolding (Fig 2-1) for bone regeneration[1] and augmentation for bony defects resulting from trauma, pathology, or surgery. They can also be used to restore bone loss resulting from dental disease; to fill extraction sites; and to preserve the height and width of the alveolar ridge through augmentation and reconstruction. Autogenous bone remains the best grafting material because of its osteogenic properties, which allow bone to form more rapidly in conditions that require significant bone augmentation or repair. The allografts most commonly used for restoring osseous defects are mineralized or demineralized freeze-dried bone allografts (FDBA). The primary alloplasts are hydroxyapatite, bioactive glasses, tricalcium phosphate (TCP) particulates, and synthetic polymers. The primary xenograft material is purified anorganic bone, either alone or enhanced with tissue-engineered molecules. These augmentation materials can be incorporated in the modeling, remodeling, or healing processes of bone to assist or to stimulate bone growth in areas where resorption has occurred and implants are needed.

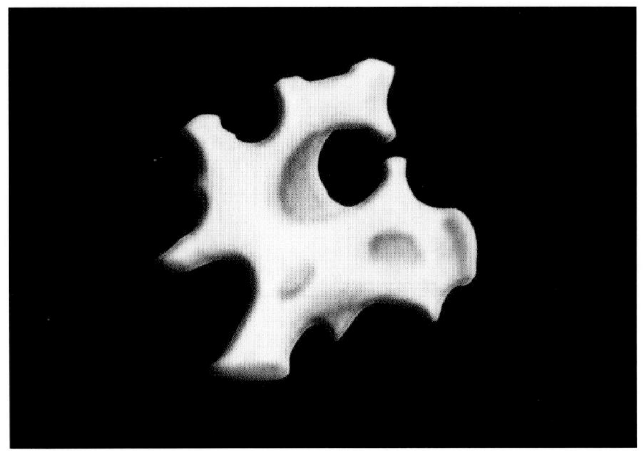

Fig 2-1
Bone-grafting materials provide a resorbing scaffold that permits osseous tissue ingrowth. Ideally, resorption is gradual enough to allow the surrounding bony tissues to occupy the recipient site completely, while still allowing dental implants to be placed in new osseous tissue as quickly as possible.

Mechanisms of Bone Regeneration and Augmentation

Three different processes are associated with successful bone grafting: osteogenesis, osteoinduction, and osteoconduction.[2–5] *Osteogenesis* is the formation and development of bone. An osteogenic graft is derived from or composed of tissue involved in the natural growth or repair of bone. Osteogenic cells can encourage bone formation in soft tissues or activate more rapid bone growth in bone sites. *Osteoinduction* is the process of stimulating osteogenesis. Osteoinductive grafts can be used to enhance bone regeneration and may even cause bone to grow or extend into an area where it is not normally found. *Osteoconduction* provides a physical matrix or scaffolding suitable for the deposition of new bone. Osteoconductive grafts are conducive to bone growth and allow bone apposition from existing bone, but they do not produce bone formation themselves when placed within soft tissue. To encourage bone growth across its surface, an osteoconductive graft requires the presence of existing bone or differentiated mesenchymal cells. All bone-grafting materials possess at least one of these three modes of action.

Types of Graft Material

As noted above, the three primary types of bone graft material are autogenous bone; allografts; and alloplasts, of which commercially available xenografts are generally considered a subgroup. The mechanism by which these graft materials work normally depends on the origin and composition of the material.[3,6] Autogenous bone, an organic material harvested from the patient, forms new bone by osteogenesis, osteoinduction, and osteoconduction. Harvested from cadavers, allografts, which may be cortical or trabecular, have osteoconductive and possibly osteoinductive properties, but they are not osteogenic. Alloplasts, which may be composed of natural or synthetic material, are typically only osteoconductive.

In determining what type of graft material to use, the clinician must consider the characteristics of the bony defect to be restored.[3] In general, the larger the defect, the greater the amount of autogenous bone required. For small defects and for those with three to five bony walls still intact, alloplasts may be used alone or with allografts. For relatively large defects or those with only one to three bony walls intact, autogenous bone must be added to any other type of graft material being considered. Soft tissue ingrowth can be a complication during augmentation procedures with any grafting materials, so guided bone regeneration (GBR) using resorbable or nonresorbable membranes is often employed.[7]

Autogenous Bone

Autogenous bone, long considered the gold standard of grafting materials, is currently the only osteogenic graft material available to clinical practitioners. Grafted autogenous bone heals into growing bone through all three modes of bone formation; these stages are not separate and distinct, but rather overlap each other.[3] Common areas from which autogenous bone can be harvested include extraoral sites such as the iliac crest or tibial plateau and intraoral sites such as the mandibular symphysis, maxillary tuberosity, ramus, or exostoses.[3,8,9] Less resorption has been associated with the use of mandibular bone grafts than with iliac crest grafts.[8] Resorption may be reduced during healing by the use of expanded polytetrafluoroethylene (e-PTFE) membranes or slowly resorbable collagen membranes.[10] Bone grafts obtained intraorally generally result in less morbidity; however, intraoral donor sites provide a significantly smaller volume of bone than do extraoral sites such as the iliac crest or tibial plateau.

The optimal donor site depends on the volume and type of regenerated bone needed for the specific case. The posterior iliac crest provides the greatest amount of bone—up to 140 mL (Table 2-1 and Fig 2-2). This compares to up to 70 mL from the anterior iliac crest, 20 to 40 mL from the tibial plateau (Fig 2-3), 5 to 10 mL from the ascending ramus, up to 5 mL from the anterior mandible (Fig 2-4), up to 2 mL from the tuberosity, and varying amounts from bone shavings (Fig 2-5) or exostoses or through the use of suction traps (Fig 2-6). Autogenous bone is highly osteogenic and best fulfills the dental grafting requirements of providing a scaffold for bone regeneration.[11] The disadvantages associated with the use of autogenous bone are the need for a second operative site, resultant patient morbidity, and in some cases the difficulty of obtaining a sufficient amount of graft material (especially from intraoral sites). These limitations led to the development of allografts and alloplasts as alternative grafting materials.[2,11,12]

Table 2-1 Graft form and maximum volume available from autogenous bone donor sites

Donor site	Form available	Maximum volume (mL)
Extraoral		
Posterior iliac crest	Block and/or particulate	140
Anterior iliac crest	Block and/or particulate	70
Tibia	Particulate	20 to 40
Cranium	Dense cortical block	40
Intraoral		
Ascending ramus	Block	5 to 10
Anterior mandible	Block and/or particulate	5
Tuberosity	Particulate	2
Miscellaneous (eg, bone shavings, suction traps)	Particulate	Varies

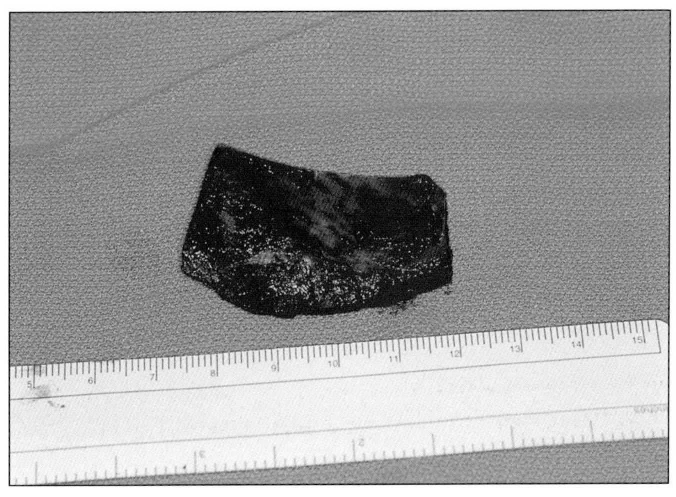

Fig 2-2
The ilium provides a greater amount of bone than do other donor sites, making it ideal when 50 mL or more is required. Harvesting is performed in a hospital operating room under general anesthesia. The harvested block is measured carefully before being divided to ensure appropriate size and dimension of the pieces.

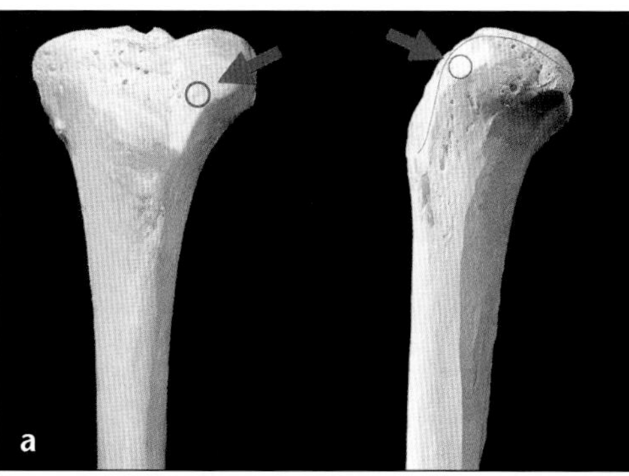
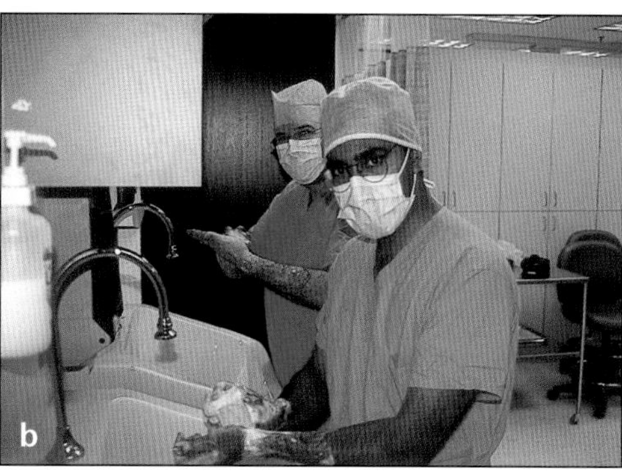
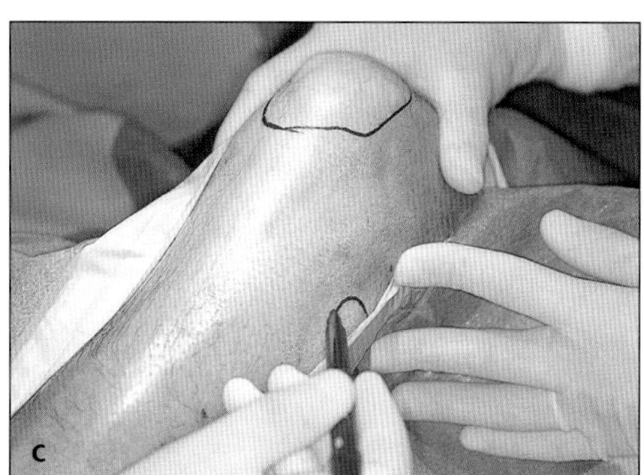
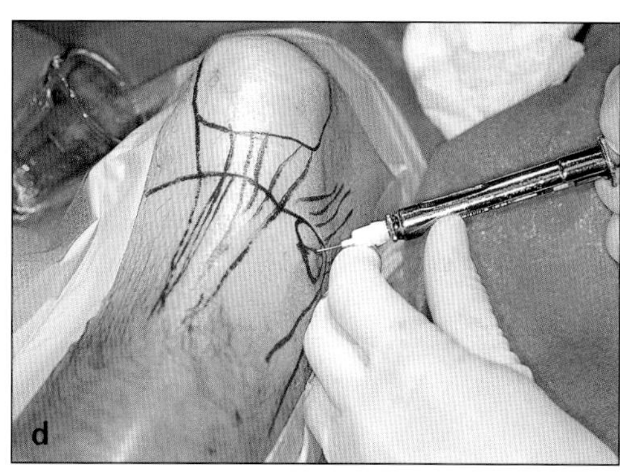
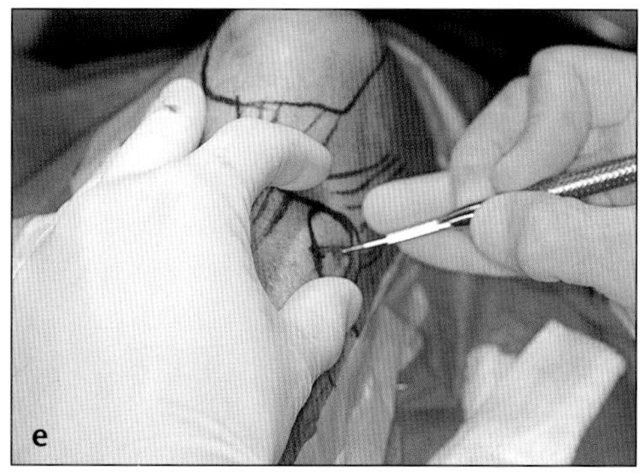
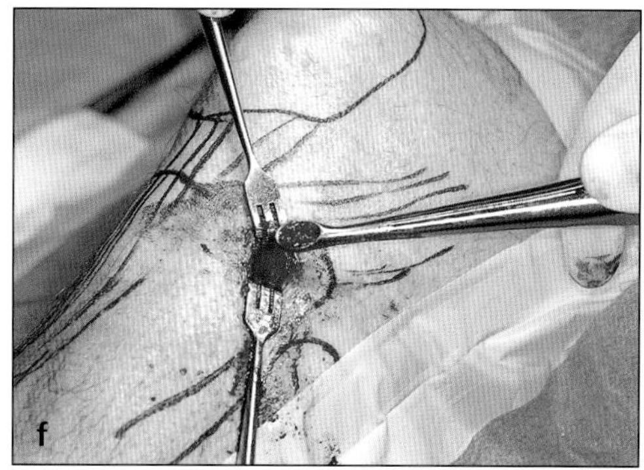
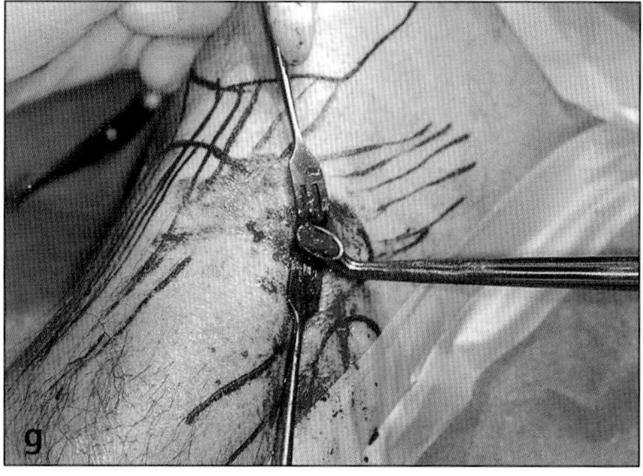
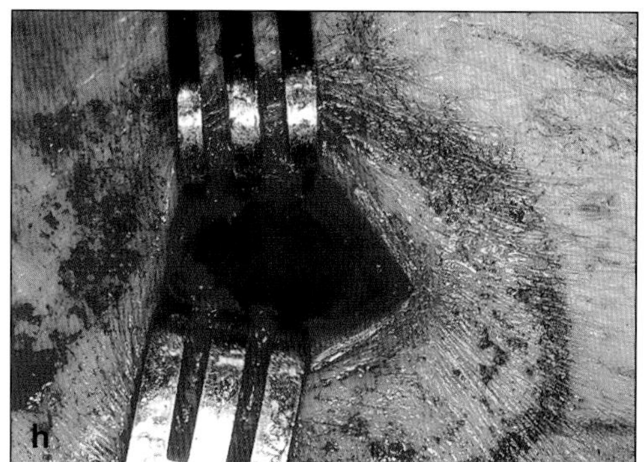

Fig 2-3 Prominent location and low morbidity make the anterior tibial plateau (with its Gerdy tubercle) ideal for bone harvesting as an outpatient procedure under intravenous (IV) sedation in the dental surgeon's office.

(a) The exact location of the osteotomy is marked with a red circle.

(b) Anterior tibial plateau bone harvesting requires full surgical scrub, Betadine preparation, and appropriate surgical drapes to maintain a sterile field and avoid contamination of the wound.

(c) The surrounding anatomy is outlined before surgery begins. This procedure is discussed in detail in chapter 7.

(d) A carpule of standard lidocaine with 1:100,000 epinephrine is administered before the incision is made.

(e) An initial oblique incision of approximately 1.5 cm is made through the skin above the Gerdy tubercle.

(f) Tissues are incised by layers to the bone; an appropriate bur is then used to create a small opening in the cortical bone. Bone is then harvested with a no. 4 Molt curette (G. Hartzell & Son, Concord, CA) or a straight orthopedic curette.

(g) Additional bone marrow can be scooped from the tibia with back-angle curettes to allow deeper access when needed.

(h) The cavity created within the bone. A hemostatic agent is placed in the cavity prior to suturing in layers. Within 3 to 4 months, the cancellous bone will naturally regenerate.

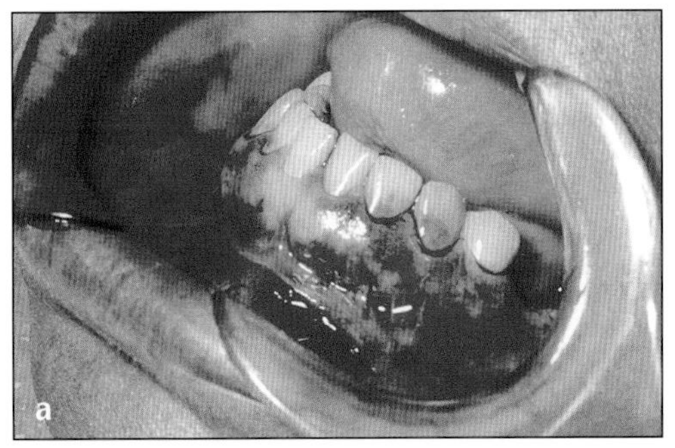

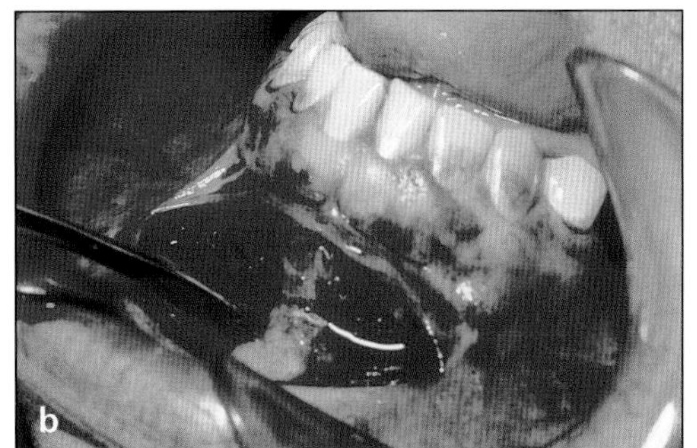

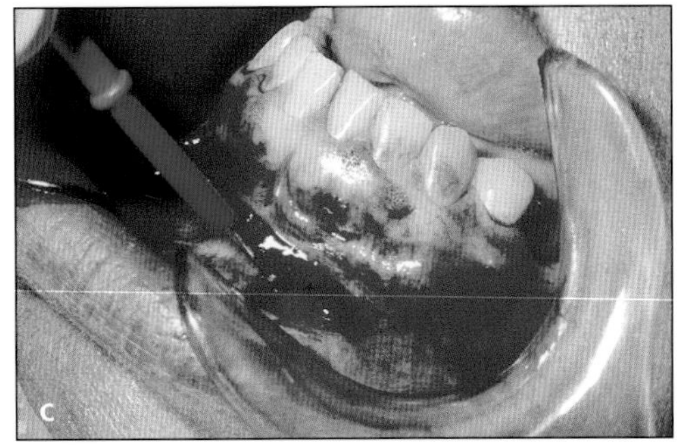

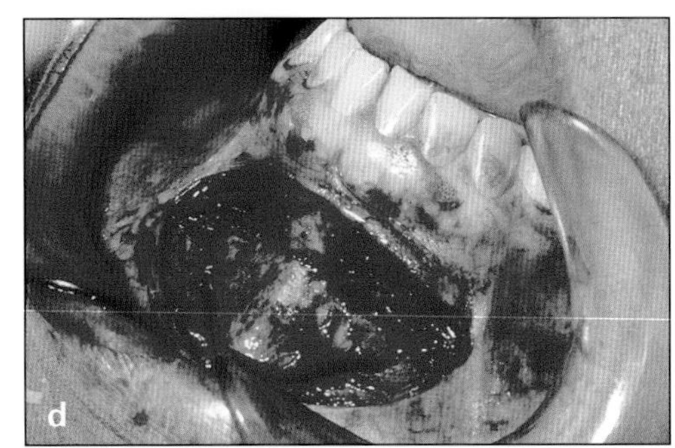

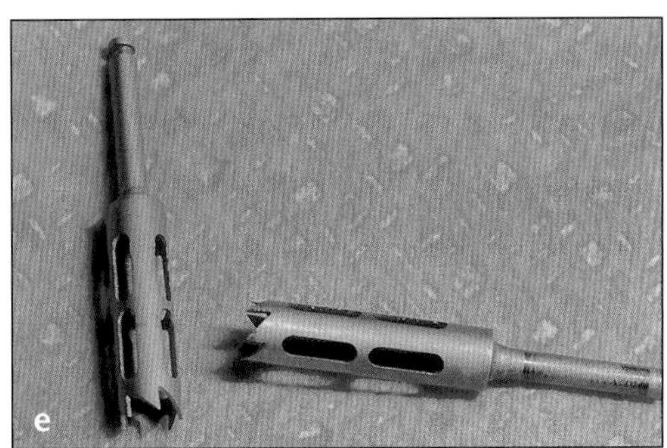

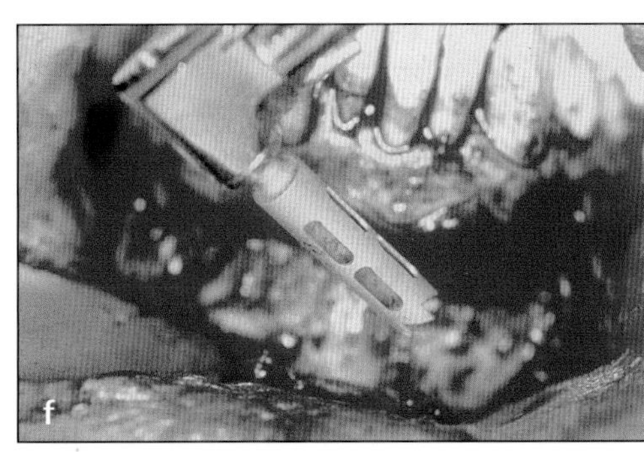

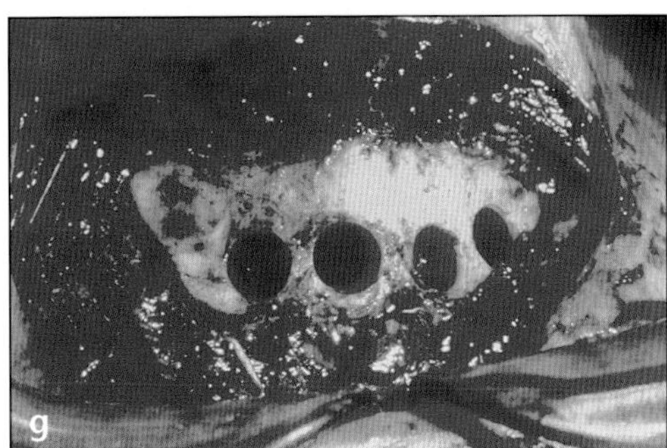

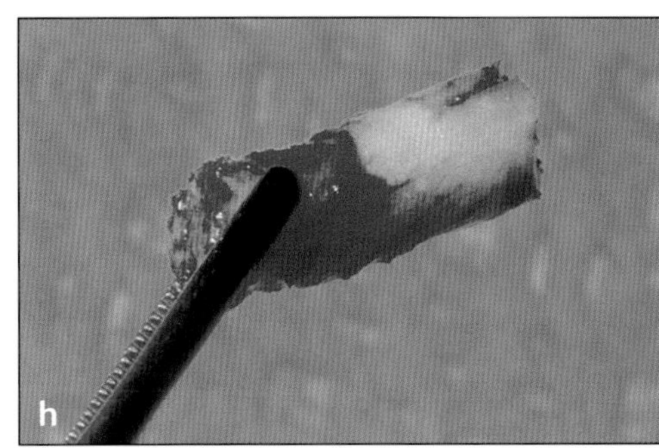

Fig 2-4 The anterior mandible may be used to harvest up to 5 mL of corticocancellous bone.

(a) A vestibular incision is made 3 to 5 mm apical to the mucogingival junction.

(b) The mentalis muscle is dissected to expose the facial aspect of the anterior mandible.

(c) The electrocautery tip is used to control bleeding, which can impair visualization of the bony wall.

(d) The mental area is exposed and ready for harvesting. This procedure is discussed in detail in chapter 6.

(e) Trephine burs of 4-mm diameter are ideal for harvesting chinbone cores that can later be crushed and used in particles. Microsaws or cylindrical burs should be used to obtain bone blocks.

(f) Trephine burs can be used effectively in either an implant drill or a straight surgical handpiece.

(g) The bone cores, generally 8 to 10 mm long, can be harvested separately with a remaining septum in between (as shown) or as a whole for larger openings.

(h) One of the harvested bone cores. The cortical portion on the right side is relatively avascular and acellular when compared to the cancellous portion on the left.

Fig 2-5 Bone shavings from adjacent areas of the surgical site or from the buccal shelf or ascending ramus can provide a more modest volume of autogenous bone.

(a) Bone-shaving devices can be used to harvest autogenous bone.

(b) The curved blade shaves bone when "raked" with appropriate pressure over the bony surface, producing very thin, curled bone strips, which are collected in a chamber that can hold up to 2 mL of bone shavings.

(c) A "pencil grip" with an angulation of 25 to 30 degrees from the bone surface is recommended during the pull stroke.

(d) The bone in the chamber is easily retrieved when the blade is retracted. The blade can then be placed back in position for additional harvesting in the same patient. The device is disposable.

(e) The osseous coagulum is placed in a receptacle in which additional allogeneic or alloplastic graft materials can be added to increase the total volume. Platelet-rich plasma (PRP) can be added to increase healing capacity.

(f) A curled strip of bone shaving seen under a scanning electron microscope reveals how multiple shavings can provide a greater exposed volume for release of cells and proteins in the recipient site than they supplied at the donor site.

(g) A nondisposable bone-shaving device can also be used with a pull stroke over the bone surface.

(h) The blade can be removed to access the bone collected in the chamber.

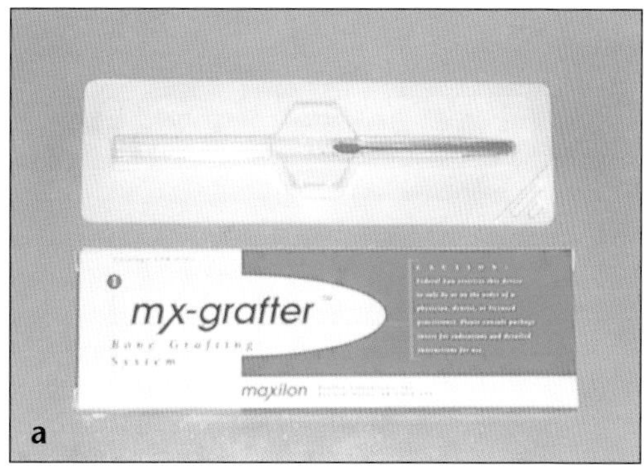

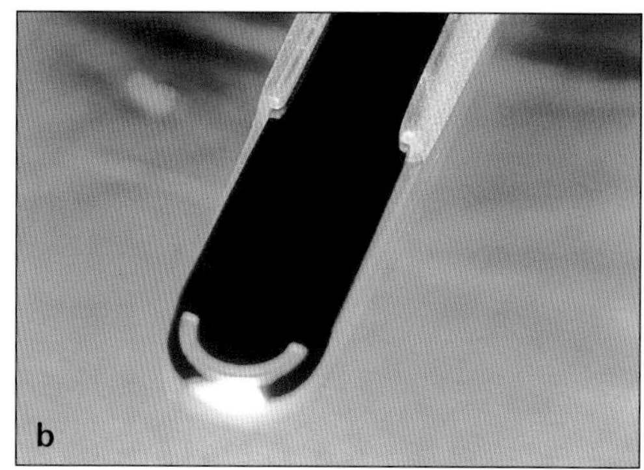

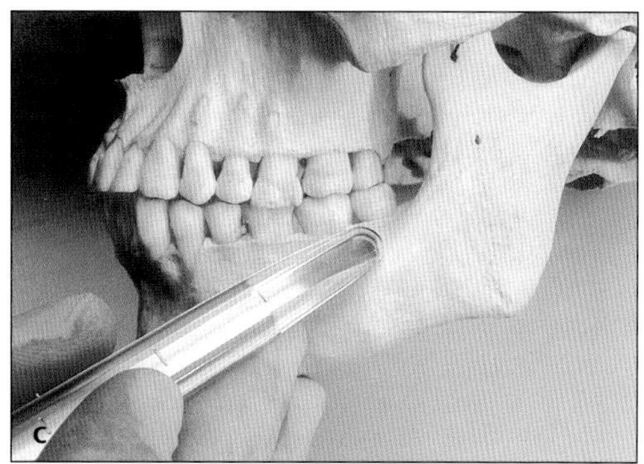

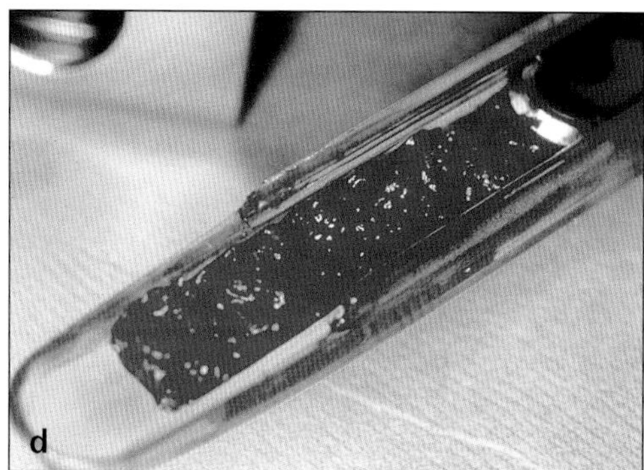

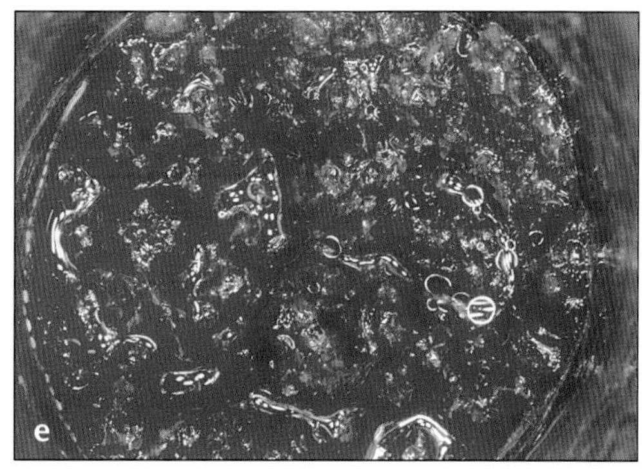

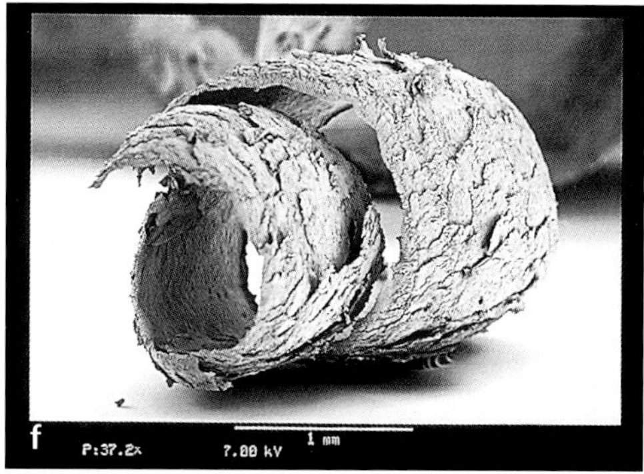

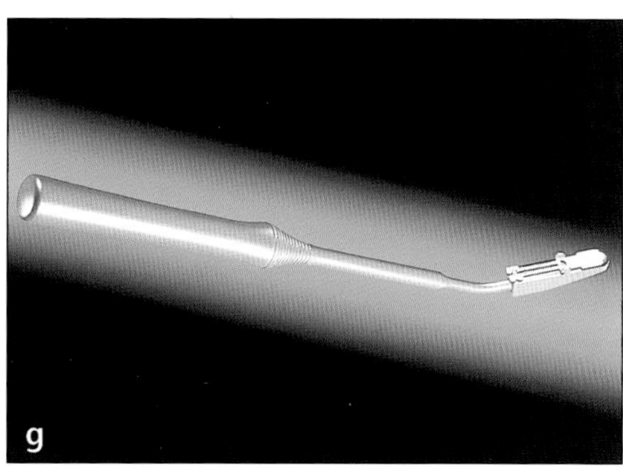

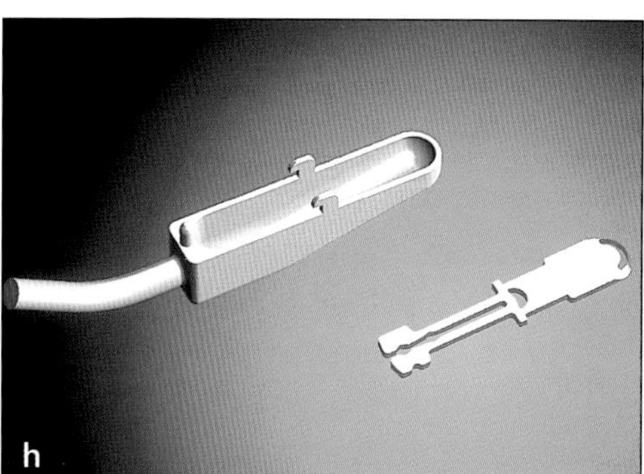

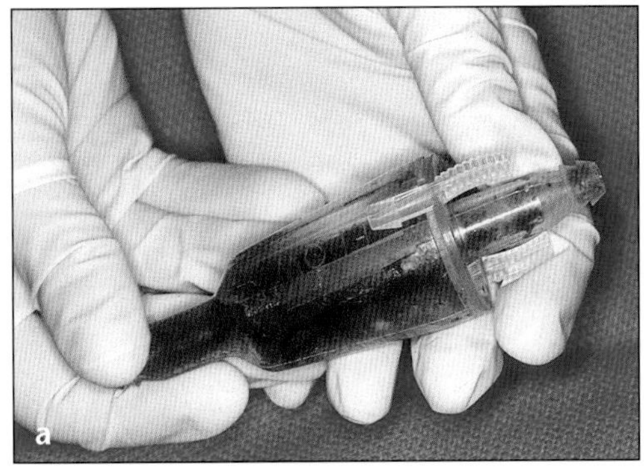

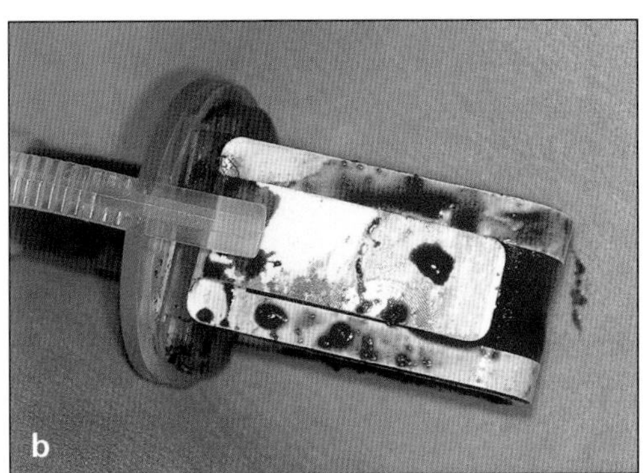

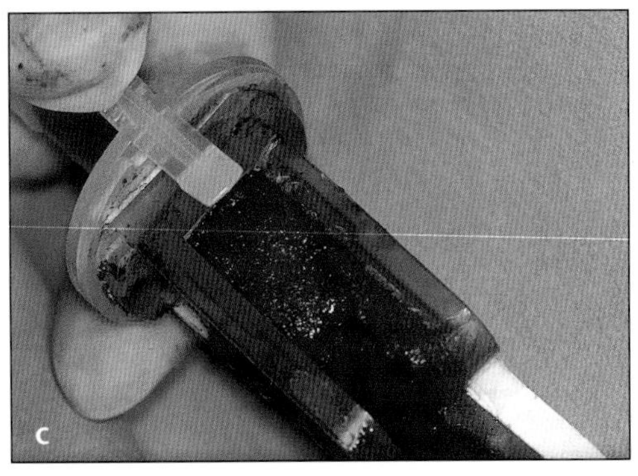

Fig 2-6 Autogenous bone collected with a suction trap while drilling osteotomies can be used to fill small defects.

(a) A commercially available, completely disposable suction trap. There are also many suction traps that can be sterilized for reuse and feature a disposable collecting screen.

(b) Bone can be harvested from a suction trap cup. The amount of bone collected in this device depends on many variables (eg, particle size obtained according to the bur used, amount of irrigation, amount of saliva, drilling speed). The viable bone cells are generally suctioned out; the autogenous bone will contain bacterial contamination.

(c) The side of this disposable trap can be opened by pulling on a tab. Inside is an osseous coagulum that can be augmented with other graft materials for small grafting procedures.

Allografts

Bone allografts are obtained from cadavers (Fig 2-7) or from patients' living relatives or nonrelatives. Those obtained from cadavers are available through tissue banks that are accredited by the American Association of Tissue Banks, which process and store the allografts under complete sterility (Fig 2-8). The advantages of allografts include ready availability, elimination of the need for a patient donor site, reduced anesthesia and surgical time, decreased blood loss, and fewer complications.[3] Disadvantages are primarily associated with the antigenicity of tissues harvested from another individual; transplanted bone may induce a host immune response. Cadaveric bone also may be rejected, as occurs with other transplanted tissues or organs.[2,3,13]

The most commonly used forms of allografts are frozen, freeze-dried (lyophilized), demineralized freeze-dried, and irradiated. Fresh allografts are the most antigenic; freezing or freeze-drying the bone significantly reduces the antigenicity.[6] Because allografts are not osteogenic, bone formation takes longer and results in less volume than can be achieved with autogenous grafts.[3] Concerns have been raised regarding the possible transmission of HIV through a bone allograft; however, when proper precautions and adequate laboratory studies are employed, the risk of using or receiving an allograft from an unrecognized early HIV–infected donor is approximately 1:1,600,000.[14]

FDBA can be used in either a mineralized or a demineralized (DFDBA) form. Demineralization removes the mineral phase

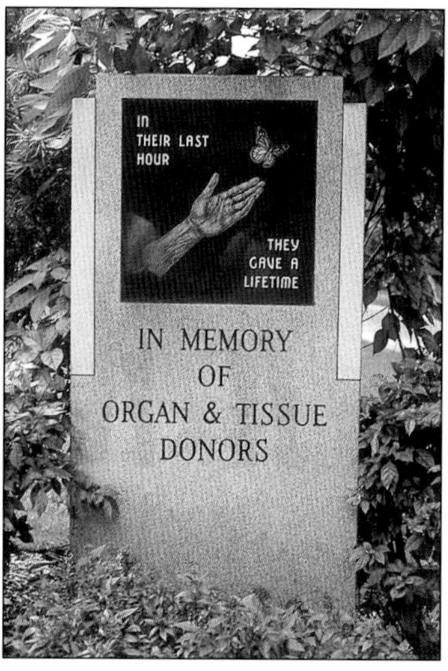

Fig 2-7
A memorial stone at the University of Miami honors organ and tissue donors. Harvesting, processing, and distribution of donated tissues are extensively regulated, limiting tissue availability.

of the graft material and purportedly exposes the underlying bone collagen and possibly some growth factors, particularly bone morphogenetic proteins (BMPs), which may increase its osteoinductive capabilities.[2,15,16] FDBA may form bone by osteoinduction and osteoconduction.[3] Because it is mineralized, it hardens faster than DFDBA. Clinical experience has shown that grafting of the sinuses with DFDBA alone results in the presence of dense connective tissue after 6 months, whereas grafting with FDBA results in the presence of new bone formation.[17] Bone is essential when treating defects in preparation for implant placement. The clinical and histologic findings of one study demonstrated that sites grafted with FDBA and complemented with an e-PTFE barrier can yield predictable results when augmenting alveolar ridges prior to the placement of implants.[18]

MTF (Dentsply Friadent CeraMed, Lakewood, CO) is an allogeneic freeze-dried bone that is available in both mineralized and demineralized forms. FDBA is more effective than DFDBA in the following situations:

1. Repair and restoration of fenestrations
2. Minor ridge augmentation
3. Fresh extraction sites (used as a fill)
4. Sinus lift cases (used as a graft)
5. Repair of dehiscences and failing implants

This particulate material is available in a variety of sizes, which should be selected according to the intended application. Similar graft results have been shown from the use of particles ranging from 200 to 1,000 μm for various cases as needed. Indications for DFDBA are limited to periodontal defects.

Puros (Zimmer Dental, Carlsbad, CA) is an allogeneic graft material that has undergone a well-tested processing method to reduce antigenicity and to minimize any risk of viral cross-contamination from donor material.[19] This type of allograft, which is solvent-preserved (as opposed to freeze-drying to extract the water component), has been shown to osseointegrate as effectively as cryopreserved material and to be equally biotolerable.[20] Animal and human studies of this material have shown good bone formation and repair

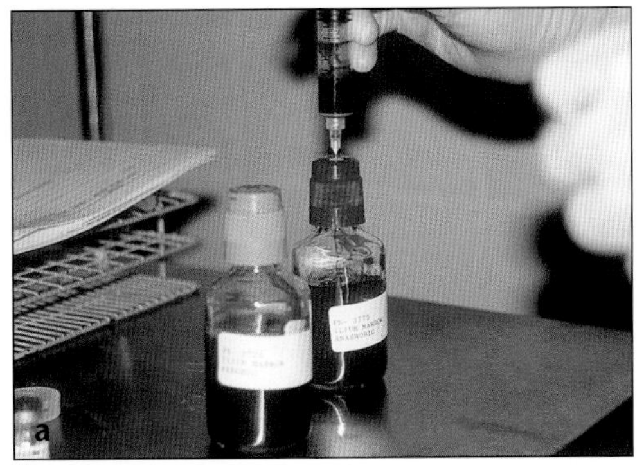

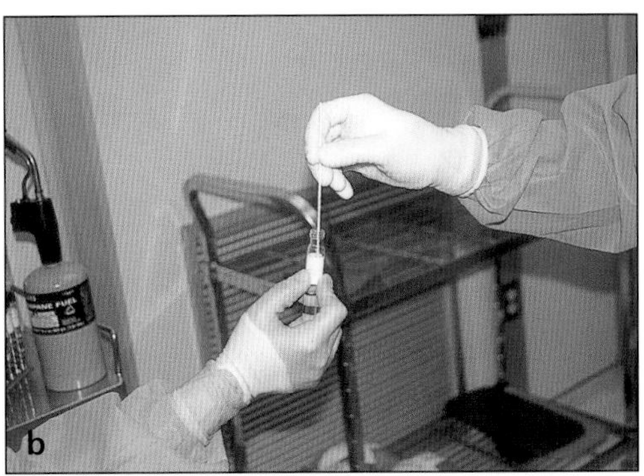

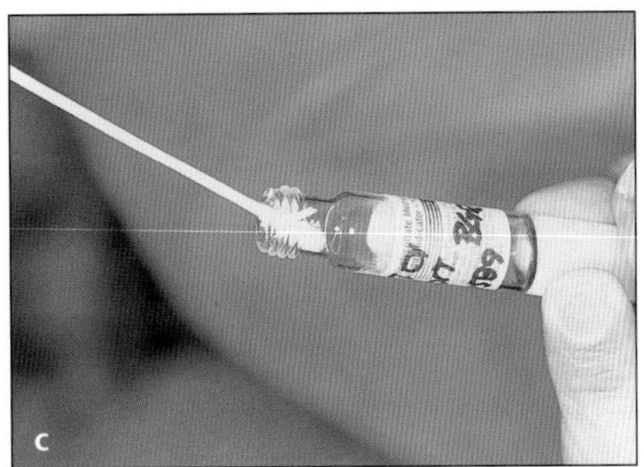

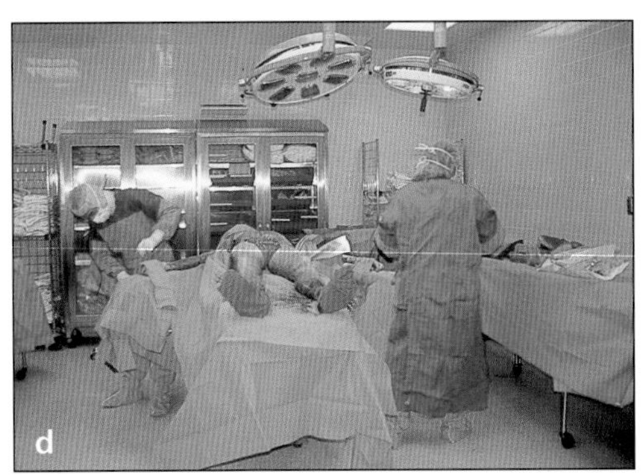

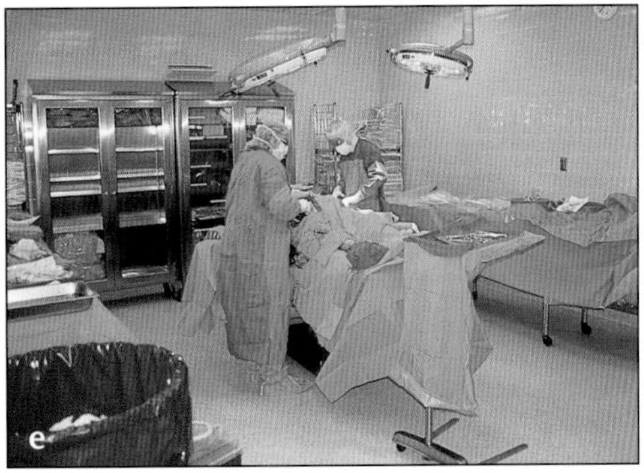

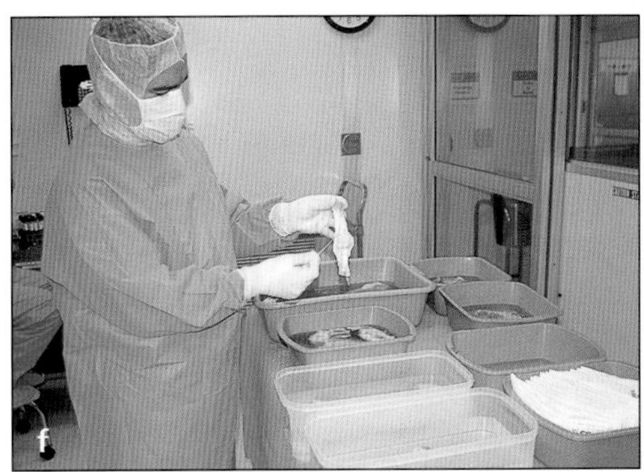

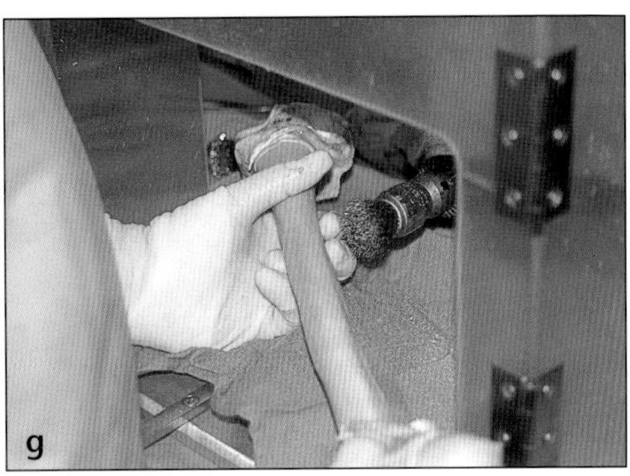

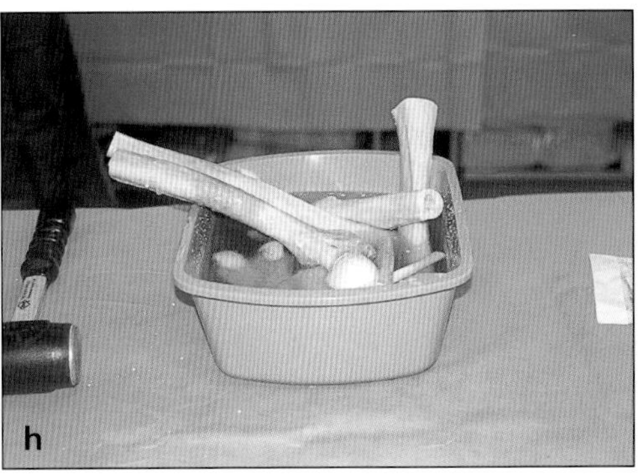

Fig 2-8 Bone allografts obtained from cadavers undergo strict screening and processing by tissue banks before they are made available to surgeons.

(a) Strict donor screening begins with blood tests.

(b) Culture studies are performed on tissue samples from the medullary canal, the specific tissues being donated, and the entire donor.

(c) Additional cultures are taken throughout the various steps of tissue processing. Material that is ready for distribution may have undergone as many as 200 cultures.

(d) High-quality tissue banks follow strict procedures for preparing and procuring specimens, beginning with a full surgical preparation within 24 hours of the donor's death.

(e) The donor is prepared in completely sterile and aseptic conditions. A detailed autopsy is conducted to ensure that there are no underlying medical conditions that could contraindicate the use of the donor's tissues.

(f) The different tissues are classified and placed in trays.

(g) The soft tissue is stripped from the bone surface, both by hand and mechanically.

(h) Large pieces of bone are cleaned and placed in separate containers.

Fig 2-8 *(cont)*
(i) Osseous tissues are cut into different configurations according to the request of various surgical specialties (eg, orthopedics, oral surgery).

(j) Bones are cut into standard sizes and shapes or, when possible, based on a surgeon's particular needs.

(k) The grafts are then ready for the removal of lipids, cells, and moisture.

(l) Tissues are soaked in sterile solutions to remove unwanted compounds.

(m) Once the lipids and cells are removed, the pieces are crushed into powders.

(n) The bone powders are passed through sifters to obtain particles of various sizes.

(o) The powders are freeze-dried in liquid nitrogen tanks or with chemical solvents to eliminate all remaining moisture.

(p) The freeze-dried bone is packaged in airtight containers and numbered for tracking before distribution. Demineralized freeze-dried bone is obtained by placing freeze-dried bone in a strong hydrochloride acid bath to remove its mineral matrix.

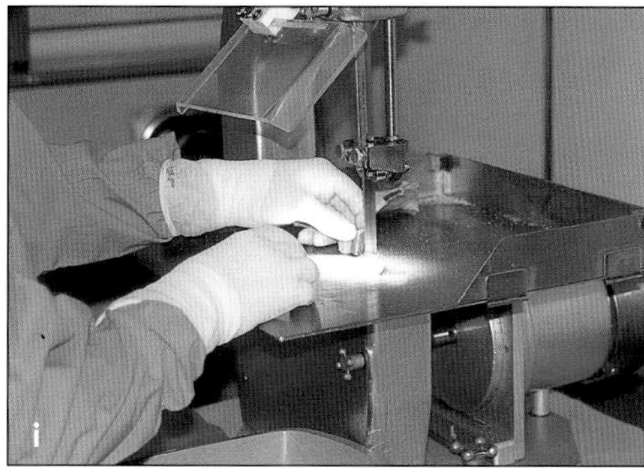

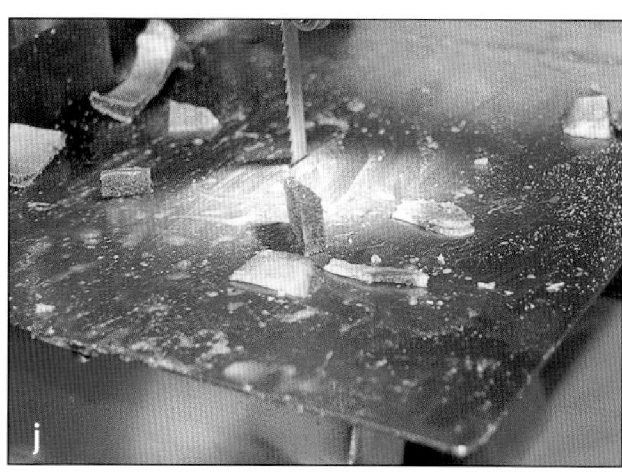

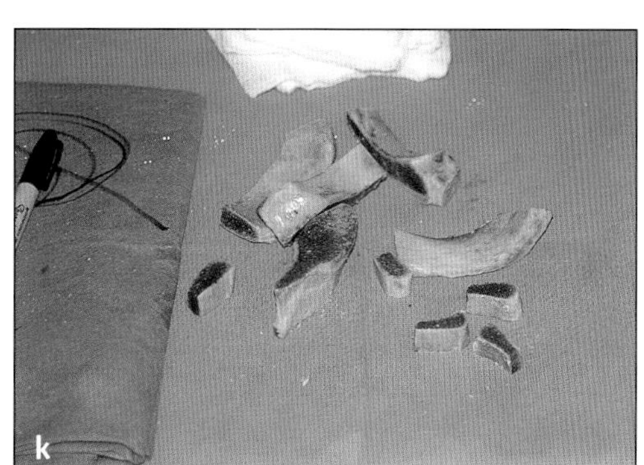

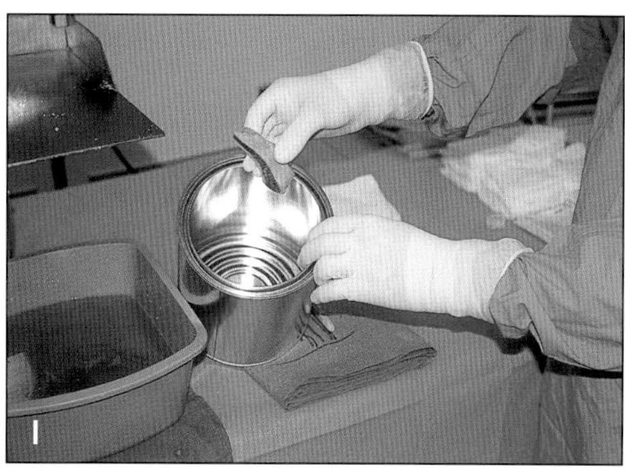

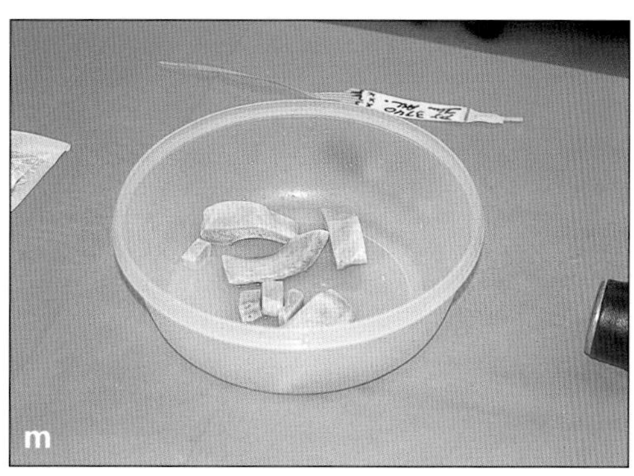

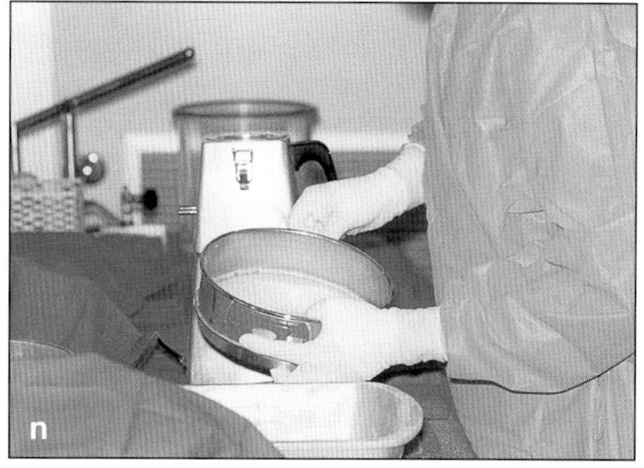

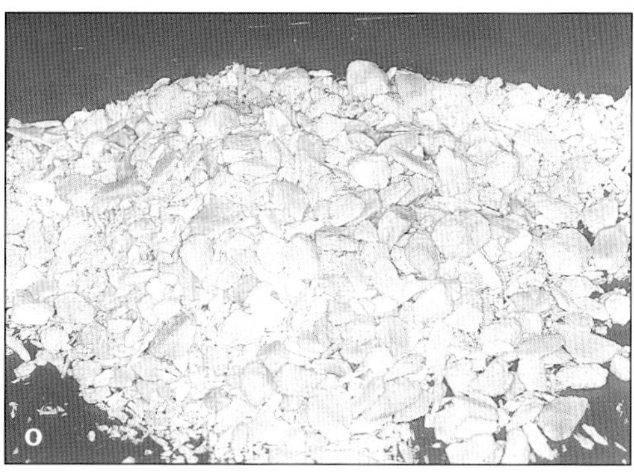

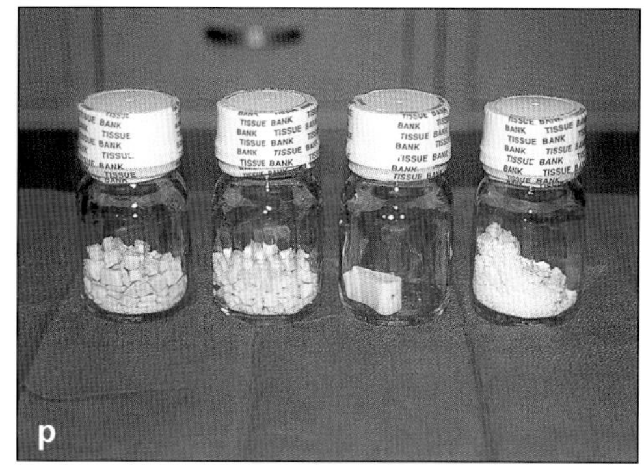

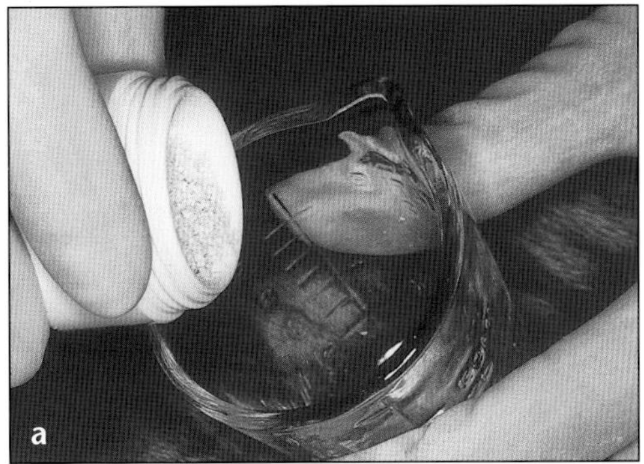

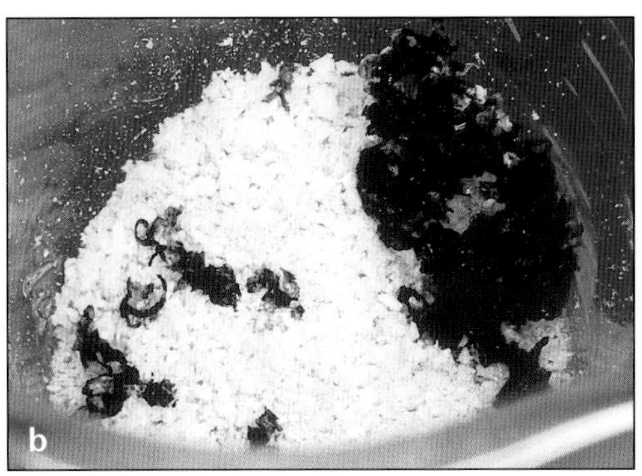

Fig 2-9
(a) A vial of Puros graft material is placed into a sterile container in a surgical field.

(b) The Puros graft material is rehydrated with nonactivated PRP to enhance healing. Blood from the patient that has been aspirated in the area of the surgical site can also be used for rehydration; alternatively, 0.9% saline solution may be used. Bone shavings from the patient have been added to the graft to provide living bone cells. Composite graft material should contain a minimum of 20% autogenous bone for best results.

results.[21-24] Moreover, because the water component is removed by solvents rather than by freeze-drying, which can potentially alter the mineral as a result of the volume expansion that occurs during the transition from the liquid to the solid phase, the mineral matrix is purported to remain more intact.[20] This material also has both the mineral and collagen phases of allogeneic tissues (Fig 2-9).

The use of DFDBA as a graft material has been questioned because of some reports that it is unpredictable in regenerating new bone. In one study in humans, for instance, the DFDBA particles were found to be surrounded by uninflamed connective tissue.[25] A later study showed positive results with the use of DFDBA and a cell-occlusive membrane. Incorporation of the DFDBA particles was observed in new bone that contained lacunae with osteocytes.[25] The results of this study might have been improved by the use of FDBA instead of DFDBA. The benefits seen in this study could also have been from the barrier membrane rather than the graft material, as it was DFDBA and not FDBA.

It is generally believed that BMPs and other noncollagenous proteins in the exposed matrix are responsible for the osteoinductivity of DFDBA. This osteoinductivity, however, depends on the quality and quantity of the bone matrix in the graft material.[26] Studies have shown that the osteoinductive activity of DFDBA may vary considerably among bone banks as well as among different samples from the same bone bank.[27] There are no widely accepted tests or guarantees to ensure that DFDBA material meets any minimum standards for osteoinductive properties. As a result, this graft material has fallen out of favor with many surgeons. In vitro and in vivo assays have been used to a limited extent to assess the osteoconductivity of DFDBA.[26]

DFDBA has been combined with other materials that have the potential to enhance bone growth. For example, the use of tetracycline with a DFDBA allograft has been studied. No significant benefit was shown to be derived from reconstituting the DFDBA particles in tetracycline hydrochloride during grafting of osseous defects.[28] Osteogenin, a bone-inductive protein isolated from human long bones, has been combined with DFDBA and studied in the regeneration of intrabony periodontal defects. While regeneration of new attachment apparatus and component tissues was significantly enhanced with this combination, new bone regeneration was not.[29]

A study using athymic rats has shown that two commercially prepared and available DFDBA preparations with gel carriers—Osteofil (Regeneration Technologies, Alachula, FL) and Grafton (Osteotech, Eatontown, NJ)—yielded similar results in bone formation via osteoconductivity at 28 days after implantation. However, significantly more bone was produced by Grafton than by Osteofil, suggesting that graft processing methods could represent a greater source of variability than do differences among donors.[30]

Irradiated cancellous bone (Rocky Mountain Tissue Bank, Denver, CO) has also been used as a substitute graft material for autogenous bone.[31,32] This bone allograft is trabecular bone obtained from the spinal column and treated with between 2.5 and 3.8 Megarads of radiation. Some authors have reported that among all available allografts, irradiated bone is most similar to autogenous bone in terms of demonstrating rapid replacement and consistent establishment of a reasonable ratio of new bone with less expense and morbidity than that associated with autogenous material.[31,32] However, because of a lack of published scientific documentation, use of this material is not recommended.

Alloplasts, Xenografts, and Tissue-Engineered Materials

The most commonly used bone substitutes are ceramic materials, including deorganified bovine bone, synthetic calcium phosphate ceramics (eg, hydroxyapatite, TCP), and calcium carbonate (eg, coralline). The mechanism of action in these ceramics is strictly osteoconduction,[3,33] with new bone formation taking place along their surfaces.[13,34] These materials are used to reconstruct bony defects and to augment resorbed alveolar ridges by providing a scaffold for enhanced bone tissue repair and growth. They can also improve probing depths and clinical attachment levels but have yet to demonstrate an ability to trigger or enhance the formation of new attachment apparatus on their own.[35] In general, these materials exhibit good compressive strength but poor tensile strength, similar to the properties of bone. Although their biologic responses differ, they have all been recommended for augmentation purposes.[3] Other currently available alloplasts include hard tissue replacement (HTR) polymer and bioactive glass ceramics.

Alloplastic and xenograft materials are available in a variety of textures, sizes, and shapes. Based on their porosity, they can be classified as dense, macroporous, or microporous, and they can be either crystalline or amorphous. Alloplasts can also be granular or molded. The specific properties of an alloplast determine which type is best for a particular application.[3,36]

Hydroxyapatite

During the past two decades, bovine-derived hydroxyapatite has received the most attention as a substitute for autogenous bone grafts. The primary inorganic, natural component of bone,[3,4,37,38] hydroxyapatite is highly biocompatible and bonds readily to adjacent hard and soft tissues.

The physical properties (ie, surface area and form of product, porosity, and crystallinity) and chemical properties (ie, calcium-to-phosphorus ratio, elemental impurities, ionic substitution in hydroxyapatite, and pH of the surrounding area) of a hydroxyapatite material determine the rate of resorption and the clinical applications of the graft.[3,39] For instance, larger particles take longer to resorb and remain longer at the augmentation site.[40] The greater the material's porosity, the more scaffolding it provides for new bone growth and the more quickly it is resorbed. The more crystalline the graft, the slower its resorption rate. Hence, amorphous grafts resorb more quickly than crystalline grafts. Solid, dense blocks of hydroxyapatite have a high compressive strength but are brittle; therefore, they are not considered suitable for load-bearing conditions. A general disadvantage of porous ceramics is that their strength decreases exponentially as their porosity increases.

In studies using hydroxyapatite for surgical reconstruction of atrophic ridges, results showed that it was superior, in terms of efficacy and morbidity, to the use of segmental osteotomies for bone grafts in which a large segment of bone is mobilized, frequently causing nerve injury.[41] An advantage of using hydroxyapatite is that it does not disturb the bone base, and the ridge is reconstructed over the residual bony structures.

Hydroxyapatite particles (approximately 1 mm in diameter) are often used for ridge augmentation and conform well to the underlying bone structure. Using particles instead of solid, dense blocks minimizes the problem of brittleness. In cases where porous hydroxyapatite blocks have been used as an alternative to hydroxyapatite particles,[4] the amount of bone ingrowth increases.[42] Another study notes a decrease in the clinical use of nonresorbable, nonporous hydroxyapatite for alveolar ridge augmentation, citing its tendency to lack cohesive strength and to migrate under stress during the healing process, as well as a concomitant increase in the use of porous hydroxyapatite.[43]

Bovine-derived anorganic bone matrix material

Bio-Oss (Osteohealth, Shirley, NY) is anorganic bovine bone that has been chemically treated to remove its organic component (Fig 2-10). After the material is sterilized, it can be used as a graft without causing a host immune response.[11] Bio-Oss is osteoconductive,[11,44] and, over time, the graft undergoes physiologic remodeling and becomes incorporated with the surrounding bone. Anorganic bone can be used alone or in combination with barrier membranes in isolated lesions such as periodontal defects, in dehiscences and fenestrations around implants, and in small sinus osteotomies. In large alveolar ridge deficiencies, anorganic bone can be combined with autogenous bone for successful augmentation. Anorganic bone has been used in a variety of treatment situations, including intrabony defects, maxillary sinus augmentation, GBR,[45] and around implants.

Augmenting the severely resorbed maxillary sinus area using Bio-Oss and Interpore 200 (Interpore International, Irvine, CA), a coralline material discussed later in this section, has also been evaluated. Predictable results were obtained with both materials, whether used alone or combined with autogenous bone from the chin and iliac crest.[46] However, Interpore 200 resorbs very slowly and thus remains in the form of hydroxyapatite rather than being replaced by host bone.

OsteoGraf/N (Dentsply Friadent CeraMed) is a popular example of this type of microporous hydroxyapatite particulate material derived from bovine bone. It is available in two varieties: OsteoGraf/N300, which has particles ranging from 250 to

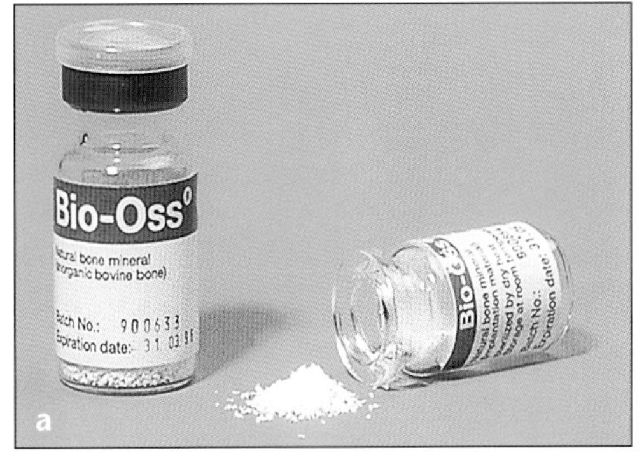

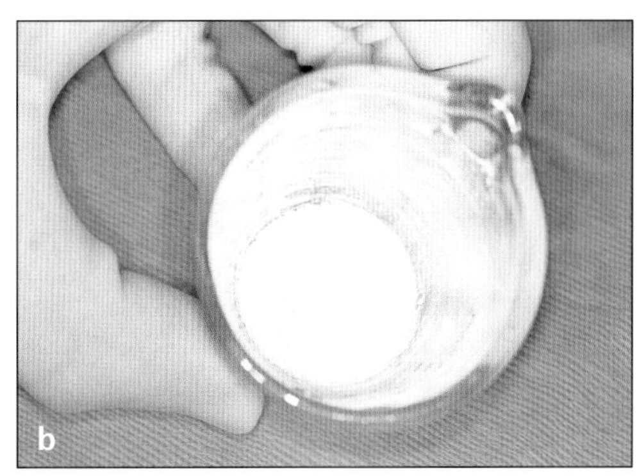
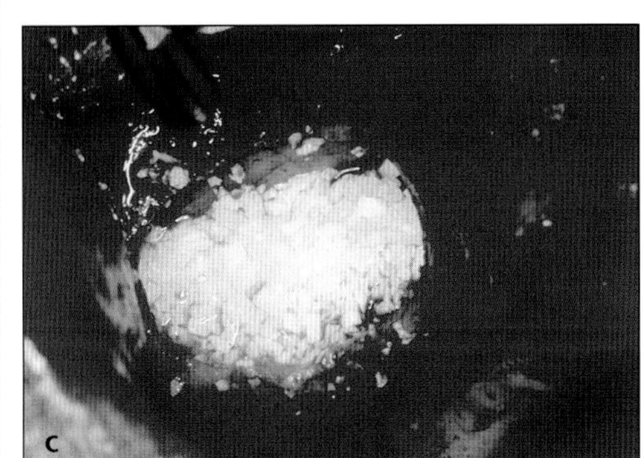
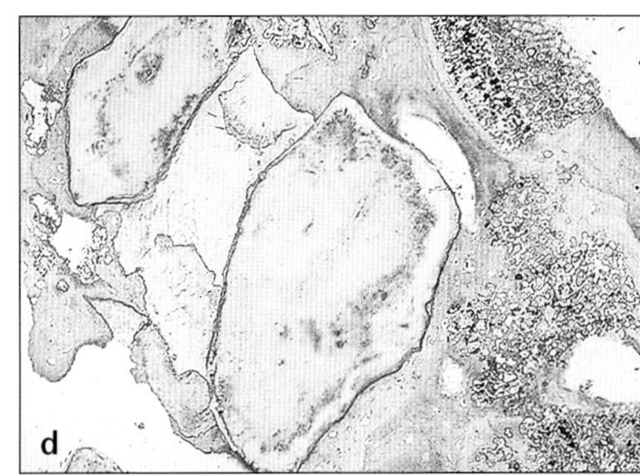

Fig 2-10 Bio-Oss, an anorganic bone graft material, can be used alone or with barrier membranes in a variety of treatment situations.

(a) Bio-Oss is packaged in 0.25-, 0.5-, 2.0-, and 5.0-g vials of cancellous granules and 0.5-, 2.0-, and 5.0-g vials of cortical granules.

(b) Bio-Oss is immersed in saline solution for rehydration.

(c) Bio-Oss graft material is used for a sinus lift procedure.

(d) Histology of an area grafted with Bio-Oss at 42 months postsurgery shows particulate bone formation around the graft material. This material will eventually resorb and be replaced by host bone.

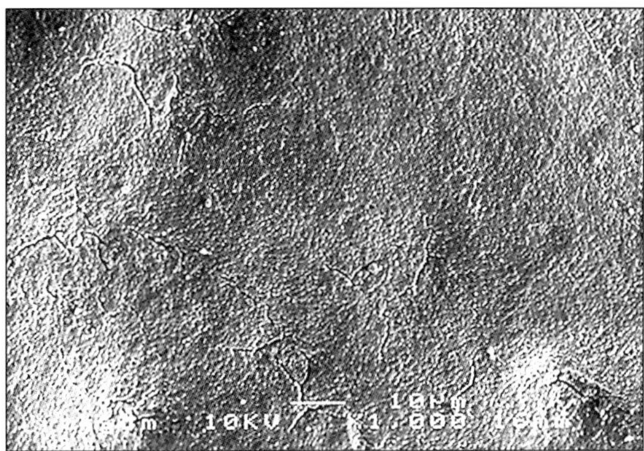

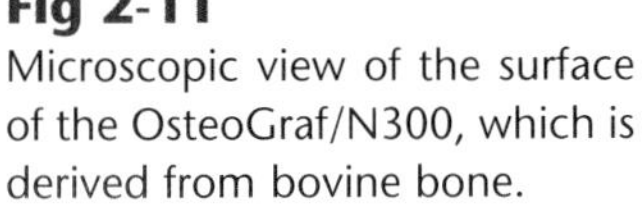

Fig 2-11
Microscopic view of the surface of the OsteoGraf/N300, which is derived from bovine bone.

420 µm, and OsteoGraf/N700, which has particles ranging from 420 to 1,000 µm (Fig 2-11). The small-particle variety has been used to treat ridge defects with good results.[47] After a healing period of slightly longer than 4 months, the grafted areas revealed overlying soft tissue color and tone similar to the nongrafted sites. In addition, the material in the grafted areas could not be dislodged from the adjacent bone without force. OsteoGraf/N has also been widely used in combination with DFDBA for sinus augmentation.[48] In a 3-year study in sinus lift cases, substantially more bone volume was achieved by mixing OsteoGraf/N with autogenous bone (80:20 ratio).[49]

PepGen P-15 (Dentsply Friadent CeraMed) is an enhanced form of bovine-derived hydroxyapatite that contains an added synthetic short-chain peptide, P-15. This com-

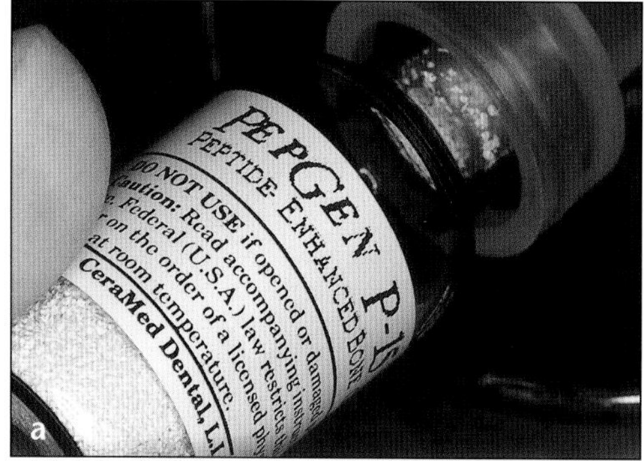

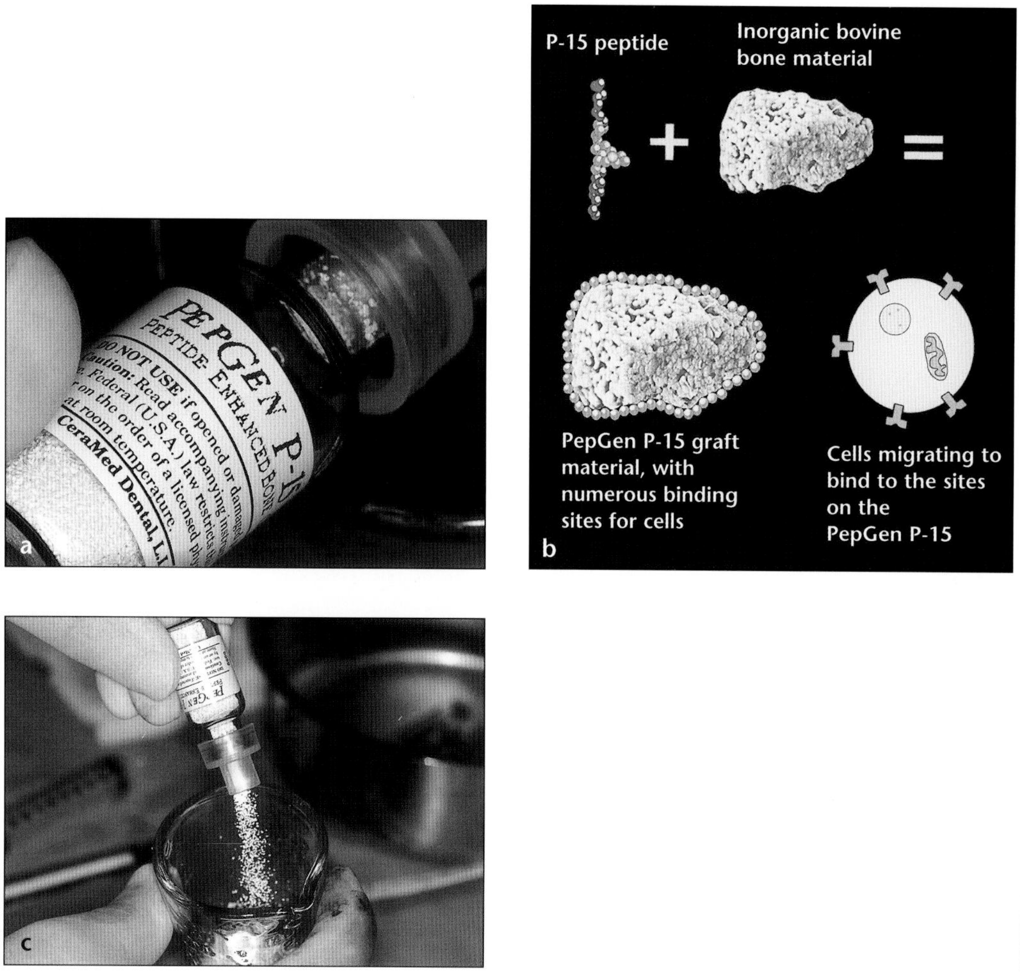

P-15 peptide

Inorganic bovine bone material

PepGen P-15 graft material, with numerous binding sites for cells

Cells migrating to bind to the sites on the PepGen P-15

b

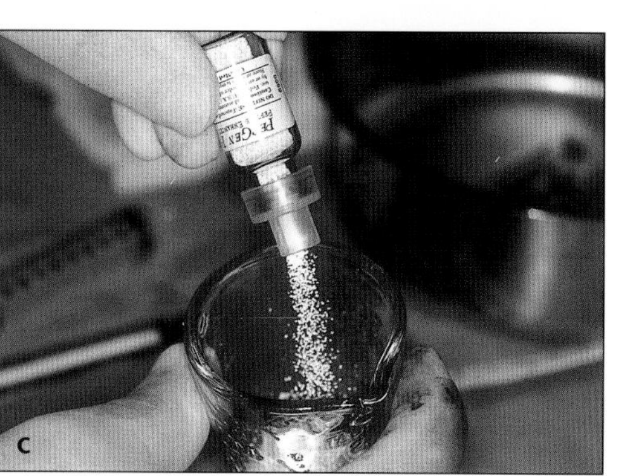

Fig 2-12
(a) PepGen P-15 graft material is a commercially available bone graft that combines OsteoGraf/N300 with a 15–amino acid peptide to attract osteoblasts.

(b) PepGen P-15 mimics autogenous bone; it has an inorganic bovine bone mineral and an organic component (the specific sequence of 15 amino acids designated as P-15). This peptide is involved in cell binding, attracting osteoblasts at a rate exponentially higher than that of the same graft material without the peptide.

(c) PepGen P-15 is available in 1- and 2-g vials. If used in a sterile manner during surgery, any remaining vial contents can be autoclaved up to three times (for up to four different patients). Adding a small amount of PepGen P-15 to harvested autogenous bone will assist in slowing the rapid resorption rate of autogenous bone and enhance the radiopacity of the graft for better definition on radiographs.

ponent mimics the cell-binding domain of type I collagen, which is responsible in natural bone for cell migration, differentiation, and proliferation.[50] This material may provide the benefit of a synthetic graft containing an inorganic and an important organic component that together may mimic autogenous bone in graft sites (Fig 2-12). It has been reported that PepGen P-15 provides enhanced bone formation in a shorter time compared with the bovine-derived hydroxyapatite plus DFDBA graft material traditionally used for sinus augmentation.[48] Similarly, other studies have reported a threefold increase in the amount of vital bone growth achieved in a sinus lift case when P-15 material is used compared with when anorganic bovine material is used alone[51] and significantly better regenerative results for periodontal bone defects grafted with the PepGen P-15 than for those treated using DFDBA or open-flap debridement.[52–54] Another study indicates that enhanced bone formation and faster particle resorption can occur with PepGen P-15 Flow (PepGen P-15 particles suspended in biocompatible inert hydrogel consisting of sodium carboxymethylcellulose, glycerol, and water) compared with the PepGen P-15 particulate.[55]

Synthetic bone material

OsteoGen (Impladent, Holliswood, NY) is a synthetic bioactive resorbable graft (SBRG). It is an osteoconductive, nonceramic graft

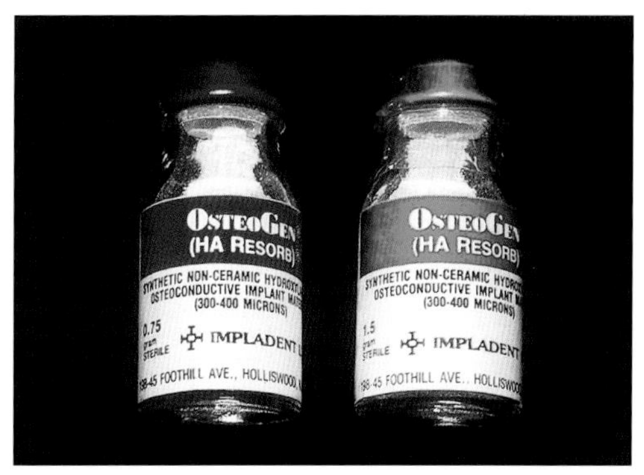

Fig 2-13
OsteoGen is a synthetic bioactive resorbable graft designed for bone augmentation or repair of alveolar defects.

material indicated for contouring and improving alveolar ridge deformities; filling extraction sockets; using around dental implants and in sinus grafts; and repairing marginal, periapical, and periodontal alveolar bony defects (Fig 2-13). A true synthetic, OsteoGen contains no organic components and can be used without fear of disease transmission.

This material's highly porous crystalline clusters act as a physical matrix to permit the infiltration of bone-forming cells and the subsequent deposition of host bone. As new bone is deposited, the material progressively resorbs over a 6- to 8-month period. Depending on the size of the defect and the patient's age and metabolism, approximately 80% of the material will be resorbed within 4 to 6 months.

OsteoGen was approved for marketing by the Food and Drug Administration in 1984 and is available in sterile crystalline cluster form (300 to 400 μm) in 0.75-, 1.5-, and 3.0-g vials and 0.3-g prefilled syringes.

Tricalcium phosphate

TCP is similar to hydroxyapatite, but it is not a natural component of bone material. In the body, TCP is converted in part to crystalline hydroxyapatite.[2] The rate of TCP resorption varies and appears to depend greatly on the material's chemical structure, porosity, and particle size. Like all bone substitute materials, TCP is osteoconductive and is intended to provide a physical matrix that is suitable for the deposition of new bone.[3] It is often used for repairing nonpathologic sites, where resorption of the graft with concurrent bone replacement might be expected.[38] TCP can also be used with osteogenic or osteoinductive materials to improve the handling characteristics of the graft during placement.[3] Both hydroxyapatite and TCP are safe and well tolerated.[56]

Cerasorb (Curasan, Kleinostheim, Germany) is a beta-tricalcium phosphate (beta-TCP) material that has been certified for use in bone defect regeneration in the entire skeletal system (Fig 2-14). In June 2000 it was certified in Europe as a synthetic material carrier for the patient's own PRP. The material is resorbed completely and is generally replaced by natural bone in a 3- to 24-month period, depending on the type of bone. During the process, collagen and blood vessels are incorporated with the Cerasorb granules (micropores) and the intergranular cavities (macropores). Collagen fibers guide capillaries and newly formed bone before resorption begins. Although highly porous, Cerasorb is stable and highly resistant to abrasion. Generally, a round-particle size of 10 to 63 μm prevents phagocytosis by macrophages.

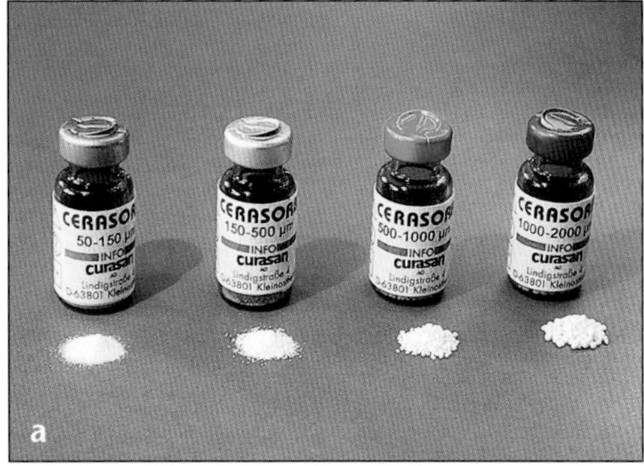

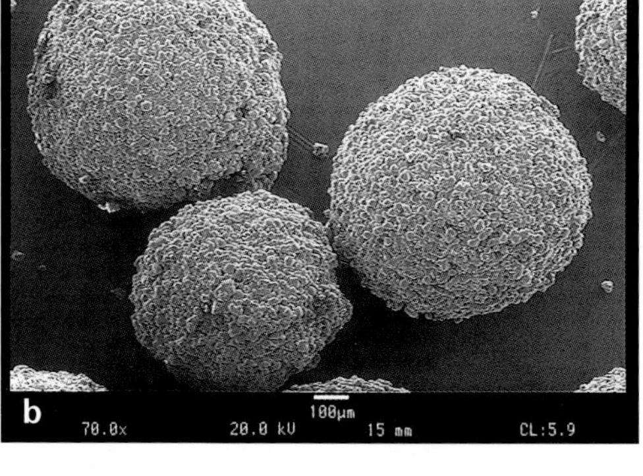

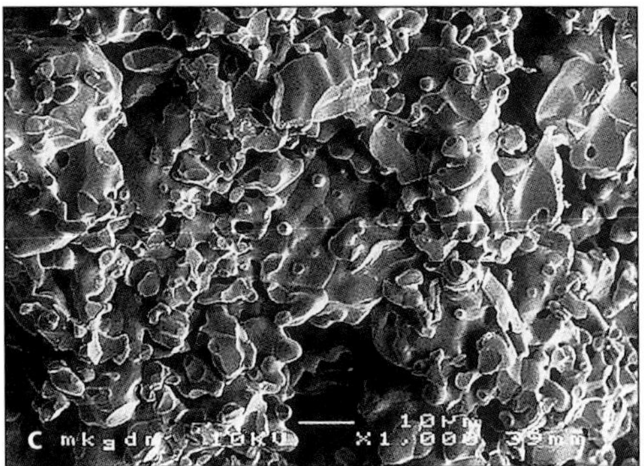

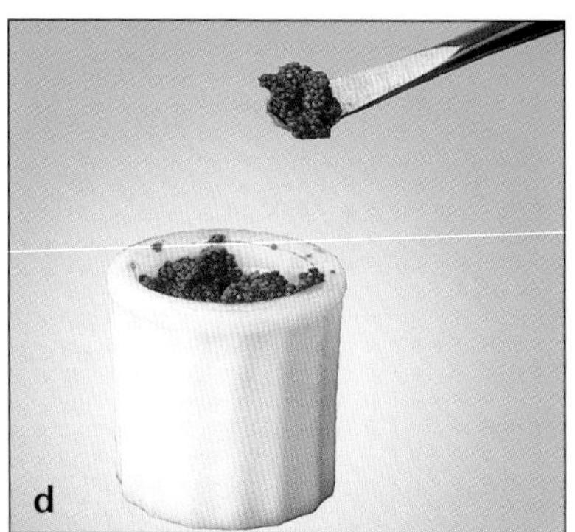

Fig 2-14
(a) Cerasorb, a beta-TCP material, was certified in Europe in 2000 for use as a PRP carrier.

(b) The porous surface of the round particles facilitates incorporation of new tissue.

(c) A microscopic view of the particles shows their spherical shape. The particles range in size from 10 to 63 µm in diameter; this size prevents them from being engulfed by macrophages.

(d) The Cerasorb material will be completely resorbed and replaced by new bone 3 to 24 months after grafting.

Calcium carbonate materials

Coralline

Coralline is a ceramic graft material synthesized from the calcium carbonate skeleton of coral. One of its advantages is that it has a three-dimensional structure similar to that of bone.[2] A recent study conducted among a population of young, growing patients demonstrated the suitability of coral granules for ridge preservation in the posterior maxilla and mandible in the presence of ankylosed primary teeth and congenitally absent permanent teeth but found it unsuitable for treatment in the traumatized anterior maxilla.[57]

As noted earlier, Interpore 200 is an example of a porous coralline hydroxyapatite. This material is essentially composed of pure hydroxyapatite and some TCP, and its mechanism of action is osteoconduction.[58] Interpore 200 (in blocks and granules) has been used as an implant graft that provides a matrix for bone ingrowth, as an onlay graft for the alveolar ridge, and as an interpositional implant in the mandible (Fig 2-15).[59] Some researchers have found the shape of this material to be easily modified during surgery to obtain an exact fit[59]; however, other investigators have found it to be brittle and difficult to handle.[36]

The resorption rate of porous ceramic graft material such as Interpore 200 has been studied.[60] Although the material was expected to degrade faster when placed in soft tissue, it was found that resorption was extremely slow, both in bone and soft tissue. Bone can grow around the material and into its porosities; however, the material takes a significant amount of time to resorb and to be replaced with bone.

Biocoral (Inoteb, LeGuernol, Saint-Gonnery, France) is another resorbable

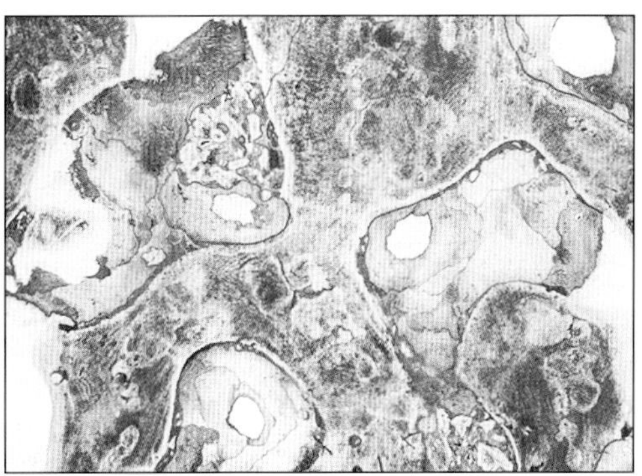

Fig 2-15
Histologic section of Interpore 200 particles with bone growth at 24 months. The particles have yet to be completely resorbed and replaced by host bone.

porous coralline graft material. It is a natural coral in the form of aragonite (more than 98% calcium carbonate) that is not altered by processing. It has been reported that the clinical response to this material, particularly related to periodontal osseous defect fill, is similar to or slightly better than the response to other hydroxyapatite graft materials.[61] The size and shape of the particles facilitate ease of handling and manipulation during surgery. This calcium carbonate also is not readily displaced from the treatment site.

Calcified algae

C-Graft (The Clinician's Preference, Golden, CO) has been used successfully for more than 10 years for grafting and remodeling bone.[62] Similar to bone in its crystalline, porous surface structure and chemical composition, C-Graft is a calcium phosphate ceramic with the hexagonal crystalline structure of hydroxyapatite and a large specific surface area with high bioactivity. C-Graft has an interconnecting microporosity that guides hard and soft tissue formation and can be very effective for filling tooth extraction sites and bone defects. It is an inorganic, biocompatible calcium phosphate material derived from calcium-encrusted sea algae, which are processed in order to develop an apatite material that is analogous to bone apatite (Fig 2-16). It is provided sterile in prefilled vials and has a granular size range of 300 to 2,000 μm. One study demonstrated that the texture of C-Graft acted as an osseoconductive scaffold for osteoblastic cells and that it also facilitated matrix deposition. The particles underwent osseointegrated as well as physiologic bone remodeling. New bone slowly replaced the resorbed biomaterial.[63]

Hard tissue replacement polymer

Bioplant HTR Polymer (Bioplant, Norwalk, CT) is a microporous composite with a calcium hydroxide graft surface.[36,64] The polymer resorbs slowly and is replaced by bone after approximately 4 to 5 years (Fig 2-17). Bioplant HTR has been reported to be an effective material for use in the following situations[36,64,65]:

1. Bone (ridge) maintenance, by preventing the anticipated loss of alveolar bone following extraction, preserving the height and width of the alveolar ridge
2. Ridge augmentation, in which immediate use following extraction increases the height and width of the alveolar ridge
3. Delayed augmentation (after extensive atrophy has already occurred), in which the dimensions of the alveolar ridge are increased and bony defects are corrected
4. Repair of periodontal and other bony defects

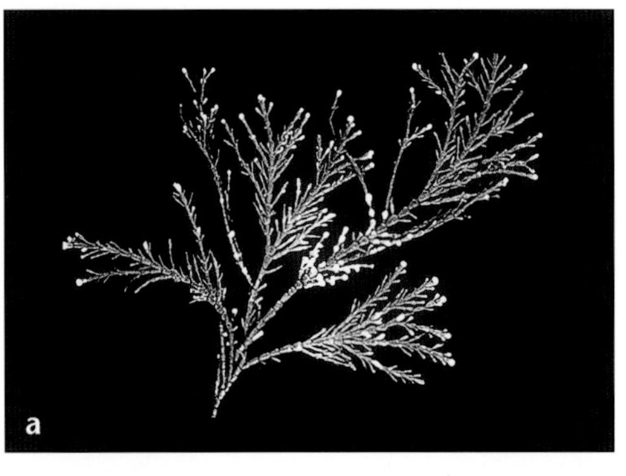

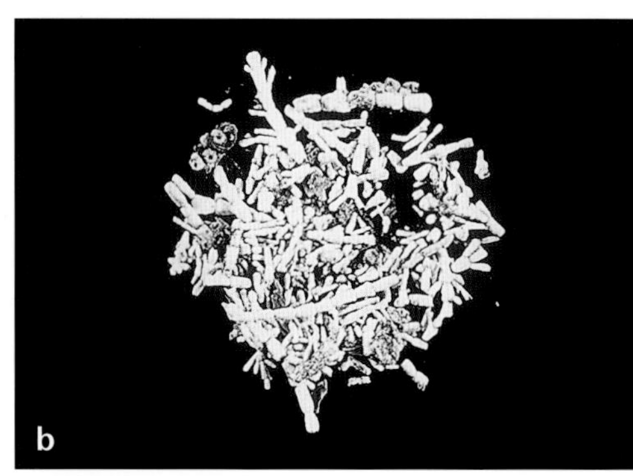

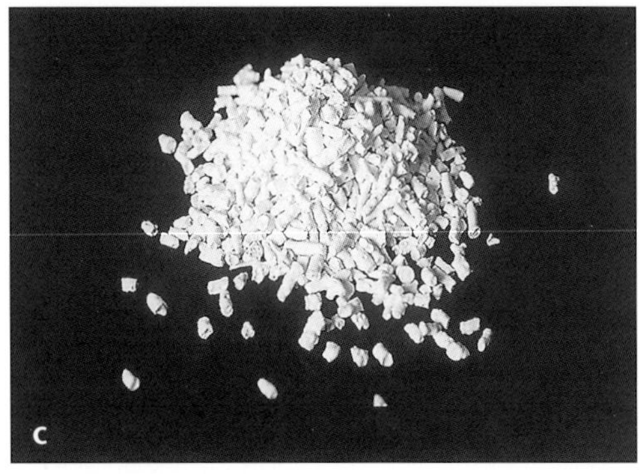

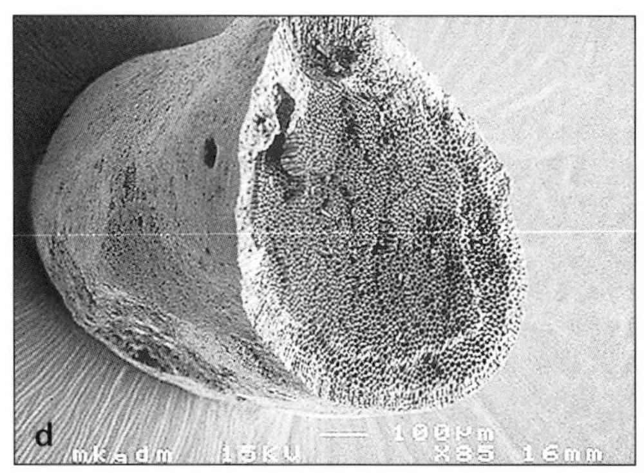

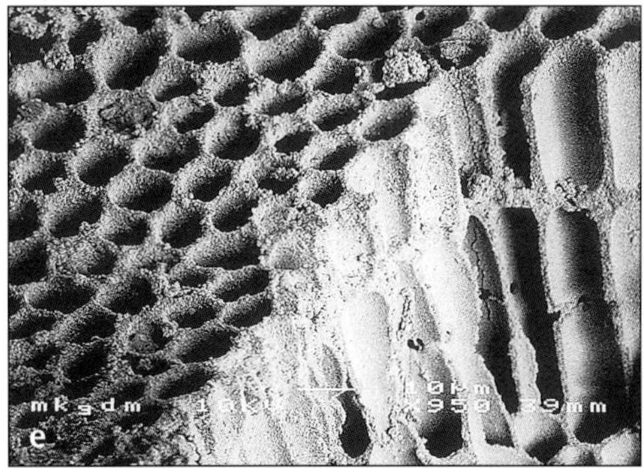

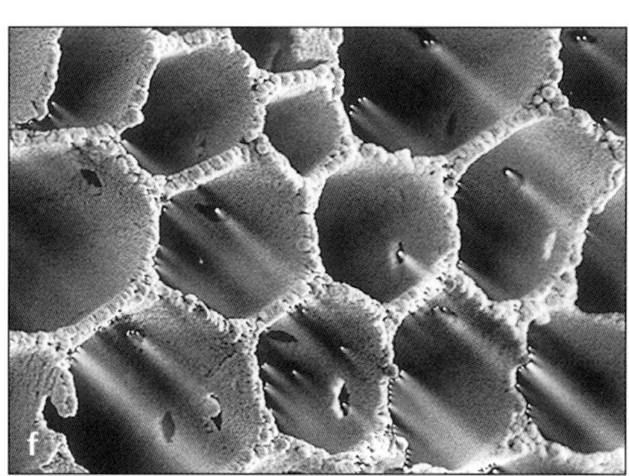

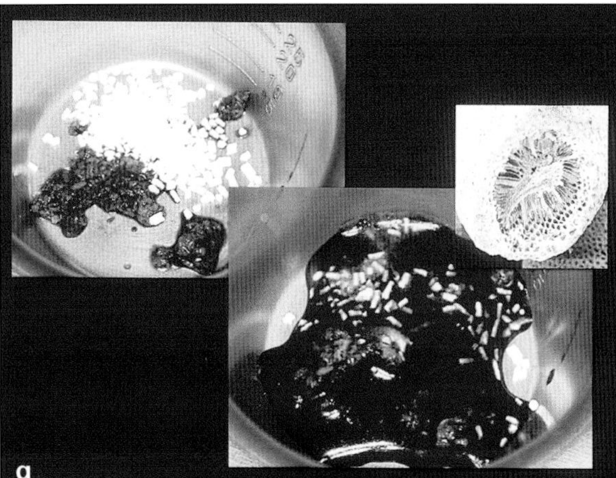

Fig 2-16 Calcified algae is an effective graft material for filling tooth extraction sites and bone defects.

(a) Sea algae used to create C-Graft is shown here in its non-calcified form.

(b) The calcified algae are crushed and prepared to be processed into graft material.

(c) The particles have been processed and are ready to be used for grafting.

(d) A crushed granule of C-Graft showing the smooth outer surface and extremely porous internal structure (85× magnification).

(e) Honeycombed inner surface. The blood-absorbing matrix these pores offer is obtained by crushing the granules is recommended prior to grafting (300× magnification).

(f) Higher magnification view of the honeycomb structure (2000× magnification).

(g) Once the C-Graft material absorbs blood, it becomes extremely cohesive and easy to handle.

Fig 2-16 *(cont)*
(h) A portion of C-Graft bonded with blood is taken to the recipient site.

(i) C-Graft in its commercially available form.

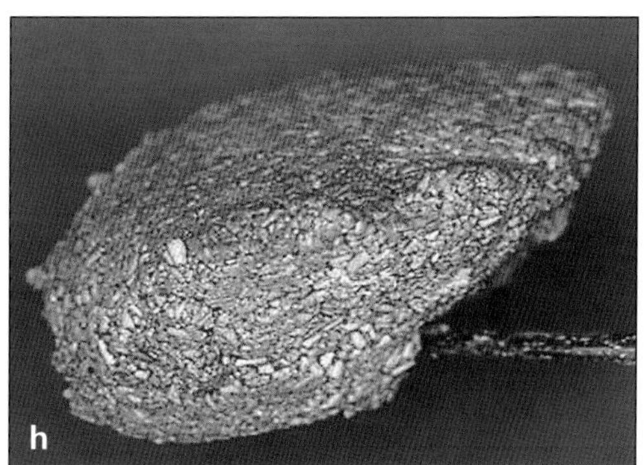

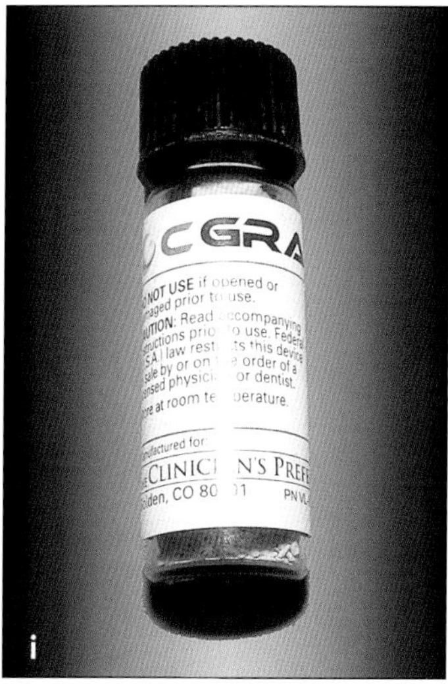

Fig 2-17
(a) Hard tissue replacement polymer material (Bioplant HTR Polymer) is available packaged in a syringe.

(b) The material resembles small microporous beads.

(c) Microscopic view of one of the beads. Its hollowness permits bone growth inside the bead as well as around it (200× magnification).

(d) Diagram showing the dimensions of an HTR bead. Note that the size of the opening in the bead permits bone to grow inside.

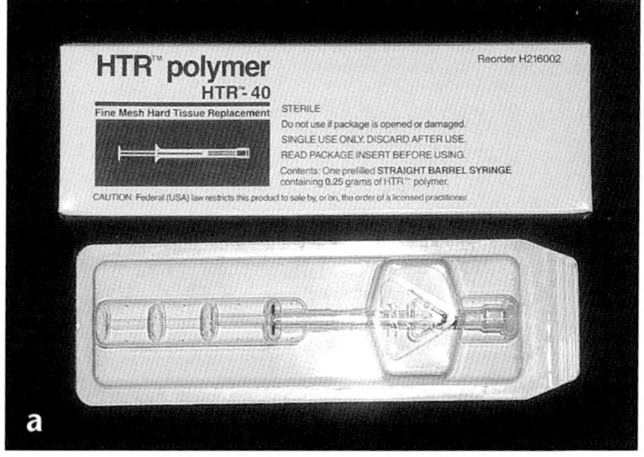

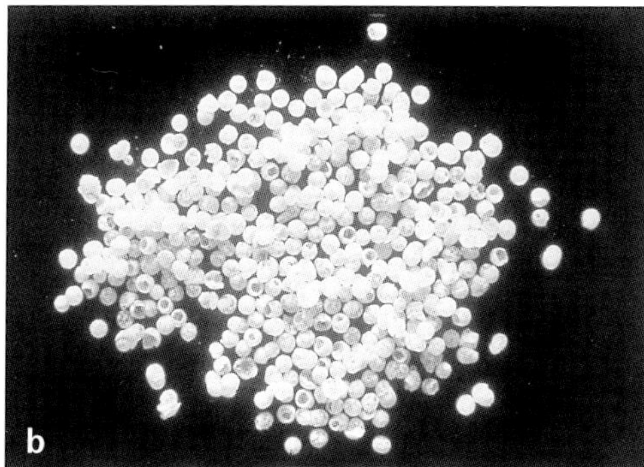

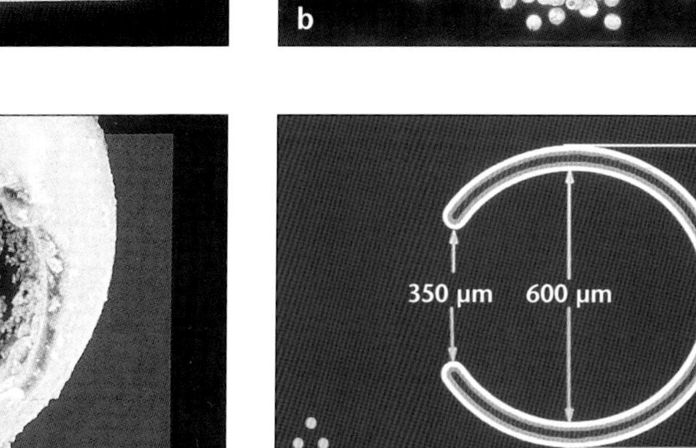

The use of HTR polymer particles in intrabony lesions has been studied, and researchers have obtained varying results within the same patient and among different patients.[66] Some sites showed an increase in closure by epithelial adhesion, while others demonstrated varying amounts of new attachment. The use of debridement alone and in addition to the placement of HTR polymer grafts for treating periodontal osseous defects has also been studied.[67] A mean defect fill of 60.8% was found in sites that received the combination treatment compared with 32.2% in sites treated with debridement alone. Another study suggests that HTR facilitates ridge width preservation when used with the immediate placement of implants in fresh extraction sockets.[68]

Bioactive glass ceramics

Bioglass (US Biomaterials, Jersey City, NJ) is composed of calcium salts and phosphate in a proportion similar to that found in bone and teeth, as well as sodium salts and silicon, which are essential for bone to mineralize. An amorphous material, bioactive glass ceramic is not available in a crystalline form (to strengthen the material) because its developers suggested that degradation of the material by tissue fluids and subsequent loss of the crystals could cause a loss of integrity. Because it is not porous, tissue and blood vessel ingrowth is prevented. The biologic impact of this property is not known, and few studies support the use of this material in periodontal and maxillofacial applications.

Bioactive glass ceramics have two properties that contribute to the successful results observed with its use: *(1)* a relatively quick rate of reaction with host cells, and *(2)* an ability to bond with the collagen found in connective tissue.[69] It has been reported that the high degree of bioactivity may stimulate the repair process and induce osteogenesis.[56] Because the bioactivity index is high, reaction layers develop within minutes of implantation. As a result, osteogenic cells in the implantation site may colonize the surface of the particles and produce collagen on these surfaces. Osteoblasts then lay down bone material on top of the collagen. The latter action may supplement the bone that grows by osteoconduction from the alveolus.

Bioglass is reported to bond not only to bone, but also to soft connective tissues.[70] Collagen produced by osteogenic and nonosteogenic cells (eg, fibroblasts) becomes embedded in the interfacial layer as it grows and may provide a compliant adherent interface with the graft material. The cells also appear to lay down collagen above the level of the particulate. This collagen attaches to the superficial particles, immobilizing them in the soft tissue. A mechanically compliant layer approximately 0.3 mm in thickness is created, which may aid in the repair of the connective tissue ligament.[71] However, much of the biologic significance of the properties of bioactive glass remains to be discovered, and there is no documentation that the material aids in periodontal regeneration.[58] For example, one study recommends against the use of bioactive glass alloplast and GBR to augment a localized ridge to place implants.[72]

The endosseous ridge maintenance implant (ERMI, US Biomaterials) is a cone-shaped device made of Bioglass that is placed in the extraction socket (Fig 2-18).[73] The manufacturer recommends this implant system for maxillary and mandibular premolars and anterior teeth; it can also be used for preserving the contour of the alveolar ridge following tooth removal. This implant acts under a time-dependent kinetic modification of its surface after placement; within 1 hour of implantation, a chemical bond appears to form within the bone tissue.[73] According to a study,

Fig 2-18 The endosseous ridge maintenance implant is indicated for ridge preservation in the anterior maxilla, for anterior mandibular teeth, and for premolars.

(a) Endosseous ridge maintenance implant kit.

(b) The shape and hardness of this cone of Bioglass material allows for easy insertion into sockets after extraction. The cones are available in eight different sizes.

(c) Eight burs of different sizes complement each of the cones.

(d) Preoperative view of flap reflection adjacent to teeth requiring extraction.

(e) After tooth extraction, the socket is prepared with a bur of the closest size to remove any residue from the periodontal ligament and to slightly contour the bone.

(f) The socket is now appropriately shaped to receive the corresponding cone of Bioglass material.

(g) After socket preparation, the cone of hard graft material should slide easily into place. The area is then closed with sutures.

(continued)

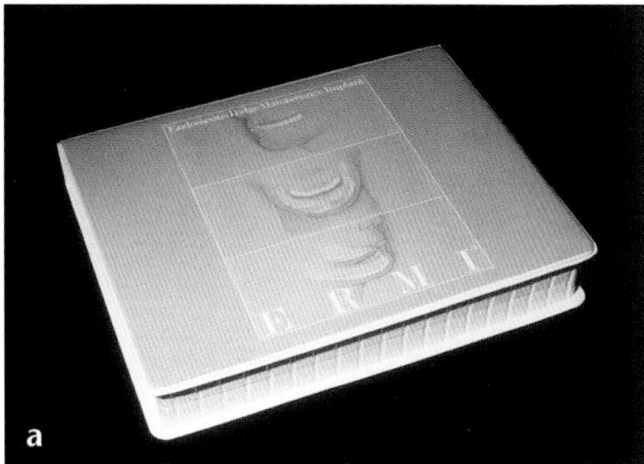

a

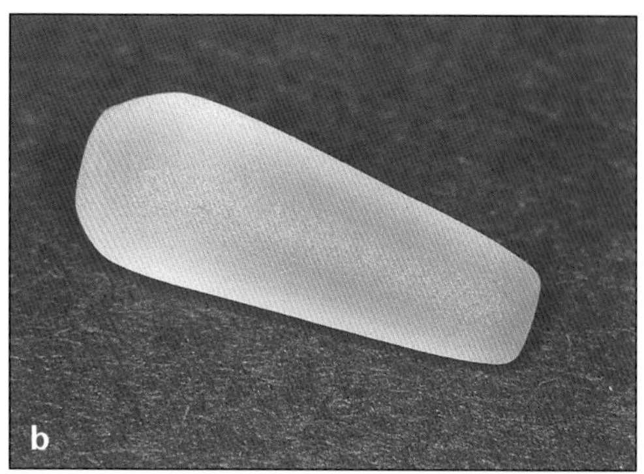
b

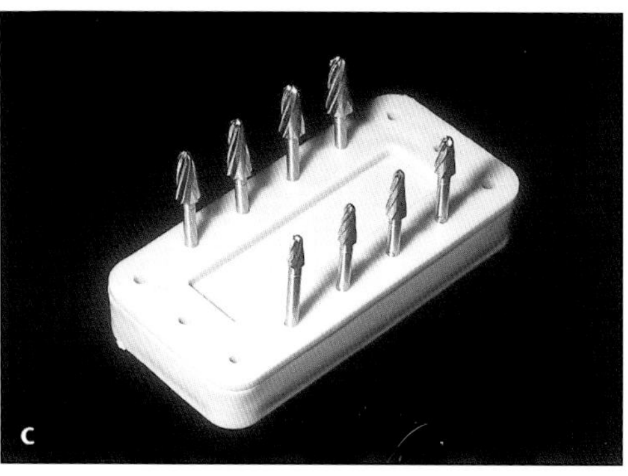
c

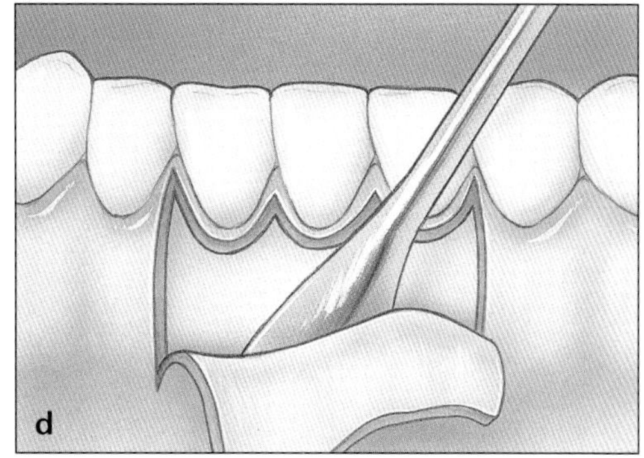
d

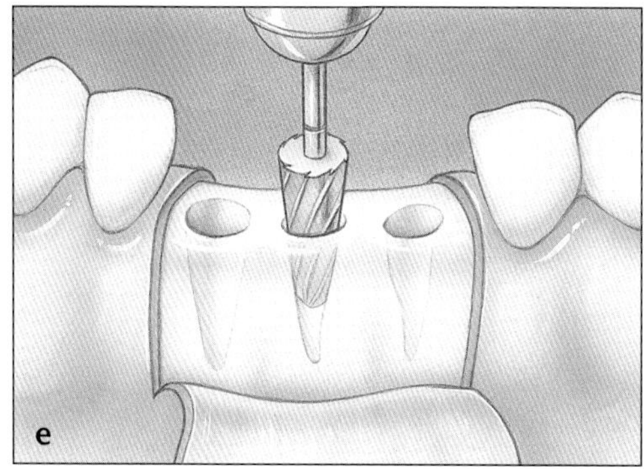
e

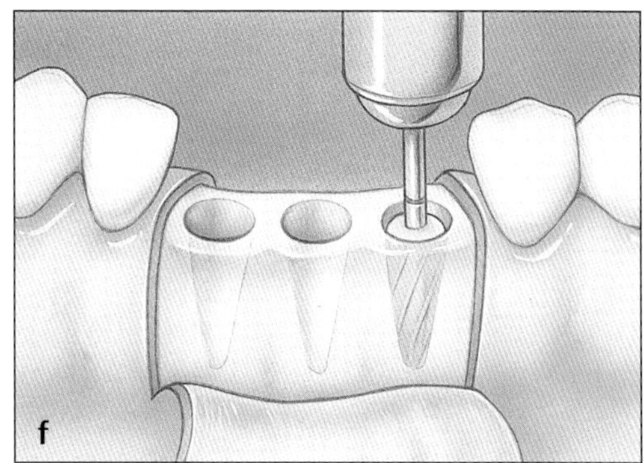
f

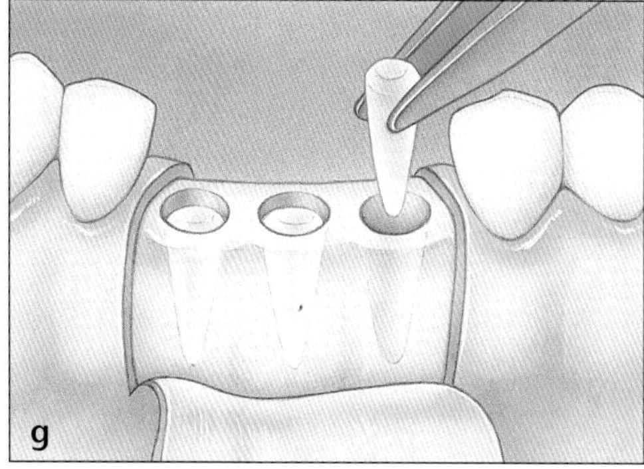
g

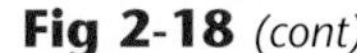

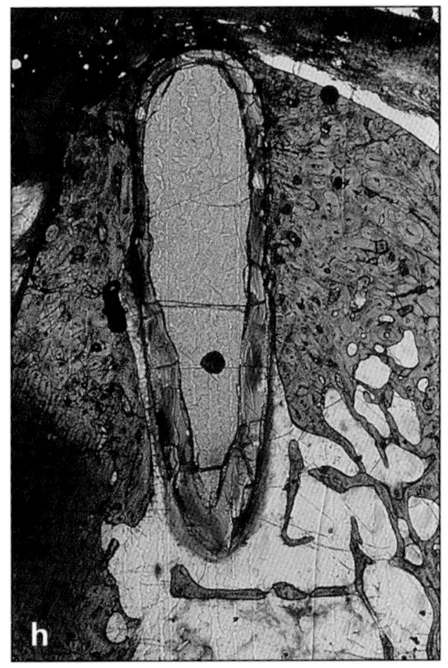

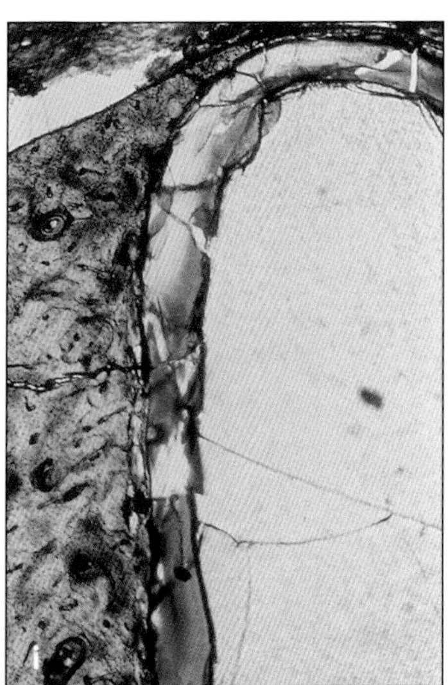

Fig 2-18 *(cont)*
(h) Histologic section showing that the center of the grafted section has not resorbed and is intact, while the outer surface of the cone is beginning to resorb and bond with the surrounding bone (10× magnification).

(i) Higher magnification reveals the intimate adaptation of bone to the surface of the Bioglass cone (100× magnification).

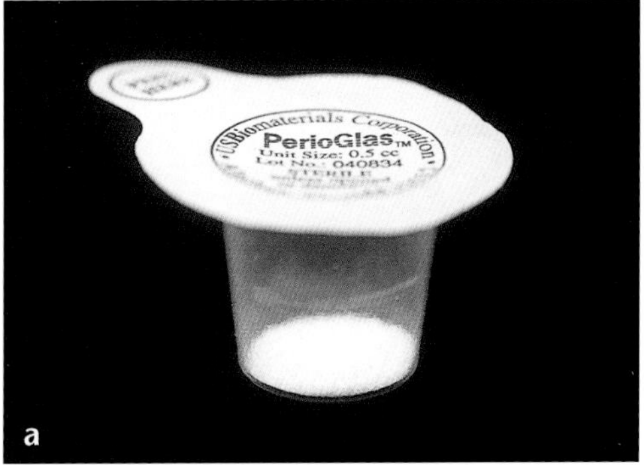

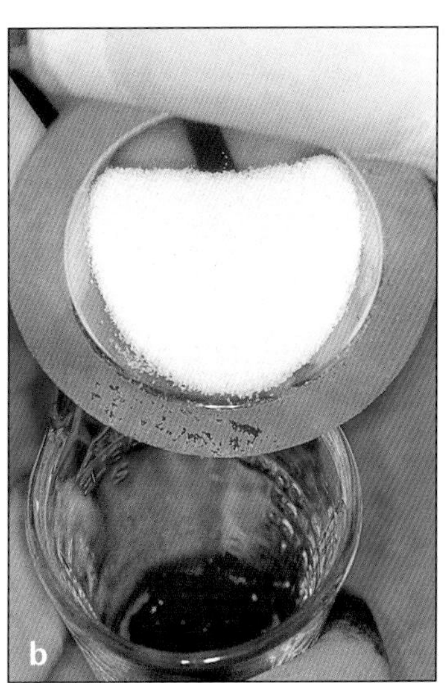

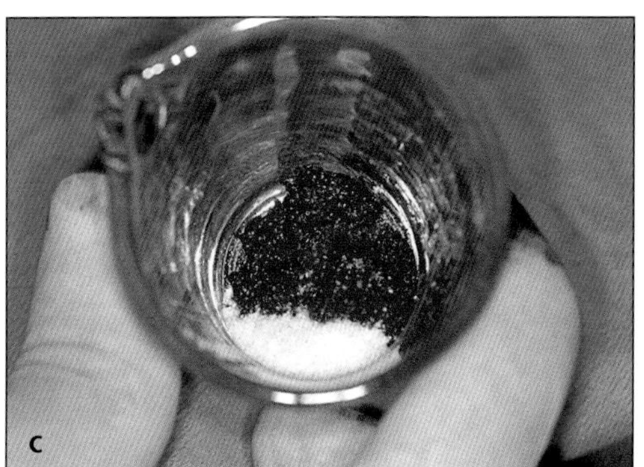

Fig 2-19 PerioGlas, a mineral-composite graft material, can be used alone or in combination with autogenous bone.

(a) PerioGlas, which consists of crushed Bioglass particles, is packaged in a sterile soft plastic cup.

(b) It can be reconstituted in saline or with blood, depending on the clinician's preferences and the defect.

(c) Mixing autogenous bone and PerioGlas enhances bone regeneration.

denture wearers showed a retention rate of approximately 90% for up to 7 years when the Bioglass implants were used for alveolar ridge maintenance.[73]

PerioGlas (NovaBone, Alachua, FL) is a synthetic particulate form of Bioglass that bonds to both bone and certain soft connective tissue.[74] PerioGlas is composed of calcium, phosphorus, silicon, and sodium.[56] The rate and density of new bone deposition may increase with the use of PerioGlas particles compared with hydroxyapatite crystals.[75] This bioactive synthetic grafting particulate is indicated for the treatment of infrabony defects. Criteria for successful PerioGlas use include pretreatment planning, debridement of the defect, preservation of soft tissue vascularity, and infection control (Fig 2-19).[76]

In animal studies, PerioGlas has demonstrated two favorable characteristics: ease of compactability and ability to promote hemostasis.[56] When well packed into osseous defects, this material was strongly adherent and appeared to harden into a solid mass after placement in the defect. After a few minutes, it remained in the osseous defect, even when a suction tip or handpiece was used in the vicinity. Hemorrhaging from the defects stopped within a few seconds after graft placement. This hemostasis is most likely related to the compactability and adhesiveness of the material.[56] The material:

1. Appeared to partially repair intraosseous defects through osteoproduction
2. Resulted in osseous and cementum repairs superior to those obtained with hydroxyapatite and TCP
3. Initiated a rapid chemical bond that appeared to impede the downgrowth of epithelium (although this finding has not been confirmed in human studies)
4. Was easily mixed, transferred, and packed and was well contained in the defect site
5. May have hemostatic attributes within intraosseous defects

Particle size was not related to the healing response. The conclusion was that by bonding to both bone and connective tissues, PerioGlas achieved improved grafting results.[56]

Biogran (3i Implant Innovations, Palm Beach Gardens, FL) is a resorbable bone graft material made of bioactive glass granules that are chemically identical to PerioGlas and are composed of calcium, phosphorus, silicon, and sodium. The difference between PerioGlas and Biogran is the size range of particles—300 to 355 μm for Biogran and 90 to 710 μm for PerioGlas. Biogran is hydrophilic and slightly hemostatic; it stays in place in the defect when bleeding occurs. When wetted with sterile saline or the patient's blood, a cohesive mass forms that can be shaped to fill the defect.[77] Bone transformation and growth occur within each granule. This osteogenesis, guided by bioactive glass particles, occurs at multiple sites, rapidly filling the osseous defect with new bone that continuously remodels in the normal physiologic manner.[13,34,78] Such controlled bioactivity reportedly permits material and bone transformation to occur simultaneously (Fig 2-20).

Calcium sulfate

CapSet (Lifecore Biomedical, Chaska, MN) is a commercially available kit containing medical-grade calcium sulfate, commonly known as plaster of Paris (Fig 2-21), that has been used after immediate implant placement as part of a bone graft placed around the implants. Grafts composed of medical-grade calcium sulfate and DFDBA have been used for bone regeneration. The sterile kits contain exact amounts of medical-grade calcium sulfate powder and

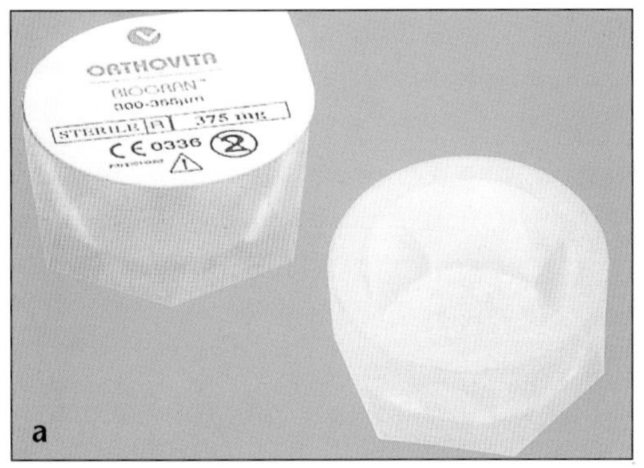

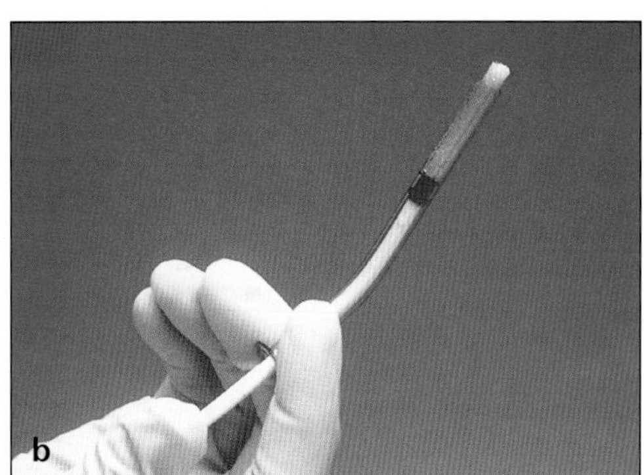

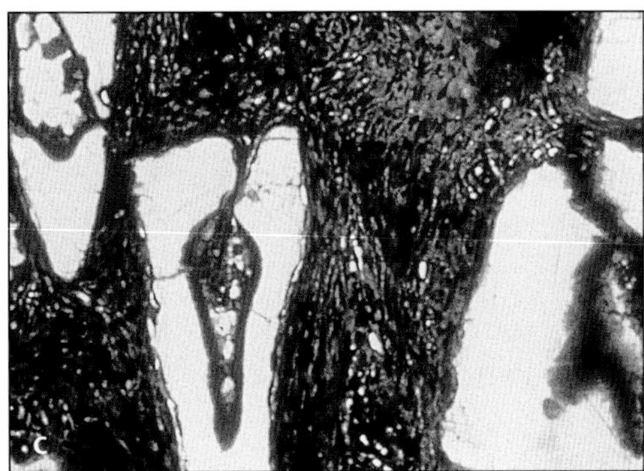

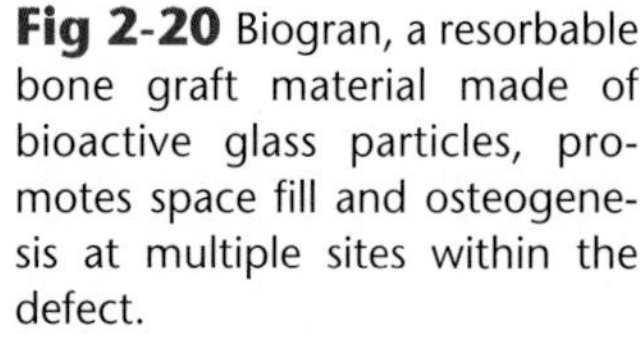

Fig 2-20 Biogran, a resorbable bone graft material made of bioactive glass particles, promotes space fill and osteogenesis at multiple sites within the defect.

(a) Biogran graft material is packaged in a disposable acrylic container that serves as a mixing well for additional material. The inside of the container is sterile.

(b) Biogran is also commercially available in a sterile syringe delivery device, the tip of which has a removable screen that permits suctioning of saline or blood in order to reconstitute the material. Once the particles have absorbed as much liquid as possible, the excess saline or blood is ejected. The screen tip is then removed and the material delivered directly to the defect.

(c) Histologic section showing bone around the particles and within cracks inside the material.

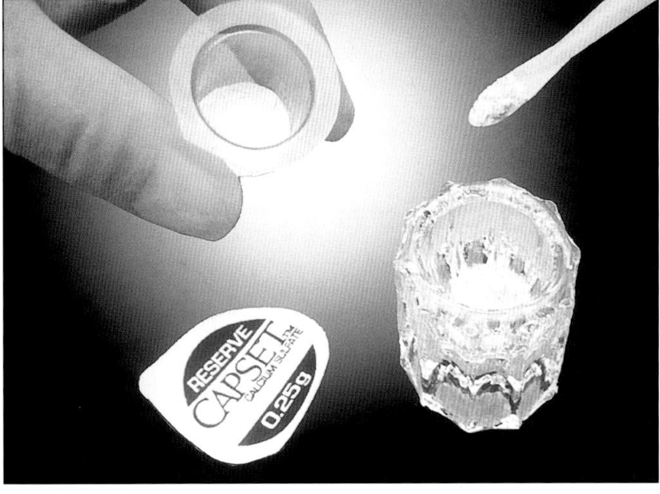

Fig 2-21
Medical-grade calcium sulfate can be used as a graft material and comes packaged in a kit that contains the calcium sulfate powder and a diluent. Mixing the powder and liquid together results in a paste that can be easily molded to form a barrier over a bone graft, or—when mixed with an allograft, autogenous bone, or synthetic bone graft—acts as a resorbable binder, making the graft easier to handle by preventing particle migration.

a syringe prefilled with a diluent. When mixed together, these substances create a moldable plaster that can conform to the desired shape, even in the presence of blood. Because this mixture is adhesive, sutures are not required. Calcium sulfate dissolves in approximately 30 days without an inflammatory reaction, and it does not attract bacteria or support infection.

Conclusion

The use of autogenous bone, allografts, alloplasts, or tissue-engineered materials, alone or in combination, should be based on the osteogenic potential of the recipient site. This decision is based on the individual's systemic healing ability (eg, age; systemic illness affecting healing, such as diabetes or autoimmune disorders like scleroderma and lupus; previous surgeries to the area; previous treatment with radiation or chemotherapy; irradiated tissue bed), local osteogenic potential of the defect (eg, defect size; ratio of host bone to graft material; number of walls of the defect; geometry of the defect; soft tissue bed; adjacent scar tissue; health of adjacent periosteum; stability of the graft material; soft tissue closure; use of interim restorative device over and around grafted site), the osteogenic potential of the graft site (eg, configuration and geometry of graft material; stability of graft material; soft tissue closure; soft tissue matrix for graft site), the surgeon's skill, and the time available for graft maturation. The composition of the grafting mix used should correspond to the material's mechanism of action, the osteogenic potential of the defect/host, and the time available for graft maturation.

In general, alloplasts can be used alone or with allografts or tissue-engineered materials for small defects in healthy patients. Autogenous bone must be added for progressively more unhealthy patients with relatively larger defects. The lower the osteogenic potential of the defect and of the patient, the greater the amount of autogenous bone required (Fig 2-22). The higher the osteogenic potential of the defect and of the patient, the smaller the amount of autogenous bone required and the more allogeneic and alloplastic materials can be used (Fig 2-23 and Table 2-2).

Table 2-3 compares the particulate graft materials described in this chapter and recommends the clinical situations and types of defect for which each material is best suited. Because each material has its own advantages and disadvantages, the clinician should carefully review the material chosen for each procedure to maximize success and minimize cost, time, and morbidity for a particular grafting situation. The higher the relative rank of a material in the table, the more predictable it is for areas with lower osteogenic potential; lower-ranked materials can be used for areas with higher osteogenic potential. Note that the numbering system that is used to rank the relative quality of graft material for bone formation was created by the author based on both clinical experience and a review of the literature.

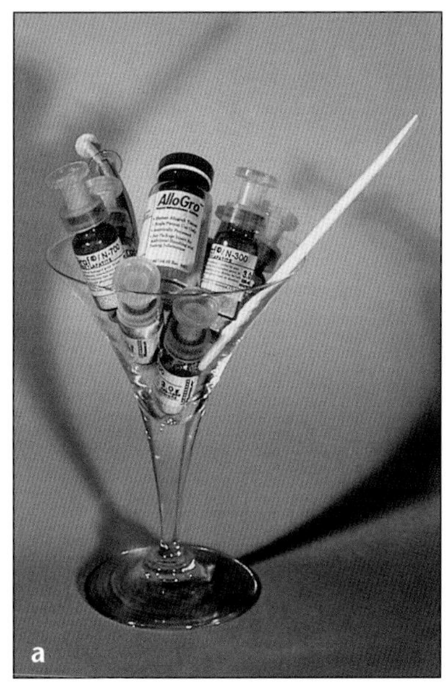
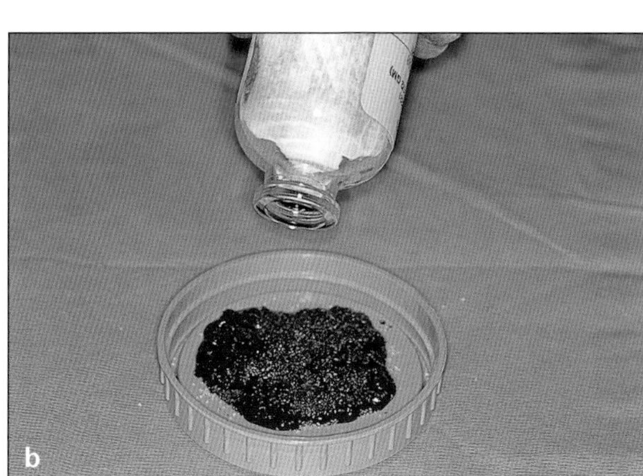

Fig 2-22 Composite grafts are used most frequently to increase the advantages of each product in the mix and minimize the disadvantages of each.

(a) Myriad regeneration materials are available, often confusing the clinician. Becoming familiar with the indications, contraindications, and mechanisms of action of the different materials is essential so that the optimal "cocktail" (ie, composite graft) can be created and utilized based on the characteristics of the patient and the recipient site.

(b) DFBA is added to previously harvested autogenous bone to create a composite graft mix. Autogenous bone, considered the gold standard of grafting materials, should be added to other grafting materials whenever possible to maximize the osteogenic potential of the graft.

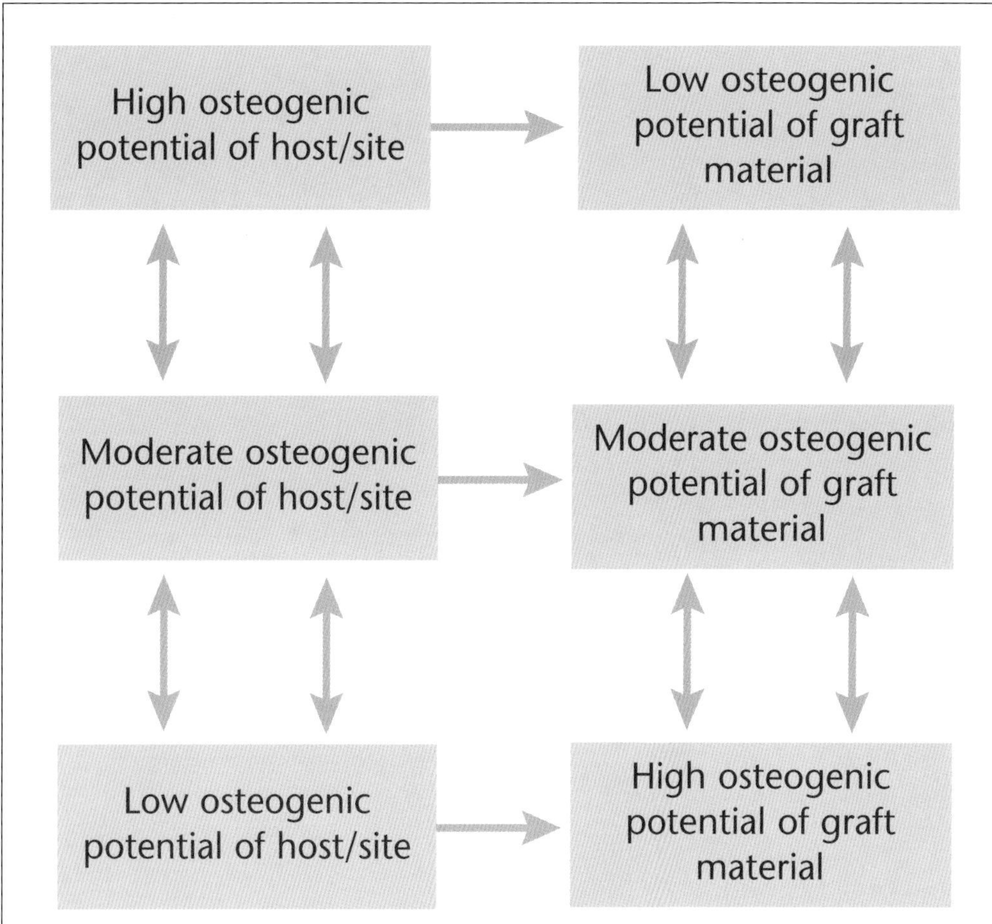

Fig 2-23
The higher the osteogenic potential of the defect based on systemic health of the patient, size and/or geometry of the defect, ratio of host bone to grafted bone, etc, the smaller the amount of autogenous bone required and the greater the amount of allogenic and alloplastic materials that can be used. The lower the osteogenic potential of the defect and of the patient, the greater the amount of autogenous bone required.

Table 2-2 Particulate graft materials to use in defects of high, medium, and low osteogenic potential

Osteogenic potential of defect	Recommended graft material
High	80% to 90% Puros; 10% to 20% any alloplast
Medium	40% autogenous bone; 40% Puros; 20% PepGen P-15, C-Graft, or Bio-Oss; and possibly PRP
Low	90% autogenous bone; 10% slow-resorbing, bone-enhancing alloplast; and PRP

Table 2-3 Comparison of particulate graft materials

Particulate graft material	Approximate resorption time	Relative quality of graft material for bone formation*	Volume available	Relative cost†	Indications/ contraindications
Autogenous bone					
Iliac crest	3–6 mo	10	70–140 mL	NA	Large reconstructions for severely atrophied bony areas. Requires hospitalization and surgery. Cost and morbidity high. Appropriate only for cases requiring large amounts and specific types of bone.
Tibial plateau	3–6 mo	10	20–40 mL	NA	Moderate to large reconstructions in defects of low or moderate osteogenic potential. Ridge reconstructions with membranes or titanium cribs, or unilateral or bilateral hyperpneumatized maxillary sinuses. Can be performed in an office setting with IV sedation by a trained surgeon.

*1 = poorest quality; 10 = best quality.
†Relative cost of graft materials based on price per unit dose. $ = low relative cost; $$ = moderate relative cost; $$$ = high relative cost.

Table 2-3 *(cont)*

Particulate graft material	Approximate resorption time	Relative quality of graft material for bone formation*	Volume available	Relative cost†	Indications/ contraindications
Mandibular symphysis	4–8 mo	10	5 mL	NA	Small reconstructions in defects with low or moderate osteogenic potential, such as hyperpneumatized unilateral maxillary sinuses, resorbed or moderately resorbed ridges, or bilateral sinuses in conjunction with other graft materials.
Maxillary tuberosity	3–6 mo	7	2–4 mL	NA	Small reconstructions in defects with low or moderate osteogenic potential, such as hyperpneumatized unilateral maxillary sinuses, moderately resorbed ridges, or bilateral sinuses in conjunction with other graft materials.
Bone shavings from adjacent areas of surgical site or from buccal shelf/ ascending ramus	3–7 mo	6	0.5–2.5 mL	$	Small reconstructions in defects with low or moderate osteogenic potential, such as hyperpneumatized unilateral maxillary sinuses, moderately resorbed ridges, or bilateral sinuses in conjunction with other graft materials.
Bone suctioned while drilling osteotomies	1–3 mo	4	0–0.5 mL	$	Very small defects, such as several exposed implant threads.
Allografts					
Puros (allogeneic bone)	6–15 mo	6	Unlimited	$$	Small reconstructions in defects with low or moderate osteogenic potential, such as hyperpneumatized unilateral maxillary sinuses, moderately resorbed ridges, or bilateral sinus grafts in conjunction with other graft materials.
FDBA	6–15 mo	5.5	Unlimited	$$	Small reconstructions in defects with low or moderate osteogenic potential, such as hyperpneumatized unilateral maxillary sinuses, moderately resorbed ridges, or bilateral sinus grafts in conjunction with other graft materials.
Irradiated cancellous bone	4–12 mo	3	Unlimited	$	Not enough supporting literature to justify clinical use.
DFDBA	2–4 mo	2	Unlimited	$	For periodontal defects only. Provides no bone, only dense connective tissue when used for bone growth.

Table 2-3 *(cont)*

Particulate graft material	Approximate resorption time	Relative quality of graft material for bone formation*	Volume available	Relative cost†	Indications/ contraindications
Alloplasts/xenografts/tissue-engineered materials, etc					
PepGen P-15 (bovine-derived hydroxyapatite with synthetic peptide)	18–36 mo	5	Unlimited	$$$	Small to moderate reconstructions in defects with moderate to high osteogenic potential, such as minimally to moderately resorbed maxillary sinuses. Very expensive; generally recommended as a part of a composite graft with other less expensive materials. Can also be used to add to a composite graft for radiographic clarity.
C-Graft (calcified algae)	6–18 mo	4	Unlimited	$	Small reconstructions in defects with high osteogenic potential, such as minimally resorbed maxillary sinuses, slightly resorbed ridges alone or in conjunction with barrier membranes, a few exposed threads on an implant, or four- to five-wall extraction sockets.
Bio-Oss (anorganic bovine bone)	15–30 mo	4	Unlimited	$$	Small reconstructions in defects with high osteogenic potential, such as minimally resorbed maxillary sinuses, slightly resorbed ridges alone or in conjunction with barrier membranes, a few exposed threads on an implant, or four- to five-wall extraction sockets. Can also be used to add to a composite graft for radiographic clarity.
OsteoGraf/N (microporous hydroxyapatite particulate)	18–36 mo	4	Unlimited	$$	Small reconstructions in defects with high osteogenic potential, such as minimally resorbed maxillary sinuses, slightly resorbed ridges alone or in conjunction with barrier membranes, a few exposed threads on an implant, or four- to five-wall extraction sockets. Can also be used to add to a composite graft for radiographic clarity.
OsteoGen (porous anorganic crystal)	4–10 mo	3	Unlimited	$	Small reconstructions in defects with high osteogenic potential, such as minimally resorbed maxillary sinuses, slightly resorbed ridges alone or in conjunction with barrier membranes, a few exposed threads on an implant, or four- to five-wall extraction sockets.
Cerasorb (beta-TCP)	4–12 mo	3	Unlimited	$	Resorbs too quickly to recommend use alone for bone grafting. Can be used as an inexpensive mix in a composite graft.

Table 2-3 *(cont)*

Particulate graft material	Approximate resorption time	Relative quality of graft material for bone formation*	Volume available	Relative cost†	Indications/ contraindications
Interpore 200 (porous coralline hydroxyapatite)	5–7 y	3	Unlimited	$$	Resorbs too slowly to recommend for bone-grafting procedures.
CapSet (medical-grade calcium sulfate)	1–2 mo	3	Unlimited	$	Requires some time to mix, and working time is limited. Works well for small four- to five-wall defects when mixed with other materials such as FDBA or DFDBA.
Bioplant HTR Polymer (microporous composite with a calcium hydroxide surface)	10–15 y	2	Unlimited	$	Resorbs too slowly to recommend for bone growth. Can be used in areas that do not require bone growth and where slow resorption is ideal, such as an extraction socket that will serve beneath the pontic of a fixed prosthetic bridge to maintain a long-term esthetic ridge beneath the pontic.
PerioGlas (synthetic particulate glass ceramic)	18–24 mo	2	Unlimited	$	Recommended for periodontal defects only. Slumps too much and resorbs too slowly for bone grafting.
Biogran (synthetic particulate glass ceramic)	20–22 mo	1	Unlimited	$	Recommended for periodontal defects only. Slumps too much and resorbs too slowly for bone grafting.

References

1. Hoexter DL. Bone regeneration graft materials. J Oral Implantol 2002;28:290–294.
2. Lane JM. Bone graft substitutes. West J Med 1995;163:565–566.
3. Misch CE, Dietsh F. Bone-grafting materials in implant dentistry. Implant Dent 1993;2: 158–167.
4. Frame JW. Hydroxyapatite as a biomaterial for alveolar ridge augmentation. Int J Oral Maxillofac Surg 1987;16:642–655.
5. Pinholt EM, Bang G, Haanaes HR. Alveolar ridge augmentation in rats by combined hydroxylapatite and osteoinductive material. Scand J Dent Res 1991;99:64–74.
6. Second-hand bones? Lancet 1992;340:1443.
7. Schopper C, Goriwoda W, Moser D, Spassova E, Watzinger F, Ewers R. Long-term results after guided bone regeneration with resorbable and microporous titanium membranes. Oral Maxillofac Clin North Am 2001;13: 449–457.
8. Koole R, Bosker H, van der Dussen FN. Late secondary autogenous bone grafting in cleft patients comparing mandibular (ectomesenchymal) and iliac crest (mesenchymal) grafts. J Craniomaxillofac Surg 1989;17(suppl 1:28–30.
9. Garg AK. Practical Implant Dentistry. Dallas: Taylor, 1996:89–101.
10. Buser D, Dula K, Hirt HP, Schenk RK. Lateral ridge augmentation using autografts and barrier membranes: A clinical study with 40 partially edentulous patients. J Oral Maxillofac Surg 1996;54:420–432.
11. Hislop WS, Finlay PM, Moos KF. A preliminary study into the uses of anorganic bone in oral and maxillofacial surgery. Br J Oral Maxillofac Surg 1993;31:149–153.
12. Rummelhart JM, Mellonig JT, Gray JL, Towle HJ. A comparison of freeze-dried bone allograft and demineralized freeze-dried bone allograft in human periodontal osseous defects. J Periodontol 1989;60:655–663.
13. Schepers EJ, Ducheyne P, Barbier L, Schepers S. Bioactive glass particles of narrow size range: A new material for the repair of bone defects. Implant Dent 1993;2:151–156.
14. Buck BE, Malinin TI, Brown MD. Bone transplantation and human immunodeficiency virus. An estimate of risk of acquired immunodeficiency syndrome (AIDS). Clin Orthop 1989;240:129–136.
15. Acil Y, Springer IN, Broek V, Terheyden H, Jepsen S. Effects of bone morphogenetic protein-7 stimulation on osteoblasts cultured on different biomaterials. J Cell Biochem 2002; 86:90–98.
16. Wikesjo UM, Sorensen RG, Kinoshita A, Wozney JM. RhBMP-2/alphaBSM induces significant vertical alveolar ridge augmentation and dental implant osseointegration. Clin Implant Dent Relat Res 2002;4:174–182.
17. Meffert RA. Current usage of bone fill as an adjunct in implant dentistry. Dent Implantol Update 1998;9:9–12.
18. Feuille F, Knapp CI, Brunsvold MA, Mellonig JT. Clinical and histologic evaluation of bone-replacement grafts in the treatment of localized alveolar ridge defects. Part 1: Mineralized freeze-dried bone allograft. Int J Periodontics Restorative Dent 2003;23:29–35.
19. Masullo C. Estimate of the theoretical risk of transmission of Creutzfeldt-Jakob disease by human dura mater grafts manufactured by the Tutoplast process: A commissioned report for Biodynamics International. Rome, Italy: Institute of Neurology, Catholic University: 1995.
20. Gunther KP, Scharf HP, Pesch HJ, Puhl W. Osteointegration of solvent-preserved bone transplants in an animal model. Osteologie 1996;5:4–12.
21. Sener BC, Tasar F, Akkocaoglu M, Özgen S, Kasapouglu O. Use of allogenic bone grafts in onlay and sandwich augmentation techniques. Presented at the XIV Congress of the European Association for Cranio-Maxillofacial Surgery, Helsinki, 1–5 September 1998.
22. Becker W, Urist M, Becker BE, et al. Clinical and histologic observations of sites implanted with intraoral autologous bone grafts or allografts. 15 human case reports. J Periodontol 1996;67:1025–1033.
23. Dalkyz M, Ozcan A, Yapar M, Gokay N, Yuncu M. Evaluation of the effects of different biomaterials on bone defects. Implant Dent 2000;9:226–235.
24. Alexopoulou M, Semergidis T, Sereti M. Allogenic bone grafting of small and medium defects of the jaws. Presented at the XIV Congress of the European Association for Cranio-Maxillofacial Surgery, Helsinki, 1–5 September 1998.

25. Brugnami F, Then PR, Moroi H, Leone CW. Histologic evaluation of human extraction sockets treated with demineralized freeze-dried bone allograft (DFDBA) and cell occlusive membrane. J Periodontol 1996;67:821–825.
26. Zhang M, Powers RM Jr, Wolfinbarger L Jr. A quantitative assessment of osteoinductivity of human demineralized bone matrix. J Periodontol 1997;68:1076–1084.
27. Schwartz Z, Mellonig JT, Carnes DL Jr, et al. Ability of commercial demineralized freeze-dried bone allograft to induce new bone formation. J Periodontol 1996;67:918–926.
28. Masters LB, Mellonig JT, Brunsvold MA, Nummikoski PV. A clinical evaluation of demineralized freeze-dried bone allograft in combination with tetracycline in the treatment of periodontal osseous defects. J Periodontol 1996;67:770–781.
29. Bowers G, Felton F, Middleton C, et al. Histologic comparison of regeneration in human intrabony defects when osteogenin is combined with demineralized freeze-dried bone allograft and with purified bovine collagen. J Periodontol 1991;62:690–702.
30. Takikawa S, Bauer TW, Kambic H, Togawa D. Comparative evaluation of the osteoinductivity of two formulations of human demineralized bone matrix. J Biomed Mater Res 2003;65A:37–42.
31. Tatum OH Jr, Lebowitz MS, Tatum CA, Borgner RA. Sinus augmentation. Rationale, development, long-term results. N Y State Dent J 1993;59:43–48.
32. Tatum OH Jr. Osseous grafts in intra-oral sites. J Oral Implantol 1996;22:51–52.
33. Meffert RM, Thomas JR, Hamilton KM, Brownstein CN. Hydroxylapatite as an alloplastic graft in the treatment of human periodontal osseous defects. J Periodontol 1985; 56:63–73.
34. Schepers E, de Clercq M, Ducheyne P, Kempeneers R. Bioactive glass particulate material as a filler for bone lesions. J Oral Rehabil 1991;18:439–452.
35. Rosen PS, Reynolds MA, Bowers GM. The treatment of intrabony defects with bone grafts. Periodontol 2000 2000;22:88–103.
36. Ashman A. The use of synthetic bone materials in dentistry. Compendium 1992;13:1020, 1022, 1024–1026, passim.
37. Stahl SS, Froum SJ. Histologic and clinical responses to porous hydroxylapatite implants in human periodontal defects. Three to twelve months postimplantation. J Periodontol 1987; 58:689–695.
38. Jarcho M. Biomaterial aspects of calcium phosphates. Properties and applications. Dent Clin North Am 1986;30:25–47.
39. Kasperk C, Ewers R, Simons B, Kasperk R. Algae-derived (phycogene) hydroxylapatite. A comparative histological study. Int J Oral Maxillofac Surg 1988;17:319–324.
40. Fucini SE, Quintero G, Gher ME, Black BS, Richardson AC. Small versus large particles of demineralized freeze-dried bone allografts in human intrabony periodontal defects. J Periodontol 1993;64:844–847.
41. Mercier P, Bellavance F, Cholewa J, Djokovic S. Long-term stability of atrophic ridges reconstructed with hydroxylapatite: A prospective study. J Oral Maxillofac Surg 1996;54:960–968.
42. Frame JW, Rout PG, Browne RM. Ridge augmentation using solid and porous hydroxylapatite particles with and without autogenous bone or plaster. J Oral Maxillofac Surg 1987; 45:771–778.
43. Boyne PJ. Advances in preprosthetic surgery and implantation. Curr Opin Dent 1991;1: 277–281.
44. Pinholt EM, Bang G, Haanaes HR. Alveolar ridge augmentation in rats by Bio-Oss. Scand J Dent Res 1991;99:154–161.
45. Artzi Z, Dayan D, Alpern Y, Nemcovsky CE. Vertical ridge augmentation using xenogenic material supported by a configured titanium mesh: Clinicohistopathologic and histochemical study. Int J Oral Maxillofac Implants 2003;18:440–446.
46. Hurzeler MB, Kirsch A, Ackermann KL, Quinones CR. Reconstruction of the severely resorbed maxilla with dental implants in the augmented maxillary sinus: A 5-year clinical investigation. Int J Oral Maxillofac Implants 1996;11:466–475.
47. Callan DP, Rohrer MD. Use of bovine-derived hydroxyapatite in the treatment of edentulous ridge defects: A human clinical and histologic case report. J Periodontol 1993;64: 575–582.
48. Krauser JT, Rohrer MD, Wallace SS. Human histologic and histomorphometric analysis comparing OsteoGraf/N with PepGen P-15 in the maxillary sinus elevation procedure: A case report. Implant Dent 2000;9:298–302.

49. Froum SJ, Tarnow DP, Wallace SS, Rohrer MD, Cho SC. Sinus floor elevation using anorganic bovine bone matrix (OsteoGraf/N) with and without autogenous bone: A clinical, histologic, radiographic, and histomorphometric analysis—Part 2 of an ongoing prospective study. Int J Periodontics Restorative Dent 1998;18:528–543.
50. Smiler DG. Comparison of anorganic bovine mineral with and without synthetic peptide in a sinus elevation: A case study. Implant Dent 2001;10:139–142.
51. Bhatnagar RS, Qian JJ, Wedrychowska A, Sadeghi M, Wu YM, Smith N. Design of biomimetic habitats for tissue engineering with P-15, a synthetic peptide analogue of collagen. Tissue Eng 1999;5:53–65.
52. Yukna RA, Krauser JT, Callan DP, Evans GH, Cruz R, Martin M. Multi-center clinical comparison of combination anorganic bovine-derived hydroxyapatite matrix (ABM)/cell binding peptide (P-15) and ABM in human periodontal osseous defects. 6-month results. J Periodontol 2000;71:1671–1679.
53. Yukna RA, Callan DP, Krauser JT, et al. Multi-center clinical evaluation of combination anorganic bovine-derived hydroxyapatite matrix (ABM)/cell binding peptide (P-15) as a bone replacement graft material in human periodontal osseous defects. 6-month results. J Periodontol 1998;69:655–663.
54. Yukna R, Salinas TJ, Carr RF. Periodontal regeneration following use of ABM/P-1 5: A case report. Int J Periodontics Restorative Dent 2002;22:146–155.
55. Hahn J, Rohrer MD, Tofe AJ. Clinical, radiographic, histologic, and histomorphometric comparison of PepGen P-15 particulate and PepGen P-15 flow in extraction sockets: A same-mouth case study. Implant Dent 2003;12:170–174.
56. Fetner AE, Hartigan MS, Low SB. Periodontal repair using PerioGlas in nonhuman primates: Clinical and histologic observations. Compendium 1994;15:932, 935–938.
57. Sandor GK, Kainulainen VT, Quieroz JO, Carmichael RP, Oikarinen KS. Preservation of ridge dimensions following grafting with coral granules of 48 post-traumatic and post-extraction dento-alveolar defects. Dent Traumatol 2003;19:221–227.
58. Schmitt JM, Buck DC, Joh SP, Lynch SE, Hollinger JO. Comparison of porous bone mineral and biologically active glass in critical-sized defects. J Periodontol 1997;68:1043–1053.
59. White E, Shors EC. Biomaterial aspects of Interpore-200 porous hydroxyapatite. Dent Clin North Am 1986;30:49–67.
60. Pollick S, Shors EC, Holmes RE, Kraut RA. Bone formation and implant degradation of coralline porous ceramics placed in bone and ectopic sites. J Oral Maxillofac Surg 1995;53:915–922.
61. Yukna RA. Clinical evaluation of coralline calcium carbonate as a bone replacement graft material in human periodontal osseous defects. J Periodontol 1994;65:177–185.
62. Schopper C, Ewers R, Moser D. Bioresorption of Algipore at human recipient sites. J Cranio Max Fac Surg 1998;26(suppl 1):172–173.
63. Schopper C, Moser D, Wanschitz F, et al. Histomorphologic findings on human bone samples six months after bone augmentation of the maxillary sinus with Algipore. J Long Term Eff Med Implants 1999;9:203–213.
64. Ashman A. Clinical applications of synthetic bone in dentistry. Part 1. Gen Dent 1992;40:481–487.
65. Ashman A. Clinical applications of synthetic bone in dentistry, Part II: Periodontal and bony defects in conjunction with dental implants. Gen Dent 1993;41:37–44.
66. Stahl SS, Froum SJ, Tarnow D. Human clinical and histologic responses to the placement of HTR polymer particles in 11 intrabony lesions. J Periodontol 1990;61:269–274.
67. Yukna RA. HTR polymer grafts in human periodontal osseous defects. I. 6-month clinical results. J Periodontol 1990;61:633–642.
68. Yukna RA, Saenz AM, Shannon M, Mayer ET. Use of HTR synthetic bone as an augmentation material in conjunction with immediate implant placement: A case report. J Oral Implantol 2003;29:24–28.
69. Wilson J, Nolletti D. Bonding of soft tissues to Bioglass. In: Yamamuro T, Hench LL, Wilson J (eds). Handbook of Bioactive Ceramics, vol 1. Boca Raton, FL: CRC Press, 1990:282–302.
70. Wilson J, Low SB. Bioactive ceramics for periodontal treatment: Comparative studies in the Patus monkey. J Appl Biomater 1992;3:123–129.
71. Greenspan DC. Bioglass bioactivity and clinical use. Presented at the Dental Implant Clinical Research Group Annual Meeting, St Thomas, VI, 27–29 Apr 1995.

72. Knapp CI, Feuille F, Cochran DL, Mellonig JT. Clinical and histologic evaluation of bone-replacement grafts in the treatment of localized alveolar ridge defects. Part 2: Bioactive glass particulate. Int J Periodontics Restorative Dent 2003;23:129–137.
73. Kirsh ER, Garg AK. Postextraction ridge maintenance using the endosseous ridge maintenance implant (ERMI). Compendium 1994;15:234, 236, 238 passim.
74. Wilson J, Clark AE, Hall M, Hench LL. Tissue response to Bioglass endosseous ridge maintenance implants. J Oral Implantol 1993;19:295–302.
75. Oonishi H, Kushitani S, Yasukawa E, et al. Bone growth into spaces between 45S5 Bioglass granules. Presented at the 7th International Symposium on Ceramics in Medicine, Turku, Finland, 28–30 July 1994.
76. Quinones CR, Lovelace TB. Utilization of a bioactive synthetic particulate for periodontal therapy and bone augmentation techniques. Pract Periodont Aesthet Dent 1997;9:1–7.
77. Bone preservation: Taking appropriate steps to maintain the alveolar ridge. Medco Forum 1997;4:1, 4.
78. Ducheyne P, Bianco P, Radin S, Schepers E (eds). Bioactive Materials: Mechanisms and Bioengineering Considerations. Philadelphia: Reed Healthcare, 1992:1–12.

CHAPTER

3 Barrier Membranes for Guided Bone Regeneration

With the advent of barrier membrane techniques and materials, more predictable restoration of the architecture and function of the bone and periodontium are being achieved through guided tissue regeneration (GTR) and guided bone regeneration (GBR). Barrier membrane techniques are based on criteria that reflect the biologic behavior of different tissues (eg, gingival epithelium, connective tissue, periodontal ligament, alveolar bone) during wound healing.[1] The purpose of barrier membrane procedures is selective cell repopulation—to guide proliferation of the different tissues during healing after therapy (Fig 3-1).[2] Cells that have the ability to form bone, cementum, and periodontal ligament must occupy the defect to stimulate tissue regeneration. The progenitor cells reside in the periodontal ligament and/or alveolar bone, both of which remain around the tooth or bony defect (Fig 3-2).[3] Placement of a physical barrier between the gingival flap and the defect before flap repositioning and suturing prevents the gingival epithelium and connective tissue (undesirable cells) from contacting the space created by the barrier. The barrier also facilitates repopulation of the defect by regenerative cells.[4-7]

Although most early studies were concerned with the treatment of periodontal defects, the principal objectives of barrier membrane techniques are to facilitate augmentation of alveolar ridge defects, improve bone healing around dental implants, induce complete bone regeneration, improve bone-grafting results, and treat failing implants.[8-14] Barrier membrane techniques, or osteopromotion procedures, use a barrier to prevent other tissues, especially connective tissue, from entering

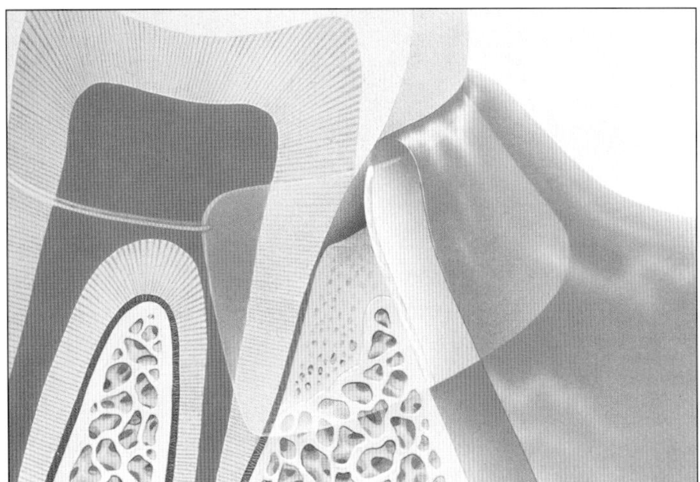

Fig 3-1
Barrier membranes are placed to prevent undesirable tissues from invading the defect and to protect and promote desirable tissue formation within the defect.

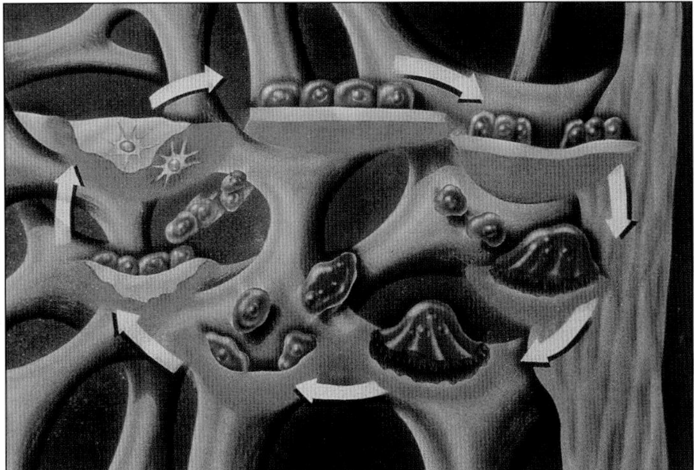

Fig 3-2
Barrier membranes can protect and isolate progenitor cells in the periodontal ligament and alveolar bone.

the intended site of bone reformation and from interfering with osteogenesis and direct bone formation.[9] Membranes may also provide additional wound coverage, acting as a duplicate surgical flap to provide added stability and protection of the blood clot and preventing ruptures along the interface between the healing tissues and the root surface.[15] In addition, membranes may also provide a tent-like area for the blood clot, creating a space under the surgical flap that will act as the scaffold for the ingrowth of cells and blood vessels from the base of the lesion.[16]

Studies have shown that interacting factors influence the predictability of periodontal procedures; tissue separation is just one of these factors.[17,18] The main objective of barrier membrane procedures is to create a suitable environment in which the natural biologic potential for functional regeneration can be maximized.[18] Creating and maintaining a blood clot–filled space, preventing inflammation as a result of bacterial invasion, isolating the regenerative space from undesirable tissues, and ensuring the mechanical stability of the resolving wound complex are some of the most important factors for creating a suitable environment for regeneration.

The final goal of barrier membrane technologies is the restitution of the supporting tissues (ie, bone) that were lost as a consequence of inflammatory disease or trauma.[19,20] Several treatment modalities have been used in an attempt to reach this goal, with or without the placement of bone grafts or bone substitutes.[19,21]

Materials Used for Barrier Membrane Techniques

Different types of membrane materials have been developed concomitant with the expansion of barrier membrane techniques and their clinical applications.[8] The biomaterial and physical characteristics of the membranes that are used can significantly influence barrier function.[18] Biocompatibility, cell occlusiveness, space making, tissue integration, and clinical manageability are criteria that must be considered in the design of materials used for regenerative procedures.[22] These materials should also be safe, efficient, cost effective, and easy to use. In addition, they must remain in place until regeneration is complete and must not interfere with newly formed tissue.[23,24]

The clinical and histologic results of studies using various barriers have generally been favorable. However, no single material has been found to be ideal for every clinical situation because each type has specific benefits and certain associated drawbacks or limitations.[18,25,26] To ensure success, it is important to know the advantages and disadvantages inherent to each material for the application in which it is being used.[18] For example, pin fixation systems can be used to stabilize membranes in some situations, whether or not bone graft procedures are included.[27,28] Generally, membrane barrier materials are divided into two categories, nonresorbable and resorbable. In addition, attempts have been made to use alternative materials, such as titanium foil, to gain the stability of a nonresorbable membrane without the need for membrane removal.[29]

Nonresorbable Membranes

The earliest studies used nonresorbable materials, such as cellulose filters (Millipore Filter, Millipore, Bedford, MA) and expanded polytetrafluoroethylene (e-PTFE) (Gore-Tex, W. L. Gore, Flagstaff, AZ). These materials were not originally manufactured for use in medical or dental procedures (Fig 3-3). Cellulose filters and e-PTFE were chosen as barrier materials because they allowed the passage of liquid and nutritional products through the barrier, but their microporosity excluded cell passage.[2] An in vitro study concluded that the Millipore filters enhanced early osteoblast (MC3T3-E1) attachment.[30] Another nonresorbable membrane barrier that has received considerable attention in the literature is a simple dental rubber dam.

Cellulose filters

Initial studies examined the use of cellulose filters in primates to exclude connective tissue and gingival epithelium, allowing cells from the periodontal ligament to repopulate the wound.[31] The periodontal ligament, cementum, and alveolar bone on the facial aspect of the canine teeth were removed, and cellulose filters were placed over the defects. Histologic examination subsequently showed regeneration of the alveolar bone and new attachment of cementum with inserting periodontal ligament fibers.

Researchers have studied the use of these filters on a human tooth.[31] Debridement and scaling/root planing were performed on a mandibular incisor with advanced periodontal disease after the elevation of full-thickness flaps. A cellulose filter was placed to cover the defect and part of the alveolar bone. Histologic examination showed new cementum with inserting collagen fibers after 3 months. Disadvantages of the use of cellulose filters include exfoliation, premature removal, and the need for a second surgical procedure for their removal.

Expanded polytetrafluoroethylene membranes

To date, the majority of studies related to membrane barriers have involved e-PTFE membranes. Widely used in many animal and human studies, these membranes have been considered the gold standard against which other types of membranes are compared.[2,24] E-PTFE membranes are composed of a matrix of polytetrafluoroethylene (PTFE) nodes and fibrils in a microstructure that varies in porosity and that addresses the clinical and biologic requirements of its intended applications. E-PTFE is known for its inertness and tissue compatibility.[32] Its porous microstructures allow the ingrowth and attachment of connective tissue for stabilization of the healing wound complex and the inhibition of epithelial migration. In addition, e-PTFE has a history of safe and effective use as an implantable medical material.[18]

E-PTFE membrane barriers consist of two parts. The first is a coronal border (open microstructure collar) that facilitates early clot formation and collagen fiber penetration to immobilize the membrane (Fig 3-4). The collar may also stop apical proliferation of epithelium through a phenomenon called *contact inhibition*. The second part is an occlusive portion that prevents gingival tissues outside the barrier from interfacing with the healing process at the defect site.[2,20] Two different configurations of e-PTFE membranes can be used according to the situation. The *transgingival design* is used to treat defects associated with structures, such as teeth, that extend through the gingiva. The *submerged design* is used to treat situations, such as bony defects, where there is no communication with the oral environment.[32]

Titanium-reinforced e-PTFE membranes were designed to increase the tent-like effect that is needed when the defect morphology does not create an adequate space.[33] Space creation and maintenance have been recognized as important prerequisites for achieving regeneration (Fig 3-5). Space making is also dependent on the mechanical ability of a membrane to resist collapse. The first membranes created for regeneration were intended to possess a certain grade of stiffness. However, the membranes had a degree of memory that limited their use to situations in which adequate membrane support would be provided by the adjacent bone.[18] Therefore, titanium-reinforced e-PTFE membranes were created for use in situations where the anatomy of the defect may cause nonreinforced material to collapse into the defect space or where more space is needed for the desired regeneration. Like traditional e-PTFE membranes, titanium-reinforced membranes are available in transgingival and submerged configurations.[32,34] Several studies have shown titanium-reinforced e-PTFE membranes to have substantial biologic potential for the regeneration of alveolar bone and periodontal structures. The space that was created was more predictable and resistant to collapse due to overlying mucosal tissue compared with the space that was created with nonreinforced membranes (Fig 3-6).[35,36]

Fig 3-3
Gore-Tex membranes are available for a variety of medical applications. This hollow, tube-shaped configuration is 12 inches long and 0.5 inches in diameter and is designed for vascular repair.

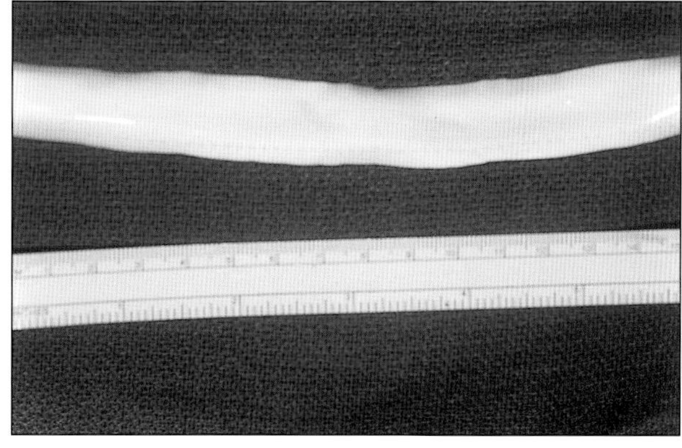

Fig 3-4
This nonresorbable e-PTFE membrane (Gore-Tex) in its submerged configuration is designed for use with defects that can be completely isolated from the oral environment by means of flap repositioning. The periphery of the membrane has an open microstructure that permits early clot formation and collagen fiber penetration to help stabilize the membrane. The open microstructure also stops apical proliferation of epithelium by contact inhibition. The occlusive center portion prevents gingival tissue invasion.

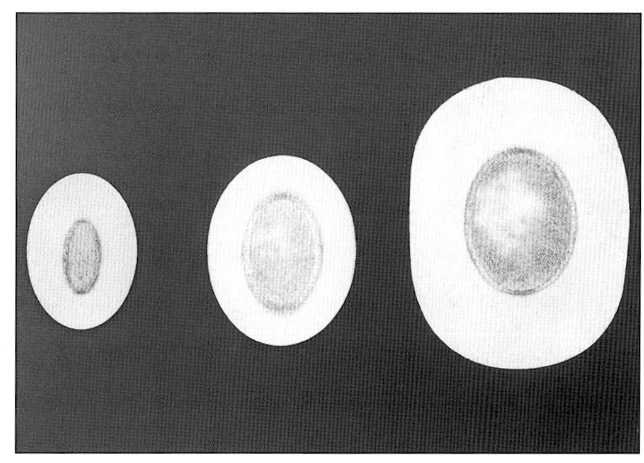

Fig 3-5
(a) Because the size of the defect in this anterior mandible site (from tooth loss due to trauma) prevents membrane collapse, an e-PTFE membrane without titanium reinforcements is indicated. Implants are placed simultaneously. One fixation screw is placed under the membrane to "tent up" the membrane. Additional screws will be used to fixate the membrane.

(b) Note the excellent ridge volume at membrane removal. The membrane was submerged, allowing for good closure and isolation to maintain the marginal tissues, as shown by the papilla.

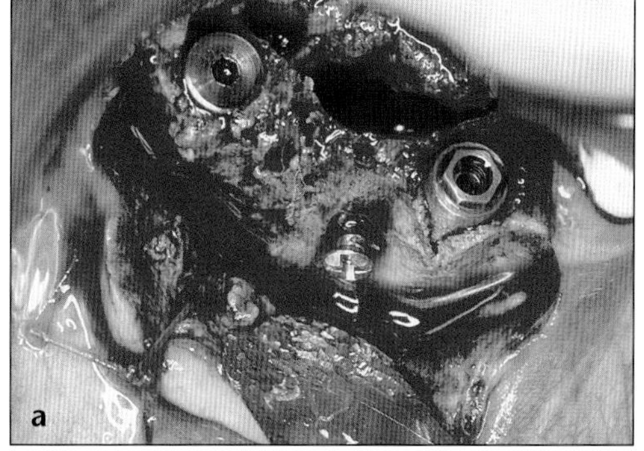

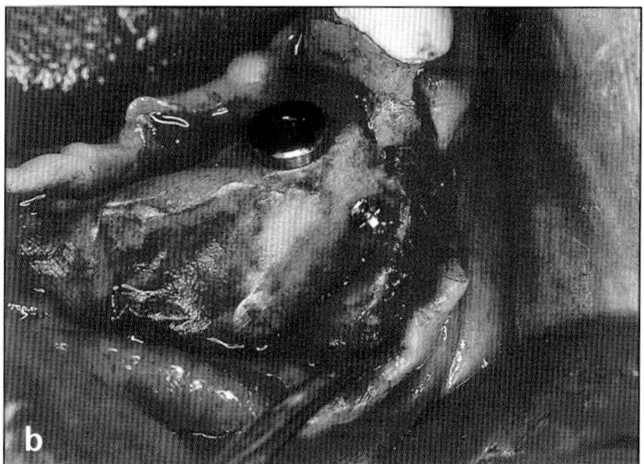

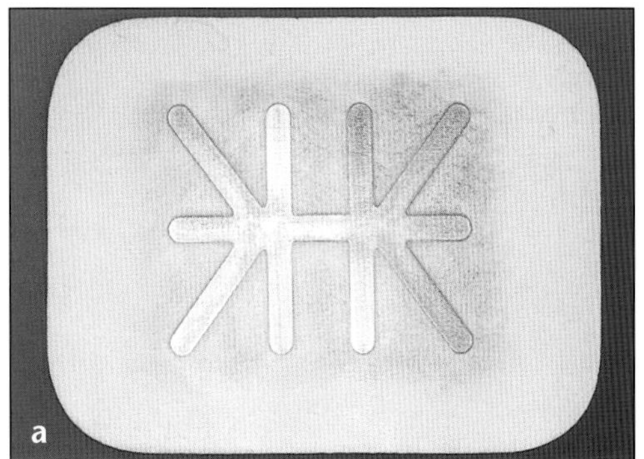

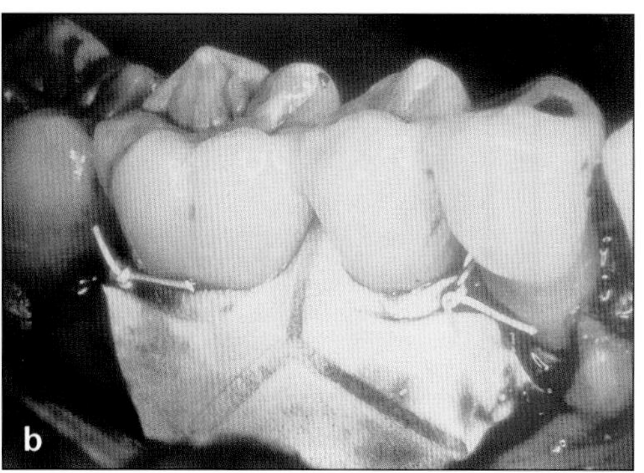

Fig 3-6
(a) This e-PTFE membrane configuration contains transversing titanium bands designed to create a noncollapsible space for healing.

(b) This transgingival nonresorbable e-PTFE membrane configuration, which contains titanium bands, is used for a defect that extends through the gingiva into the oral cavity.

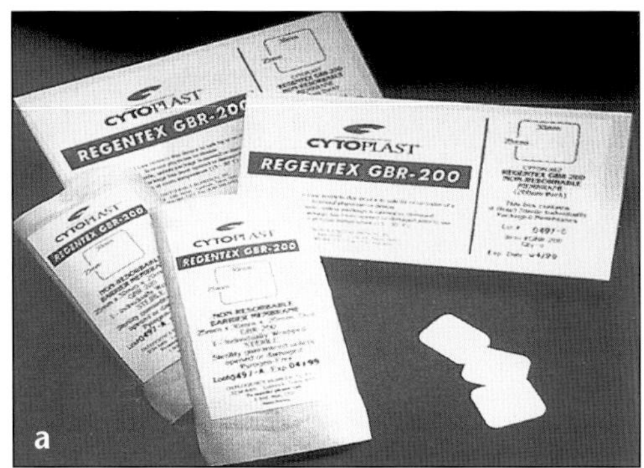

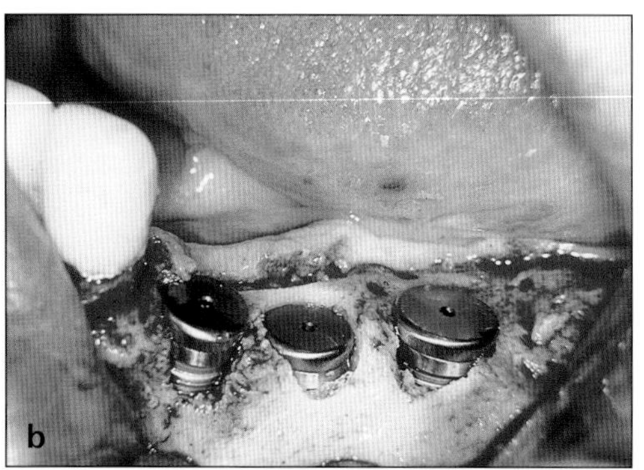

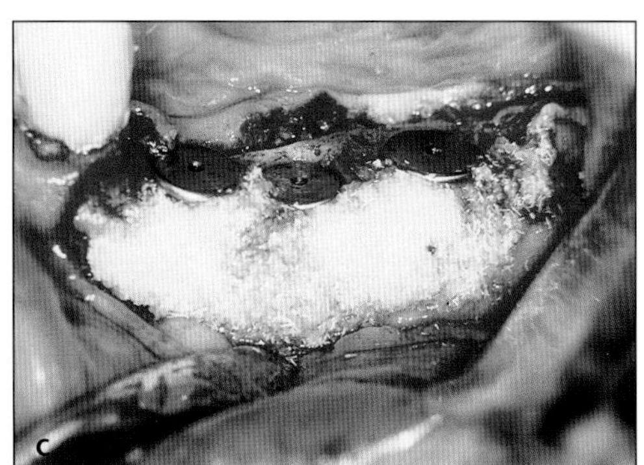

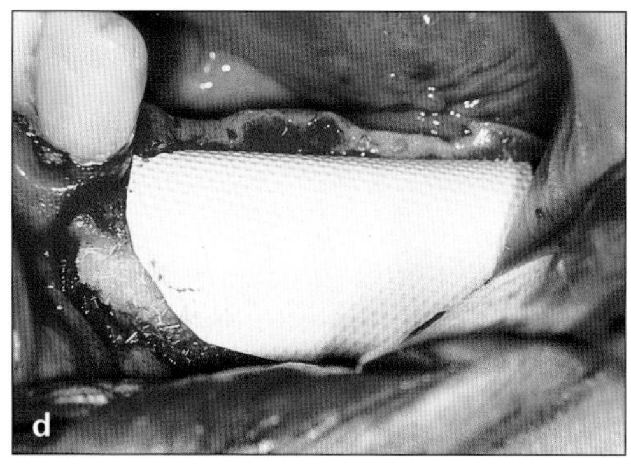

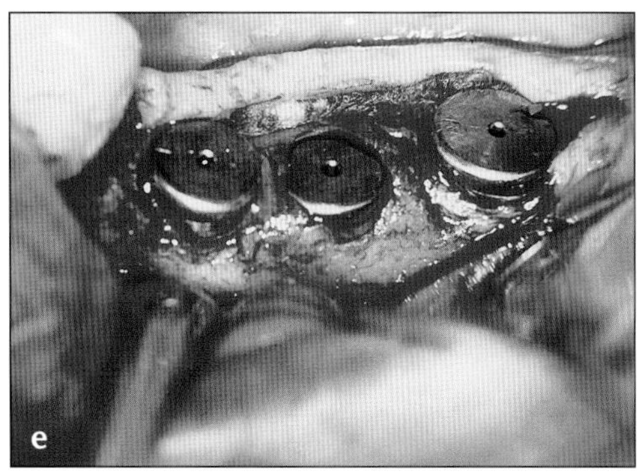

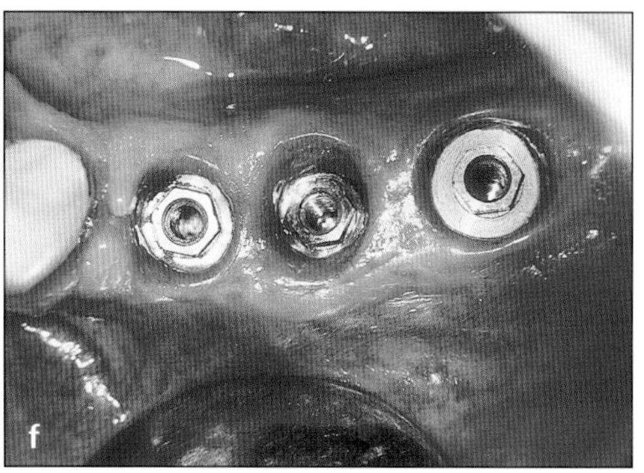

Fig 3-7 Nonexpanded, high-density PTFE membranes have shown promise as effective barriers that allow bone deposition in osseous defects, but further studies are needed to evaluate their effect.

(a) Regentex GBR-200, made of nonexpanded PTFE, is purportedly designed to be used as a nonresorbable membrane barrier.

(b) A defect in the bone leaves three implants slightly exposed on the buccal side.

(c) Covering the defect with a graft does not guarantee graft dispersal or that undesirable soft tissue will not migrate and fill the defect.

(d) Membrane is cut to an appropriate size to cover the grafted site.

(e) Optimal bone coverage means that the membrane helps contain the particulate graft, encouraging bony tissue regeneration.

(f) Good hard and soft tissue contours 15 days after implant exposure demonstrate the value of using bone graft and a barrier membrane.

The main disadvantage of the use of e-PTFE membranes is that a second surgical procedure is required for their removal, which increases the cost and surgical trauma to the patient.[2] With the use of these membranes, clinicians can control the length of time that the membrane remains in place. It has been suggested that healing times may vary among different types or sizes of defects, especially bony defects of the alveolar ridge.[18,36] The principal advantage of the use of this membrane is that it retains its functional characteristics long enough for adequate healing to occur and then it can be eliminated immediately. After removal, there is no possibility of breakdown products interfering with the maturation of the regenerated tissues.[24]

In some situations, nonresorbable membranes provide a more predictable performance, with less risk for long-term complications and with simplified clinical management.[18] The use of e-PTFE membranes may be advantageous in situations where soft tissue management problems are anticipated and complete flap closure cannot be achieved. If premature removal of the membrane is required, it can be accomplished without interfering with the regenerated tissues.[24]

The use of a nonexpanded, high-density PTFE barrier (Regentex GBR-200, Oraltronics, Bremen, Germany) for barrier membrane techniques has also been evaluated.[25] The membrane appeared to be well tolerated by the soft tissue, caused no inflammation or drainage, and provided an effective barrier that allowed bone deposition in the osseous defects (Fig 3-7). However, additional clinical studies are needed to evaluate the effect of this type of membrane.[25] The purported advantage of its use is that it can be left exposed in the oral cavity without risk of compromising the bone regeneration process (Fig 3-8).

Dental rubber dam

A number of studies have suggested the suitability of using dental rubber dam as a barrier membrane for GTR in periodontal procedures.[37–41] For example, a 1994 study documented five cases in which rubber dam was used as a barrier in the GTR treatment of infrabony defects.[37] According to this study, the barrier was placed subsequent to flap elevation, debridement, and root planing. Rubber dam covered the defect and surrounding bone; the surgical flap covered rubber dam, which was removed after 5 weeks. Clinical measurements and a reentry procedure at 1 year showed the suitability of the rubber dam barrier. A 1998 study concluded that dental rubber dam can be used as a barrier membrane for GTR procedures but that e-PTFE membranes provide better probing, attachment level, and vertical bone gains. This is probably because of rubber dam's inability to cover the regenerated tissue completely as a result of consistent recession of gingival tissues in dam-treated sites.[40] A 2002 study compared the connective tissue and bacterial deposits on rubber dam sheets and e-PTFE membranes used as barrier membranes in GTR and found no significant difference in the total number of connective tissues on both types of membranes.[41] In fact, the total amount of bacteria on rubber dam sheets was statistically lower than the amount on the e-PTFE membranes. The comparability in the number of connective tissues found on both types of membranes suggests the suitability of using rubber dam sheets as barrier membranes in GTR. These results reflect the conclusions of earlier studies that suggested no significant healing differences between rubber dam and e-PTFE membranes.[38,39]

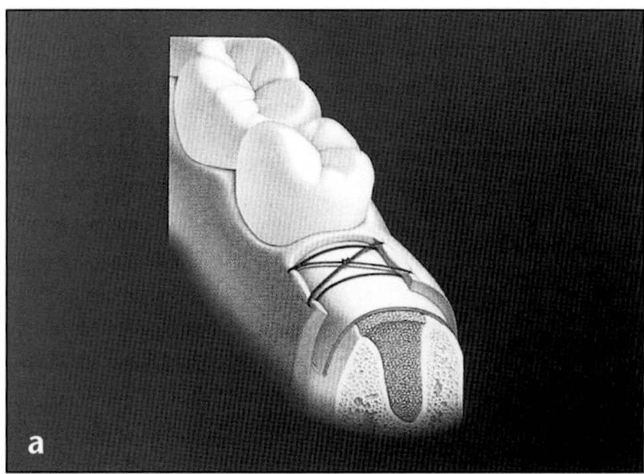
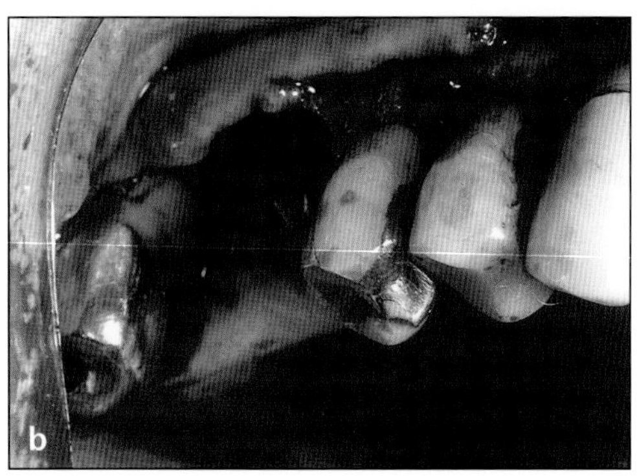
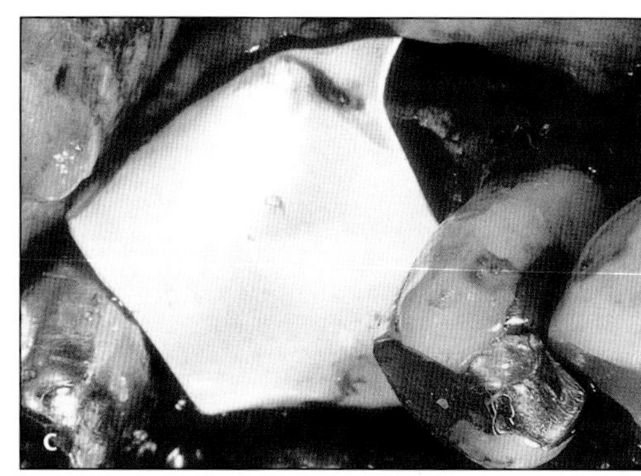
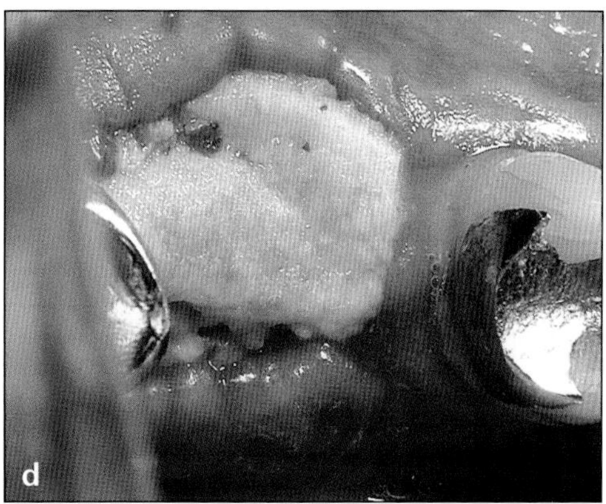
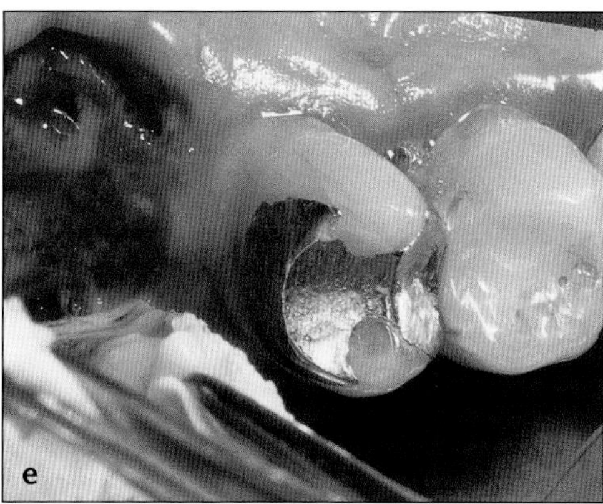

Fig 3-8 Nonexpanded, high-density PTFE membranes have the purported advantage of permitting exposure to the oral cavity without risk of compromising the bone regeneration process.

(a) The Regentex GBR-200 membrane permits exposure while preventing bacteria from seeping into the defect.

(b) A large defect after tooth extraction requires the use of a barrier membrane to retain grafting material and to prevent epithelial tissues from growing into the socket. Because of this, primary closure will be difficult. The socket is grafted with bone graft material.

(c) A Regentex membrane is then placed to extend a few millimeters beyond the defect margins.

(d) Despite the lack of complete closure, gingival epithelium did not enter the socket but instead migrated over the site. The layer of yellowish plaque that formed over the membrane can be easily removed. The absence of inflammation suggests that no infection has occurred.

(e) After the membrane is removed, the epithelium that formed over the socket and under the membrane can be seen. Beneath this tissue, the desired osteoid tissue continues to mature.

Titanium membranes

Titanium membranes can also be used for GTR/GBR in oral implant applications. These membranes are totally inert and osteophyllic. It has been reported that in a series of 42 patients using a 22-µm-thick titanium membrane in conjunction with composite grafting of autologous bone and demineralized freeze-dried bone for treatment of peri-implant bony defects at the time of implant placement, satisfactory augmentation was achieved in 90% of cases, surpassing the success rate of Gore-Tex membranes.[42]

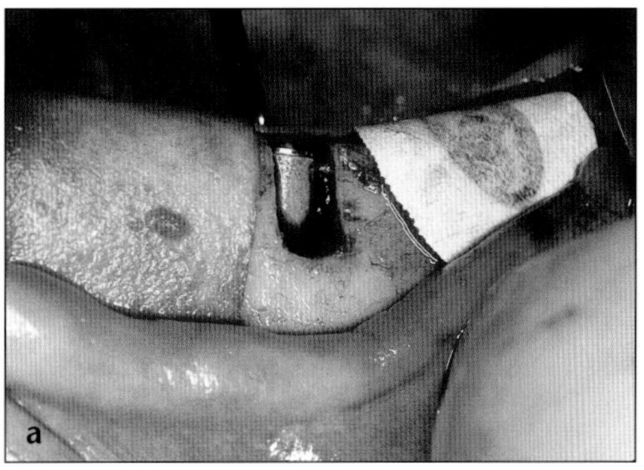

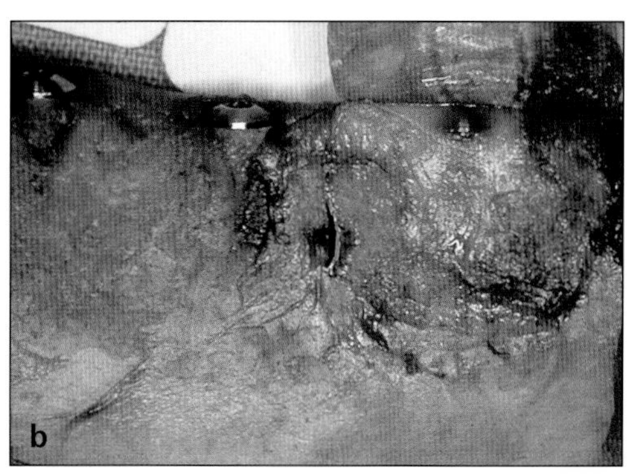

Fig 3-9
(a) Three defect areas in the same alveolar ridge, similar in extension and configuration, were left to heal under different conditions: one covered with a resorbable membrane *(left)*, the second covered with a nonresorbable membrane *(right)*, and the third left uncovered as a control *(center)*.

(b) Different levels of bone formation can be observed at each site. The site covered with the nonresorbable membrane shows the greatest amount of bone formation.

Resorbable Materials and Devices

The main advantage of using resorbable membranes is the avoidance of a second surgical procedure, thus reducing patient morbidity and expense.[26] A disadvantage is that material exposure or flap dehiscence can cause postoperative tissue management problems. Material exposure after surgery can lead to bacterial growth, alteration of fibroblast morphology, and migration, all of which may jeopardize the success of the regeneration process. Another common problem is the difficulty of preventing membrane collapse into the defect, which can result in inadequate space making.[43]

The use of resorbable barriers is based on criteria similar to those for nonresorbable membranes, and the degradation process should not negatively affect the regenerative outcome (Fig 3-9).[2,18] Resorbability may be associated with degradation through enzymatic activity (biodegradation) or hydrolyzation (bioabsorption) as a cellular response from the surrounding tissue. The inflammatory response should be minimal and reversible and must not interfere with regeneration.[2] A large number of resorbable barrier materials exist, some more popular than others.

Collagen membranes

Collagen is a physiologically metabolized macromolecule of the periodontal connective tissue that has two different properties: chemotaxis (for fibroblasts) and hemostasis. It is also a weak immunogen and may act as a scaffold for migrating cells (Fig 3-10).[26,44] Collagen possesses several characteristics that make it a suitable barrier material, including favorable effects on coagulation and wound healing, controlled cross-linking, low antigenicity and extensibility, high tensile strength, and fiber orientation. Collagen can also be produced in various forms such as sheets, gels, tubes, powders, and sponges (Fig 3-11).[45]

Since the mid-1990s, several collagen-based materials have been used as a barrier membrane in periodontal and oral and maxillofacial surgery. Processed bovine type I collagen membranes, originating both from tendons (Fig 3-12) and from dermal sites, have been evaluated for barrier membrane procedures in animals and humans with positive results.[26] Multicenter studies have shown results that are equivalent to those obtained using nonresorbable membranes in periodontal defects.[26]

Early studies established the potential for reabsorption of collagen membranes.[46,47]

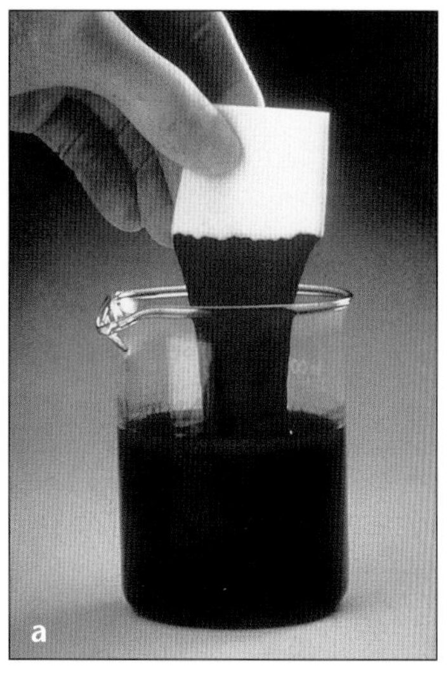

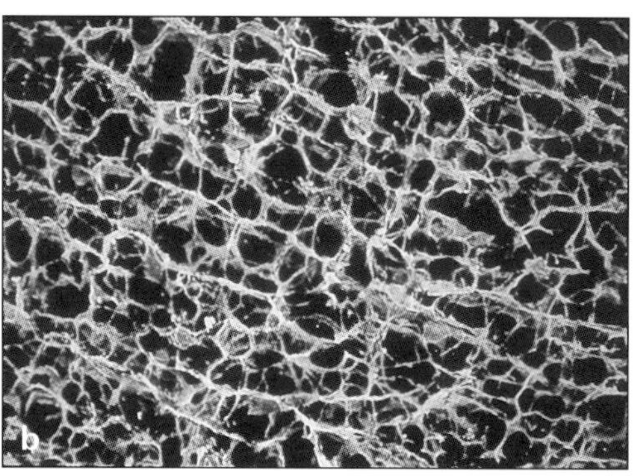

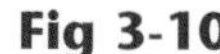

Fig 3-10
(a) A collagen membrane such as CollaTape (Zimmer Dental, Carlsbad, CA) is an ideal carrier for substances such as antibiotics or platelet-rich plasma (PRP). Because collagen enhances platelet aggregation, this membrane helps stabilize blood clots.

(b) More than 90% of the sponge-like surface of CollaTape (a collagen material obtained from bovine Achilles tendon) consists of open pores that retain fluids.

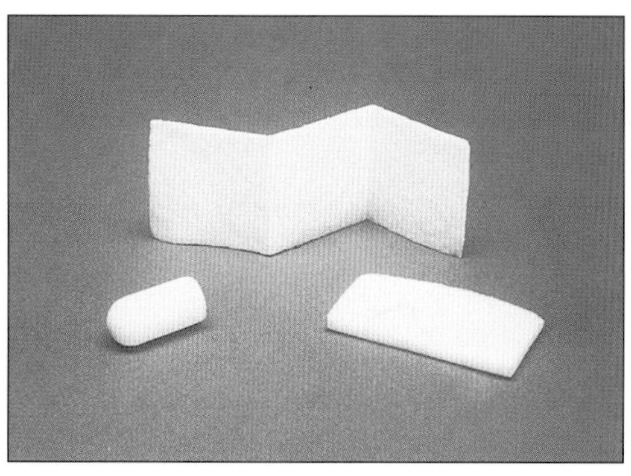

Fig 3-11
Absorbable collagen dressings are available in different configurations and sizes. CollaTape (*center*) can be used to cover and stabilize graft materials, CollaPlug (Zimmer Dental; *left*) can be placed into or over extraction sockets, and CollaCote (Zimmer Dental; *right*) can be used to fill in harvested soft tissue sites, such as the palate.

Results were limited because of rapid degradation (30 days) caused by enzymes found in plaque and healing wounds. Because of these findings, researchers improved the quality of collagen membranes through the use of bilayered barriers to compensate for the premature degradation of the external barrier and by adding heparin sulfate and fibronectin to the internal barrier. Fibronectin acts as a chemotactic factor for fibroblasts and is able to bind the heparin sulfate to the collagen membrane. The inner barrier is designed to act as a second barrier for the migrating epithelium and to serve as a delivery system for fibronectin and heparin sulfate. The results of this study demonstrated that the enriched collagen barrier had improved properties to retard apical migration of epithelium compared with nonenriched membranes.[48]

A multicenter study that evaluated the use of bovine tendon type I collagen membranes for membrane barrier procedures in human Class II furcation defects compared the efficacy of bioabsorbable collagen membranes with that of surgical debridement or e-PTFE membranes.[26] The results of the study showed that collagen membranes were clinically effective and safe for use in periodontal barrier membrane procedures. The gain in attachment using collagen membranes was equal to or greater than that obtained with the use of surgical debridement or e-PTFE membranes.

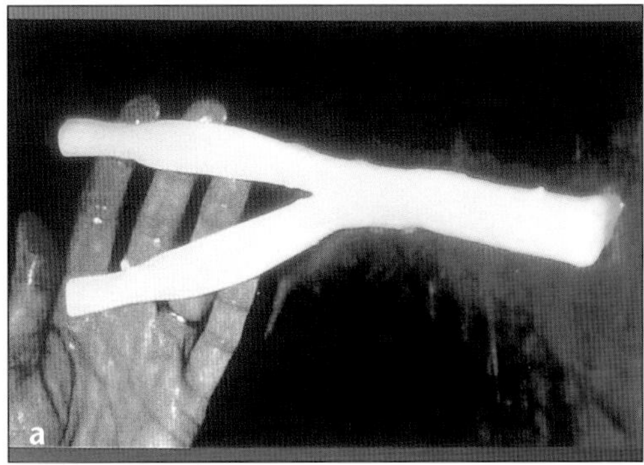

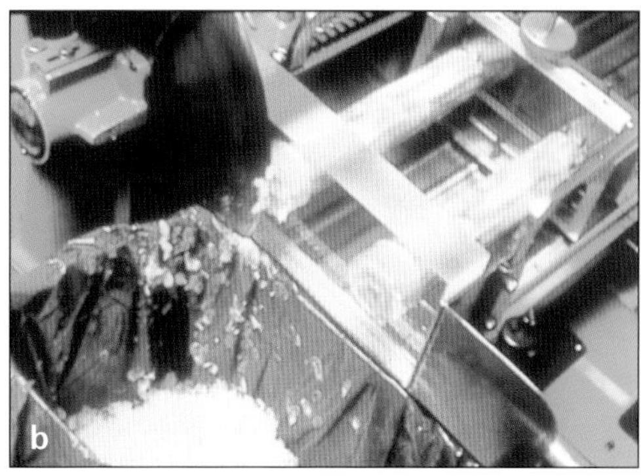

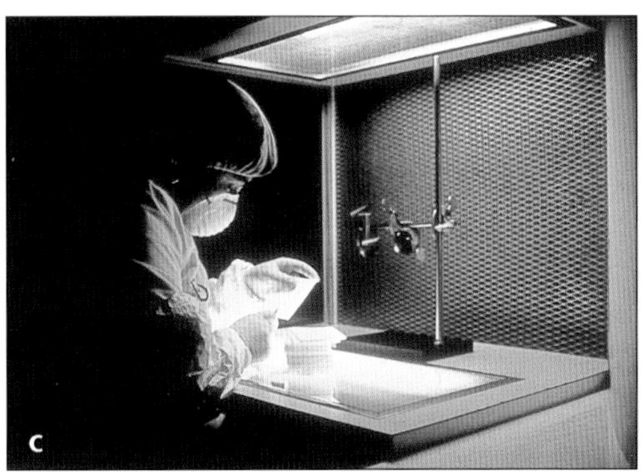

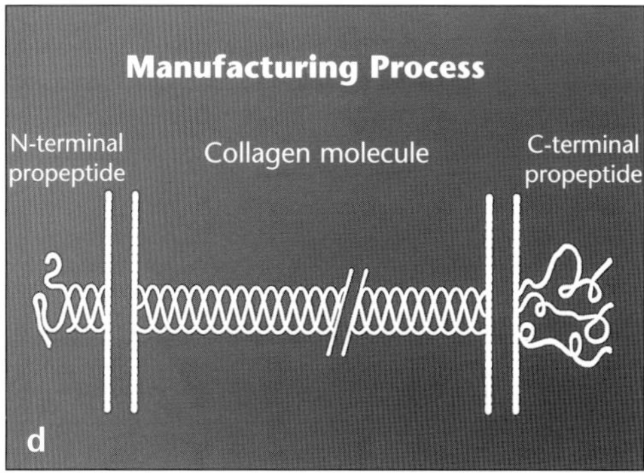

Fig 3-12 Processed bovine type I collagen membranes have shown results equivalent to those obtained using nonresorbable membranes in periodontal defects.

(a) Bovine deep flexor (Achilles) tendon is the type I collagen source for the BioMend (Zimmer Dental) resorbable membrane.

(b) Careful processing of the tendon includes the removal of antigenic portions.

(c) The entire manufacturing process involves rigorous inspection of the material.

(d) The removal of antigenic portions of the polypeptide chain increases the biocompatibility and recipient tolerance of the BioMend membrane.

Another study showed successful treatment of one-, two-, and three-wall defects via a collagen membrane combined with antigen-extracted allogeneic bone and collagen gel.[49] In this study, a 1- to 2-mm film of collagen gel was placed in the base of the defect, the allogeneic bone was packed into the defect, and a collagen membrane was placed over the defect. Another study compared e-PTFE membranes with type I collagen in GTR of Class II mandibular molar furcation defects; healing intervals were 1 year, and clinical assessments took place at 8 months. Reentry occurred at 1 year.[50] The researchers observed no significant differences between the two types of membranes with regard to reduction of pocket depth, attachment gain, or horizontal defect filling. The collagen membrane outperformed the e-PTFE membrane with regard to vertical fill.

The advantages of collagen membrane use include minimal postoperative complications, a good healing rate, and no incidence of material dehiscence, tissue perforation, sensitivity reactions, immune response, tissue sloughing, delayed healing, or postoperative infection.[51] Collagen appears to be a useful and beneficial membrane material for regenerative therapy because collagen membranes meet the criteria for membrane barrier techniques—space creation, tissue integration, cell occlusivity, biocompatibility, and clinical manageability.[51]

One collagen product, CollaTape, has been used for minor oral wounds, to close graft sites, and to repair schneiderian membranes. Its benefits include controlling bleeding and stabilizing blood clots, protecting wound beds, and providing a matrix for tissue ingrowth associated with

GTR. It fully resorbs in 10 to 14 days. Another product, Paroguide (Coletica, Lyon, France), is made of cross-linked bovine collagen from calfskin. It is composed of 96% type I collagen and 4% chondroitin-4-sulfate and has a resorption rate of 4 to 8 weeks.[52] Paroguide is an opaque, off-white substance of medium rigidity. It comes packaged in two double-chambered blister packs, one of which holds the membrane, the other of which contains two modeling membranes used to fashion models for the actual membrane to be placed. Paroguide can be used to reconstruct osseous defects, to repair bone furcations, to augment the alveolar ridge, and to cover peri-implantation spaces and extraction sites. Resorbable sutures can be used to hold the membrane in place.

BioMend is an absorbable collagen membrane derived from bovine Achilles tendon that has been shown to be effective in bone regeneration procedures.[53] An in vitro study concluded that the BioMend membrane enhanced early osteoblast (MC3T3-E1) attachment.[30]

BioMend is a compressed, nonfriable type I collagen matrix. Paper-white when dry and leather-like in its surface texture, its condensed composition of laminated sheets can be seen in cross section. When wet, the membrane becomes translucent, but it is not slippery and can be adapted to the tooth structure. Antigenic portions of the collagen molecule are removed when the product is manufactured, increasing its biocompatibility and tissue tolerance. Its immune response has been clinically verified, and separate production lots are verified as nonpyrogenic.[53] BioMend resorbs into gingival connective tissue via enzyme (collagenase) degradation. It is designed to remain intact for 4 weeks and has an average life span of 6 to 7 weeks. Full resorption takes place within 8 weeks (Fig 3-13).

Results from eight centers and 133 patients compared BioMend absorbable collagen membranes with e-PTFE membranes or surgical debridement used to treat furcation defects.[54] A statistically significant decrease in probing depth and clinical gain in probing attachment were noted in patients treated with BioMend versus e-PTFE membranes. Only the BioMend membrane patients experienced complete furcation closures. BioMend Extend is a longer-lasting version of BioMend that is thicker, more pliable, and tear-resistant. It is resorbed within 18 weeks and thus able to maintain a regenerative barrier for a longer period (Fig 3-14).

Ossix (ColBar R&D, Herzliya, Israel) is a resorbable collagen membrane that functions as a regenerative barrier for 6 months after placement. Its durability addresses a problem associated with successful bone regeneration using collagen membranes—namely, the degradation of such membranes by mammalian collagenase when submerged or by bacterial collagenase when exposed.[55] A group of researchers explored the barrier membrane potential of Ossix for bone augmentation.[56] For clinical purposes, both primary and, in particular, secondary healing patterns were studied. Researchers documented soft tissue healing photographically; image analysis on digitized photographs was then used to calculate the size of dehiscences. Researchers dissected and histologically evaluated the barrier remnants during reentry. The study indicated that the mean value for dehiscences was 35.5 mm; after evidence of exposure, all dehiscences healed within 4 weeks. Statistically significant differences were noted between weeks 2 and 6 for previously exposed sites. Histologically, the study showed direct apposition of fibrous and bone tissues on the membrane surface. The researchers concluded that when the membrane was

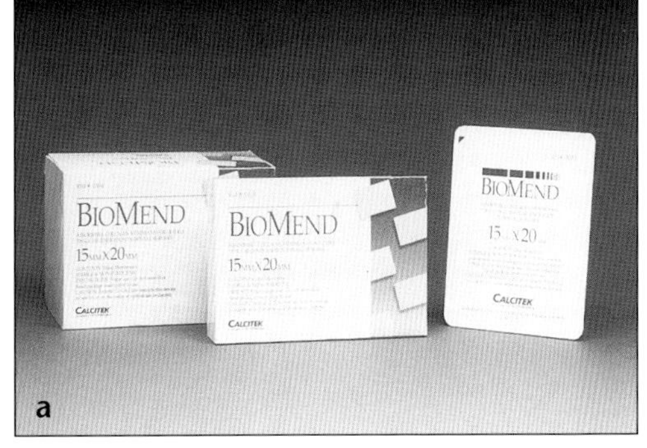

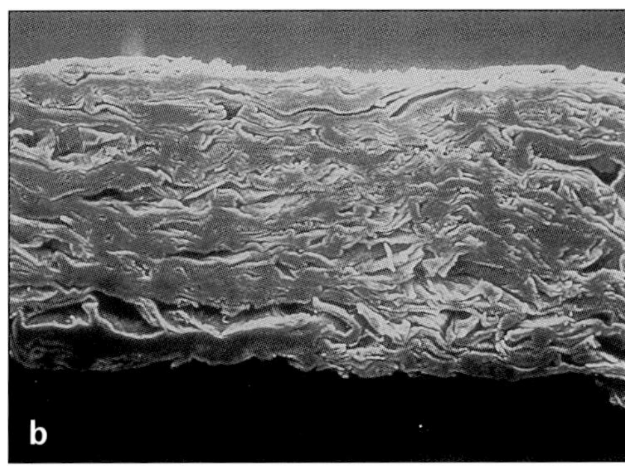

Fig 3-13
(a) The BioMend membrane is packaged in an envelope with templates to accommodate defects of different sizes and shapes.

(b) Under a scanning electron microscope, the BioMend membrane appears as a condensed laminated sheet in cross-section (200× magnification).

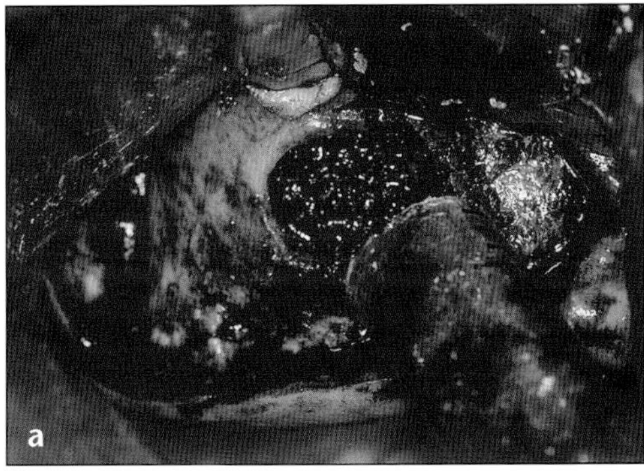

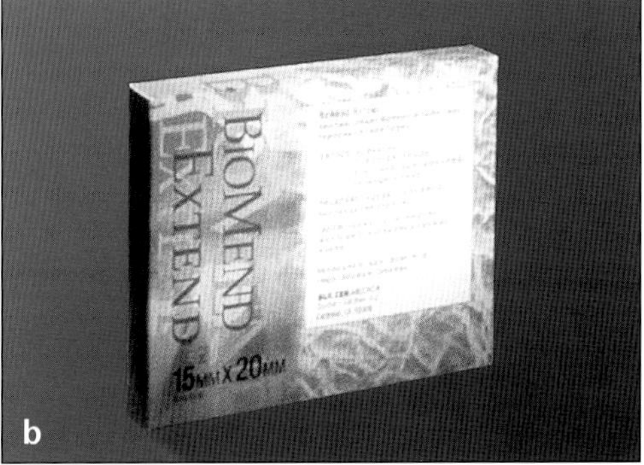

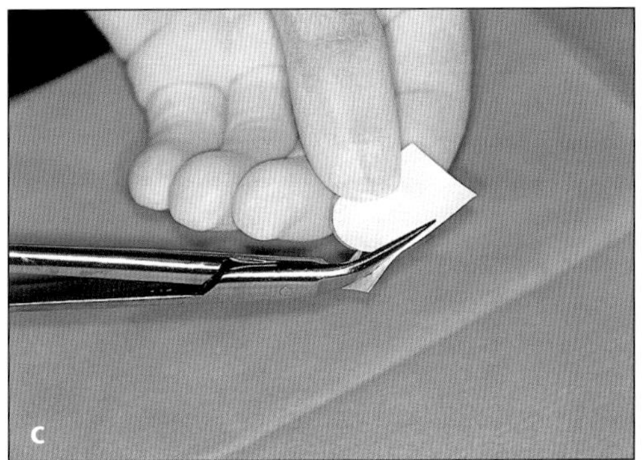

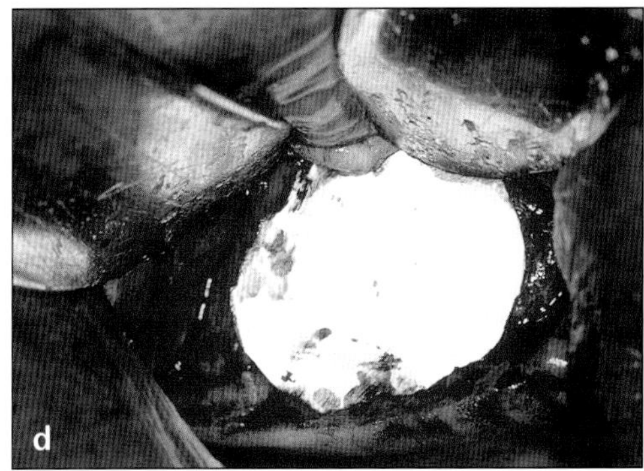

Fig 3-14 BioMend Extend, a longer-lasting absorbable collagen membrane, is fully absorbed within 18 weeks and maintains a regenerative barrier for a longer period of time.

(a) A sinus cavity window that has been fully grafted during a sinus lift is covered with a barrier membrane to protect and isolate the graft from epithelial downgrowth.

(b) The pore size (0.004 μm) of the BioMend Extend membrane, which resorbs more slowly than BioMend, effectively retards epithelial invasion during early healing phases.

(c) The BioMend Extend membrane is rigid enough to be trimmed to the desired shape.

(d) The material's stiffness makes it ideal for the semi-flat configuration over the sinus window. The membrane should be trimmed 2 to 3 mm beyond the periphery of the window.

exposed, gingival dehiscences always disappeared in subsequent weeks with no effect on healing. Bone regeneration occurred during barrier stability over 6 months, according to the histologic results (Fig 3-15).

Another study compared qualitative histologic results from the use of Ossix and deproteinized bovine bone mineral (DBBM) as a space maintainer versus the standard e-PTFE membrane (Gore-Tex) and the same bone substitute, with the latter used as the control group.[57] According to the Mann-Whitney test, differences in results were not statistically significant. When barrier exposure occurred, it did not interfere with the histologic outcome in either group. Thus, bone regeneration re-

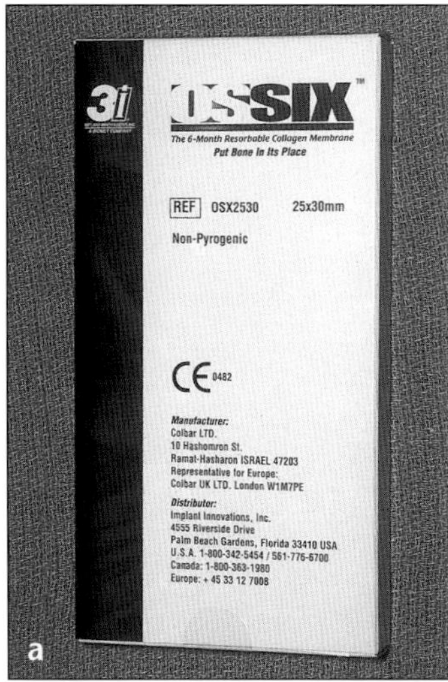

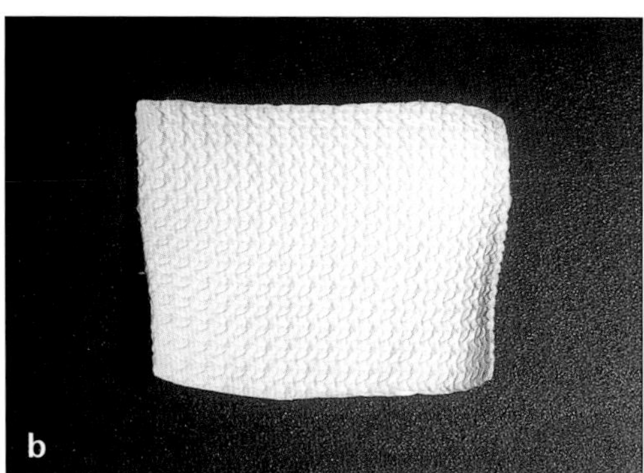

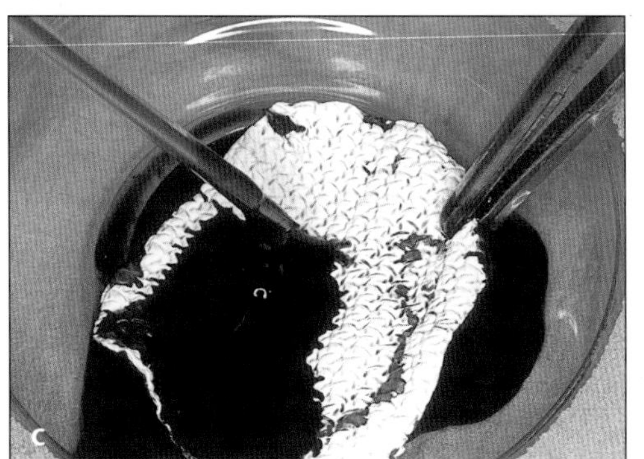

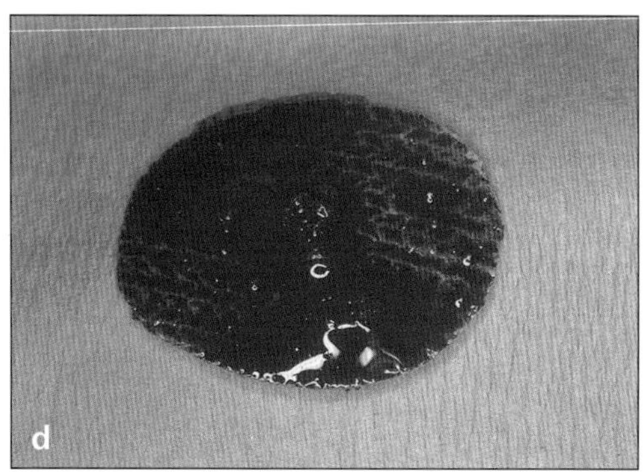

Fig 3-15 Ossix, a resorbable collagen membrane, can remain for up to 6 months after placement.

(a) The collagen in the Ossix membrane is cross-linked with glucose metabolites to help reduce inflammation and resist absorption even after exposure.

(b) Easy to cut and shape, this collagen membrane's flexibility helps it adhere to tissues during application without tacking or suturing.

(c) PRP growth factors will enhance the function of the collagen membrane; the PRP easily adheres to both sides of the membrane. The Ossix membrane remains manageable even after wetting.

(d) An Ossix membrane saturated with PRP for the recipient site will retain its malleability.

sults were comparable for Ossix and the e-PTFE barrier.

Bio-Gide (Geistlich Biomaterials, Wohlhusen, Switzerland) is a slow-resorbing (taking at least 4 months), pure (no organic residue or additional chemicals) bilayer collagen membrane composed of porcine collagen types I and III. Any possibility of viral or bacterial contamination has been eliminated from the product by means of an alkaline treatment, among other procedures. Developed specifically for periodontal and peri-implant procedures (as well as for facilitation of bone defect ossification), Bio-Gide is composed of one compact, smooth layer covered by a dense film. The smooth side is designed to prevent soft tissue encroachment during GBR. The other side is rough and designed to be placed facing the bone defect to facilitate bone ingrowth (Fig 3-16).[58] Numerous studies have demonstrated the effectiveness of Bio-Gide in bone regeneration procedures—often in conjunction with Bio-Oss porous bovine bone mineral (Osteohealth, Shirley, NY)—including augmentation around simultaneously placed implants; GBR in dehiscence defects; localized ridge augmentation prior to the placement of implants; reconstruction of the alveolar ridge prior to prosthetic treatment; and bone defect filling subsequent to root resection, cystectomy, or tooth removal (Fig 3-17).[28,53,59–65]

Reguarde (The Clinician's Preference, Golden, CO) is a type I bovine collagen

Fig 3-16 Bio-Gide is a slow-resorbing collagen membrane developed for periodontal and peri-implant procedures.

(a) The Bio-Gide membrane is manufactured from type I and type II porcine collagen. This bilayered membrane has undergone an alkaline treatment to prevent the transmission of viruses or bacteria.

(b) Bio-Gide has two distinct sides, one of which faces the flap and is designed to facilitate flap formation.

(c) The other, rougher side faces the bone and facilitates bone formation.

(d) The side of the membrane that faces the oral cavity is marked *up*.

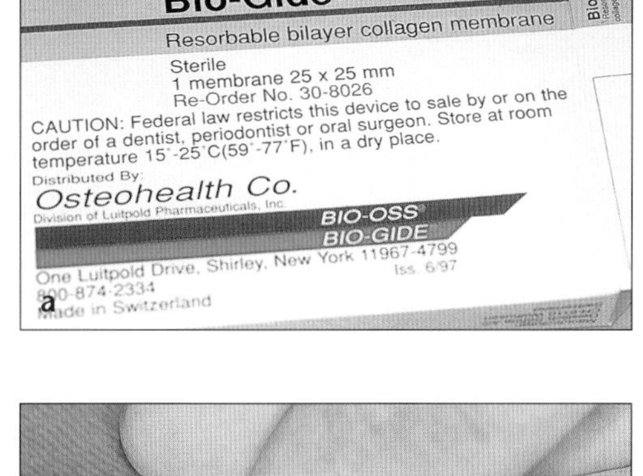

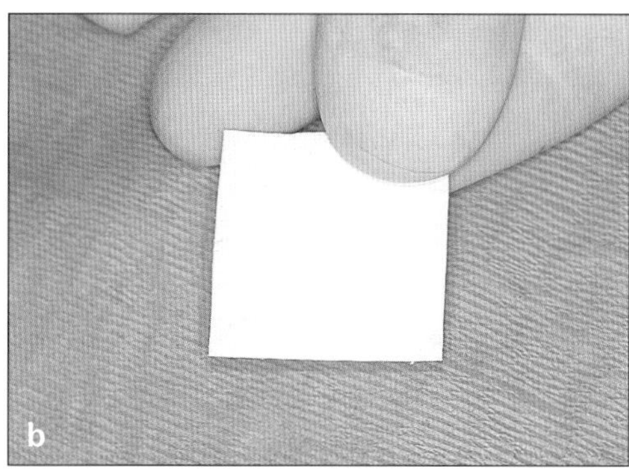

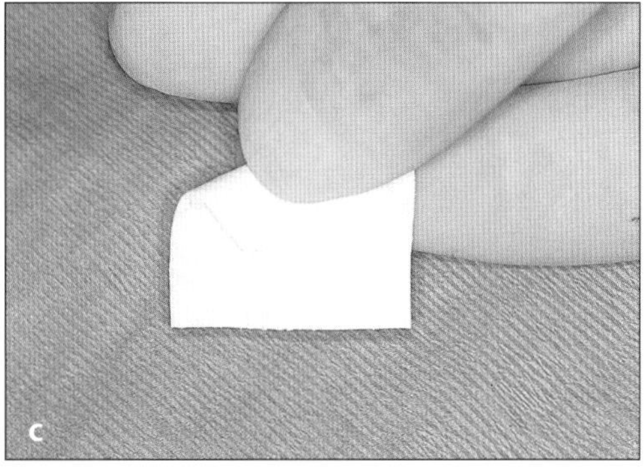

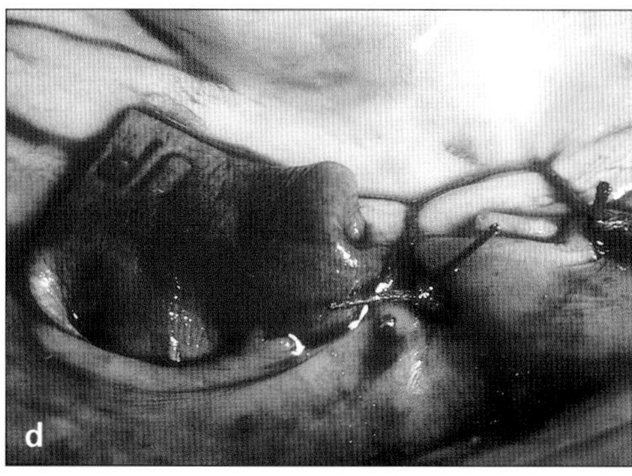

Fig 3-17 Bio-Gide's effectiveness in bone regeneration procedures has been established in numerous studies.

(a) Like other membranes, this PRP-saturated membrane carries growth factors. PRP is applied to the membrane immediately before placement to take advantage of growth factor–releasing platelets.

(b) Bio-Gide used in a ridge augmentation procedure. This membrane is extremely pliable and must be supported by bony walls, graft materials, or fixation screws for tenting.

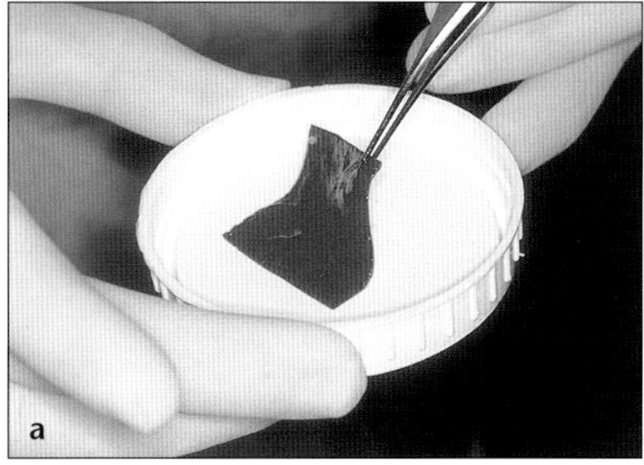

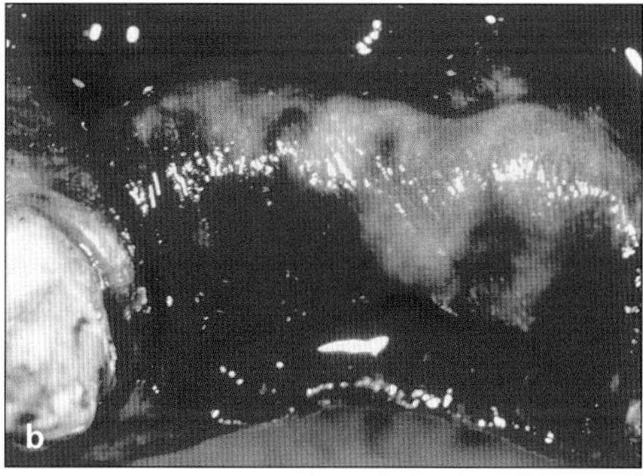

membrane indicated for use in both GBR and GTR procedures. This cross-linked, nonpyrogenic membrane retards epithelium downgrowth while the macromolecular pore size allows nutrient transfer. Its mechanical strength ensures membrane stabilization with a resorption time of 26 to 38 weeks. This occlusive membrane is available in three flexible sizes: 15 × 20 mm, 20 × 30 mm, and 30 × 40 mm.

Other collagen membranes include Periogen (Collagen, Palo Alto, CA), which is derived from bovine dermis and composed of types I and III collagen and has a resorption rate of 4 to 8 weeks; Biostite (Coletica), which is derived from calfskin and composed of 88% hydroxyapatite, 9.5% type I collagen, and 2.5% chondroitin-4-sulfate and has a resorption rate of 4 to 8 weeks; and Tissue Guide (Koken, Tokyo, Japan), which is derived from bovine dermis and tendon and composed of atelocollagen and tendon collagen and has a resorption rate of 4 to 8 weeks.[52]

Polylactic acid and polyglycolic acid

The first resorbable barrier to be approved by the Food and Drug Administration (FDA) for barrier membrane techniques was Guidor (Guidor, Huddinge, Sweden), a bioresorbable matrix barrier composed of a blend of polylactic acid that was softened with citric acid for malleability and to facilitate clinical handling. This product is a multilayered matrix designed for ingrowth of gingival connective tissue, preventing apical downgrowth of gingival epithelium.[2] The inner layer, which is in contact with the bone or tooth, features small circular perforations and several space holders to ensure sufficient room for the formation of new attachment, whereas the outer layer, which is in contact with the gingival tissue, has larger rectangular perforations to allow rapid growth of gingival tissue into the interspace between the two layers, preventing or minimizing epithelial downgrowth.[8,66,67] The resorption process of the material is programmed to ensure that it will function as a barrier for a minimum of 6 weeks, after which time it slowly resorbs. Complete resorption occurs at approximately 12 months (Fig 3-18).[67,68]

Several studies have demonstrated the efficacy of polylactic acid (PLA) membranes to produce the formation of new attachment and bone in the treatment of interproximal defects and gingival recession in primates, as well as infrabony defects and Class II furcation defects in humans.[68–72] The results obtained in these studies showed that the use of this matrix barrier around teeth resulted in reduced probing depths; a gain in clinical attachment; and a very low incidence of gingival pathologic disease, gingival recession, and device exposure.[68]

However, some researchers failed to demonstrate any advantage in the use of PLA membranes in the treatment of circumferential periodontal defects in dogs, contradicting the results of their previous study that used the same membranes in dogs.[16,73] The reason for the difference in the results may be related to the defect type—surgically created dehiscence defects on the buccal aspects of maxillary and mandibular premolars versus surgically created circumferential (one-wall vertical and horizontal) defects on maxillary premolars.[16,73] A later study also failed to show adequate regeneration with the use of PLA membranes (with a nonspecific design) in circumferential periodontal lesions in primates.[74] The membrane failed to produce new attachment, and gingival recession and device exposure were common. In addition, an epithelial layer was found in these membranes. These results suggest that the membrane had exfoliated rather than reabsorbed in the tissue. However, it was concluded that the material

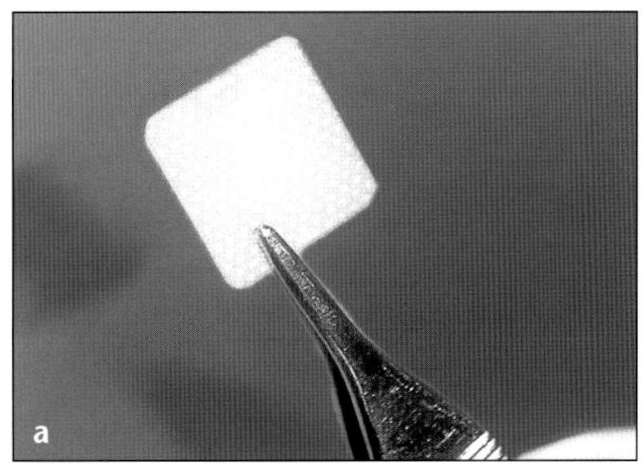

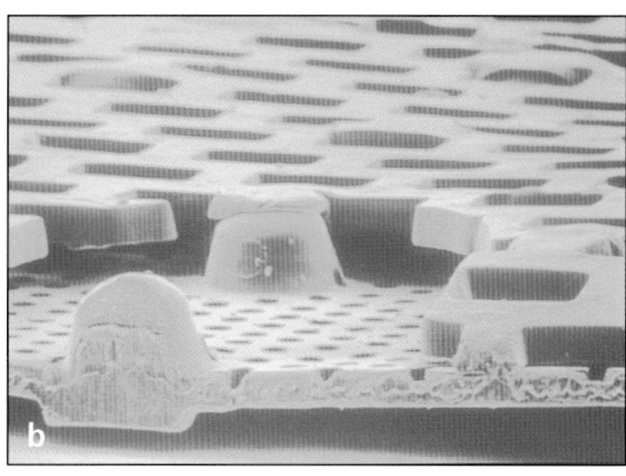

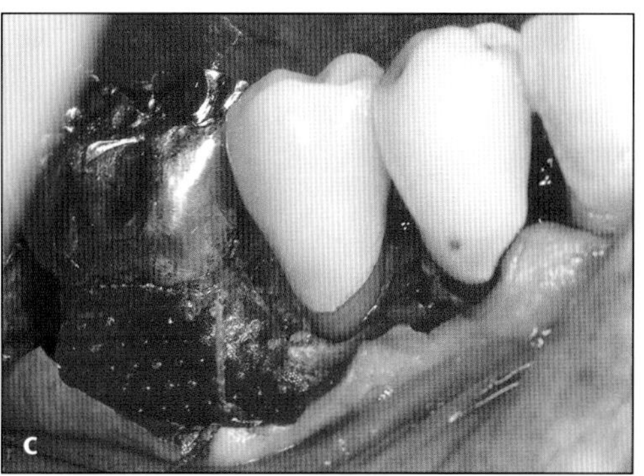

Fig 3-18 PLA membranes are designed for ingrowth of gingival connective tissue, preventing apical downgrowth of gingival epithelium.

(a) A PLA membrane (Guidor) is treated with citric acid to make it malleable and adaptable to the defects.

(b) Guidor consists of two layers. The inner layer, which contacts the surface where connective tissue is desired, has small circular perforations; the outer layer, which contacts the gingival tissue, has larger rectangular perforations that allow the growth of epithelium between the layers.

(c) GBR is used to treat bone resorption around a crowned molar. A Guidor membrane attached with resorbable sutures will act as a barrier for 6 weeks and will completely resorb after 12 months.

should not be considered inapplicable for use in barrier membrane techniques; further modification and transformation were required to create a membrane that possesses all of the properties necessary to obtain better results.

Another clinical study in primates compared PLA membranes with PLA mesh barriers.[75] The results demonstrated the superiority of the membranes in the production of new attachment and biocompatibility compared with the mesh barriers, which showed downgrowth of the epithelium along or around the device, gingival recession, device exposure, and pronounced soft tissue inflammation. A third clinical study compared the effectiveness of bioresorbable PLA membranes with e-PTFE membranes in the treatment of Class II furcation defects in humans.[76] This study showed that although there was a significant gain in clinical attachment with the use of both barriers, the use of bioresorbable membranes resulted in a significantly greater gain in clinical horizontal attachment and less gingival recession. Postoperative complications, such as swelling and pain, occurred more frequently after the use of e-PTFE barriers, usually during the first month of healing.

Researchers compared the reliability of resorbable PLA barriers and nonresorbable e-PTFE membranes for root coverage and clinical attachment gain in the treatment of human recession defects and reported no differences for any of the clinical variables assessed.[66] However, the advantages of the bioresorbable barrier included reduced discomfort, stress, and expense because of the single-step procedure. Others showed significantly more new attachment formation and less gingival inflammation and device exposure with the use of PLA membranes when compared with e-PTFE membranes.[77]

With respect to treatment outcome variables related to the use of PLA barrier membranes, a 2003 study determined that colonization of periodontal pathogens at sites treated by GTR may correlate with the presence of those pathogens in the mouth before surgery; the study concluded that prevention of colonization may require suppression or eradication of the pathogens before surgery.[78] Later that year, a study by the same researchers concluded that active smoking was the strongest predictor variable negatively affecting alveolar bone gain following GTR in the treatment of periodontal defects.[79]

Epi-Guide (Kensey Nash, Exton, PA) bioresorbable barrier membrane is a porous, three-dimensional hydrophilic matrix made from D, D-L, L-polylactic acid. Constructed in three layers, it is designed to attract and retain fibroblasts and epithelial cells while maintaining space around a bony defect for GTR. Epi-Guide acts as a barrier membrane for up to 20 weeks; complete bioresorption occurs between 6 and 12 months. It quickly absorbs blood and facilitates healthy clot formation, is easily handled, and can be trimmed to fit the defect site. An in vitro study concluded that the Epi-Guide membrane enhanced early osteoblast (MC3T3-E1) attachment.[30]

Bioresorbable membranes made of polyglycolic acid (PGA) and PLA (Resolut, W. L. Gore) have been tested in animals and proven to be safe with minimal inflammatory response and good promotion of periodontal regeneration.[24] These membranes consist of an occlusive film with a bonded, randomly oriented fiber matrix located on each surface. The film bonds and fibers separate the soft tissue from the defect. The random arrangement of the fibers and the openness of the fibrous matrix encourage the ingrowth of connective tissue and inhibit apical migration of the epithelium. The fiber matrix is the primary structural component that provides adequate strength for space making during the initial phases of healing (2 to 4 weeks for periodontal defects) (Fig 3-19).[18]

A multicenter clinical study was conducted to evaluate the capacity of the combination of PGA and PLA membranes to promote clinical periodontal regeneration of Class II furcation defects and two- and three-wall infrabony defects.[24] After 1 year, the defects had healed with favorable changes in the measured clinical parameters (ie, decrease in probing depths and horizontal probing for the furcations and a gain in attachment levels). An in vitro study concluded that the Resolut membrane enhanced early osteoblast (MC3T3-E1) attachment.[30] The slow-resorbing form (Resolut XT) also showed promise for barrier membrane techniques.

Other researchers studied the use of a biodegradable barrier made of polylactide:polyglycolide (50:50) copolymer (DL-PLGA, Boehringer, Ingelheim, Germany) in patients with severe horizontal bone loss and active periodontal disease.[80] Historically, this combination has been used for sutures and implant material and in a drug-delivery control system. Inflammatory tissue response after the implantation of copolymers was found to be minimal, and no adverse host tissue responses were observed. The results of this study showed that the barrier did not enhance connective tissue attachment or prevent epithelial migration. After placement, the material was clinically evident at 10 days to 2 weeks but not after 17 days.[80]

Another study compared the use of resorbable membranes made of PGA and PLA with e-PTFE membranes for barrier membrane procedures.[81] This study showed that there was a significantly greater amount of bone regeneration obtained with the use of e-PTFE membranes compared with the resorbable membranes. According to the authors, this difference may be the result of several factors: *(1)*

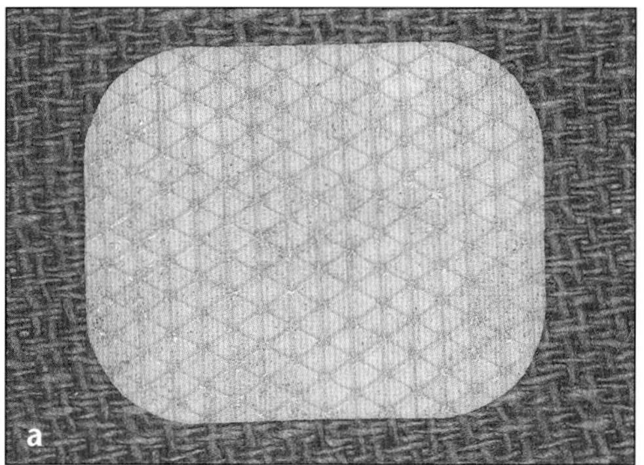

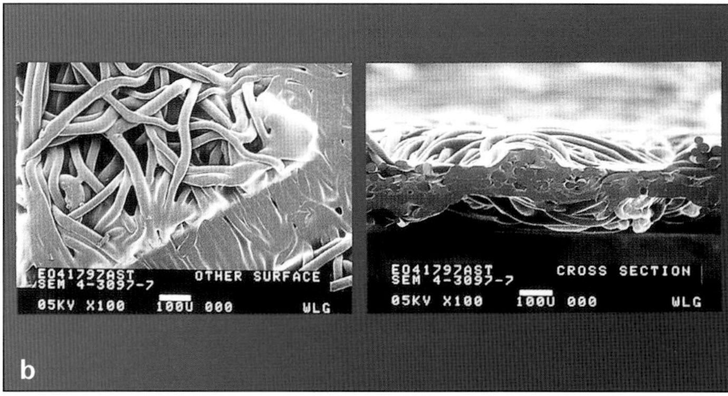

Fig 3-19
(a) Resolut is a synthetic resorbable membrane made of PLA and PGA. The Resolut membrane consists of an occlusive middle layer with a randomly oriented fiber layer on each surface that encourages ingrowth of connective tissue and prevents epithelial cells from migrating into the defect.

(b) (Left) Surface of the Resolut membrane (65× magnification). Note the randomly oriented fibers. *(Right)* Cross-sectional view of the membrane (65× magnification). Note its occlusive nature.

the fixation screws may have acted as tent poles to prevent e-PTFE membrane collapse, increasing the space for bone regeneration; *(2)* the stiffness of the resorbable material was not sufficient to maintain adequate space between the defect and the membrane; and *(3)* as the membrane resorbed, the space-making capability of the barrier decreased.

Other softer and easier to manipulate membranes of a similar composition have become available, such as Resolut Adapt. This regenerative, synthetic membrane can remain virtually intact for 8 to 10 weeks; its features include softness, suppleness, and drapeability. Resolut Adapt LT (long term) can stay virtually intact for 16 to 24 weeks. It is composed of the same types of bioabsorbable polymers that have been used safely for a considerable length of time in sutures, surgical meshes, and implantable devices.

OsseoQuest (W. L. Gore) is another synthetic membrane that remains substantially intact for 16 to 24 weeks. It consists of a three-layer structure with two random fiber matrices on either side of a cell-occlusive film. The membrane is composed of PGA, PLA, and trimethylene carbonate (Fig 3-20).

Synthetic liquid polymer

A polymer of lactic acid, poly(DL-lactide) (PLA), dissolved in N-methyl-2 pyrrolidone (NMP), has been studied as a resorbable barrier material. The material begins as a solution that sets to a firm consistency on contact with water or another aqueous solution (Atrisorb, Atrix Laboratories, Fort Collins, CO). The polymer composition is similar to that of Vicryl sutures (Ethicon, Somerville, NJ).[82,83] When outside the oral cavity, the membrane is a partially set solution, which allows it to be trimmed to

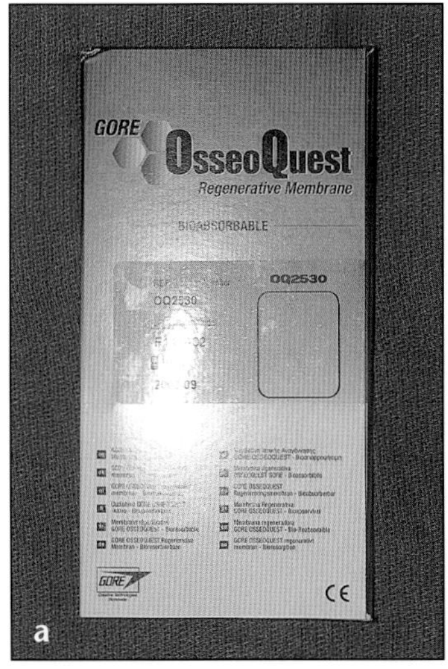

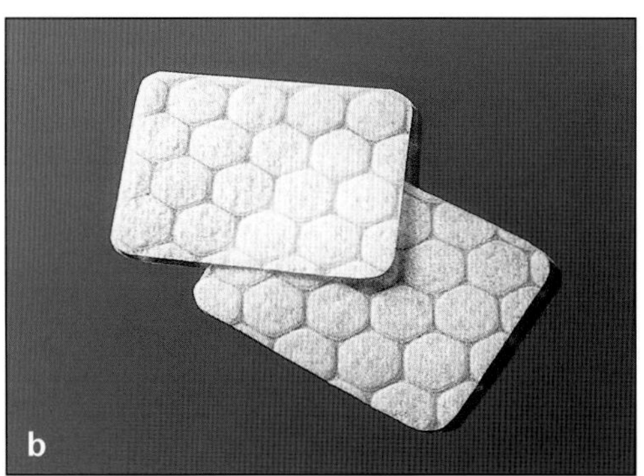

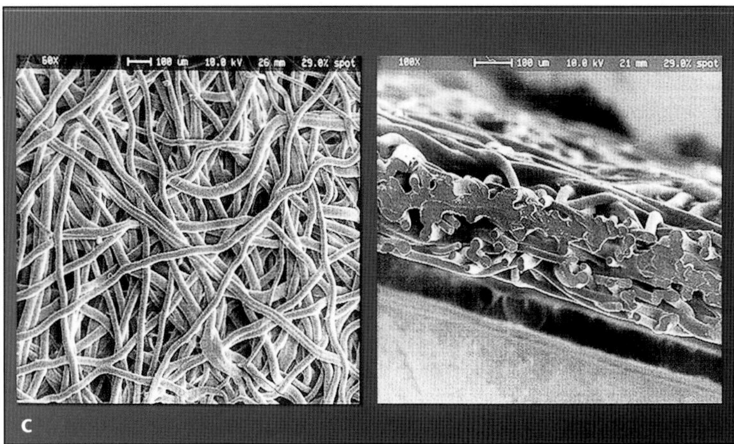

Fig 3-20

(a) OsseoQuest is a synthetic membrane that consists of three different polymers: PGA, PLA, and trimethylene carbonate.

(b) The membrane displays a macrohexametric pattern and resorbs after 16 to 24 weeks. The OsseoQuest membrane consists of a cell-occlusive middle layer with randomly arranged fiber layers on each side.

(c) (Left) Occlusal view of the surface of the OsseoQuest membrane (65× magnification). Note the randomly oriented fibers. *(Right)* Cross section of the membrane. Note the occlusive nature. Although the arrangement of fibers is similar to Resolut, OsseoQuest has a slightly different chemical composition; which accounts for its slower resorption rate.

the dimensions of the defect before intraoral placement. The barrier is then adapted to the defect and sets in a firm consistency in situ. Because of its semi-rigid consistency in the extraoral environment, this barrier has the advantage of being rigid enough for placement but flexible enough to be adapted to the defect. The barrier adheres directly to dental structures; therefore, sutures are not required.[82,83] Chemically, the material is a polymer component that is resorbed through the process of hydrolysis. The rate of resorption is controlled, and the membrane is present during the critical period of healing, preventing epithelial migration and isolating the periodontal defect compartment.[83] Alternatively, the clinician can place graft material in the defect to ensure a tent-like position of the membrane, apply the liquid polymer directly to the surgical site, and then allow contact with surrounding fluids, which initiates the setup of polymer in a firm consistency (Fig 3-21).

Several authors have studied the efficacy of this barrier. Early investigations in dogs demonstrated that the material is safe, nontoxic, and resorbable, and that it efficiently produces regeneration.[84] The animal model allowed histologic analysis 9 to 12 months after baseline surgery, which showed that formation of new ce-

Fig 3-21 Synthetic liquid polymers exist as a liquid-gel outside the oral cavity. The liquid polymer will set into a solid membrane upon placing it onto a sponge wetted with saline, water, or saliva to faciliate setting. The barrier membrane can then be adapted to the defect and placed.

(a) The liquid Atrisorb membrane, composed of PLA dissolved in NMP, becomes rigid after contact with another liquid. Here, it is opened in preparation for use.

(b) This synthetic liquid polymer membrane is packaged with a plastic case that serves as a stent; saline is dripped over the white sponge pad in order to provide a wet surface. Once wetted, the Atrisorb gel will be injected onto the wet pad and will set into a solid membrane.

(c) Two blue plastic bands (spacers) of a predetermined thickness prevent complete closure. The Atrisorb is injected onto the wetted white sponge pad between the two blue bands, and the lid of the device is closed.

(d) The space on the wetted sponge pad created by the spacers is filled with the liquid polymer, which becomes rigid upon contact with the wet surface. After several minutes, the device is opened and the newly formed solid membrane is lifted out.

(e) The newly formed membrane is now ready for use. The membrane's rigidity facilitates cutting and shaping, while its malleability allows it to adapt to the defect.

(f) Alternatively, a much more practical method of using this material is to simply attach an 18-gauge needle onto the vial of Atrisorb. The Atrisorb can be placed or injected directly onto the defect and will set into a solid membrane after wetting with water or saliva.

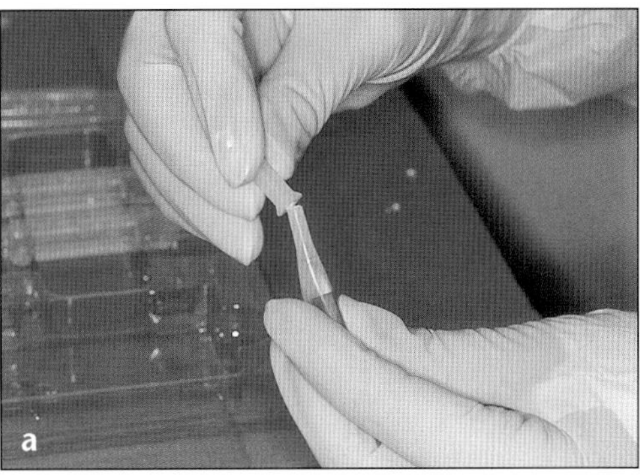
a

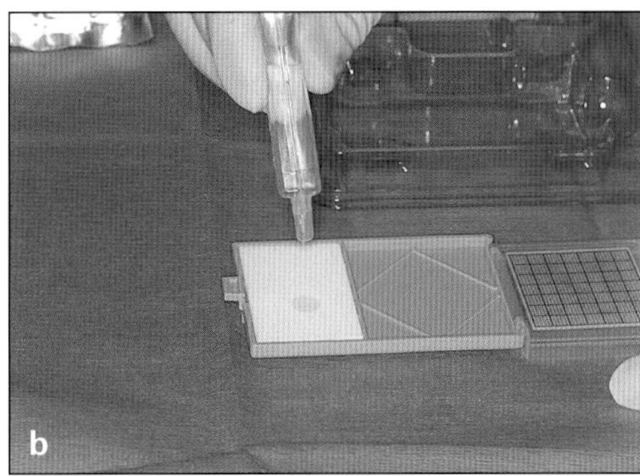
b

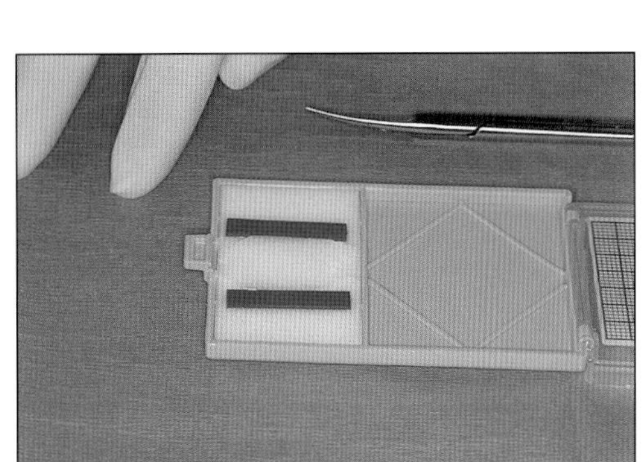
c

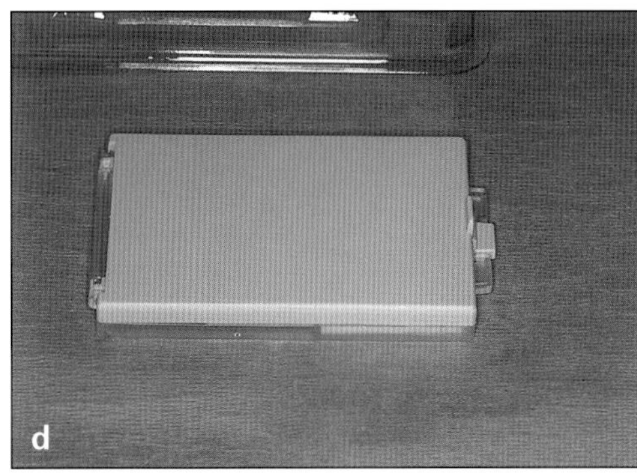
d

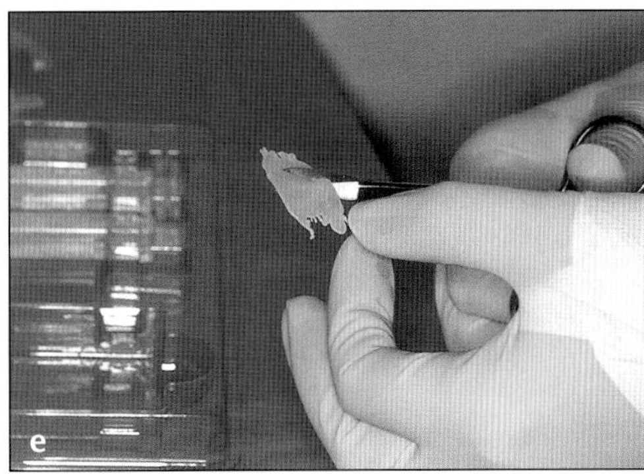
e

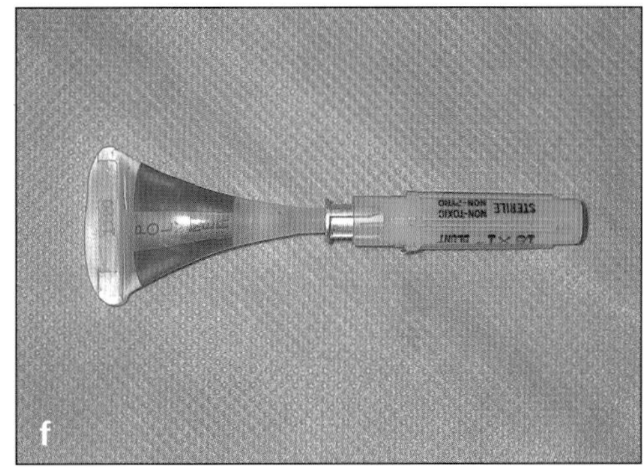
f

mentum, periodontal ligament, and alveolar bone occurred after the placement of this membrane. Studies in humans also showed the efficacy of this material to produce periodontal regeneration in Class II furcation defects.[83] The results obtained in this study were reconfirmed in a later multicenter study by the same researchers.[82]

Polyglactin

Another bioresorbable material that has been developed as a barrier membrane is a woven mesh barrier made of polyglactin 910 (Vicryl Periodontal Mesh), a copolymer of PGA and PLA with a resorption rate of 30 to 90 days. The results of several studies have questioned the use of polyglactin for GTR procedures, reporting that the mesh provides an insufficient barrier because of fragmentation of the material. The integrity of the mesh is lost after 14 days, and the cervical seal between the mesh and the adjacent tooth may not be perfect, allowing for the growth of connective tissue and epithelium between the root surface and the barrier (Fig 3-22).[67,85]

A clinical and histologic study in primates that compared the design of the mesh barrier with a matrix barrier concluded that the healing processes differed considerably. Histologically, complete integration with the surrounding tissue was found with a majority of the matrix barriers, preventing epithelial downgrowth and pocket formation around the barrier. However, advanced epithelial downgrowth was found on the mesh barriers. Based on these findings, the use of mesh barriers was not recommended for barrier membrane procedures.[67] These results were similar to those of previous studies in which epithelial downgrowth, gingival recession, device exposure, and pronounced soft tissue inflammation were observed with the use of mesh barriers.[75]

Calcium sulfate

Medical-grade calcium sulfate, commonly known as plaster of Paris, has been used after immediate implant placement as part of a bone graft placed around the implants. Barriers composed of medical-grade calcium sulfate can be placed over bone grafts for clot stabilization and to exclude undesirable tissue (gingival connective tissue and epithelium). The advantages of this material include providing a source of calcium in the early mineralization process and aiding particle retention.[86,87]

One study compared the bone regeneration capability of demineralized freeze-dried bone allograft (DFDBA) in the treatment of mandibular Class II furcation defects using an e-PTFE membrane versus a barrier of calcium sulfate.[88] The results obtained with both barriers were comparable in selected defects. Other studies showed successful results using medical-grade calcium sulfate and DFDBA for regeneration of periodontal defects.[43,89]

Calcium sulfate has been shown to facilitate complete closure in situations where wound closure over the barrier membrane is not possible. An in vitro experiment comparing the capacity of human gingival fibroblasts to migrate along a chemotactic gradient over the three different forms of barrier membrane materials (e-PTFE, polylactic acid, calcium sulfate) showed that the mean migration distance, as well as cell attachment and spreading, was significantly greater with the calcium sulfate barriers.[8] It was concluded that calcium sulfate as a membrane appeared to offer greater potential than other membranes for healing by secondary intention in surgical sites where primary closure cannot be obtained.

Calcium sulfate is available in sterile kits that contain premeasured amounts of

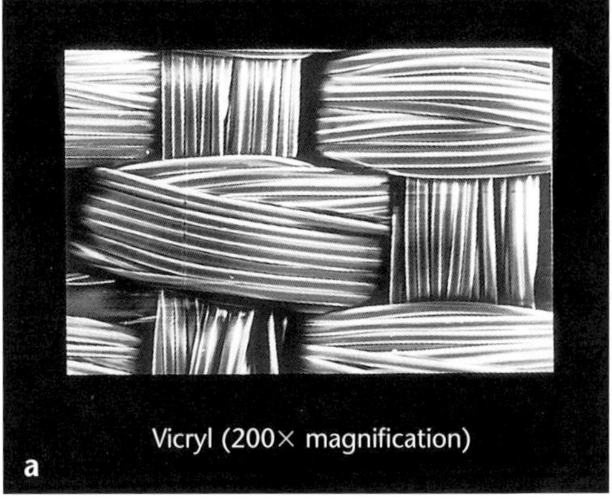

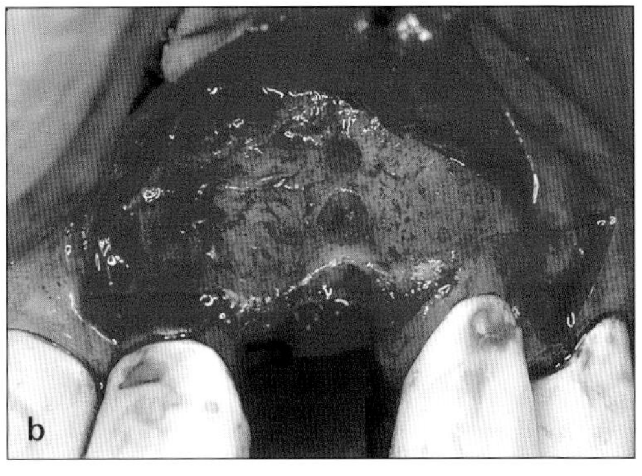

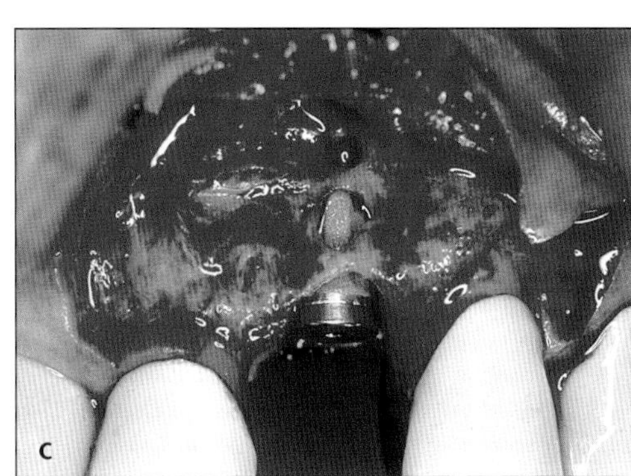

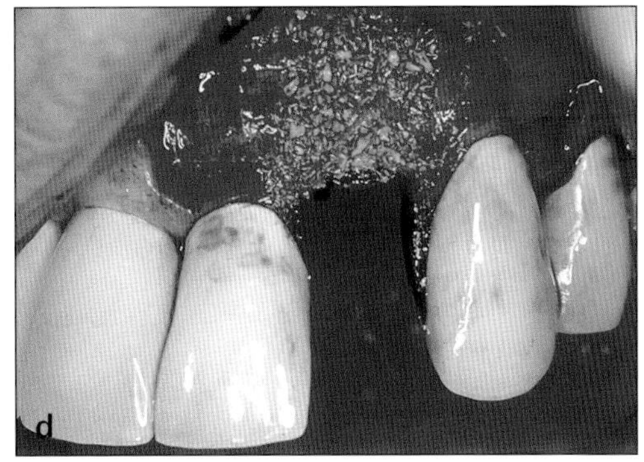

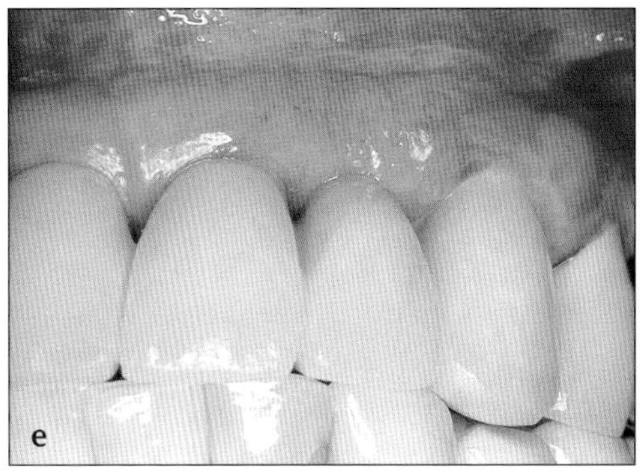

Fig 3-22 Polyglactin barrier membranes have a resorption rate of 30 to 90 days, but their use has been questioned because of fragmentation of the material and should be limited to areas requiring minimal benefit of a membrane barrier.

(a) The Vicryl mesh membrane consists of woven polyglactin 910, a copolymer of PGA and PLA.

(b) Immediate implant placement is planned after the removal of this residual root with dehiscence in the buccal bone.

(c) The root is extracted, and an implant is placed during the same procedure. Correction of the bone defect will optimize implant osseointegration.

(d) Particulate alloplast is placed over the defect, which is then covered with a Vicryl mesh membrane. Much of the benefit here is from the bone graft itself.

(e) The final restoration shows successful implant integration with good bone formation at the buccal wall.

medical-grade calcium sulfate powder and a syringe that is prefilled with an accelerating diluent (CapSet, Lifecore Biomedical, Chaska, MN). When mixed together, these substances create a moldable plaster that can conform to the desired shape, even in the presence of blood. Sutures are not required because this mixture is adhesive. Calcium sulfate dissolves in approximately 30 days without an inflammatory reaction, and it does not attract bacteria or support infection (Fig 3-23).[86]

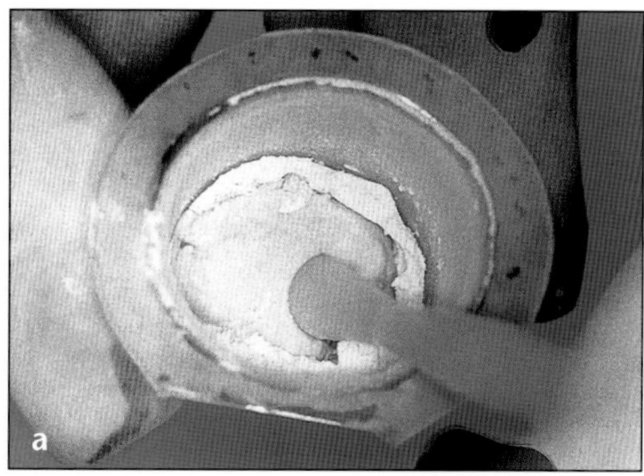

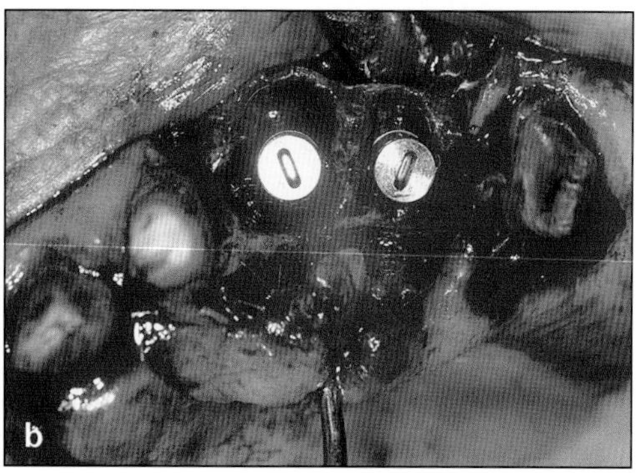

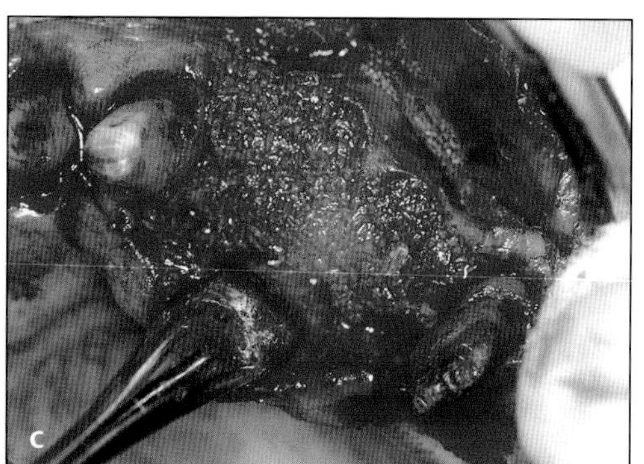

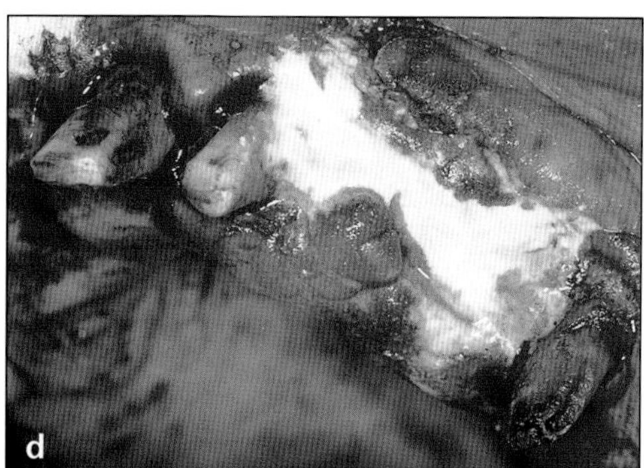

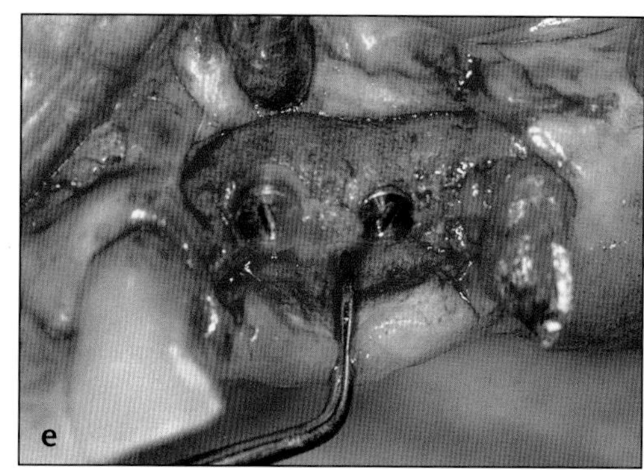

Fig 3-23 Calcium sulfate has been shown to facilitate GBR in periodontal and oral surgery procedures.

(a) The medical-grade calcium sulfate and diluent contained in the CapSet kit are mixed to form a moldable plaster.

(b) These implants were immediately placed in extraction sites in the anterior maxilla. They are stable because of good apical bone anchorage, but the coronal portion exhibits bone deficit.

(c) A mixture of DFDBA and CapSet is used to graft the area around and over the implants.

(d) A layer of pure CapSet is placed over the graft as a barrier membrane to prevent epithelial downgrowth and to protect the graft. Primary closure is not possible in this case.

(e) Good epithelial coverage occurred over the calcium sulfate barrier. At stage 2 surgery, good bone formation can be observed around the implants.

The rationale for using medical-grade calcium sulfate for GTR procedures is as follows[42,90,91]:

1. Complete resorption within 3 to 4 weeks
2. Biocompatibility (causes no increase in inflammation)
3. Adaptability (does not need to be cut before placement)
4. Porosity (allows fluid exchange, but excludes the passage of epithelium and connective tissue)
5. Minimal postoperative discomfort
6. Clot protection during the early stages of healing
7. Soft tissue growth over exposed calcium sulfate
8. Lack of infection with material exposure
9. Minimal effect on cellular morphology

Acellular dermal allografts

A relatively new type of bioresorbable grafting material is acellular human cadaver skin obtained from tissue banks (AlloDerm, LifeCell, Branchburg, NJ). The material has undergone a process of de-epithelialization and decellularization to eliminate the targets of rejection response, leaving an immunologically inert avascular connective tissue.[92] Dermal allografts have been successfully used for the treatment of third-degree burns and are currently used as a barrier membrane for mucogingival defects,[93] for formation of attached gingival tissue,[94] and for soft tissue development around dental implants[95] and as a biologic bandage after osseous resection.[96]

In one study, the material appeared to become completely and permanently incorporated into the surrounding tissue after 6 weeks when used as a barrier membrane.[97] With the use of dermal allografts, clinically normal healing and no inflammatory infiltration have been observed, indicating that this material is compatible with human oral tissue.[98] A number of studies indicate the efficacy of using acellular dermal allografts to combat gingival recession and to provide root coverage,[99–105] including its use as a viable alternative to connective tissue grafting,[106] thus helping to avoid donor-site morbidity in the palate.[107–109]

Acellular dermal allografts have desirable properties for a barrier membrane material, such as being memory free, easy to place and adapt, biocompatible, and able to be covered by soft tissue and remain covered. If the material is bioresorbable, it must be predictable and remain intact as a barrier for 6 weeks, with complete resorption occurring in less than 6 months.[23]

The use of acellular dermal allografts has several advantages. They contain no cellular material, which eliminates the possibility of rejection because of the presence of major histocompatibility complex class I and II antigens. In addition, the unlimited supply, color match, thickness, lack of degradation if primary closure is not achieved, and formation of additional attached gingiva make this material a good choice for barrier membrane techniques (Fig 3-24).

Laminar bone membranes

Lambone (Pacific Coast Tissue Bank, Los Angeles, CA) membrane is composed of flexible sheets of demineralized freeze-dried human laminar cortical bone. A number of studies have examined the efficacy of using laminar bone as a barrier membrane in GTR procedures.[110–114] For example, in one study, laminar bone sheets were used as barrier membranes for GTR around implants and for ridge augmentation.[110] Hard tissue regeneration was significant, and there were no complications. Another study compared clinical changes and osseous regeneration in comparable Class II mandibular molar furcation invasion defects when either a laminar bone allograft membrane or an e-PTFE membrane was used for GTR.[111] Results suggested that the laminar bone membrane was as suitable as e-PTFE when both were used in conjunction with demineralized freeze-dried bone allografts. A third study showed similar GTR effects when laminar bone was compared to Gore-Tex Augmentation Membranes (GTAM) (W. L. Gore).[112]

Freeze-dried dura mater

Lyodura (B. Braun, Melsungen, Germany) is a human tissue product harvested from cadavers as an alternative to the patient's own tissue for the repair of wounds. First developed in 1969, Lyodura is harvested from dura mater, the tough membrane that covers the brain. From 1969 to 1996, the product was distributed internationally;

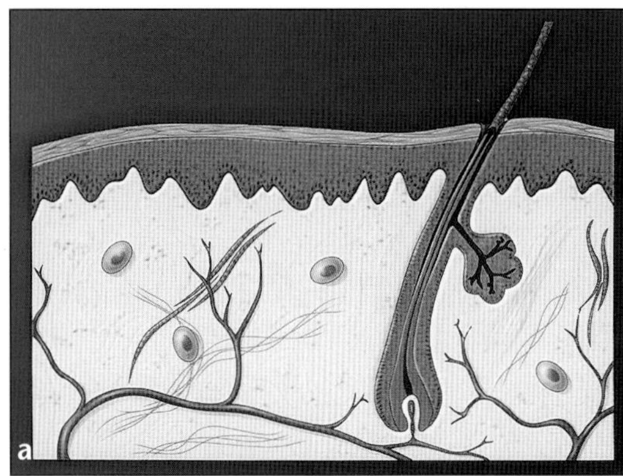

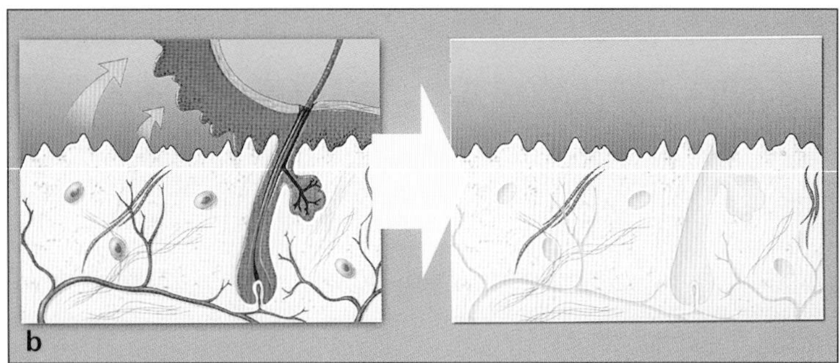

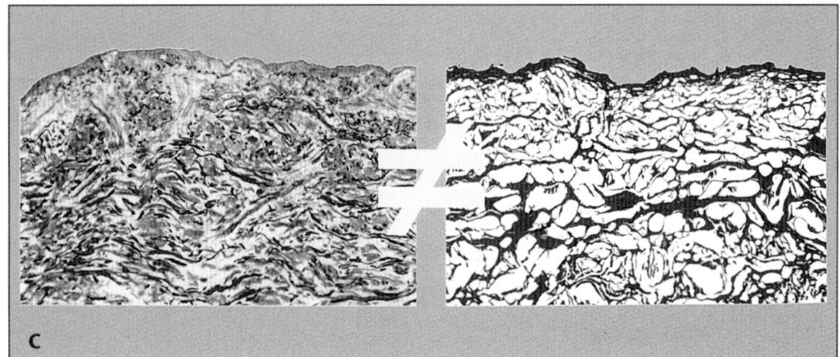

Fig 3-24 As barrier membranes, acellular allografts have desirable properties such as being memory free, easy to place and adapt, biocompatible, and able to be covered by soft tissue and remain covered.

(a) AlloDerm, derived from human cadaver skin obtained from tissue banks, is carefully screened for diseases such as hepatitis B and C, HIV, and syphilis.

(b) The cadaver skin undergoes dermal cell solubilization, or elimination of the epithelium and the underlying hair follicles, sebaceous glands, vascular network, etc, that can trigger an immunologic response.

(c) AlloDerm *(left)* maintains its collagen, elastin, and proteoglycans, providing an undamaged acellular dermal matrix, unlike freeze-dried skin *(right)*.

it was not FDA-approved but was available in the United States via Canadian distributors. Although currently FDA-approved and available for use, it is rarely used as a membrane barrier because contamination problems with recipients have been documented, the most serious of which links Lyodura and Creutzfeldt-Jakob disease.[115–117] A 1999 study concluded that the product is safe and effective when used as a resorbable barrier around dental implants for GBR at extraction sites and for dehiscence defects (Fig 3-25)[118]; however, concerns remain about its safety, especially in comparison to the many other choices that are available.

Fig 3-24 *(cont)*
(d) At the start of the surgery, the AlloDerm graft is placed in saline solution for rehydration.

(e) Once rehydrated, AlloDerm tissue is indistinguishable from a dermal autograft. It is important to follow the product's instructions carefully to ensure that the correct side of the tissue is placed.

(f) This tooth extraction case requires optimal bone formation for future implant placement.

(g) The AlloDerm membrane is cut to fit the site and then placed.

(h) Primary closure is not possible without damaging the gingival architecture. The AlloDerm tissue can be left exposed to the oral cavity or covered with periodontal cement.

(i) Early healing (3 weeks postsurgery) shows that epithelium has completely migrated over and into the AlloDerm membrane. Pigment and texture match those of the surrounding tissues. The soft tissue graft will continue to mature over the next several weeks and the color and texture will improve further.

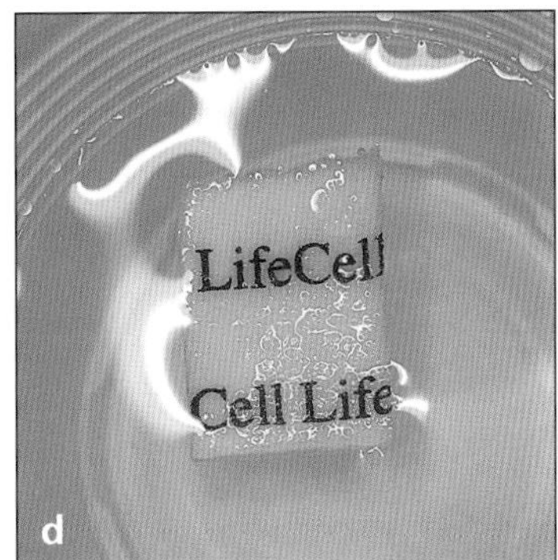

d

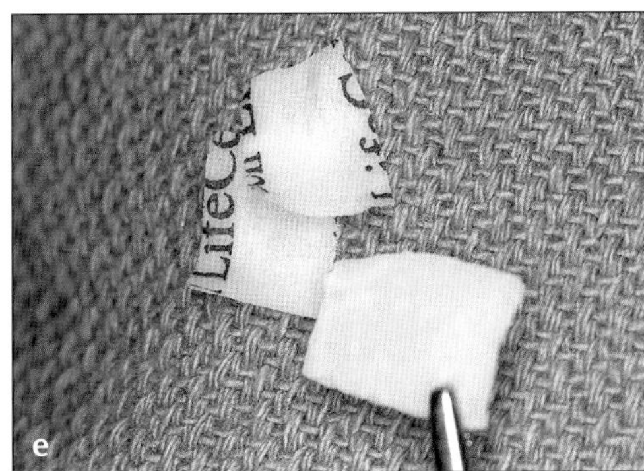

e

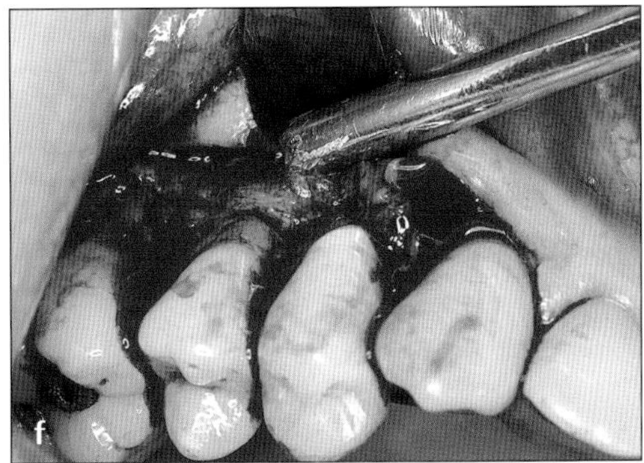
f

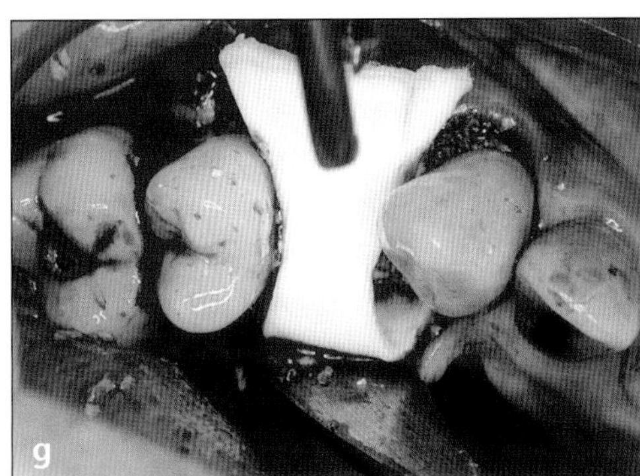
g

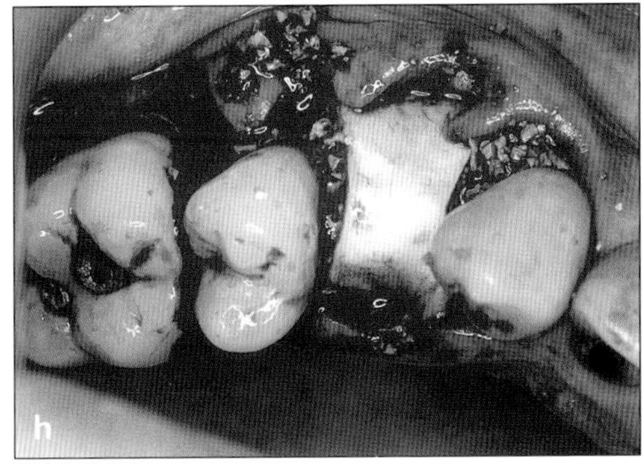
h

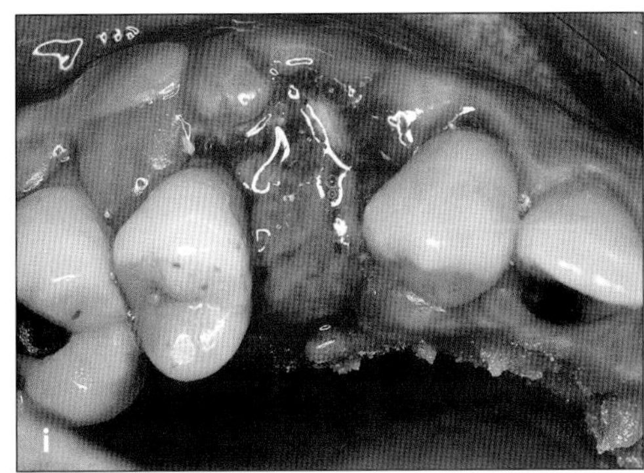
i

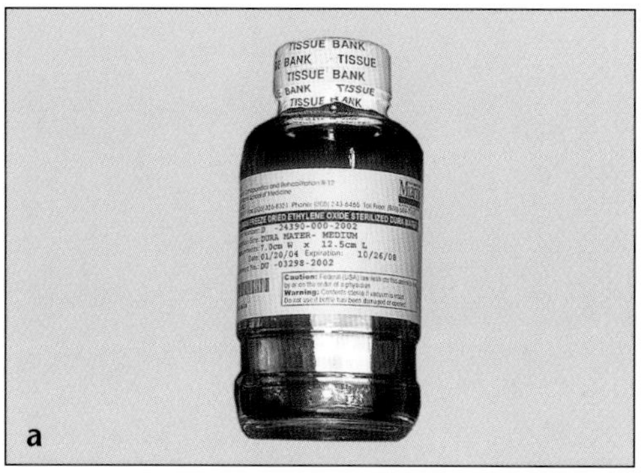

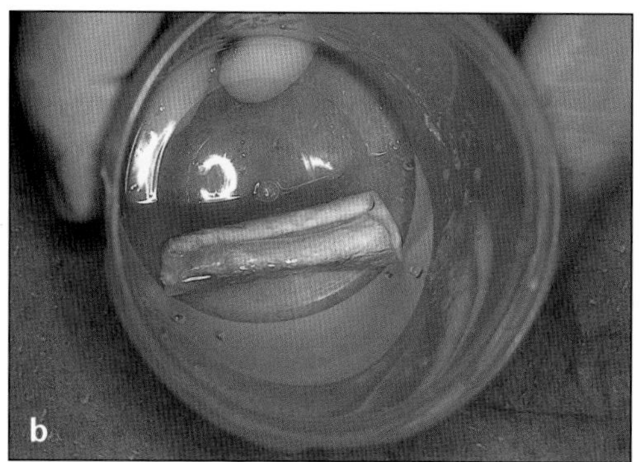

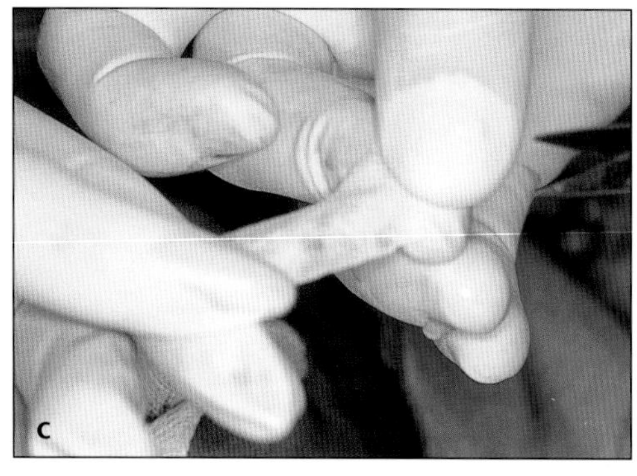

Fig 3-25
(a) Lyodura, which is freeze-dried dura mater (the meningeal layer that lies closest to the cranial bone), is harvested from human cadavers.

(b) The dura mater membrane is rehydrated in saline solution prior to delivery.

(c) The seemingly fragile dura mater tends to roll in on itself, actually facilitating placement.

Oxidized cellulose mesh

Early studies of oxidized cellulose showed that this material resorbs without harmful effects on the healing process and has antibacterial properties.[119] A more recent study was conducted to evaluate the use of an oxidized cellulose mesh (Surgicel, Johnson & Johnson, New Brunswick, NJ) as a biodegradable membrane to produce GTR in furcation and infrabony defects.[120] The oxidized material is a resorbable hemostatic dressing that converts to a gelatinous mass and incorporates the blood clot to form a membrane. Most of the mesh resorbed at 1 week postoperatively. The defects in this case demonstrated normal healing, crevicular depths of 2 mm in most sites, and no evidence of bleeding with gentle probing. It was concluded, however, that a single case report was not sufficient to make judgments regarding the efficacy and advantages of oxidized cellular mesh for the purposes of a barrier membrane.[119]

PRP membranes

In addition to being a useful adjunct to grafts and membrane materials, PRP can itself be formed into a quasi-membrane. Besides delivering additional quantities of PRP into the general graft site, a PRP membrane also helps to stabilize the particulate graft and may act as a short-acting biologic barrier. Because it is generally accepted that all available platelets will degranulate within 3 to 5 days and that their initial growth activity will expire by 10 days, a PRP membrane will not be an effective barrier to epithelial tissue invasion. It can, however, be used to enhance short-term tissue healing. For areas requiring a true barrier membrane, another type of membrane can be infused with PRP gel to retard epithelial migration as well as to deliver localized growth factors that can accelerate hard and soft tissue maturation.

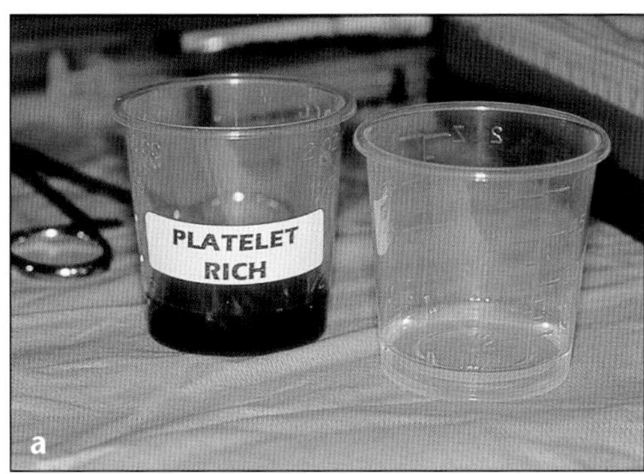

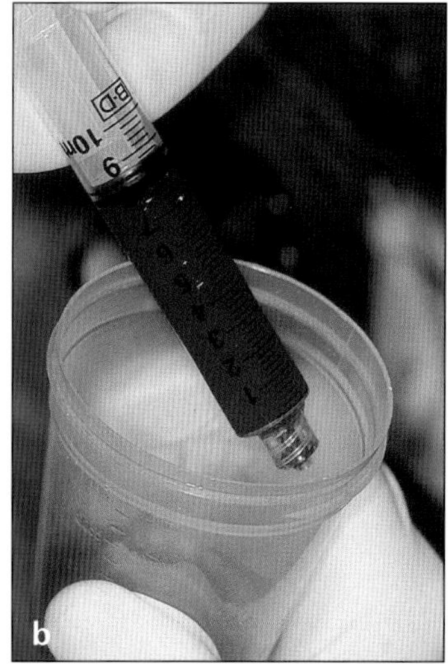

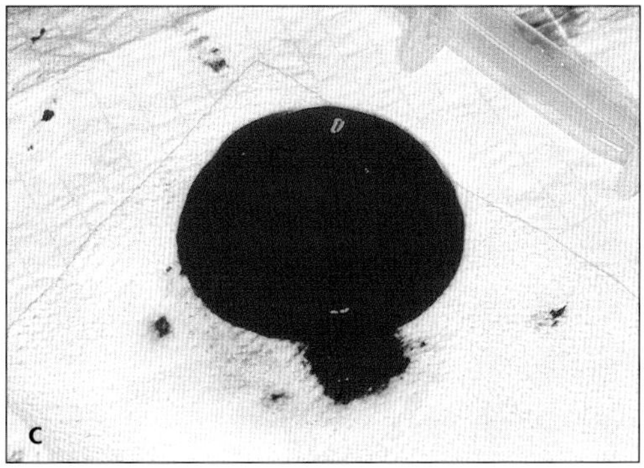

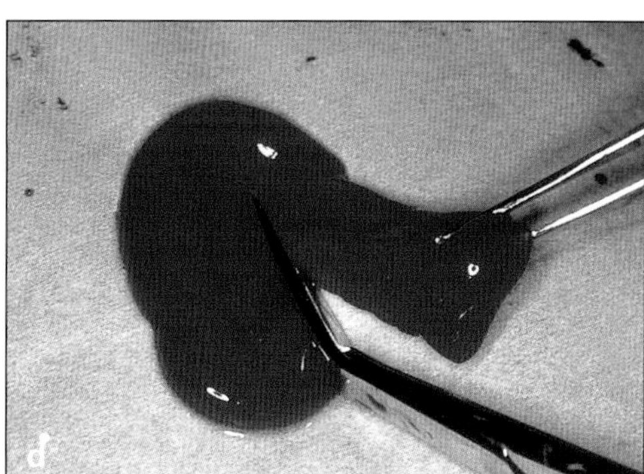

Fig 3-26 PRP can be used as a quasi-membrane to deliver additional quantities of PRP to the graft site, to stabilize the particulate graft, and to act as a short-term biologic barrier.

(a) Prior to delivery, PRP is placed in a sterile container next to the bovine thrombin and calcium chloride that will be used for activation.

(b) At the time of delivery, PRP is activated by adding calcium chloride and thrombin to facilitate the delivery of growth factors by the platelets.

(c) PRP can be injected onto a sterile, smooth surface to form a biologic membrane within a few minutes.

(d) This PRP membrane can be manipulated and cut to fit a desired area. While it is not a true barrier membrane, it nevertheless stabilizes the graft and provides valuable growth factors.

Preparing PRP gel and membranes

Once the PRP is drawn off, it must be activated to begin the gelling for application to the surgical site. This activator should consist of 5 mL of 10% calcium chloride with 5,000 units of topical bovine thrombin. A small amount of activated PRP can be placed on a flat surface or, preferably, in a small mold. Allowing the PRP to set for 2 to 4 minutes will create a quasi-membrane that can be used to deliver additional growth factors to the surgical site and as a short-term barrier membrane.

To infuse a traditional barrier membrane with the PRP preparation, a collagen-based membrane should be selected, trimmed to the size and shape appropriate for the defect, and then sprayed on each side with activated PRP prior to placement at the recipient site (Fig 3-26).

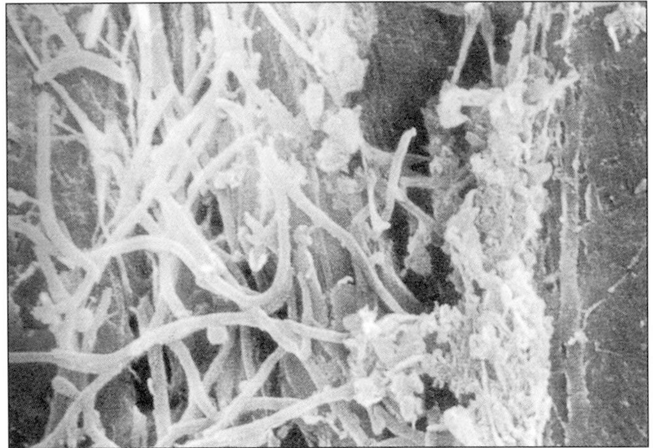

Fig 3-27
Microscopic view showing that membrane filaments can be invaded by different types of bacteria as a result of premature exposure of membranes that are incompatible with the environment of the oral cavity.

Microbiology Associated with Barrier Membranes

Failure of barrier membrane procedures may be caused by infectious bacteria and related complications.[121] Many of the bacterial cells that have been found on membranes have been linked to a gain in probing attachment.[122] The successful regenerative results that have been obtained in animal studies using membranes may be partly explained by the experimental procedure, which involved coronal repositioning of the flaps or complete submersion of the teeth. However, in clinical use, the barrier may become partially exposed during the early stages of healing, leading to contamination by oral microorganisms (Fig 3-27). Therefore, the material that is used may become a pathway for infection, jeopardizing the regenerative process.[121] In addition, one study documented accelerated epithelial invagination into periodontal incisional wounds at plaque-infected sites.[123]

Clinical and microbiologic studies of early (1-week) exposure of titanium-reinforced PTFE membranes in primates determined that the sequelae of membrane exposure included redness, edema, and tissue slough. *Bacteroides fragilis, Streptococcus pneumoniae, Prevotella intermedia,* and *Staphylococcus intermedius* microorganisms were found at all sites with prematurely exposed membranes. The results of this study emphasized the importance of studying microbiota because of their potential implications in the regenerative process.[124]

Porphyromonas gingivalis is a common microorganism found in patients with periodontal disease, especially those with the rapidly progressive type. In addition, the combination of *P gingivalis* and *Streptococcus mutans* has been found to have the strongest affinity to the membranes used for periodontal regeneration.[125]

An in vitro study evaluated the ability of *P gingivalis* to colonize and to adhere to six different types of membranes (resorbable and nonresorbable).[126] The results showed that *P gingivalis* cells passed through all six membranes analyzed at 48 hours. PLA and PGA barriers (Resolut) and lactide copolymer membranes (Guidor) showed the lowest adherence with the microorganism, whereas Vicryl fibers were heavily colonized by cell aggregates. Another study reported that the collagenase activity of *P gingivalis* degraded the collagen membrane completely within 4 to 5 days.[125] Other research concluded that essential factors, such as the host defense mechanisms and bacterial competition, were completely excluded because an in vitro study cannot represent the complex system of the oral cavity.[126]

Based on the research available, the complete effects of bacteria on exposed membranes are unclear. However, clinical experience has shown that the majority of membrane barriers, with the exception of AlloDerm and CapSet, cannot be left exposed through the soft tissue and still provide their intended benefits.

Conclusion

After considering all of the different factors associated with the variety of membranes available, clinicians must choose the type of barrier that is appropriate for each patient and each defect.[24] In some clinical situations, such as repair of sinus membrane tears, the use of nonresorbable barriers is contraindicated; in other situations, where membrane exposure is possible, the use of resorbable membranes is contraindicated.[25] The observations of various studies indicate that the procedure is sensitive and dependent on the characteristics of the membrane used. However, the capacity to prevent or retard epithelial migration along tooth surfaces is essential.

Because each barrier membrane material has specific benefits and limitations, and none has been found to be ideal for every clinical situation, the clinician must have a fundamental understanding of the different membranes available and use them selectively, based on the indications of each case. Table 3-1 compares the barrier membrane materials described in this chapter and recommends the procedures and types of defects for which each material is best suited. Because each material has its own advantages and disadvantages, the clinician should carefully review the material being used for each procedure to maximize success and minimize cost, time, and morbidity for a particular situation. The higher the relative rank of a material, the more predictable it is for areas with lower osteogenic potential; lower-ranked materials can be used for areas with higher osteogenic potential. Note that the numbering system used to rate the relative quality of each membrane for bone and/or soft tissue growth was created by the author based on his clinical experience and a review of the literature.

Table 3-1 Comparison of barrier membranes

Membrane (commercial name)	Composition	Relative effectiveness for bone and/or soft tissue growth*	Approximate resorption time	Relative cost†	Recommended indications/contraindications
BioMend Extend	Bovine tendon collagen	9	4 mo	$$	To cover the lateral window after a maxillary sinus graft procedure, or for small to moderate ridge deficiencies with pin fixation and underlying graft material with or without simultaneous implants.
GTAM	e-PTFE with titanium reinforcement	9	NA	$$$	For additional ridge width or height in conjunction with particulate graft materials and pin fixation in small to large defects.
AlloDerm	Acellular freeze-dried cadaver skin	8	4 mo	$$	Best choice for difficult or impossible primary closure of soft tissues, or when tissue opening is likely. Also recommended (when patient acceptance is not a factor) for large schneiderian membrane tears, three- or four-wall extraction sockets over a graft material, or small ridge deficiencies with or without simultaneous implants.
Atrisorb	Liquid PLA	8	4 mo	$$	For periodontal application in conjunction with a graft material; material consistency allows for intimate connection with root surfaces.
BioMend	Bovine tendon collagen	8	2 mo	$$	For large schneiderian membrane tears, three- or four-wall extraction sockets over a graft material, or small ridge deficiencies with or without simultaneous implants.
Gore-Tex	e-PTFE	8	NA	$$$	One of the original membrane barriers. Many more effective/inexpensive options now available.
Resolut Adapt	PLA/PGA	8	3 mo	$$$	To cover the lateral window after a maxillary sinus graft procedure. Not stiff enough for ridge augmentation procedures.
Resolut Adapt LT	PLA/PGA	8	4 mo	$$$	To cover the lateral window after a maxillary sinus graft procedure. Not stiff enough for ridge augmentation procedures.
BioGide	Porcine dermal collagen	7	3–4 mo	$$–$$$	To cover the lateral window after a maxilliary sinus graft procedure. Not stiff enough for ridge augmentation procedures.
Epi-Guide	PLA/PGA	7	4 mo	$$	For small ridge deficiencies with or without simultaneous implants.

*1 = least effective; 10 = most effective.

†Relative cost of barrier membranes based on price per unit. $ = low relative cost; $$ = moderate relative cost; $$$ = high relative cost.

Table 3-1 *(cont)*

Membrane (commercial name)	Composition	Relative effectiveness for bone and/or soft tissue growth*	Approximate resorption time	Relative cost†	Recommended indications/ contraindications
Ossix	Bovine tendon collagen	7	6 mo	$$	To cover the lateral window after a maxillary sinus graft procedure. Not stiff enough for ridge augmentation procedures.
Reguarde	Bovine tendon collagen	7	4 mo	$$	For large schneiderian membrane tears, three- to four-wall extraction sockets over a graft material, or small ridge deficiencies with or without simultaneous implants.
Resolut	PLA/PGA	7	3 mo	$$	For small ridge deficiencies with or without simultaneous implants.
Resolut XT	PLA/PGA	7	4 mo	$$	For small ridge deficiencies with or without simultaneous implants.
Titanium	Titanium	6–7	NA	$$	For additional ridge width or height in conjunction with particulate graft materials and pin fixation, but only in highly experienced hands because of risks associated with material manipulation and possible soft tissue dehiscence.
CapSet	Medical-grade calcium sulfate	6	2 mo	$	To cover grafted three- to five-wall extraction sockets. Also recommended for periodontal application in conjunction with a graft material; material consistency allows for intimate connection with root surfaces.
Lambone	Thin sheet of DFDBA	6	5 mo	$$	For additional ridge width or height in conjunction with particulate graft materials and pin fixation in small to large defects. Material trademarked but similar products available at many American Association of Tissue Banks–endorsed tissue banks.
Lyodura	Freeze-dried human dura mater	5	2–3 mo	$$	Not recommended for clinical use because of concerns about possible Creutzfeldt-Jakob disease transmission.
OsseoQuest	PLA/PGA	5	6 mo	$$$	Not recommended for clinical use: high exposure rate, too stiff, and too costly.
Regentex GBR-200	PTFE	4	NA	$	Not recommended; limited documented success.
Vicryl Periodontal Mesh	Woven Vicryl	2	1 mo	$	Not recommended because of fast resorption and wicking effect.
CollaTape	Bovine tendon collagen	NA	2 wk	$	For small and moderate schneiderian membrane tears, or over small particulate grafts to keep particles from migrating. Not a barrier membrane in the true sense because of short resorption time.

References

1. Melcher AH. On the repair potential of periodontal tissues. J Periodontol 1976;47:256–260.
2. Gottlow J. Guided tissue regeneration using bioresorbable and non-resorbable devices: Initial healing and long-term results. J Periodontol 1993;64(11 suppl):1157–1165.
3. Caton JG, Greenstein G. Factors related to periodontal regeneration. Periodontol 2000 1993; 1:9–15.
4. Rowe DJ, Leung WW, Del Carlo DL. Osteoclast inhibition by factors from cells associated with regenerative tissue. J Periodontol 1996;67:414–421.
5. Pecora G, Baek SH, Rethnam S, Kim S. Barrier membrane techniques in endodontic microsurgery. Dent Clin North Am 1997;41:585–602.
6. Caffesse RG. Regeneration of soft and hard tissue defects. Medicine Meets Millennium: World Congress on Medicine and Health, 21 July–31 August 2000, Hanover, Denmark. Available at: http://www.mhhannover.de/aktuelles/projekte/mmm/englishversion/fs_programme/speech/Caffesse_V.html. Accessed 6 Aug 2003.
7. Froum SJ, Gomez C, Breault MR. Current concepts of periodontal regeneration. A review of the literature. N Y State Dent J 2002;68:14–22.
8. Payne JM, Cobb CM, Rapley JW, Killoy WJ, Spencer P. Migration of human gingival fibroblasts over guided tissue regeneration barrier materials. J Periodontol 1996;67:236–244.
9. Linde A, Alberius P, Dahlin C, Bjurstam K, Sundin Y. Osteopromotion: A soft-tissue exclusion principle using a membrane for bone healing and bone neogenesis. J Periodontol 1993;64(11 suppl):1116–1128.
10. Assenza B, Piattelli M, Scarano A, Lezzi G, Petrone G, Piattelli A. Localized ridge augmentation using titanium micromesh. J Oral Implantol 2001;27:287–292.
11. Hammerle CH, Jung RE, Feloutzis A. A systematic review of the survival of implants in bone sites augmented with barrier membranes (guided bone regeneration) in partially edentulous patients. J Clin Periodontol 2002; 29(suppl 3):226–231.
12. Lorenzoni M, Pertl C, Polansky RA, Jakse N, Wegscheider WA. Evaluation of implants placed with barrier membranes. A retrospective follow-up study up to five years. Clin Oral Implants Res 2002;13:274–280.
13. Nemcovsky CE, Artzi Z. Comparative study of buccal dehiscence defects in immediate, delayed, and late maxillary implant placement with collagen membranes: Clinical healing between placement and second-stage surgery. J Periodontol 2002;73:754–761.
14. Kohal RJ, Hurzeler MB. Bioresorbable barrier membranes for guided bone regeneration around dental implants [in German]. Schweiz Monatsschr Zahnmed 2002;112:1222–1229.
15. Mellonig JT, Triplett RG. Guided tissue regeneration and endosseous dental implants. Int J Periodontics Restorative Dent 1993;13: 108–119.
16. Magnusson I, Stenberg WV, Batich C, Egelberg J. Connective tissue repair in circumferential periodontal defects in dogs following use of a biodegradable membrane. J Clin Periodontol 1990;17:243–248.
17. Blumenthal NM. A clinical comparison of collagen membranes with e-PTFE membranes in the treatment of human mandibular buccal class II furcation defects. J Periodontol 1993; 64:925–933.
18. Hardwick R, Hayes BK, Flynn C. Devices for dentoalveolar regeneration: An up-to-date literature review. J Periodontol 1995;66:495–505.
19. Karring T, Nyman S, Gottlow J, Laurell L. Development of the biological concept of guided tissue regeneration—animal and human studies. Periodontol 2000 1993;1:26–35.
20. Caffesse RG, Quinones CR. Guided tissue regeneration: Biologic rationale, surgical technique, and clinical results. Compendium 1992; 13:166, 168, 170 passim.
21. Lang NP, Karring T. Proceedings of the 1st European Workshop on Periodontology. London: Quintessence, 1994.
22. Scantlebury TV. 1982-1992: A decade of technology development for guided tissue regeneration. J Periodontol 1993;64(11 suppl): 1129–1137.
23. Meffert RM. Guided tissue regeneration/guided bone regeneration: A review of the barrier membranes. Pract Periodontics Aesthet Dent 1996;8:142–144.
24. Becker W, Becker BE, Mellonig J, et al. A prospective multi-center study evaluating periodontal regeneration for Class II furcation invasions and intrabony defects after treatment with a bioabsorbable barrier membrane: 1-year results. J Periodontol 1996;67: 641–649.

25. Bartee BK. The use of high-density polytetrafluoroethylene membrane to treat osseous defects: Clinical reports. Implant Dent 1995;4:21–26.
26. Yukna CN, Yukna RA. Multi-center evaluation of bioabsorbable collagen membrane for guided tissue regeneration in human Class II furcations. J Periodontol 1996;67:650–657.
27. Adachi M, Yamada T, Kimura Y, Fukaya M, Enomoto M, Yamada S. Mandibular reconstruction using the skeletal pin fixation system. Aichi Gakuin Dent Sci 1991;4:45–52.
28. Juodzbalys G. Instrument for extraction socket measurement in immediate implant installation. Clin Oral Implants Res 2003;14:144–149.
29. Gaggl A, Schultes G. Titanium foil-guided tissue regeneration in the treatment of peri-implant bone defects. Implant Dent 1999;8:368–375.
30. Wang HL, Miyauchi M, Takata T. Initial attachment of osteoblasts to various guided bone regeneration membranes: An in vitro study. J Periodontal Res 2002;37:340–344.
31. Nyman S, Lindhe J, Karring T, Rylander H. New attachment following surgical treatment of human periodontal disease. J Clin Periodontol 1982;9:290–296.
32. Gore-Tex Regenerative Material Manual. Flagstaff, AZ: W. L. Gore; 1986:6–12.
33. Tinti C, Vincenzi GP. Expanded polytetrafluoroethylene titanium-reinforced membranes for regeneration of mucogingival recession defects. A 12-case report. J Periodontol 1994;65:1088–1094.
34. Lins LH, de Lima AF, Sallum AW. Root coverage: Comparison of coronally positioned flap with and without titanium-reinforced barrier membrane. J Periodontol 2003;74:168–174.
35. Sigurdsson TJ, Hardwick R, Bogle GC, Wikesjo UM. Periodontal repair in dogs: Space provision by reinforced ePTFE membranes enhances bone and cementum regeneration in large supraalveolar defects. J Periodontol 1994;65:350–356.
36. Schenk RK, Buser D, Hardwick WR, Dahlin C. Healing pattern of bone regeneration in membrane-protected defects: A histologic study in the canine mandible. Int J Oral Maxillofac Implants 1994;9:13–29.
37. Cortellini P, Prato GP. Guided tissue regeneration with a rubber dam: A five-case report. Int J Periodontics Restorative Dent 1994;14:8–15.
38. Salama H, Rigotti F, Gianserra R, Seibert J. The utilization of rubber dam as a barrier membrane for the simultaneous treatment of multiple periodontal defects by the biologic principle of guided tissue regeneration: Case reports. Int J Periodontics Restorative Dent 1994;14:16–33.
39. D'Archivio D, Di Placido G, Tumini V, Paolantonio M. Periodontal guided tissue regeneration with a rubber dam: Short term clinical study [in Italian]. Minerva Stomatol 1998;47:103–110.
40. Paolantonio M, D'Archivio D, Di Placido G, et al. Expanded polytetrafluoroethylene and dental rubber dam barrier membranes in the treatment of periodontal intrabony defects. A comparative clinical trial. J Clin Periodontol 1998;25(11 pt 1):920–928.
41. Apinhasmit W, Swasdison S, Tamsailom S, Suppipat N. Connective tissue and bacterial deposits on rubber dam sheet and ePTFE barrier membranes in guided periodontal tissue regeneration. J Int Acad Periodontol 2002;4:19–25.
42. Schopper C, Goriwoda W, Moser D, Spassova E, Watzinger F, Ewers R. Long-term results after guided bone regeneration with resorbable and microporous titanium membranes. Atlas Oral Maxillofac Surg Clin North Am 2001;13:3–12.
43. Anson D. Calcium sulfate: A 4-year observation of its use as a resorbable barrier in guided tissue regeneration of periodontal defects. Compend Contin Educ Dent 1996;17:895–899.
44. Greenstein G, Caton JG. Biodegradable barriers and guided tissue regeneration. Periodontol 2000 1993;1:36–45.
45. Hyder PR, Dowell P, Singh G, Dolby AE. Freeze-dried, cross-linked bovine type I collagen: Analysis of properties. J Periodontol 1992;63:182–186.
46. Pitaru S, Tal H, Soldinger M, Grosskopf A, Noff M. Partial regeneration of periodontal tissues using collagen barriers. Initial observations in the canine. J Periodontol 1988;59:380–386.
47. Pitaru S, Tal H, Soldinger M, Noff M. Collagen membranes prevent apical migration of epithelium and support new connective tissue attachment during periodontal wound healing in dogs. J Periodontal Res 1989;24:247–253.

48. Pitaru S, Noff M, Grosskopf A, Moses O, Tal H, Savion N. Heparan sulfate and fibronectin improve the capacity of collagen barriers to prevent apical migration of the junctional epithelium. J Periodontol 1991;62:598–601.
49. Blumenthal N, Steinberg J. The use of collagen membrane barriers in conjunction with combined demineralized bone-collagen gel implants in human infrabony defects. J Periodontol 1990;61:319–327.
50. Pruthi VK, Gelskey SC, Mirbod SM. Furcation therapy with bioabsorbable collagen membrane: A clinical trial. J Can Dent Assoc 2002;68:610–615.
51. BioMend Absorbable Collagen Membrane Manual. Carlsbad, CA: Calcitek, 1995:12–18.
52. Bunyaratavej P, Wang HL. Collagen membranes: A review. J Periodontol 2001;72:215–229.
53. Oh TJ, Meraw SJ, Lee EJ, Giannobile WV, Wang HL. Comparative analysis of collagen membranes for the treatment of implant dehiscence defects. Clin Oral Implants Res 2003;14:80–90.
54. Zimmer Dental (formerly Centerpulse) website. Available at: http://www.calcitek.com/rg_bmMaterial.asp. Accessed 5 Apr 2004.
55. Sela MN, Kohavi D, Krausz E, Steinberg D, Rosen G. Enzymatic degradation of collagen-guided tissue regeneration membranes by periodontal bacteria. Clin Oral Implants Res 2003;14:263–268.
56. Friedmann A, Strietzel FP, Maretzki B, Pitaru S, Bernimoulin JP. Observations on a new collagen barrier membrane in 16 consecutively treated patients. Clinical and histological findings. J Periodontol 2001;72:1616–1623 [erratum 2002;73:352].
57. Friedmann A, Strietzel FP, Maretzki B, Pitaru S, Bernimoulin JP. Histological assessment of augmented jaw bone utilizing a new collagen barrier membrane compared to a standard barrier membrane to protect a granular bone substitute material. Clin Oral Implants Res 2002;13:587-94.
58. Schlegel AK, Mohler H, Busch F, Mehl A. Preclinical and clinical studies of a collagen membrane (Bio-Gide). Biomaterials 1997;18:535–538.
59. Zitzmann NU, Naef R, Scharer P. Resorbable versus nonresorbable membranes in combination with Bio-Oss for guided bone regeneration. Int J Oral Maxillofac Implants 1997;12:844–852 [erratum 1998;13:576].
60. Camelo M, Nevins ML, Schenk RK, et al. Clinical, radiographic, and histologic evaluation of human periodontal defects treated with Bio-Oss and Bio-Gide. Int J Periodontics Restorative Dent 1998;18:321–331.
61. Hockers T, Abensur D, Valentini P, Legrand R, Hammerle CH. The combined use of bioresorbable membranes and xenografts or autografts in the treatment of bone defects around implants. A study in beagle dogs. Clin Oral Implants Res 1999;10:487–498.
62. Camelo M, Nevins ML, Lynch SE, Schenk RK, Simion M, Nevins M. Periodontal regeneration with an autogenous bone–Bio-Oss composite graft and a Bio-Gide membrane. Int J Periodontics Restorative Dent 2001;21:109–119.
63. Tawil G, El-Ghoule G, Mawla M. Clinical evaluation of a bilayered collagen membrane (Bio-Gide) supported by autografts in the treatment of bone defects around implants. Int J Oral Maxillofac Implants 2001;16:857–863.
64. Carmagnola D, Adriaens P, Berglundh T. Healing of human extraction sockets filled with Bio-Oss. Clin Oral Implants Res 2003;14:137–143.
65. Dietrich T, Zunker P, Dietrich D, Bernimoulin JP. Periapical and periodontal healing after osseous grafting and guided tissue regeneration treatment of apicomarginal defects in periradicular surgery: Results after 12 months. Oral Surg Oral Med Oral Pathol Oral Radiol Endod 2003;95:474–482.
66. Roccuzzo M, Lungo M, Corrente G, Gandolfo S. Comparative study of a bioresorbable and a non-resorbable membrane in the treatment of human buccal gingival recessions. J Periodontol 1996;67:7–14.
67. Lundgren D, Laurell L, Gottlow J, et al. The influence of the design of two different bioresorbable barriers on the results of guided tissue regeneration therapy. An intra-individual comparative study in the monkey. J Periodontol 1995;66:605–612.
68. Laurell L, Falk H, Fornell J, Johard G, Gottlow J. Clinical use of a bioresorbable matrix barrier in guided tissue regeneration therapy. Case series. J Periodontol 1994;65:967–975.
69. Gottlow J, Lundgren D, Nyman S, Laurell L, Rylander H. New attachment formation in the monkey using Guidor, a bioresorbable GTR-device [abstract 1535]. J Dent Res 1992;71:297.

70. Gottlow J, Nyman S, Laurell L, Falk H, Fornell J, Johard G. Clinical results of GTR-therapy using a bioabsorbable device (Guidor) [abstract 1537]. J Dent Res 1992;71:298.
71. Laurell L, Gottlow J, Nyman S, Falk H, Fornell J, Johard G. Gingival response to Guidor, a bioresorbable device in GTR-therapy [abstract 1536]. J Dent Res 1992;71:298.
72. Christgau M, Bader N, Felden A, Gradl J, Wenzel A, Schmalz G. Guided tissue regeneration in intrabony defects using an experimental bioresorbable polydioxanon (PDS) membrane. A 24-month split-mouth study. J Clin Periodontol 2002;29:710–723.
73. Magnusson I, Batich C, Collins BR. New attachment formation following controlled tissue regeneration using biodegradable membranes. J Periodontol 1988;59:1–6.
74. Warrer K, Karring T, Nyman S, Gogolewski S. Guided tissue regeneration using biodegradable membranes of polylactic acid or polyurethane. J Clin Periodontol 1992;19(9 pt 1):633–640.
75. Laurell L, Gottlow J, Rylander H, Lundgren D, Rask M, Norlindh B. Gingival response to GTR therapy in monkeys using two bioresorbable devices [abstract 824]. J Dent Res 1993;72:206.
76. Hugoson A, Ravald N, Fornell J, Johard G, Teiwik A, Gottlow J. Treatment of class II furcation involvements in humans with bioresorbable and nonresorbable guided tissue regeneration barriers. A randomized multicenter study. J Periodontol 1995;66:624–34.
77. Gottlow J, Laurell L, Rylander H, Lundgren D, Rudolfsson L, Nyman S. Treatment of infrabony defects in monkeys with bioresorbable and nonresorbable GTR devices [abstract 823]. J Dent Res 1993;72:206.
78. Rudiger SG, Ehmke B, Hommens A, Karch H, Flemmig TF. Guided tissue regeneration using a polylactic acid barrier. Part I: Environmental effects on bacterial colonization. J Clin Periodontol 2003;30:19–25.
79. Ehmke B, Rudiger SG, Hommens A, Karch H, Flemmig TF. Guided tissue regeneration using a polylactic acid barrier. J Clin Periodontol 2003;30:368–374.
80. Vuddhakanok S, Solt CW, Mitchell JC, Foreman DW, Alger FA. Histologic evaluation of periodontal attachment apparatus following the insertion of a biodegradable copolymer barrier in humans. J Periodontol 1993;64: 202–210.
81. Simion M, Scarano A, Gionso L, Piattelli A. Guided bone regeneration using resorbable and nonresorbable membranes: A comparative histologic study in humans. Int J Oral Maxillofac Implants 1996;11:735–742.
82. Polson AM, Garrett S, Stoller NH, et al. Guided tissue regeneration in human furcation defects after using a biodegradable barrier: A multi-center feasibility study. J Periodontol 1995;66:377–385.
83. Polson AM, Southard GL, Dunn RL, Polson AP, Billen JR, Laster LL. Initial study of guided tissue regeneration in Class II furcation defects after use of a biodegradable barrier. Int J Periodontics Restorative Dent 1995;15:42–55.
84. Polson AM, Southard GL, Dunn RL, et al. Periodontal healing after guided tissue regeneration with Atrisorb barriers in beagle dogs. Int J Periodontics Restorative Dent 1995;15: 574–589.
85. Fleisher N, de Waal H, Bloom A. Regeneration of lost attachment apparatus in the dog using Vicryl absorbable mesh (Polyglactin 910). Int J Periodontics Restorative Dent 1988;8:44–55.
86. Sottosanti JS. Calcium sulfate: A valuable addition to the implant/bone regeneration complex. Dent Implantol Update 1997;8:25–29.
87. Sottosanti J, Anson D. Using calcium sulfate as a graft enhancer and membrane barrier [interview]. Dent Implantol Update 2003;14:1–8.
88. Maze GI, Hinkson DW, Collins BH, Garbin C. Bone regeneration capacity of a combination calcium sulfate-demineralized freeze dried bone allograft. Presented at the American Academy of Periodontology Annual Meeting, October 1994, San Francisco, CA.
89. Couri CJ, Maze GI, Hinkson DW, Collins BH 3rd, Dawson DV. Medical grade calcium sulfate hemihydrate versus expanded polytetrafluoroethylene in the treatment of mandibular class II furcations. J Periodontol 2002;73: 1352–1359.
90. LifeCell Biomedical Manual. Woodland, TX: LifeCell, 1995:4–7.
91. Sottosanti JS. Calcium sulfate-aided bone regeneration: A case report. Periodontal Clin Investig 1995;17:10–15.
92. Livesey SA, Herndon DN, Hollyoak MA, Atkinson YH, Nag A. Transplanted acellular allograft dermal matrix. Potential as a template for the reconstruction of viable dermis. Transplantation 1995;60:1–9.

93. Batista EL Jr, Batista FC, Novaes AB Jr. Management of soft tissue ridge deformities with acellular dermal matrix. Clinical approach and outcome after 6 months of treatment. J Periodontol 2001;72:265–273.
94. Wei PC, Laurell L, Geivelis M, Lingen MW, Maddalozzo D. Acellular dermal matrix allografts to achieve increased attached gingiva. Part 1. A clinical study. J Periodontol 2000;71:1297–1305.
95. The acellular dermal matrix: Soft tissue development for dental implants. Dent Implantol Update 2001;12:65–71.
96. AlloDerm Universal Soft Tissue Graft Manual. Woodland, TX: LifeCell Corporation, 1996:7.
97. Shulman J. Clinical evaluation of an acellular dermal allograft for increasing the zone of attached gingiva. Pract Periodontics Aesthet Dent 1996;8:201–208.
98. Mishkin DJ, Shelley LR Jr, Neville BW. Histologic study of a freeze-dried skin allograft in a human. A case report. J Periodontol 1983;54: 534–537.
99. Harris RJ. Root coverage with a connective tissue with partial thickness double pedicle graft and an acellular dermal matrix graft: A clinical and histological evaluation of a case report. J Periodontol 1998;69:1305–1311.
100. Woodyard AG, Greenwell H, Hill M, Drisko C, Iasella JM, Scheetz J. The clinical effect of acellular dermal matrix on gingival thickness and root coverage compared to coronally positioned flap alone. J Periodontal 2004;75:44–56.
101. Tal H. Subgingival acellular dermal matrix allograft for the treatment of gingival recession: A case report. J Periodontol 1999;70:1118–1124.
102. Henderson RD, Greenwell H, Drisko C, et al. Predictable multiple site root coverage using an acellular dermal matrix allograft. J Periodontol 2001;72:571–582.
103. Harris RJ. Clinical evaluation of 3 techniques to augment keratinized tissue without root coverage. J Periodontol 2001;72:932–938.
104. Mahn DH. Treatment of gingival recession with a modified "tunnel" technique and an acellular dermal connective tissue allograft. Pract Proced Aesthet Dent 2001;13:69–74.
105. Harris RJ. Cellular dermal matrix used for root coverage: 18-month follow-up observation. Int J Periodontics Restorative Dent 2002;22:156–163.
106. Tozum TF. A promising periodontal procedure for the treatment of adjacent gingival recession defects. J Can Dent Assoc 2003;69:155–159.
107. Harris RJ. A comparative study of root coverage obtained with an acellular dermal matrix versus a connective tissue graft: Results of 107 recession defects in 50 consecutively treated patients. Int J Periodontics Restorative Dent 2000;20:51–59.
108. Novaes AB Jr, Grisi DC, Molina GO, Souza SL, Taba M Jr, Grisi MF. Comparative 6-month clinical study of a subepithelial connective tissue graft and acellular dermal matrix graft for the treatment of gingival recession. J Periodontol 2001;72:1477–1484.
109. Aichelmann-Reidy ME, Yukna RA, Evans GH, Nasr HF, Mayer ET. Clinical evaluation of acellular allograft dermis for the treatment of human gingival recession. J Periodontol 2001;72:998–1005.
110. Fugazzotto PA. The use of demineralized laminar bone sheets in guided bone regeneration procedures: Report of three cases. Int J Oral Maxillofac Implants 1996;11:239–244.
111. Scott TA, Towle HJ, Assad DA, Nicoll BK. Comparison of bioabsorbable laminar bone membrane and non-resorbable ePTFE membrane in mandibular furcations. J Periodontol 1997;68:679–686.
112. Majzoub Z, Cordioli G, Aramouni PK, Vigolo P, Piattelli A. Guided bone regeneration using demineralized laminar bone sheets versus GTAM membranes in the treatment of implant-associated defects. A clinical and histological study. Clin Oral Implants Res 1999;10:406–414.
113. Kassolis JD, Bowers GM. Supracrestal bone regeneration: A pilot study. Int J Periodontics Restorative Dent 1999;19:131–139 [erratum 1999;19:314].
114. Chogle S, Mickel AK. An in vitro evaluation of the antibacterial properties of barriers used in guided tissue regeneration. J Endod 2003;29:1–3.
115. Federal Drug Administration website. Available at: http://www.fda.gov/ora/fiars/ora_import_ia8403.html. Accessed 5 Apr 2004.
116. Croes EA, Jansen GH, Lemstra AW, Frijns CJ, van Gool WA, van Duijn CM. The first two patients with dura mater associated Creutzfeldt-Jakob disease in the Netherlands. J Neurol 2001;248:877–880.

117. Hamada C, Sadaike T, Fukushima M. Projection of creutzfeldt-jakob disease frequency based on cadaveric dura transplantation in Japan. Neuroepidemiology 2003;22:57–64.
118. Peleg M, Chaushu G, Blinder D, Taicher S. Use of Lyodura for bone augmentation of osseous defects around dental implants. J Periodontol 1999;70:853–860.
119. Degenshein G, Hurwitz A, Ribacoff S. Experience with regenerated oxidized cellulose. N Y State J Med 1963;63:2639-2643.
120. Galgut PN. Oxidized cellulose mesh used as a biodegradable barrier membrane in the technique of guided tissue regeneration. A case report. J Periodontol 1990;61:766–768.
121. Selvig KA, Nilveus RE, Fitzmorris L, Kersten B, Khorsandi SS. Scanning electron microscopic observations of cell populations and bacterial contamination of membranes used for guided periodontal tissue regeneration in humans. J Periodontol 1990;61:515–520.
122. Nowzari H, Slots J. Microorganisms in polytetrafluoroethylene barrier membranes for guided tissue regeneration. J Clin Periodontol 1994;21:203–210.
123. Yumet JA, Polson AM. Gingival wound healing in the presence of plaque-induced inflammation. J Periodontol 1985;56:107–119.
124. Fritz ME, Eke PI, Malmquist J, Hardwick R. Clinical and microbiological observations of early polytetrafluoroethylene membrane exposure in guided bone regeneration. Case reports in primates. J Periodontol 1996;67: 245–249.
125. Wang HL, Yuan K, Burgett F, Shyr Y, Syed S. Adherence of oral microorganisms to guided tissue membranes: An in vitro study. J Periodontol 1994;65:211–218.
126. Ricci G, Rasperini G, Silvestri M, Cocconcelli PS. In vitro permeability evaluation and colonization of membranes for periodontal regeneration by Porphyromonas gingivalis. J Periodontol 1996;67:490–496.

CHAPTER 4

Alveolar Ridge Preservation After Tooth Extraction

Maintaining bone quality and quantity in the alveolar ridge during and after tooth removal is critical for assuring good esthetic and functional results and minimizing the need for grafting procedures prior to implant placement.[1–3] Furthermore, preserving the existing bone helps support both fixed and removable prostheses and ensure successful osseointegration of dental implants. Soft tissue contours follow hard tissue contours, so the clinician must not only prevent bone defects but also repair any defects early in the treatment phase. When grafts are necessary, proper technique is critical to the success of the grafts and the final ridge contours.

Alveolar Ridge Resorption

Routine tooth extractions normally result in extraction sockets that heal without any significant difficulties. However, a defect can result from bone naturally growing into the socket and resorbing in height and width during the process.[4] A number of different types of bone resorption related to tooth extraction have been identified in the mandible[5]; however, resorption is most often a concern in the esthetic zone or in areas where the quantity of alveolar bone was minimal before the extraction. The anterior maxillary area is at particular risk because the bone plates are thin and subject to irreversible trauma during tooth removal.[6,7] In the posterior region, the alveolus has thicker walls and is less prone to resorption.

The crucial issue is how quickly the extraction socket heals and how much connective tissue invades the socket during the process. The eventual shrinkage of the alveolar ridge seems to be related not only to the removal of the tooth, but also to the environment within which the natural healing process of the alveolar defect must occur. Clot retraction and connective tissue regeneration preclude the formation of adequate bone, causing a collapse of the socket and resulting in lost bone contour and poor esthetics.

Atraumatic Tooth Removal

Avoiding tissue loss during tooth removal can help preserve alveolar bone. This goal should be given the highest priority because it may eliminate the need for bone regeneration or grafting later. Additionally, the preservation of hard tissues both complements and bears directly on therapies associated with the treatment of soft tissue defects.[8] Some situations can make tooth removal extremely difficult, including the brittle endodontically treated tooth, the severely dilacerated root, and the fractured tooth with little coronal portion to elevate. Most of these indications do not allow for removal and immediate implant placement. Proper instrumentation and technique, however, will allow for the best possible result.

Essential criteria should be followed during tooth removal. A small, sharp periotome should be used to incise the periodontal ligament attaching the tissue and tooth. When possible, the interdental papilla should not be reflected, particularly in the esthetic zone. During actual tooth removal, the clinician should use elevators and forceps properly to reduce bony involvement and thus preserve the bone contour. Luxation and controlled force become important allies; however, sectioning the tooth also helps to prevent bone loss. Once the tooth is removed from the socket, soft tissue fragments or pathosis must be removed. The formation of a good blood clot will induce the first stages of bone healing and proper bone fill.

Ridge Preservation

The residual socket can heal uneventfully if the surrounding bone is appropriately thick, tooth removal has been atraumatic, and thick interseptal residual bone is present. In fact, the literature recognizes the legitimacy of implant placement immediately after tooth extraction, given acceptable conditions.[9] Many sockets can heal without suturing, but suturing should be accomplished when necessary to avoid damaging or adversely altering the papilla contours. When the socket is compromised, whether as a result of extraction or trauma,[10] its walls may be supported with osteoconductive or osteoinductive grafting material.[11–13] Furthermore, a good blood supply is necessary, and obtaining it may require trephining the socket lightly with a small bur to induce bleeding, which can provide a source of osteoprogenitor cells.

When bone grafting is chosen as a restorative method for ridge augmentation, the clinician must decide whether to place the graft and implant together at the time of extraction or to place the implant after the graft has had time to mature. While Becker et al suggest that ridge resorption may not be prevented when implants are placed along with barrier membranes immediately after extraction,[9] other research suggests that resorption may be prevented.[14,15] Individual patient conditions will determine when to place the implant and whether barrier membranes should accompany the graft.

Bone-Grafting Materials

As discussed in detail in chapter 2 and extensively in the literature,[16] bone-grafting materials can be divided into three groups: autogenous, allogeneic, and alloplastic or xenograft material. Bone-grafting materials can further be categorized based on four characteristics, all of which are found in the ideal bone graft: osteointegration (ability to bond chemically to bone surface with no layer of fibrous tissue in between), osteoconduction (ability to support surface bone growth), osteoinduction (ability to encourage pluripotential stem cell differentiation), and osteogenesis (ability to form new bone from osteoblastic cells).[17] Autogenous bone material, used with or without the application of complementary therapies such as platelet-rich plasma (PRP),[18–22] is the best and most reliable source for predictable results. Often referred to as the gold standard for grafting, autogenous bone is unmatched in the amount of osteogenic cell viability it offers for bone regrowth and avoidance of histocompatibility problems. For the ridge preservation technique, autogenous bone is often harvested from a secondary intraoral site, such as the mandibular symphysis or ramus or the maxillary tuberosity.[23–27] Although not a practical approach for small recipient sites, extraoral harvest sites include the iliac crest, rib, cranium, and tibial plateau.[28,29]

Allografts, such as demineralized or mineralized freeze-dried bone (DFDBA and FDBA), are often used in place of the autograft because they eliminate the need for a donor site and a second incision and work well when there is a large ratio of host bone to graft material. Allografts are available in powder or putty-like forms; the latter are especially convenient for this application. These materials may induce healing through osteoconduction, osteoinduction, or possibly a combination of both processes.

The third category of graft materials includes alloplasts, which are synthetic bone substitute materials, and xenografts, which are harvested from other species. Alloplastic materials include bioactive glass, glass ionomers, aluminum oxide, calcium sulfate, calcium phosphates, beta tricalcium phosphate, synthetic hydroxyapatite, coralline hydroxyapatite, and calcium phosphate cements.[17,30] Synthetic bone has been shown to prevent ridge resorption after immediate grafting in extraction sites.[31–34] Currently, the most popular xenograft material is bovine in origin. These materials are deproteinated to eliminate their organic properties and to reduce any antigenic potential. Xenografts heal through a process of osteoconduction, acting as a scaffold upon which the patient's own bone can grow through cellular differentiation from the host blood cells. Xenografts and alloplasts have no inductive potential, meaning they do not induce bone growth on their own. However, a newer variety has been introduced that consists of bovine-derived bone mineral combined with a synthetic short-chain peptide, PepGen P-15 Flow (Dentsply Friadent CeraMed, Lakewood, CO),[35–39] which mimics the cell-binding domain of type I collagen, and is responsible in natural bone for cell migration, differentiation, and proliferation. This material (a hydrogel for easy handling in ridge preservation)

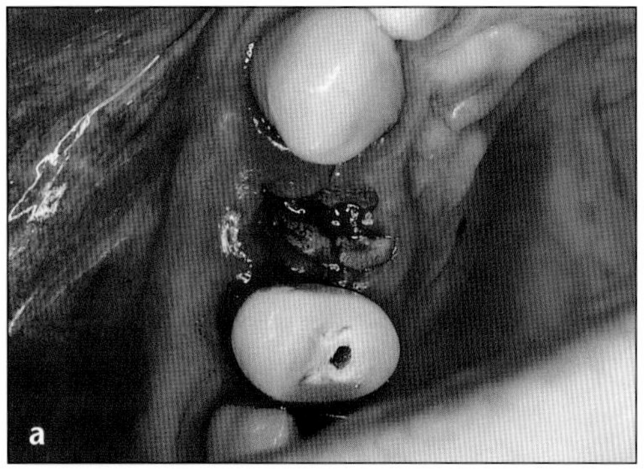

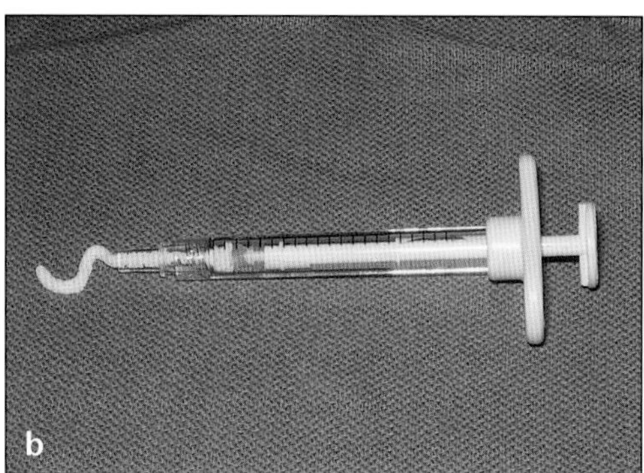

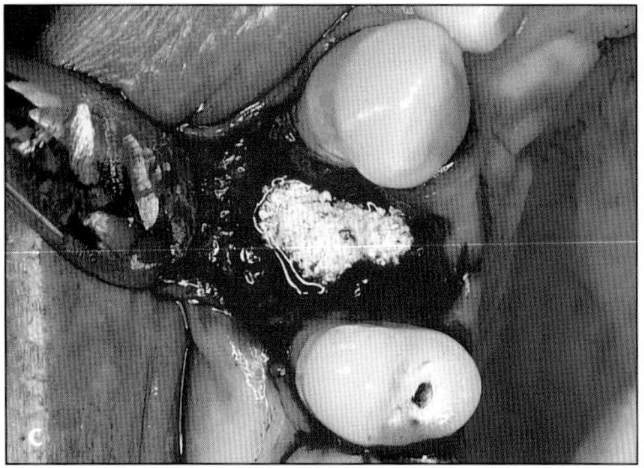

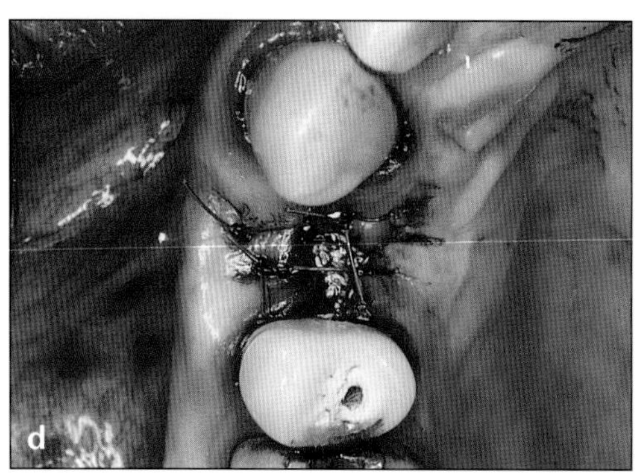

Fig 4-1 Tissue-engineered xenograft (bovine) material in a hydrogel carrier (eg, PepGen P-15 Flow) is a popular grafting material for five-wall defects.

(a) Occlusal aspect of a residual root that should not be removed by conventional procedures such as osteotomy or blunt elevator force, which can fracture the socket walls. Atraumatic extraction is preferred in such cases.

(b) Extraction is performed atraumatically, leaving the bony walls surrounding the socket intact. PepGen P-15 Flow (particles suspended in a hydrogel) is chosen to graft this socket because there is adequate bony support for the material.

(c) The socket is completely filled to the bone level.

(d) Sutures are used to approximate the flaps as closely as possible. Due to the gel consistency of the material, primary closure is not necessary.

may provide the benefits of a synthetic graft containing both an inorganic and an organic component, thus mimicking an autogenous graft material.

Choosing a Graft Material

One of the difficult aspects of ridge preservation is choosing an appropriate graft material for the specific site. To determine which material is needed, the clinician should evaluate the size and configuration of the defect and then calculate the amount of bone needed to replace the missing tissue. Larger defects require autogenous bone because it provides the maximum amount of cellularity and structure and contains proteins and cells that can cause osteoinduction of new tissue. On the other hand, smaller defects may be appropriate candidates for allografts, alloplasts, or xenografts.

The best time to preserve a ridge or to augment a tooth socket is at the time of tooth removal. Often what seems to be a simple procedure can lead to complicated problems with bone missing from the labial aspect and a compromised esthetic contour. If the lack of bone contour can be determined at the time of initial examination, then scheduling the patient for surgical removal of the tooth and grafting in a single appointment is appropriate. However, tooth extraction and grafting should not be attempted in the presence of suppuration, neoplasms, cysts, or conditions that could cause infection or graft failure.

When evaluating a patient, the clinician must identify the type of defect present; this determination strongly influences the

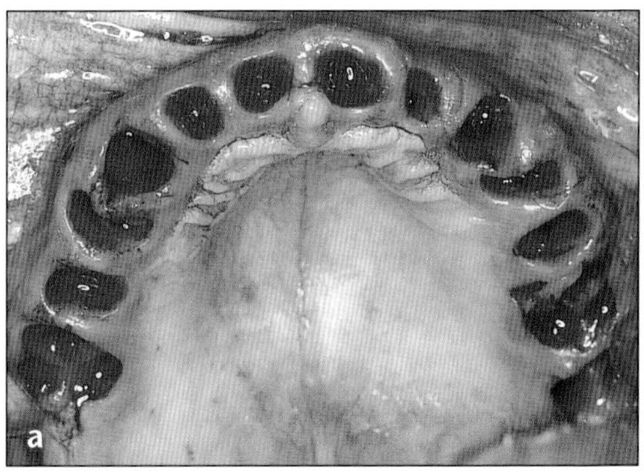

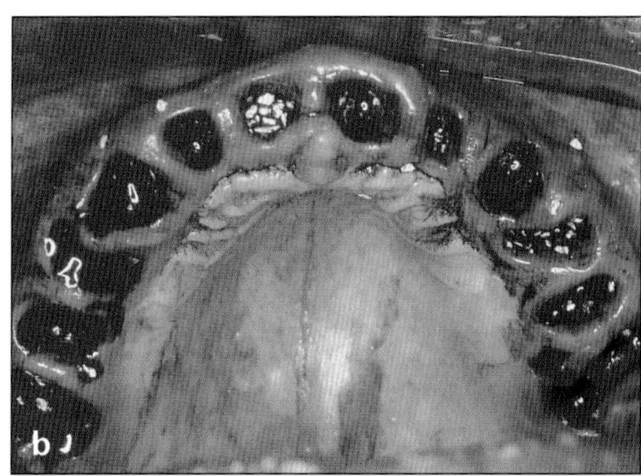

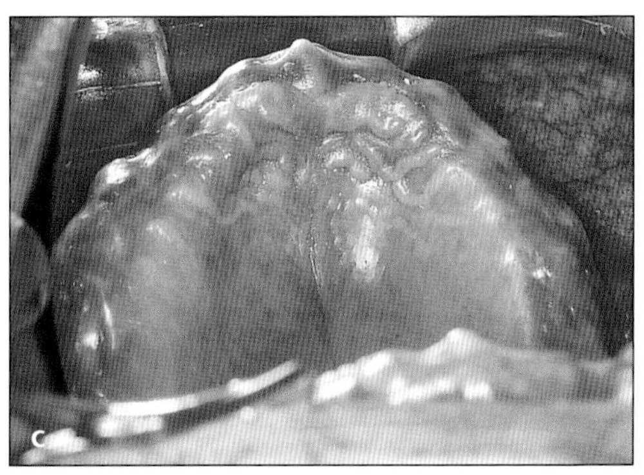

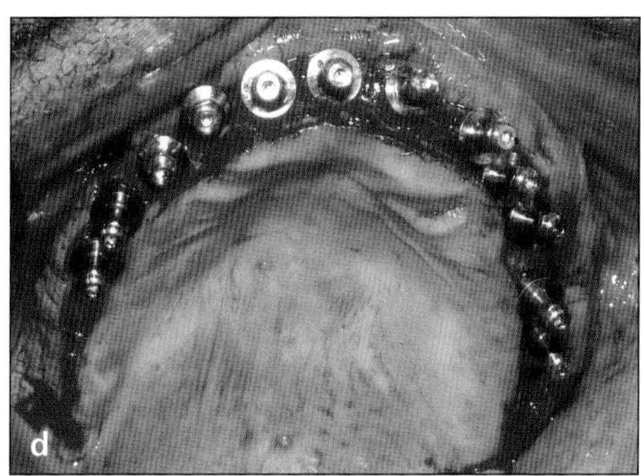

Fig 4-2 Bone grafting at the time of extraction is advised for defects with extremely thin walls.

(a) When planning for future implant placement, multiple extractions show the importance of proper grafting in the healing of sockets.

(b) Filling sockets with PepGen P-15 Flow helps maintain the width and height of the alveolar ridge.

(c) Although some swelling is present 10 days postoperatively, the areas where the implants will be placed appear to be ideal. Ideal ridge width and height for implant placement could not have been maintained without a procedure as simple as socket grafting.

(d) Socket grafting enables 12 implants to be placed in their correct three-dimensional positions that will later carry fixed restorations.

choice of procedure. For example, the clinician can categorize the defect based on the number of walls remaining in the socket, since each of these defect types requires a unique approach to ridge preservation and treatment.

Five-Wall Defects

Extraction sites with five thick bony walls intact may not require any grafting if there is a large amount of interseptal bone present. However, if grafting is indicated or desired at the time of tooth removal, any of the grafting materials in putty or gel consistency may be used for wall support. One of the most popular methods is to use tissue-engineered xenograft (bovine) material in a hydrogel carrier (eg, PepGen P-15 Flow).[38] This treatment allows for osteoconductive healing and preserves the tissue contour. The technique requires the clinician to carefully inject the graft material from its dispenser to fill the socket only to the level of bone and then to achieve good closure of the socket's cervical portion, either by advancement of the soft tissues and closure or by using a collagen plug or barrier. There is typically a 2- to 6-month waiting period before implant placement.

A recent study indicates that enhanced bone formation and faster particle resorption can occur with PepGen P-15 Flow, which consists of particles suspended in a biocompatible inert hydrogel of sodium carboxymethylcellulose, glycerol, and water, compared to the PepGen P-15 particulate (Figs 4-1 to 4-3).[40]

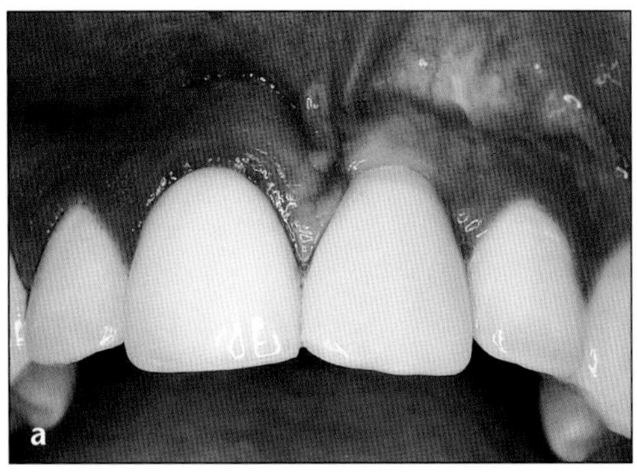

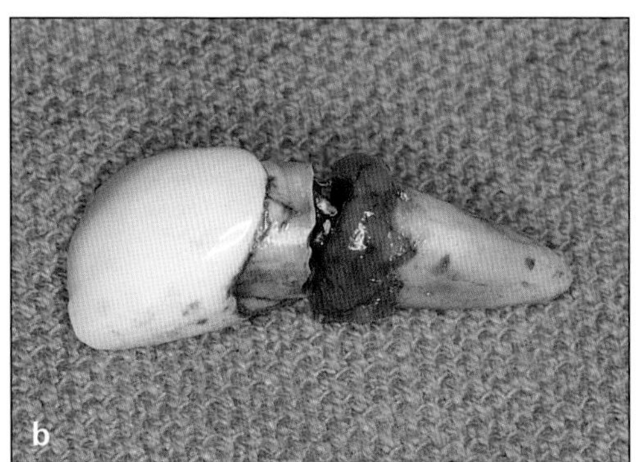

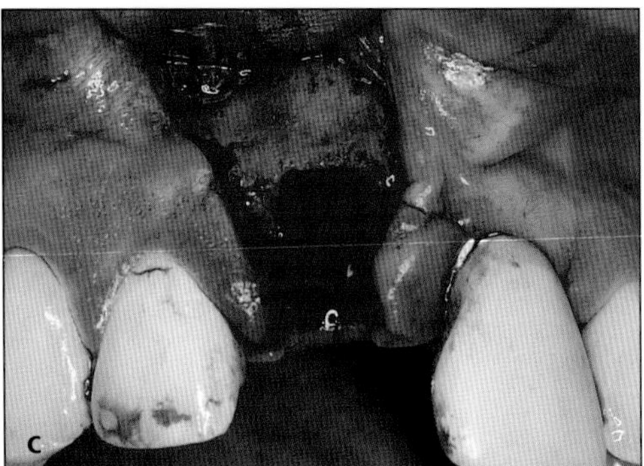

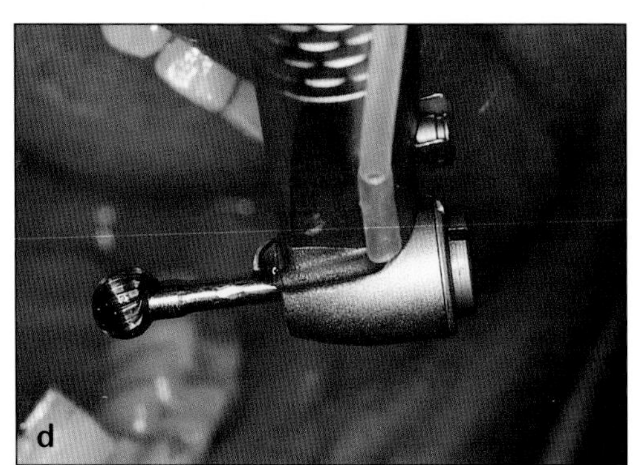

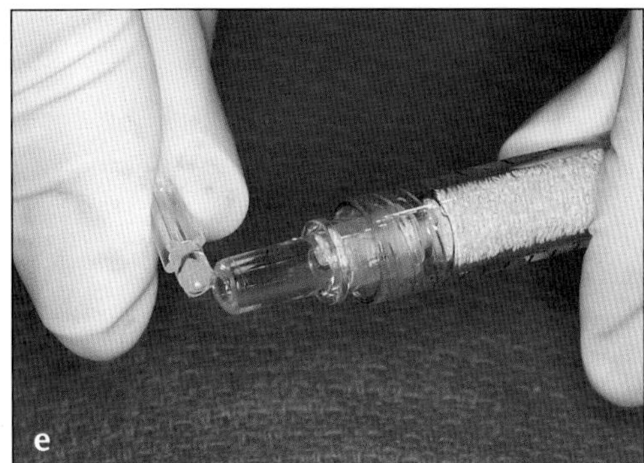

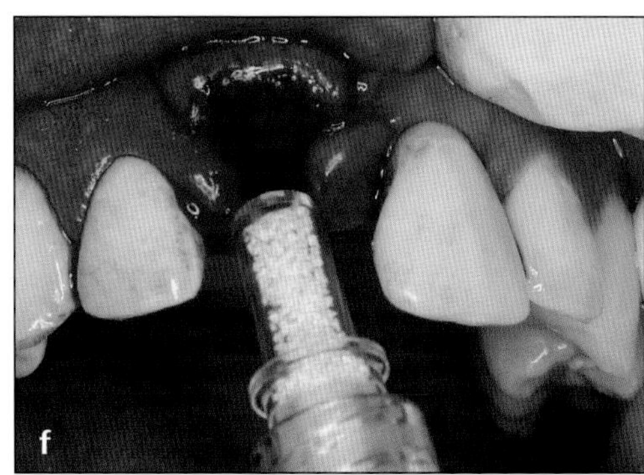

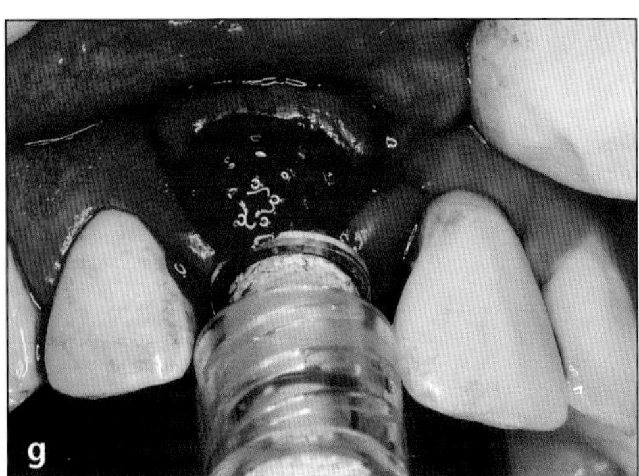

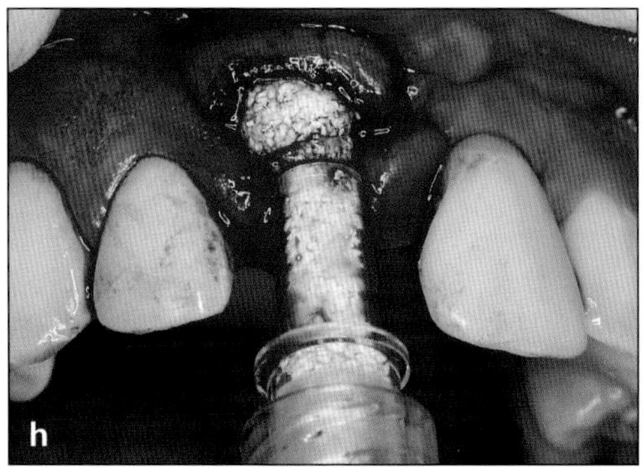

Fig 4-3 PepGen P-15 Flow is used for socket grafting prior to implant placement. This material is reported to enhance bone formation and cause faster particle resorption.

(a) Maxillary right central incisor that requires extraction due to fracture of the root. The maxillary left central incisor is a prosthetic crown over an implant placed 4 years previously.

(b) The fracture is at the cervical third of the root.

(c) After extraction, the socket walls are carefully evaluated to choose the appropriate graft material.

(d) A large, round carbide bur is used inside the socket to eliminate periodontal ligament residue attached to the internal walls.

(e) The cover on the tip of the Flow syringe is removed.

(f) The tip of the syringe easily fits into the defect, allowing the socket to be filled from a more apical position before moving coronally.

(g) The material flows into the socket, facilitating the procedure.

(h) The syringe tip is slowly withdrawn while the Flow is injected to the top of the socket bony walls.

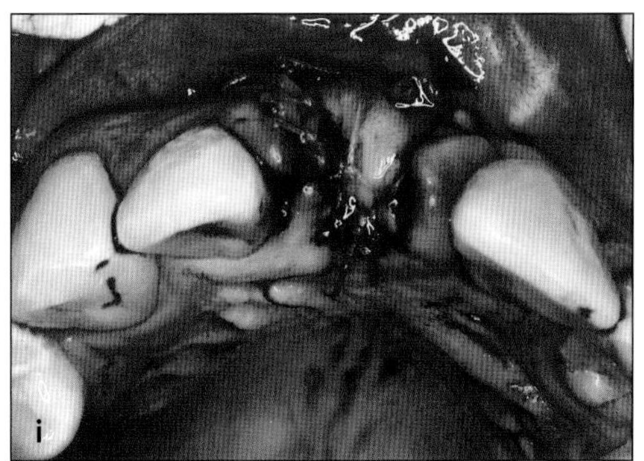

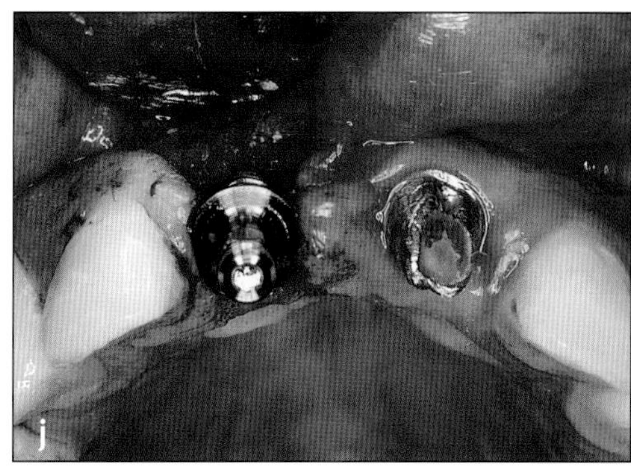

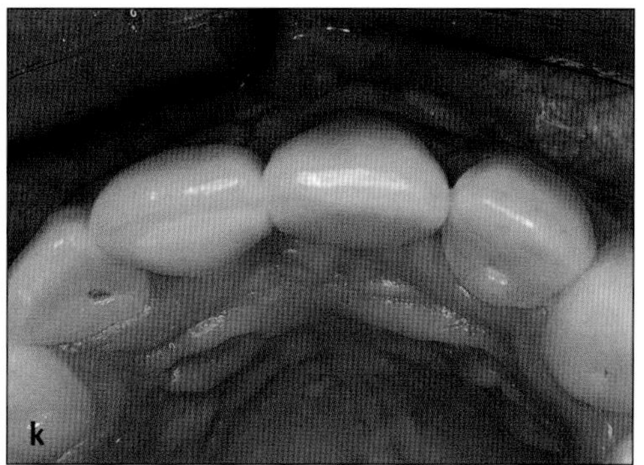

Fig 4-3 *(cont)*
(i) The sutures approximate the flaps that were previously released to avoid dehiscence caused by tension.

(j) Implant placement is successful as a result of previous socket grafting. The buccal wall of the right central incisor will match that of the left central incisor.

(k) Final restoration in place on the implant in the grafted site. Note the maintenance of buccal-palatal width of the ridge.

Four-Wall Defects

For a site that is missing one or two socket walls or that has one or more extremely thin walls, bone grafting is generally advised at the time of extraction. If not grafted, the bone typically narrows as the wound heals, leaving inadequate width for implant placement. Autogenous bone is a good choice for four-wall defects because entire bony walls often must be regenerated. If a sufficient amount of autogenous bone is not available, however, allogeneic bone putty (OrthoBlast II [The Clinician's Preference, Golden, CO], DBX [Musculoskeletal Transplant Foundation, Edison, NJ], Dyna-Graft II [IsoTis OrthoBiologics, Irvine, CA], or Grafton [Osteotech, Eatontown, NJ]), or a combination of allogeneic bone putty and autogenous bone, can be used (Figs 4-4 to 4-8).[41–48] The clinician must use a graft material with sufficient body to reconstruct the missing or thin wall (typically the facial wall) and to support the overlying soft tissues. Some clinicians use a barrier for guided bone regeneration (GBR) in an attempt to enhance the graft and prevent soft tissue ingrowth, but simply advancing the flap to obtain primary closure is generally sufficient.[49]

OrthoBlast II is a synergistic combination of demineralized bone and cancellous bone in a reverse-phase medium. OrthoBlast II is made of demineralized human bone that has passed a validated in vitro assay for osteoinduction. Because it is made of cancellous bone, it can provide an osteoconductive scaffold for bone deposi-

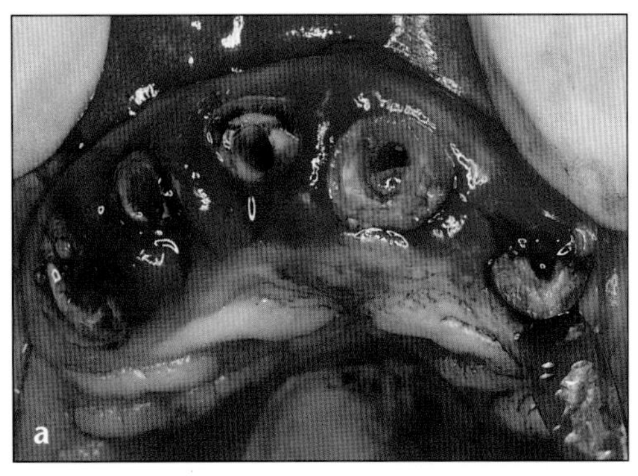

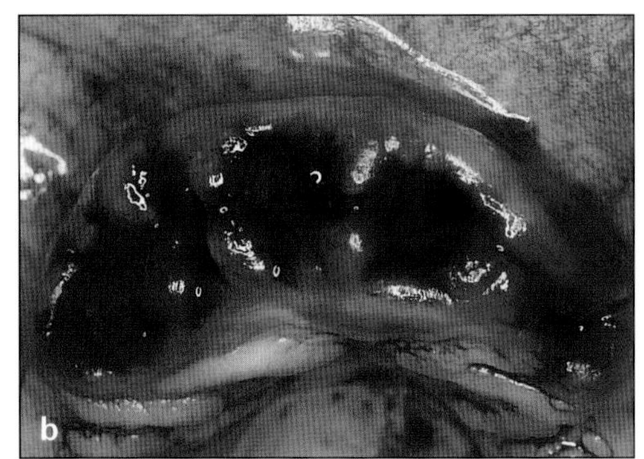

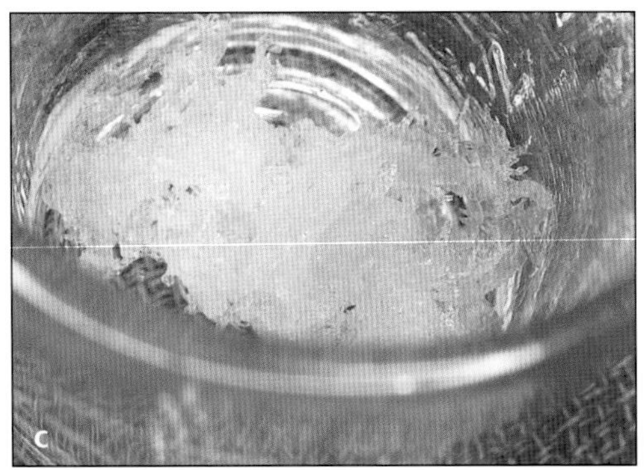

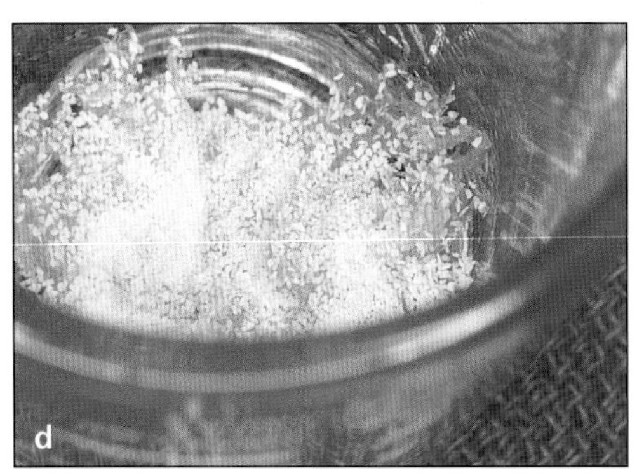

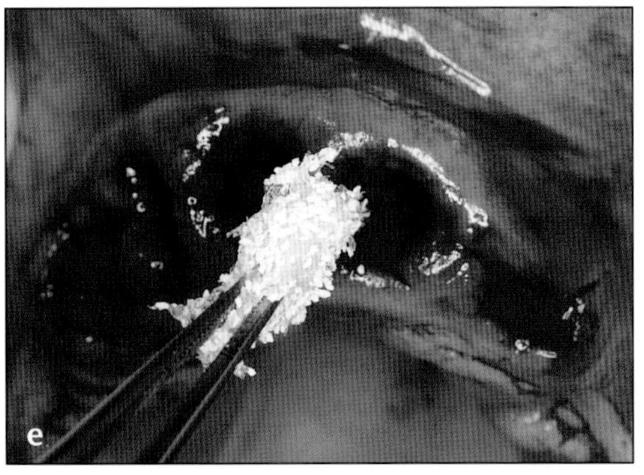

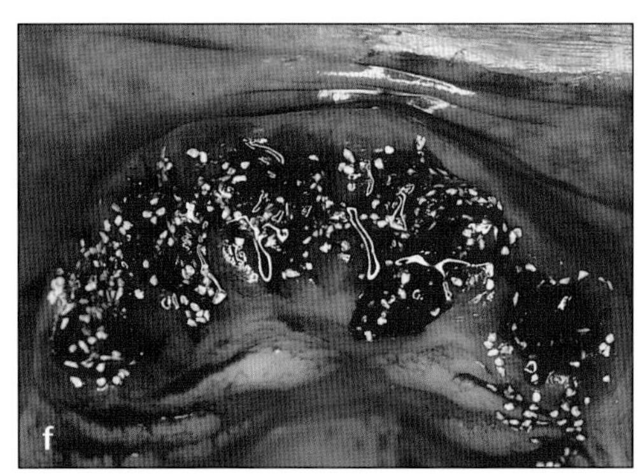

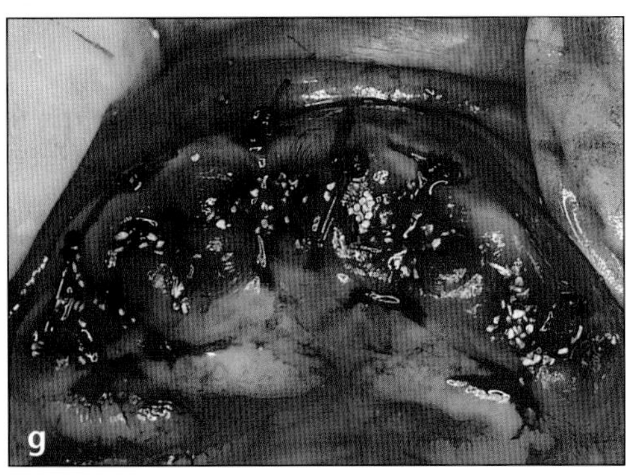

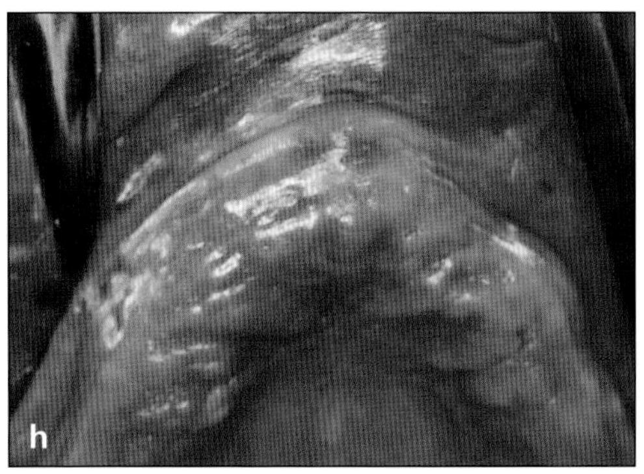

Fig 4-4 Allogeneic bone putty is used for socket grafting of a four-wall defect.

(a) A failing fixed partial denture is removed, revealing unrestorable roots. A closer look reveals that atraumatic root extractions and socket grafting are needed.

(b) Thin buccal walls will undoubtedly resorb over time if socket grafting is not performed.

(c) A DFDBA bone putty (Grafton) is used.

(d) The putty is mixed with an alloplastic mineral material to provide for a local mineral matrix in addition to the DFDBA. The consistency of the material after mixing enables easy handling.

(e) Graft material is easily transported to the sockets, where it will be gently condensed into place.

(f) Any excess material is removed to ensure that the graft material extends only to the top of the bony walls.

(g) Primary closure is not critical if the patient is using a transitional immediate denture to keep the material from washing out.

(h) The ridge has been preserved for implant placement. Grafting at an early phase and in a simple manner avoids potentially more involved grafting procedures later. This case may have required autogenous block grafts if socket grafting had not been performed at the time of extractions.

Fig 4-5 At four-wall defect sites, if socket walls are not grafted, the bone will narrow during wound healing, leaving inadequate width for implant placement.

(a) This residual root must be extracted. To prevent ridge resorption, socket grafting is needed to allow for future implant placement.

(b) Atraumatic extraction helps maintain as much bone as possible; nevertheless, a portion of the buccal wall is missing, and the remaining wall is extremely thin.

(c) DBX putty material is chosen to graft the extraction socket.

(d) In its putty form, this allograft has enough body to be molded into a shape closely approximating that of the extracted root.

(e) Giving the graft material this root-like shape helps ensure that the cavity is filled more completely and avoids leaving any dead space in the extraction socket.

(f) An adequate amount of bone can already be predicted because grafting was performed using an ideal material. The graft material is placed only to the top of the bony walls.

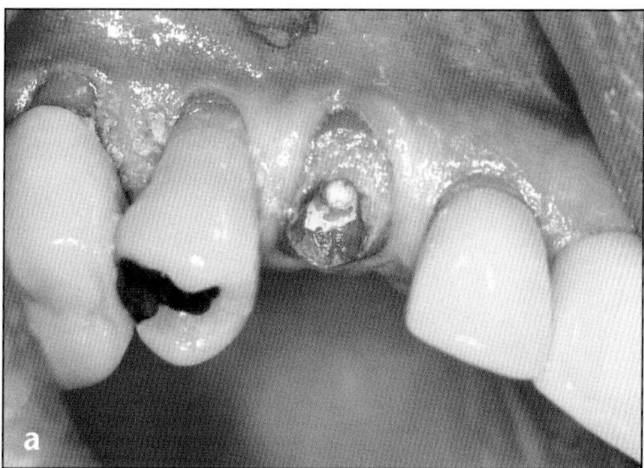
a

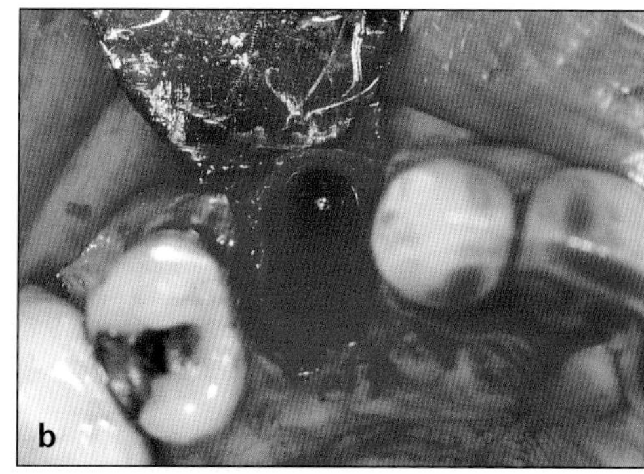
b

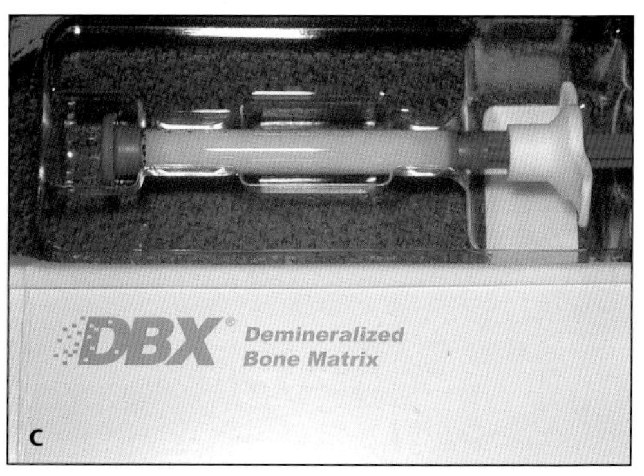

c

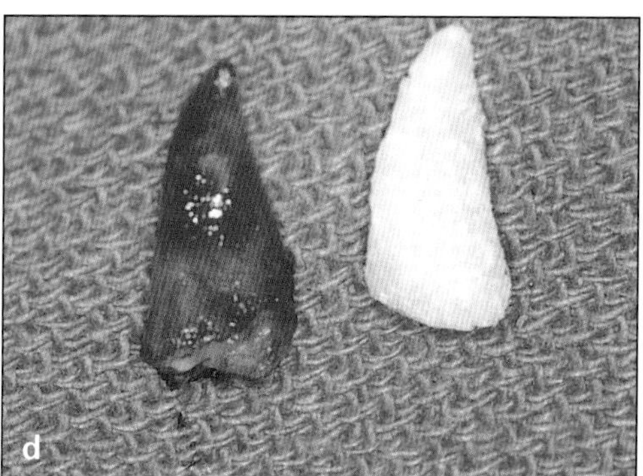
d

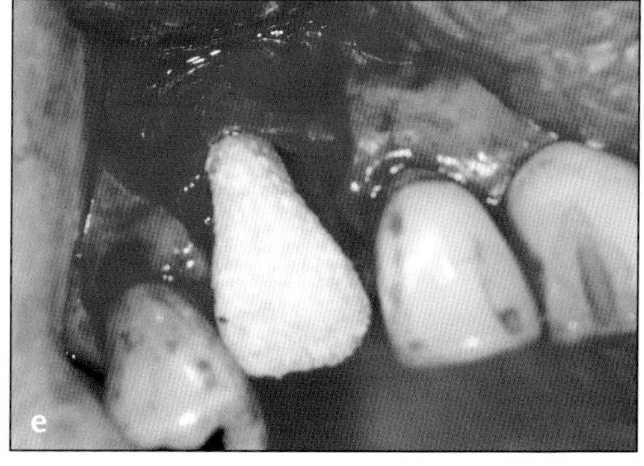
e

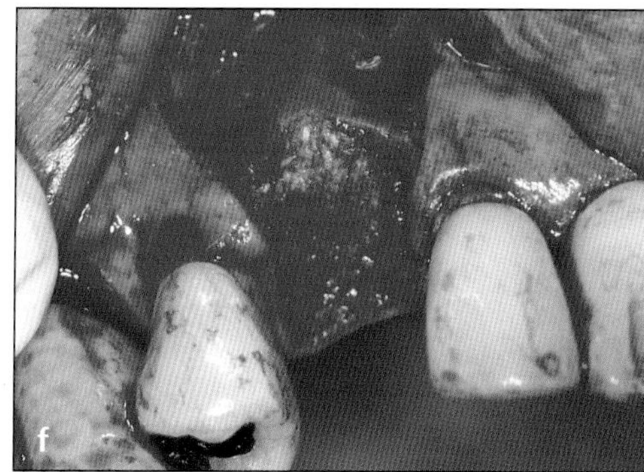
f

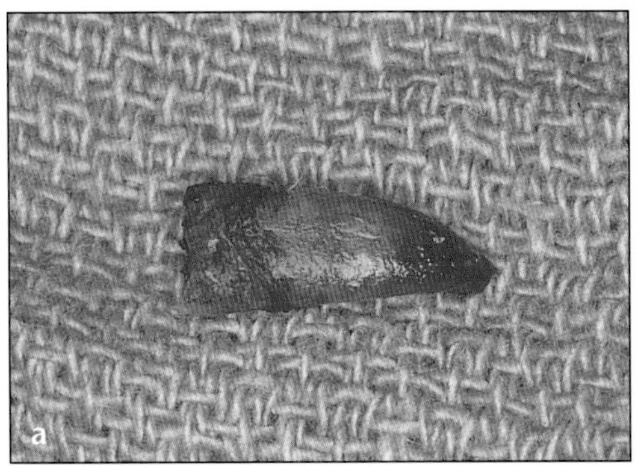

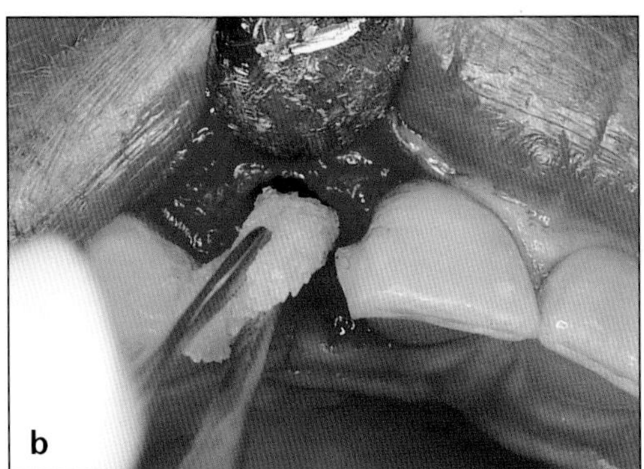

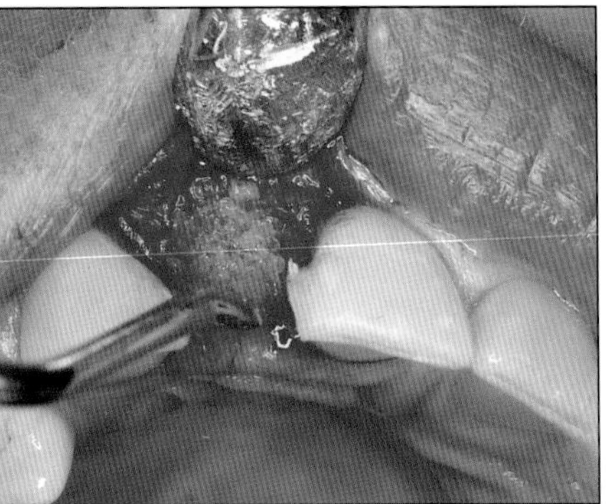

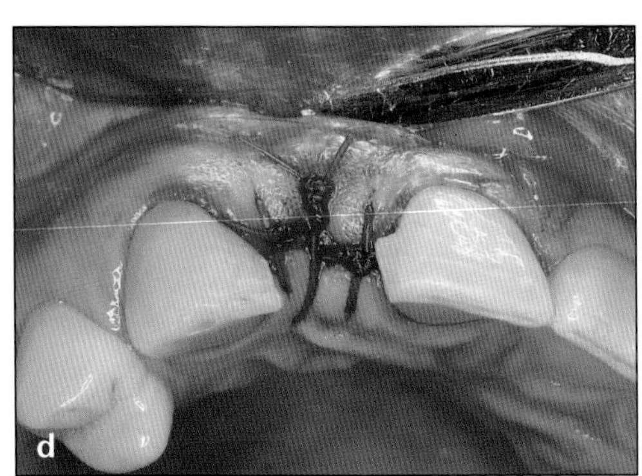

Fig 4-6 OrthoBlast II, an allograft putty composed of both mineralized and demineralized allogeneic bone, is the graft material chosen for this four-wall defect.

(a) This maxillary right lateral incisor root was extracted, and the site will be grafted in preparation for future implants.

(b) OrthoBlast II is placed in the socket. Without grafting, the socket is very likely to undergo resorption and thus jeopardize the successful placement of an implant.

(c) The socket is filled to the level of the bone crest.

(d) Primary closure is achieved with some scoring of the periosteum, although this is not critical.

tion and remodeling. Moreover, its unique reverse-phase medium carrier becomes more viscous at body temperature, providing exceptional handling and ease of use with minimal loss through irrigation and suction. OrthoBlast II is available in 1- and 3-mL prefilled syringes and in a 5-mL container for larger grafting procedures.

DynaGraft II is composed of DFDBA in a reverse phase medium. Each lot of the DFDBA is tested in a quantitative in vitro assay for its ability to stimulate new bone formation. It is highly malleable and easy to mold and pack into a defect. DynaGraft II thickens at body temperature and resists irrigation to minimize the likelihood of migration from the surgical site.

The decision to use GBR is based on the defect type and the choice of graft material.[50–53] GBR can also be used alone to prevent ridge deformities in postextraction sites that have sufficient alveolar bone.[54] Because autogenous grafts revascularize relatively quickly, leaving less time for soft tissue to invade, barrier membranes are not always necessary for predictable results. Nonetheless, some clinicians use membranes even when they are not essential; others avoid them with autogenous grafts because such barriers increase the risk of wound infection. When these defects are grafted with allogeneic or xenogenic materials, healing occurs more slowly, and barrier membranes can be useful to

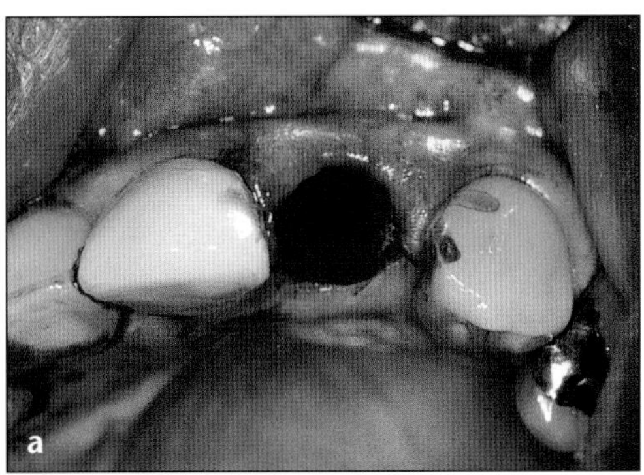

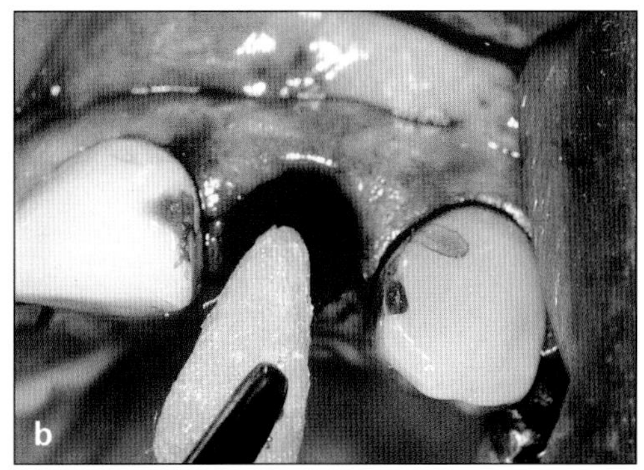

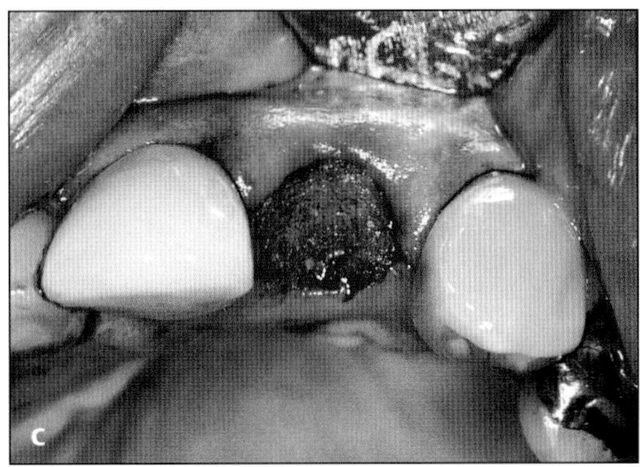

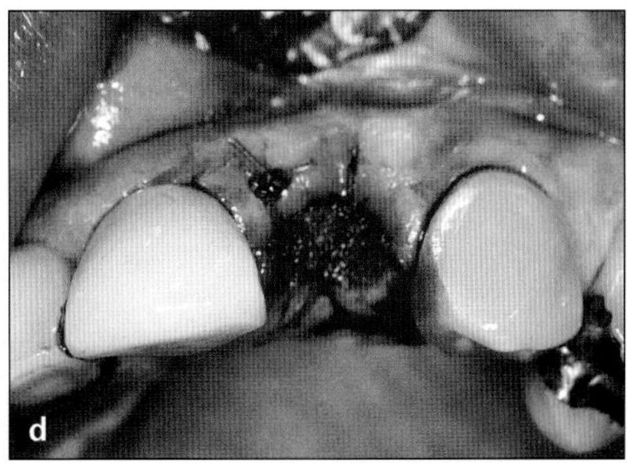

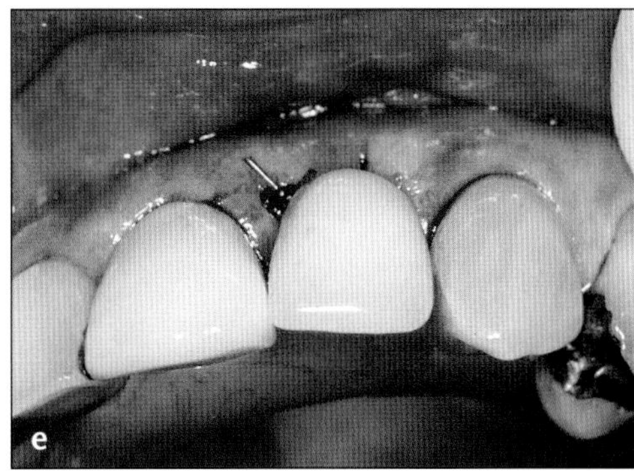

Fig 4-7 DynaGraft II, an allograft putty, is used to graft the extraction socket of a maxillary central incisor.

(a) Socket of an extracted maxillary left central incisor.

(b) The DynaGraft II is molded into the shape of the extracted root and placed so as to maximize the filling of the extraction socket.

(c) After the socket is completely filled, any graft material above the bony walls will be removed and the area will be sutured.

(d) A figure-eight suture is placed to approximate the tissues and to maintain the gingival architecture.

(e) An interim prosthesis is placed to help protect the graft. It is modified and adjusted to mold and maintain the gingival architecture.

maintain space for bone growth. Resorbable membranes reduce the incidence of wound infection, but they also decrease the predictability of graft volume. When GBR is used, the membrane should be placed away from the incision. Chapter 3 provides a comprehensive review of the large variety of barrier materials that are available.[53,55–66]

Primary closure is desirable but may not always be possible in a fresh extraction site. For most extraction sockets, simply approximating the gingival margins with sutures is adequate. For molar sockets, however, it is recommended that the flap be released and advanced or a soft tissue graft be used to obtain soft tissue closure. A tension-free closure, however, is always indicated.[67,68] Good approximation of the soft tissues allows for soft tissue closure that supports fibroblasts and optimal healing. There is typically a 3- to 6-month waiting period before implant placement.

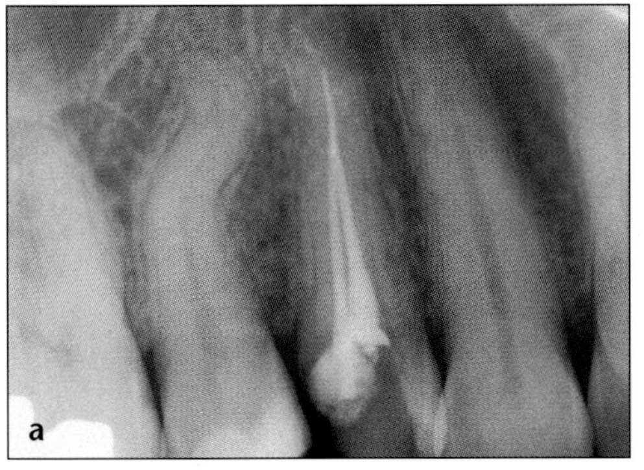

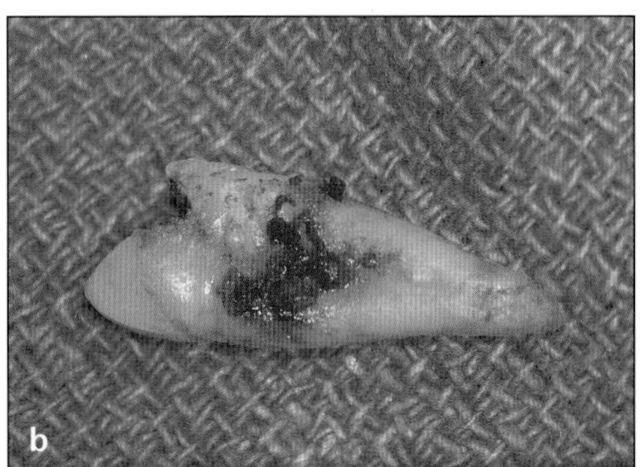

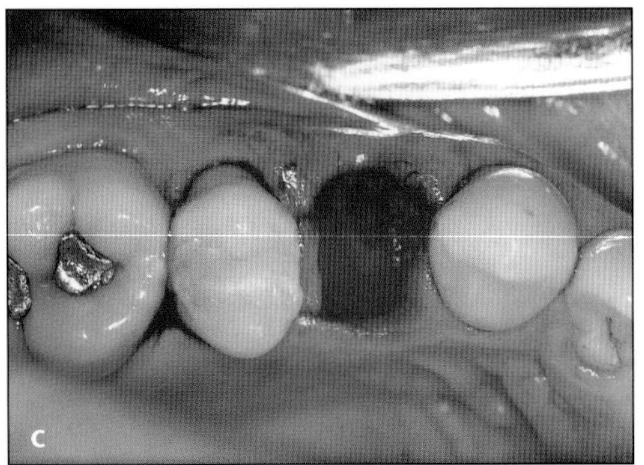

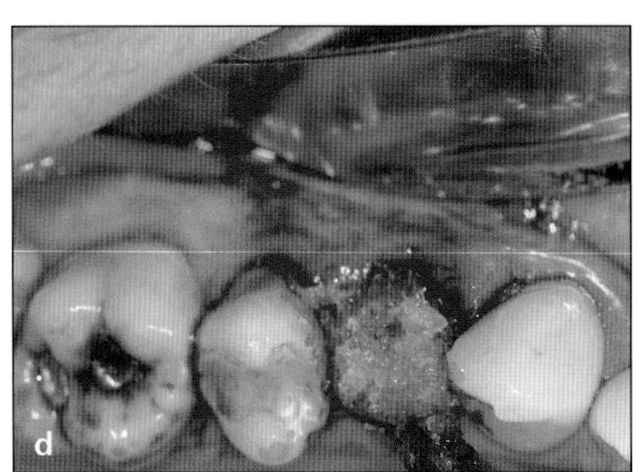

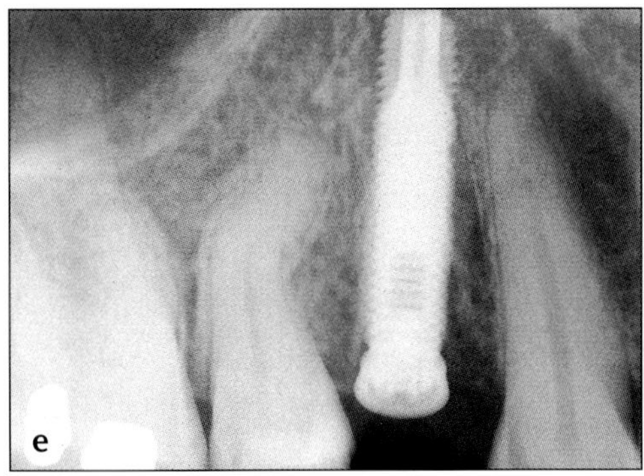

Fig 4-8 Socket grafting is indicated at the time of extraction in order to retain adequate width for implant placement.

(a) An endodontically treated first premolar is diagnosed as unrestorable; extraction, socket grafting, and subsequent implant placement are indicated.

(b) Extracting the premolar atraumatically will take longer because extensive luxation of the tooth should be avoided to reduce the possibility of socket wall fractures.

(c) The socket exhibits thin buccal and palatal walls that require grafting.

(d) For large extraction sockets, grafting can be performed in layers, starting with the apicalmost portion, where graft material is condensed with a wide amalgam plugger. The grafting material is OrthoBlast II.

(e) Note the ideal bone height around the implant 6 weeks after placement.

Three-Wall Defects

For a site that has lost two socket walls or that has two or more extremely thin walls, bone grafting is strongly advised at the time of extraction. If the socket is not grafted, the bone often narrows as the wound heals, leaving inadequate width to accommodate implant placement. Autogenous bone is again the preferred material for these defects because entire bony walls must be regenerated. If insufficient autogenous bone is available, allogeneic bone blocks mortised around the margins and within the socket with putty (eg, Grafton DBM Flex) or, alternatively, J-Block (Zimmer Dental) mortised with Puros (Zimmer Dental), OrthoBlast II, Grafton, DynaGraft II, or DBX, can be used (Fig 4-9). When using blocks of allogeneic bone graft material, the clinician places the block graft material in the appropriate

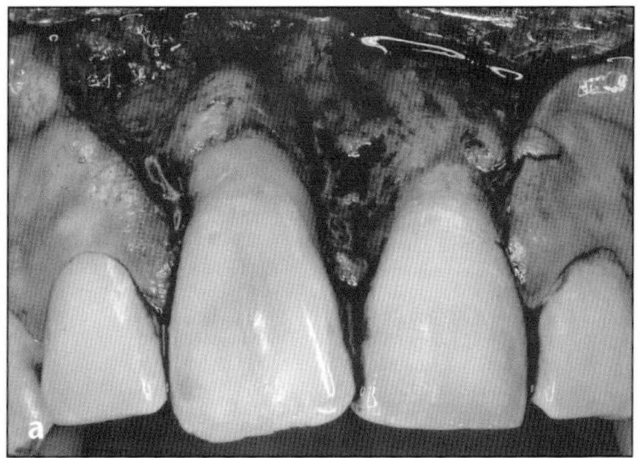

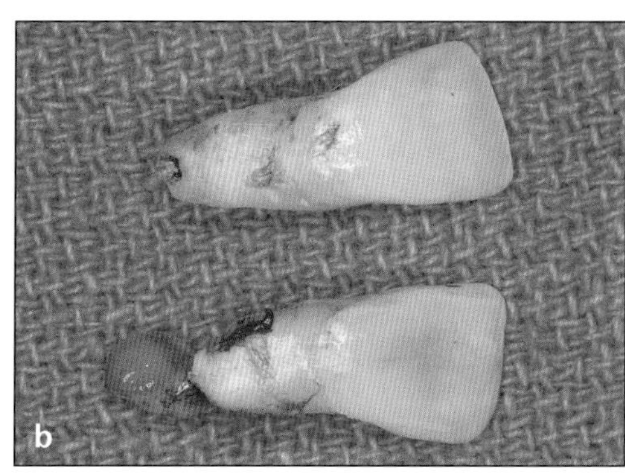

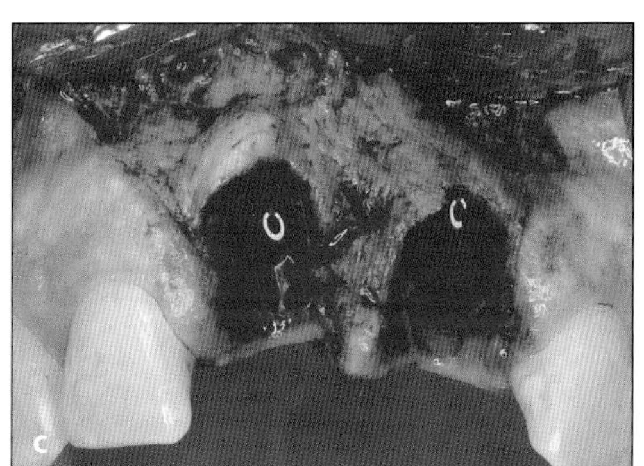

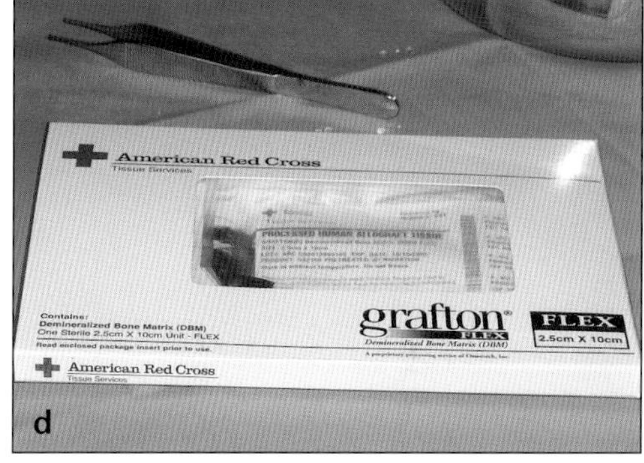

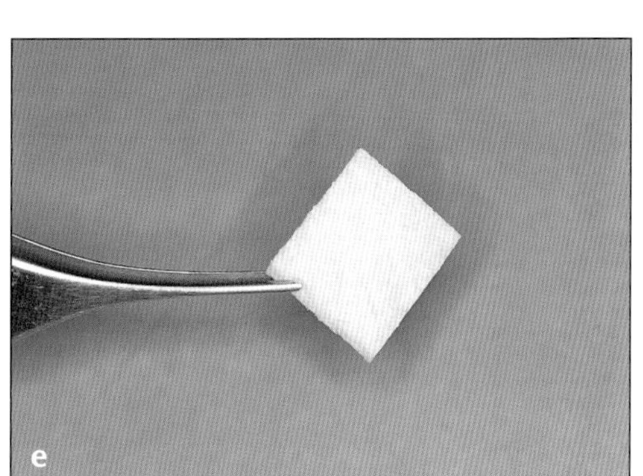

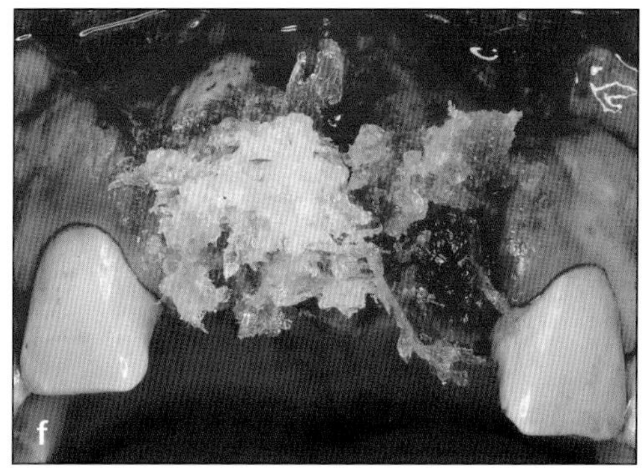

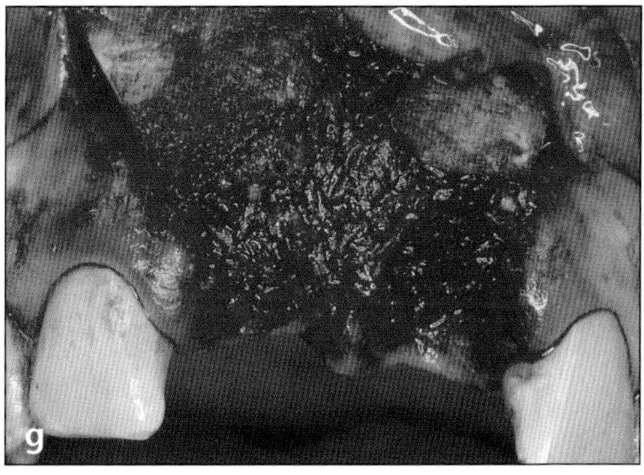

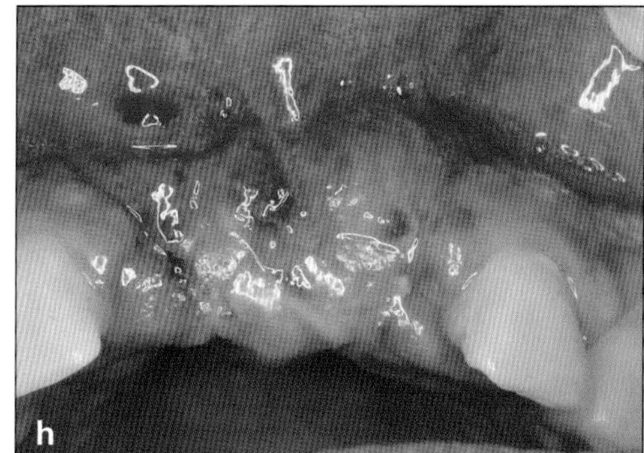

Fig 4-9 Allogeneic bone blocks mortised with putty can be used to graft three-wall defects at the time of extraction.

(a) These maxillary central incisors had been reimplanted after avulsion 5 years earlier. Flap reflection is critical for three-wall defects. In this case, a high flap reflection helps determine the amount of bone loss.

(b) The central incisors had resorbed and developed residual infection.

(c) Despite bone resorption around the sockets, good interdental crest height remains. The sockets are thoroughly curetted, irrigated, and debrided with a large bur to eliminate any granulation tissues.

(d) An allogeneic bone matrix (Grafton DBM Flex) is chosen to build up the buccal bone and to provide a matrix for the allogeneic bone putty (Grafton DBM Putty). The bone block matrix is used to build up the buccal bone, and the putty form is used to mortar around the blocks and to fill in the extraction socket.

(e) The Flex is measured and trimmed to the appropriate sizes and configurations for the defect.

(f) The putty is placed and condensed into the sockets.

(g) The Flex is placed on the buccal aspect. It is important to use periosteal sling sutures to stabilize the Flex. Note the physiologic appearance assumed by the graft material almost immediately after placement. When grafting with blocks of allogeneic bone, the clinician must obtain primary closure.

(h) Optimal ridge height and width have been achieved for future implant placement.

position over and around the defect and then uses the allogeneic bone putty to fill the defect, to "mortar" the voids, and to seal the margins. Some clinicians use a barrier membrane to enhance the graft and induce bone regeneration by preventing soft tissue ingrowth, but simply advancing the flap to obtain primary closure is typically sufficient. However, it is important to stabilize the allogeneic block. Depending on the consistency of the material being used, stabilization may require screw fixation or sling sutures. There is typically a 5- to 6-month waiting period before implant placement.

Two-Wall Defects

Patients who exhibit two-wall defects after extraction require a two-stage treatment with bone-grafting techniques. The graft material of choice for this group of patients is particulate autogenous bone with a barrier membrane (GTAM [Gore-Tex, W.L. Gore, Flagstaff, AZ]) or other stiff membrane secured in place with pins or screws (Fig 4-10). This type of grafting procedure requires careful surgical planning, and soft tissue flap design is of the utmost importance.[69] The small amount of autogenous bone required for this procedure typically can be harvested from adjacent sites or from the tuberosity area with the use of a trephine bur, MX-Grafter (Maxilon Laboratories, Hollis, NH), or Ebner grafter (Maxilon Laboratories). If larger volumes are needed for the defect, other alternative sites can be selected as discussed in chapters 5, 6, and 7. Primary stability is of paramount importance to the result and can generally be achieved by appropriately repositioning the reflected periosteum. Membranes can and generally should be used to maximize the predictability of this graft. Primary closure must be accomplished with absolutely tension-free suturing. There is typically a 5- to 6-month waiting period before implant placement.

One-Wall Defects

One-wall defects are often referred to as *knife-edge defects* and require a two-stage treatment with bone-grafting techniques. The graft material of choice for these patients is an autogenous block graft, usually obtained from the patient's mandibular ramus or anterior symphysis. The graft is placed in block rather than particulated form for added structural support. Cortical fixation screws maintain graft stability (Fig 4-11). Again, this type of graft requires careful surgical planning; the design of the soft tissue flap is the most important part of the procedure. The block graft requires the harvesting of autogenous bone of adequate size and uniform thickness to place into the defect. This procedure is described in detail in chapters 5 and 6. Primary stability is of paramount importance for achieving a predictable result. The graft must be closed primarily, and a healing period of 5 to 6 months is required before further treatment.

Fig 4-10 Two-wall defects require a two-stage treatment with bone-grafting techniques. The material of choice is particulate autogenous bone with a barrier membrane.

(a) After flap reflection and root tip extraction, the residual bone can be examined. Because of the deficiency of the ridge and the extractions required, particulate autogenous bone and a membrane with pin fixation are required.

(b) Particulate autogenous bone for grafting is placed into a sterile plastic syringe to allow for compression and to facilitate delivery to the recipient site. The tip of the syringe is cut off after the bone is compressed with the plunger. This graft will be mixed with PRP to enhance healing and malleability.

(c) The graft material has been placed with some overcontouring because a certain degree of resorption is anticipated. The barrier membrane, which must be stiff for this application, is also in place, with the palatal aspect already tacked down.

(d) The stiff barrier membrane is wrapped over the graft and tacked into place on the buccal aspect.

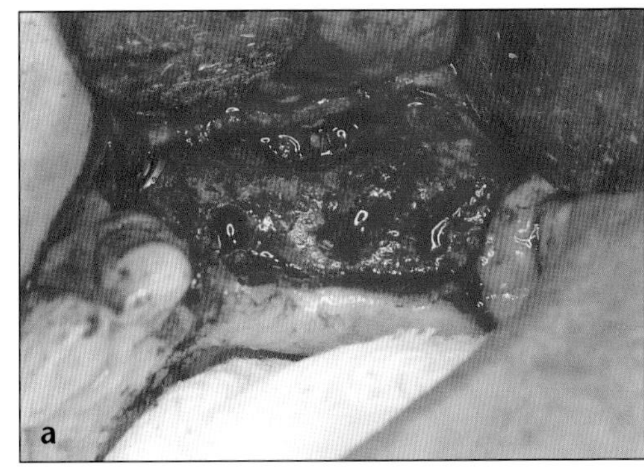

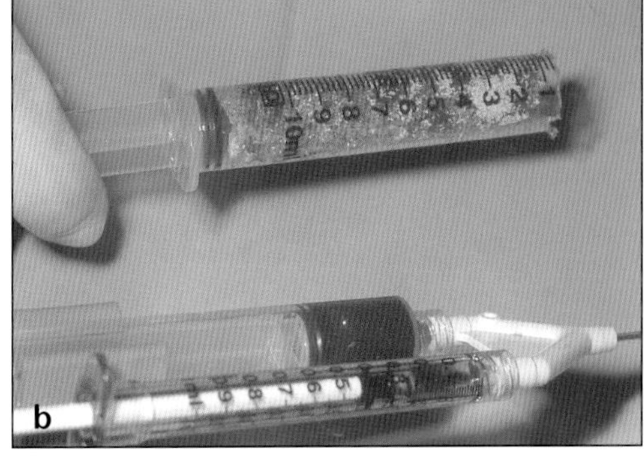

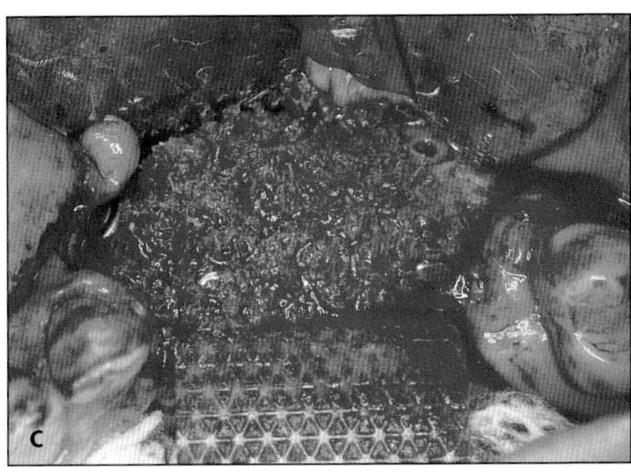

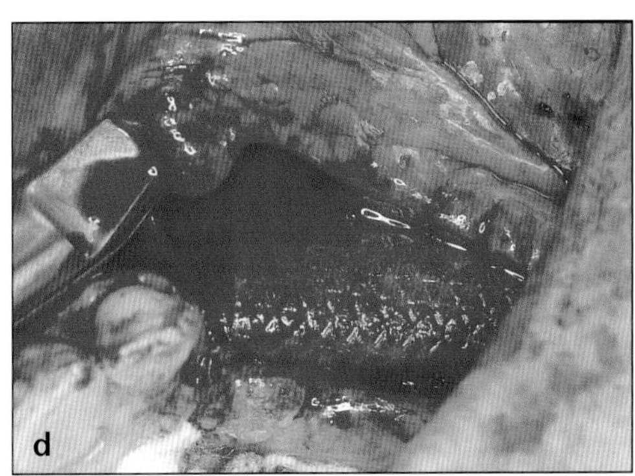

Fig 4-11
(a) For a one-wall defect after extraction, the only possibility of returning to an optimal volume for implant placement is grafting with a block graft from the anterior mandible or ramus or allogeneic bone. In this case, a monocortical block from the symphysis is used.

(b) The block of bone is fixed in place and the surrounding areas are mortared with particulate bone.

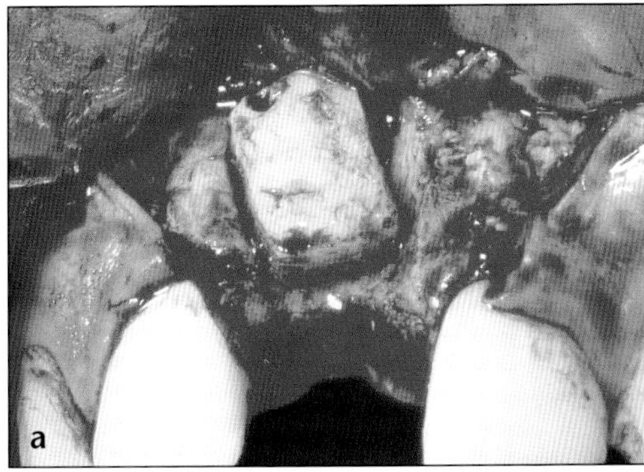

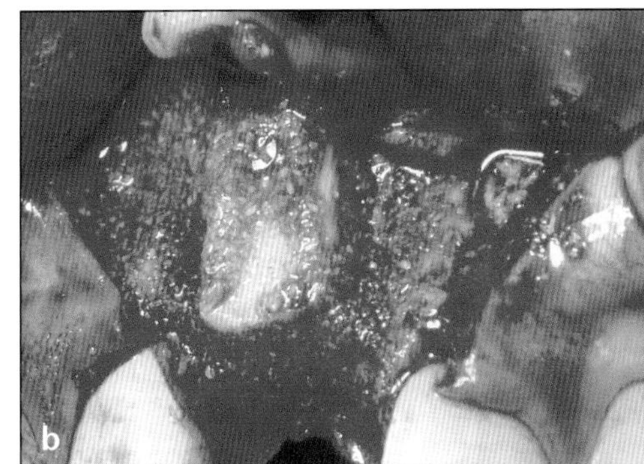

Prosthetic Management of the Ridge Preservation Process

Once surgical removal of the tooth is completed and the ridge has been restored through primary or secondary procedures, proper management of the overlying prosthesis is crucial. A well-fitted provisional restoration, either fixed or removable, will help dictate the final tissue contours. Many patients wear some type of removable provisional restoration, either a ridge-lap design or an ovate pontic shape that fits into the extraction site. An appliance with a ridge-lap design must be fabricated to avoid compressing the underlying tissue and flattening the ridge contour. The ovate pontic design is preferred because it allows the restoration to fit into the socket site and to compress the graft material, which may eliminate the need for extensive suturing.

The goal of the prosthetic restoration should be to mimic the contours of the natural tooth. Appliance stability is important because movement interferes with the adequate consolidation of bone and increases the likelihood of a failed graft. Contacts with adjacent teeth should be approximately 5 mm above the interproximal bone level for optimal bone and soft tissue maturation, esthetics, and predictability. Both vertical and horizontal movement should be minimized.

Another approach to the provisional restoration is the resin-bonded fixed partial denture. Using the crown of the extracted tooth can fulfill the necessary esthetic and functional requirement. Most patients are particularly pleased with this approach because it eliminates the need for a removable appliance. The disadvantage is that the fixed partial denture is more difficult to construct and place. It is also more difficult to monitor the soft tissue contours, and a soft tissue dehiscence may occur.

Soft Tissue Considerations in Ridge Preservation

To optimize the ridge for future implant placement, it is important to preserve and maintain not only the hard tissue structure but also the soft tissues. For this reason, the extractions must be absolutely atraumatic and maintain the bony architecture as well as the soft tissue architecture. For closure after grafting the socket, the flaps are pulled together slightly with sutures, but several millimeters can be left exposed when using gel or putty configuration materials. However, if the graft material is autogenous bone, the grafted material is only particulate material and not in a putty or gel configuration, or if the extraction socket is wide, primary soft tissue closure is critical. This can be accomplished by reflection and advancement of the flap (see Figs 4-10 and 4-11) or, alternatively, by using a harvested connective tissue graft (Fig 4-12).

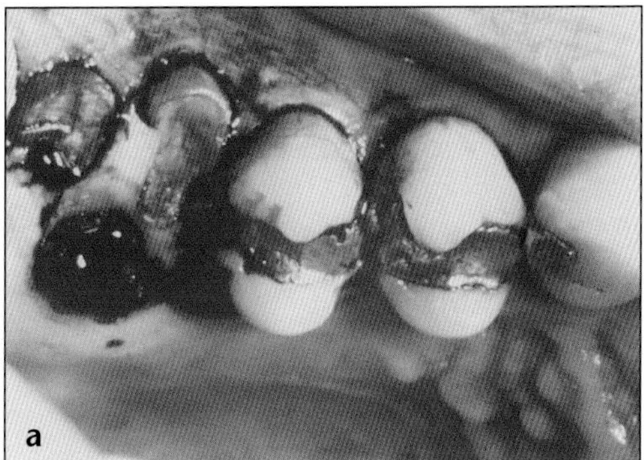
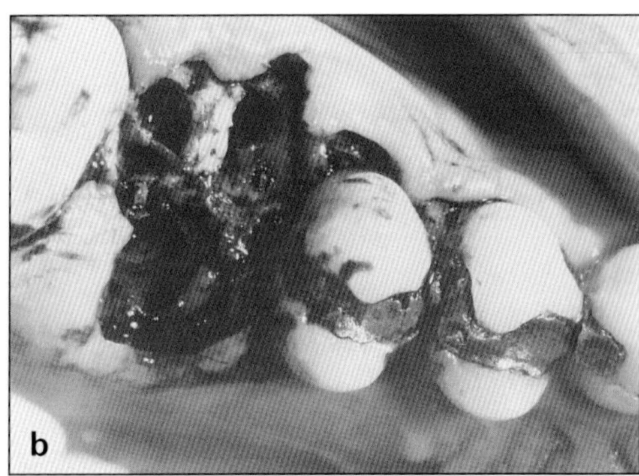
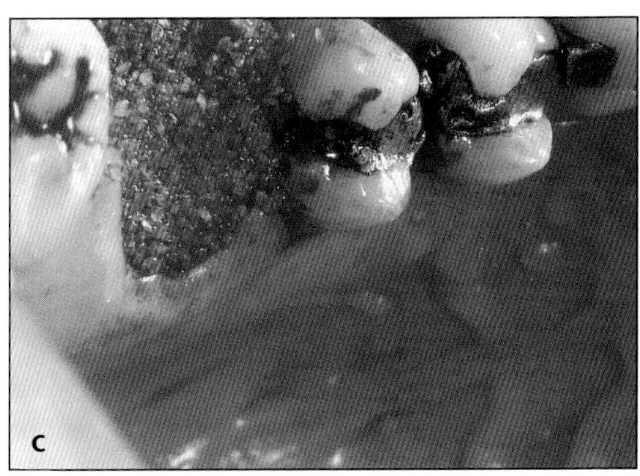
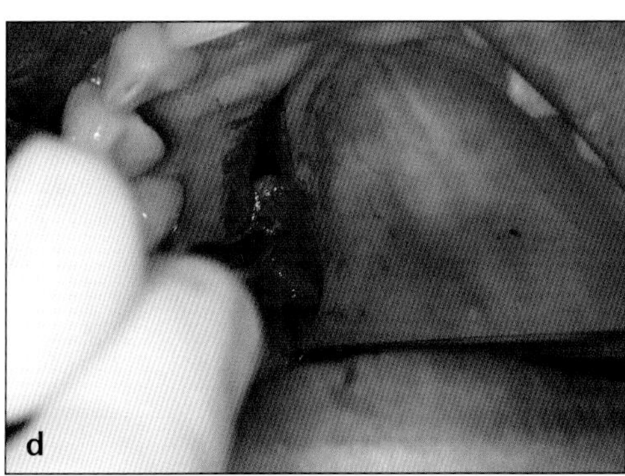
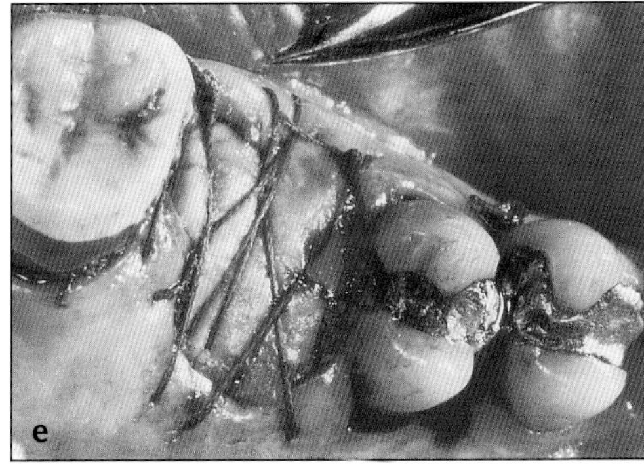
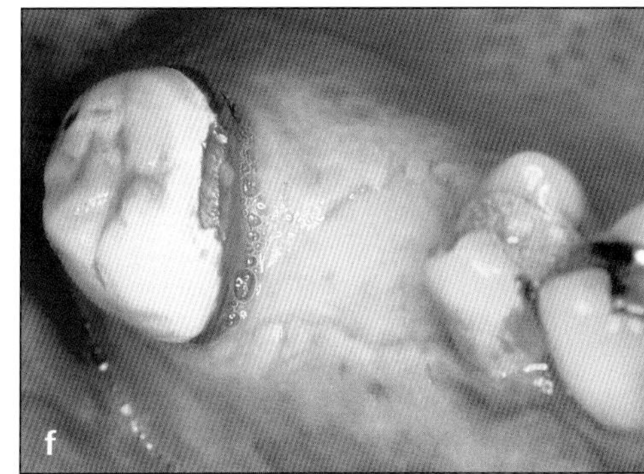

Fig 4-12 When more than several millimeters of the grafted socket will be exposed by simply suturing the buccal and palatal tissue, a soft tissue graft is important. This minimizes the amount of graft material that will wash out and also allows for excellent soft tissue contour and color.

(a) Residual maxillary first molar roots requiring extraction.

(b) After extraction, the sockets will require grafting. The soft tissue is also deficient.

(c) Although the socket is completely filled, soft tissue approximation is not possible.

(d) A connective tissue graft is harvested from the palate.

(e) The connective tissue graft, which is placed over the bone graft and under the buccal and palatal flaps of the extraction socket, is held in place with several sutures.

(f) Ridge volume is maintained and attached gingiva has formed with excellent color match to provide good hard and soft tissue formation in the area for future implant placement.

Ridge Preservation During Implant Placement

Once the ridge has been prepared or maintained, placing the implant is the final important step in the overall treatment plan. The incision technique and flap design are extremely important in achieving the best result. Proper blood flow to the surgical area will dictate the success of the flap design and, ultimately, osseointegration of the implant.

The midcrestal incision with a full-thickness mucoperiosteal flap is most often used to access the area. This technique allows for the best visualization of the osteotomy site and for positioning the implant with good bone contours. The incision can include or exclude the papilla, but the potential for scarring in a vertical direction must be addressed.

At the time of reentry there should be adequate soft tissue, and the recipient grafted site may yield dense bone material if adequate time has elapsed for bone maturation. The time frame of the reentry often influences the degree of graft consolidation. Incision design should allow for primary closure over the implant site and provide for a tight closure of the soft tissue, ensuring the best early environment for the implant to osseointegrate.

Maintaining the keratinized tissue is important for protecting the implant restoration and to allow for good hygiene. Any technique that reduces the keratinized tissue will potentially compromise the implant restoration. Some clinicians advocate the blind punch technique; however, poor visualization can create problems relating to soft and hard tissue contours and provide for bony dehiscence or fenestrations. This approach may also lead to the loss of the keratinized tissue zone. However, if the residual ridge is of adequate thickness (generally a 10-mm buccopalatal width) and there is adequate attached gingiva, this approach is simple and efficient.

Future Directions

The future of alveolar ridge preservation is exciting. Many questions remain unanswered about GBR, including success rates in implants placed with barrier membranes as well as the use of bone substitutes and growth factors.[51] Further studies involving the expanded use of traditional barrier membranes, such as calcium sulfate, are also in order.[61] Some researchers believe that regeneration research in general and bone regeneration research in particular will advance through studies involving stem cell transplantation and tissue engineering.[70,71]

As explained in chapter 11, newly identified and developed techniques for autologous proteins to be used in conjunction with graft materials can enhance the graft and decrease the maturation time.[17,30] For example, Geesink et al demonstrated bone induction through the use of a human recombinant osteogenic protein (OP-1), although further research involving the dosage and most effective types of carriers, among other concerns, is necessary.[72] Furthermore, recombinant DNA has been developed using the principles of genetic engineering to provide bone proteins that can induce bone growth in localized defects resulting from tooth removal. These proteins can be placed when the primary defect is created and can induce pluripotential or precursor cells in the host wall to regrow bone that completely fills the defect. As explained in chapter 11, although these proteins are not currently available for commercial use for dental/oral surgery purposes, they may hold promise for the future of ridge preservation, bone healing, and bone grafting.

References

1. Seibert JS, Salama H. Alveolar ridge preservation and reconstruction. Periodontol 2000 1996;11:69–84.
2. Garg AK. Alveolar ridge preservation during and after surgical tooth removal. Dent Implantol Update 2001;11:57–62.
3. Garg AK. Preservation, augmentation, and reconstruction of the alveolar ridge. Dent Implantol Update 2001;12:81–85.
4. Bartee BK. Extraction site reconstruction for alveolar ridge preservation. Part 1: Rationale and materials selection. J Oral Implantol 2001; 27:187–193.
5. Atwood D. Post-extraction changes in adult mandible as illustrated by microradiograph of midsagittal section and serial cephalometric roentgenograms. J Prosthet Dent 1963;13: 810–824.
6. Carlsson H, Thilander H, Hedegard B. Histologic changes in the upper alveolar process after extractions with or without insertion of an immediate full denture. Acta Odontol Scand 1967;25:21–43.
7. John V, Gossweiler M. Implant treatment planning and rehabilitation of the anterior maxilla: Part 1. J Indiana Dent Assoc 2001;80:20–24.
8. Caffesse RG, de la Rosa M, Mota LF. Regeneration of soft and hard tissue periodontal defects. Am J Dent 2002;15:339–345.
9. Becker W, Hujoel P, Becker BE. Effect of barrier membranes and autologous bone grafts on ridge width preservation around implants. Clin Implant Dent Relat Res 2002;4:143–149.
10. Oikarinen KS, Sandor GK, Kainulainen VT, Salonen-Kemppi M. Augmentation of the narrow traumatized anterior alveolar ridge to facilitate dental implant placement. Dent Traumatol 2003;19:19–29.
11. Froum SJ, Gomez C, Breault MR. Current concepts of periodontal regeneration. A review of the literature. N Y State Dent J 2002;68:14–22.
12. Gaggl A, Schultes G, Rainer H, Karcher H. Immediate alveolar ridge distraction after tooth extraction—A preliminary report. Br J Oral Maxillofac Surg 2002;40:110–115.
13. Garcia AG, Martin MS, Vila PG, Maceiras JL. Minor complications arising in alveolar distraction osteogenesis. J Oral Maxillofac Surg 2002;60:496–501.
14. Hoexter DL. Osseous regeneration in compromised extraction sites: A ten-year case study. J Oral Implantol 2002;28:19–24.
15. Lorenzoni M, Pertl C, Polansky RA, Jakse N, Wegscheider WA. Evaluation of implants placed with barrier membranes. A retrospective follow-up study up to five years. Clin Oral Implants Res 2002;13:274–280.
16. Hoexter DL. Bone regeneration graft materials. J Oral Implantol 2002;28:290–294.
17. Moore WR, Graves SE, Bain GI. Synthetic bone graft substitutes. ANZ J Surg 2001;71: 354–361.
18. Garg AK. The future role of growth factors in bone grafting. Dent Implantol Update 1999; 10:5–7.
19. Garg AK. The use of platelet-rich plasma to enhance the success of bone grafts around dental implants. Dent Implantol Update 2000; 11:17–21.
20. Shanaman R, Filstein MR, Danesh-Meyer MJ. Localized ridge augmentation using GBR and platelet-rich plasma: Case reports. Int J Periodontics Restorative Dent 2001;21:345–355.
21. Sanchez AR, Sheridan PJ, Kupp LI. Is platelet-rich plasma the perfect enhancement factor? A current review. Int J Oral Maxillofac Implants 2003;18:93–103.
22. Wojtowicz A, Chaberek S, Kryst L, Urbanowska E, Ciechowicz K, Ostrowski K. Fourier and fractal analysis of maxillary alveolar ridge repair using platelet rich plasma (PRP) and inorganic bovine bone. Int J Oral Maxillofac Surg 2003;32:84–86.
23. Misch CE, Dietsh-Misch F, Misch CM. A modified socket seal surgery with composite graft approach. J Oral Implantol 1999;25: 244–250.
24. Bedrossian E, Tawfilis A, Alijanian A. Veneer grafting: A technique for augmentation of the resorbed alveolus prior to implant placement. A clinical report. Int J Oral Maxillofac Implants 2000;15:853–858.
25. Zeiter DJ, Ries WL, Sanders JJ. The use of a bone block graft from the chin for alveolar ridge augmentation. Int J Periodontics Restorative Dent 2000:20:618–627.

26. Sethi A, Kaus T. Ridge augmentation using mandibular block bone grafts: Preliminary results of an ongoing prospective study. Int J Oral Maxillofac Implants 2001;16:378–388.
27. John V, Gossweiler M. Implant treatment planning and rehabilitation of the anterior maxilla, part 2: The role of autogenous grafts. J Indiana Dent Assoc 2002;81:33–38.
28. Maiorana C, Santoro F, Rabagliati M, Salina S. Evaluation of the use of iliac cancellous bone and anorganic bovine bone in the reconstruction of the atrophic maxilla with titanium mesh: A clinical and histologic investigation. Int J Oral Maxillofac Implants 2001;16:427–432.
29. Lozada J, Proussaefs P. Clinical radiographic, and histologic evaluation of maxillary bone reconstruction by using a titanium mesh and autogenous iliac graft: A case report. J Oral Implantol 2002;28:9–14.
30. Vaccaro AR. The role of the osteoconductive scaffold in synthetic bone graft. Orthopedics 2002;25(5 suppl):s571–s578 [erratum 2002;25: 1224].
31. Ashman A, Bruins P. Prevention of alveolar bone loss postextraction with HTR grafting material. Oral Surg Oral Med Oral Pathol 1985;60:146–153.
32. Grisdale J. The clinical applications of synthetic bone alloplast. J Can Dent Assoc 1999;65:559–562.
33. Bolouri A, Haghighat N, Frederiksen N. Evaluation of the effect of immediate grafting of mandibular postextraction sockets with synthetic bone. Compend Contin Educ Dent 2001;22:955–958, 960, 962 passim.
34. Sy IP. Alveolar ridge preservation using a bioactive glass particulate graft in extraction site defects. Gen Dent 2002;50:66–68.
35. Krauser JT, Rohrer MD, Wallace SS. Human histologic and histomorphometric analysis comparing OsteoGraf/N with PepGen P-15 in the maxillary sinus elevation procedure: A case report. Implant Dent 2000;9:298–302.
36. Lallier TE, Yukna R, St Marie S, Moses R. The putative collagen binding peptide hastens periodontal ligament cell attachment to bone replacement graft materials. J Periodontol 2001;72:990–997.
37. Acil Y, Springer IN, Broek V, Terheyden H, Jepsen S. Effects of bone morphogenetic protein-7 stimulation on osteoblasts cultured on different biomaterials. J Cell Biochem 2002;86:90–98.
38. Yukna R, Salinas TJ, Carr RF. Periodontal regeneration following use of ABM/P-1 5: A case report. Int J Periodontics Restorative Dent 2002;22:146–155.
39. Barboza EP, de Souza RO, Caula AL, Neto LG, Caula Fde O, Duarte ME. Bone regeneration of localized chronic alveolar defects utilizing cell binding peptide associated with anorganic bovine-derived bone mineral: A clinical and histological study. J Periodontol 2002; 73:1153–1159.
40. Hahn J, Rohrer MD, Tofe AJ. Clinical, radiographic, histologic, and histomorphometric comparison of PepGen P-15 particulate and PepGen P-15 flow in extraction sockets: A same-mouth case study. Implant Dent 2003; 12:170-174.
41. Feighan JE, Davy D, Prewett AB, Stevenson S. Induction of bone by a demineralized bone matrix gel: A study in a rat femoral defect model. J Orthop Res 1995;13:881–891.
42. Martin GJ Jr, Boden SD, Titus L, Scarborough NL. New formulations of demineralized bone matrix as a more effective graft alternative in experimental posterolateral lumbar spine arthrodesis. Spine 1999;24:637–645.
43. Callan DP, Salkeld SL, Scarborough N. Histologic analysis of implant sites after grafting with demineralized bone matrix putty and sheets. Implant Dent 2000;9:36–44.
44. Callan DP. Regenerating the ridge: Performance of the Grafton allograft. Dent Implantol Update 2000;11:9–14.
45. Shermak MA, Wong L, Inoue N, Nicol T. Reconstruction of complex cranial wounds with demineralized bone matrix and bilayer artificial skin. J Craniofac Surg 2000;11:224–231.
46. Russell JL. Grafton demineralized bone matrix: Performance consistency, utility, and value. Tissue Eng 2000;6:435–440.
47. Leatherman BD, Dornhoffer JL, Fan CY, Mukunyadzi P. Demineralized bone matrix as an alternative for mastoid obliteration and posterior canal wall reconstruction: Results in an animal model. Otol Neurotol 2001; 22:731–736.
48. Takikawa S, Bauer TW, Kambic H, Togawa D. Comparative evaluation of the osteoinductivity of two formulations of human demineralized bone matrix. J Biomed Mater Res 2003; 65A:37–42.

49. Hammerle CH, Jung RE, Feloutzis A. A systematic review of the survival of implants in bone sites augmented with barrier membranes (guided bone regeneration) in partially edentulous patients. J Clin Periodontol 2002; 29(suppl 3):226–231.
50. Fugazzotto PA. Ridge augmentation with titanium screws and guided tissue regeneration: Technique and report of a case. Int J Oral Maxillofac Implants 1993;8:335–339.
51. Hermann JS, Buser D. Guided bone regeneration for dental implants. Curr Opin Periodontol 1996;3:168–77.
52. Peleg M, Chaushu G, Blinder D, Taicher S. Use of lyodura for bone augmentation of osseous defects around dental implants. J Periodontol 1999;70:853–60.
53. Sottosanti J, Anson D. Using calcium sulfate as a graft enhancer and membrane barrier [interview]. Dent Implantol Update 2003;14:1–8.
54. O'Brien TP, Hinrichs JE, Schaffer EM. The prevention of localized ridge deformities using guided tissue regeneration. J Periodontol 1994;65:17–24.
55. Lekovic V, Kenney EB, Weinlaender M, et al. A bone regenerative approach to alveolar ridge maintenance following tooth extraction. Report of 10 cases. J Periodontol 1997;68:563–570.
56. Lekovic V, Camargo PM, Klokkevold PR, et al. Preservation of alveolar bone in extraction sockets using bioabsorbable membranes. J Periodontol 1998;69:1044–1049.
57. Yang J, Lee HM, Vernino A. Ridge preservation of dentition with severe periodontitis. Compend Contin Educ Dent 2000;21:579–583.
58. Rosen PS, Reynolds MA. Guided bone regeneration for dehiscence and fenestration defects on implants using an absorbable polymer barrier. J Periodontol 2001;72:250–256.
59. Bartee BK. Extraction site reconstruction for alveolar ridge preservation. Part 2: Membrane-assisted surgical technique. J Oral Implantol 2001;27:194–197.
60. Wang HL, Carroll MJ. Guided bone regeneration using bone grafts and collagen membranes. Quintessence Int 2001;32:504–515.
61. Yoshikawa G, Murashima Y, Wadachi R, Sawada N, Suda H. Guided bone regeneration (GBR) using membranes and calcium sulphate after apicectomy: A comparative histomorphometrical study. Int Endod J 2002; 35:255–263.
62. Donos N, Kostopoulos L, Karring T. Alveolar ridge augmentation by combining autogenous mandibular bone grafts and non-resorbable membranes. Clin Oral Implants Res 2002;13: 185–191.
63. Patino MG, Neiders ME, Andreana S, Noble B, Cohen RE. Collagen as an implantable material in medicine and dentistry. J Oral Implantol 2002;28:220–225.
64. Pruthi VK, Gelskey SC, Mirbod SM. Furcation therapy with bioabsorbable collagen membrane: A clinical trial. J Can Dent Assoc 2002; 68:610–615.
65. Degidi M, Scarano A, Piattelli A. Regeneration of the alveolar crest using titanium micromesh with autologous bone and a resorbable membrane. J Oral Implantol 2003;29:86–90.
66. Oh TJ, Meraw SJ, Lee EJ, Giannobile WV, Wang HL. Comparative analysis of collagen membranes for the treatment of implant dehiscence defects. Clin Oral Implants Res 2003;14:80–90.
67. Nemcovsky CE, Artzi Z. Split palatal flap. I. A surgical approach for primary soft tissue healing in ridge augmentation procedures: Technique and clinical results. Int J Periodontics Restorative Dent 1999;19:175–181.
68. Nemcovsky CE, Artzi Z. Split palatal flap. II. A surgical approach for maxillary implant uncovering in cases with reduced keratinized tissue: Technique and clinical results. Int J Periodontics Restorative Dent 1999;19:385–393.
69. Pripatnanont P, Nuntanaranont T, Chungpanich S. Two uncommon uses of Bio-Oss for GTR and ridge augmentation following extractions: Two case reports. Int J Periodontics Restorative Dent 2002;22:279–285.
70. Boyne PJ. Current developments with growth factors and bone proteins. Dent Implantol Update 1999;10:25–27.
71. Jadlowiec JA, Celil AB, Hollinger JO. Bone tissue engineering: Recent advances and promising therapeutic agents. Expert Opin Biol Ther 2003;3:409–423.
72. Geesink RG, Hoefnagels NH, Bulstra SK. Osteogenic activity of OP-1 bone morphogenetic protein (BMP-7) in a human fibular defect. J Bone Joint Surg Br 1999;81:710–718.

PART

II

Bone Harvesting

CHAPTER

5 Harvesting Bone from the Ramus

Significant amounts of bone can be procured from the symphysis or ramus regions of the mandible. These mandibular bone grafts have been used with extremely favorable results for alveolar repair prior to implant placement. Mandibular cortical bone grafts provide very predictable increases in bone volume with a short healing time and yield a highly dense osseous architecture for implant placement.[1] The close proximity of the donor and recipient sites reduces the duration of surgery and anesthesia and also decreases patient discomfort and morbidity from the graft harvest.[2,3] Moreover, the surgical procedure can be performed on an outpatient basis utilizing intravenous sedation and local anesthesia. This chapter focuses on the harvesting of mandibular ramus bone for grafting.

Bone harvested from the ramus is essentially cortical in nature and thus is appropriate for augmenting areas that require block grafts for structural support rather than particulated graft material from cancellous marrow harvests. In general, the ramus yields a rectangular piece of bone approximately 4 mm thick, 3 cm or more in length, and up to 1 cm in height (Fig 5-1). This graft morphology is especially well suited for use as a veneer graft to increase ridge width from one to four tooth sites.[3] Twice this amount of bone can be obtained if it is harvested bilaterally. The ascending ramus has been used for bone augmentation before implant placement,[3-8] sinus grafting,[9,10] facial augmentation,[11,12] orthognathic surgery,[13] and immediate reconstruction following tumor resection.[14]

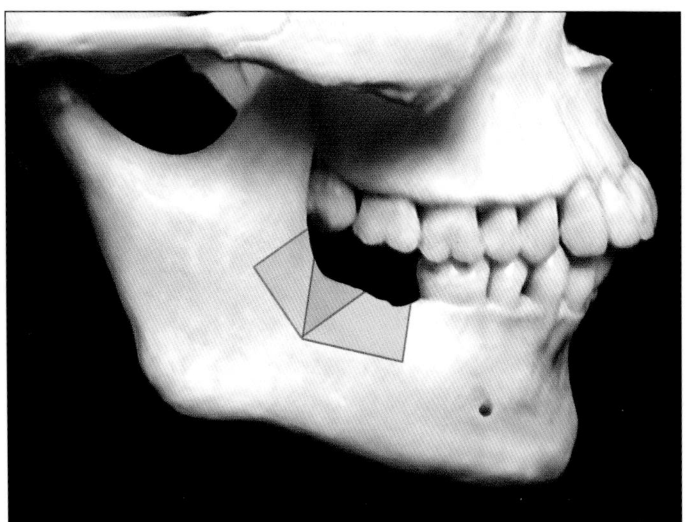

Fig 5-1
The ramus is one of the areas in the oral cavity that serves as a donor site for harvesting cortical bone. It can be used in place of or together with the anterior mandible when larger amounts of bone are needed. The area marked in red and gray represents the ideal sites for harvesting. Depending on the patient's needs, bone can be harvested from one or both of the marked areas.

Surgical Technique

The recipient site for the graft should be carefully evaluated and prepared before donor bone is harvested. This allows the surgeon to determine the size and shape of the graft required to restore ridge contour, keeping in mind that, ideally, the size of the block graft should completely restore the bone defect. It also minimizes the amount of time between graft harvest and placement (Fig 5-2).

Two key factors to consider before undertaking this technique are that *(1)* in certain patients, gaining access to the ramus can be somewhat more challenging than gaining access to the symphysis, and thus it is important to extend the initial incision to a sufficient height to reach the ascending ramus and *(2)* care must be taken to avoid injuring the neurovascular bundle.

The incision access to the ramus area for bone harvest begins in the buccal vestibule medial to the external oblique ridge and extends anteriorly and lateral to the retromolar pad. Starting the incision on the ascending ramus no higher than the level of the occlusal plane minimizes the possibility of cutting the buccal artery or exposing the buccal fat pad. The incision continues anteriorly into the buccal sulcus of the molar teeth, if present, and to the midcrestal area if the patient is edentulous in the area. The mucoperiosteal flap is then reflected from the mandibular body on the lateral aspect of the ramus. With a notched ramus retractor, the flap is elevated superiorly along the external oblique ridge to the base of the coronoid process.

The ramus osteotomy is started at the level of the occlusal plane or at a point where the ramus is adequately thick (Fig 5-3). A reciprocating saw or a no. 1702 fissure bur (Brasseler, Savannah, GA) in a straight handpiece is used to make a cut through the cortex along the anterior border of the ramus about 3 to 4 mm medial to the external oblique ridge. The osteotomy can be extended anteriorly as far as the distal aspect of the first molar. A vertical cut is then made in the mandibular body extending inferiorly from the anterior aspect of the cut. The length of this cut depends on the size of the graft required and the position of the inferior alveolar canal. The cut should be made only

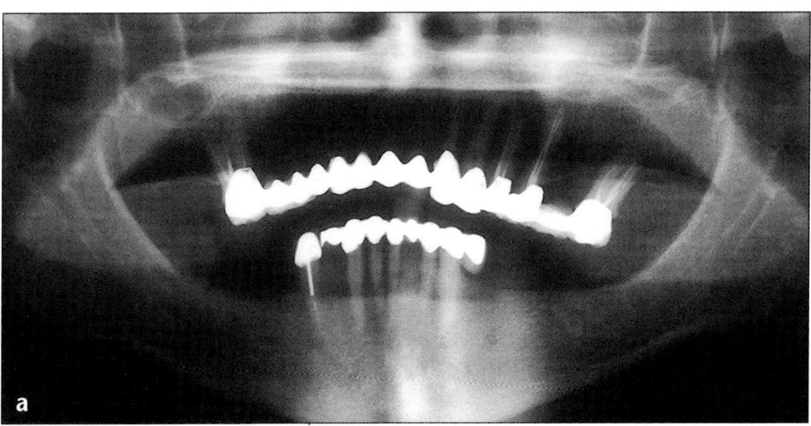

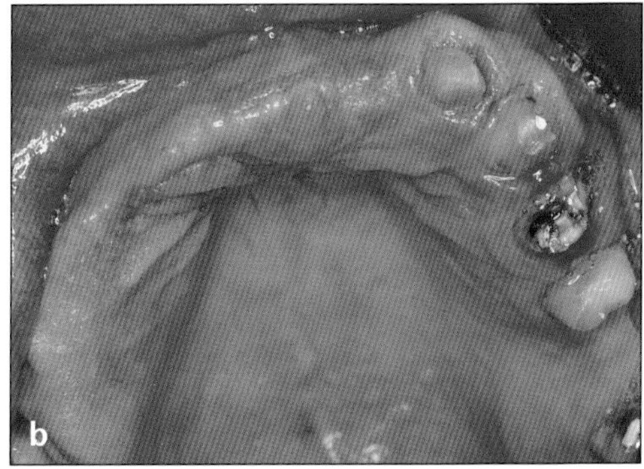

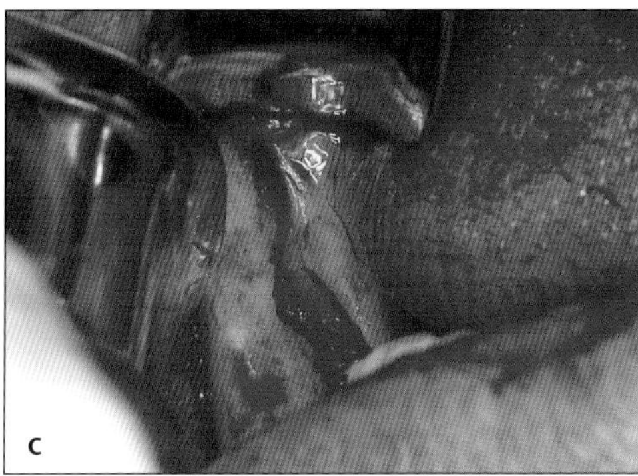

Fig 5-2 The recipient site for the graft should be carefully prepared and evaluated before donor bone is harvested.

(a) This patient is an ideal candidate for ramus bone harvesting for use in grafting of the maxilla. The fixed partial denture is failing because of the extensive unsupported pontic area. The position of the inferior alveolar nerve will permit removal of bone blocks; a chin block harvest is not indicated because of excessive tension of the orbicularis oris muscle at the lower lip and the mentalis muscle.

(b) Over time, the unilateral edentulous area that extends beyond the midline has created a buccopalatal contour deficiency that is greater than 5 mm.

(c) The incision starts over the anterior border of the ascending ramus at the level of the occlusal plane of the superior molar and continues anterior and lateral to the retromolar triangle. This incision will continue in a midcrestal fashion for an edentulous posterior mandible or intrasulcularly if molars are present. The anterior extension should provide a flap that ensures good visibility as well as working space according to the desired size of the block to be harvested.

through the cortical bone. The posterior vertical cut is made on the lateral aspect of the ramus, perpendicular to the external oblique osteotomy. The inferior osteotomy connecting the posterior and anterior vertical cuts may be performed with an oscillating saw or a no. 8 round carbide bur in a straight handpiece. Because access and visibility are limited when making the inferior osteotomy, a shallow cut can be made into the cortex, creating a line of fracture along which the bone will break once the block is tapped with a chisel.

A thin chisel is gently tapped along the entire length of the external oblique osteotomy; care should be taken to parallel the lateral surface of the ramus and to avoid inadvertent injury to the inferior alveolar nerve. A wider wedge chisel or Potts elevator may then be inserted and levered to pry the buccal segment free and to complete the splitting of the graft from the ramus. After removal of the bone graft, any sharp edges around the ramus are smoothed with a bur or file (Fig 5-4). The donor site can be quickly and easily filled

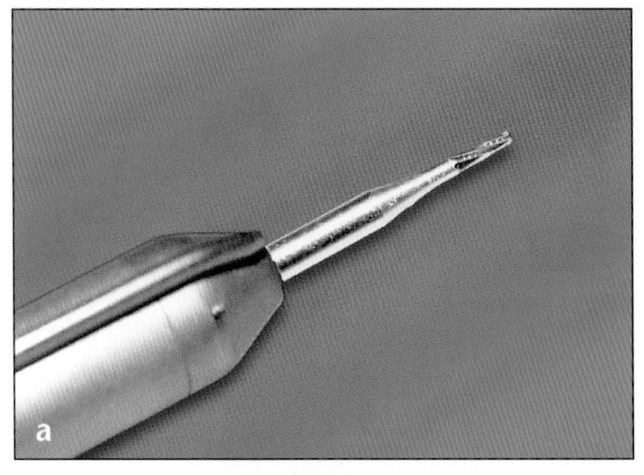

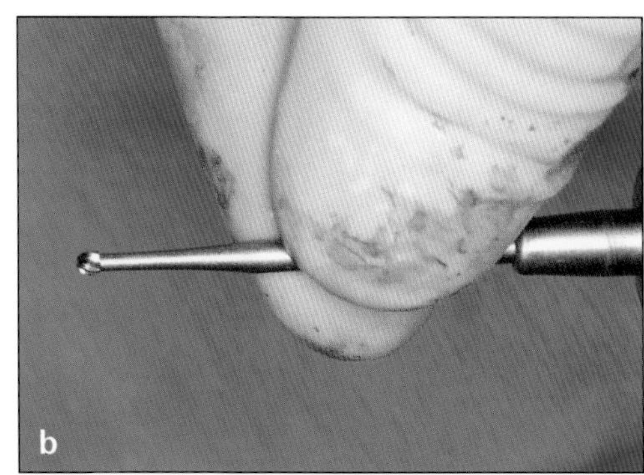

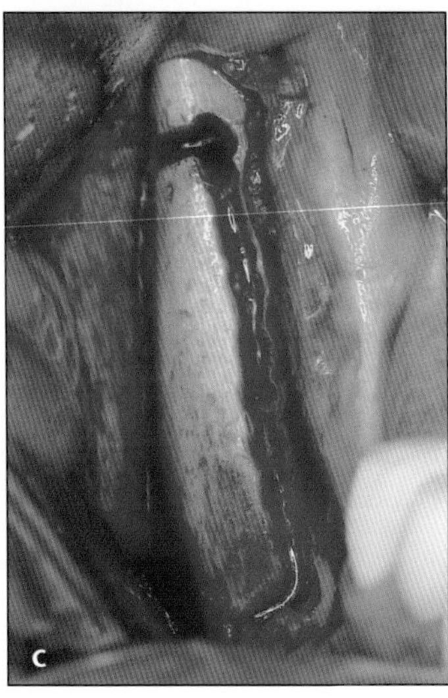

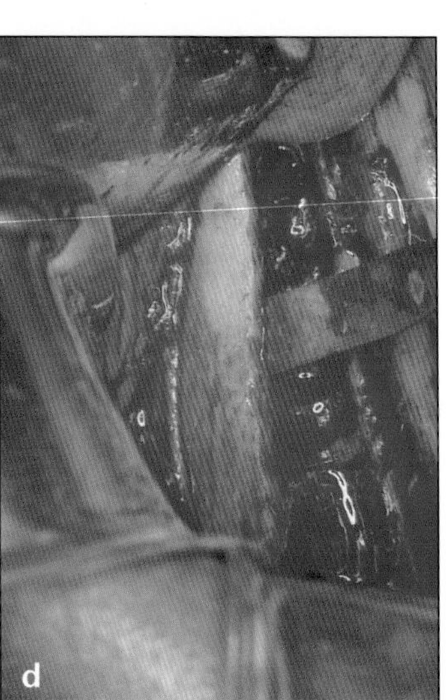

Fig 5-3 The ramus osteotomy should be started at the level of the occlusal plane or at a point where the ramus is adequately thick.

(a) A no. 1702 fissure bur in a straight handpiece provides an efficient cutting action in cortical bone.

(b) A no. 8 round carbide bur in a straight handpiece is the perfect choice for the inferior osteotomy. Because of the limited ability of the flap to stretch, the bur cannot be placed perpendicular to the lateral wall of the ramus; however, this type of bur can be used parallel to the wall, thus creating a scoring groove.

(c) The osteotomy is performed with consideration given to the size necessary to return the volume lost in the maxilla. The working area should be kept away from the lingual cortex to avoid jeopardizing the lingual nerve. The height of the block should also be determined according to the position of the inferior alveolar nerve. The superior, posterior, and anterior cuts are made with a no. 1702 bur.

(d) All surrounding tissues are retracted and protected as a chisel is slid through the superior cut. Careful, controlled tapping with a mallet on the end of the chisel will cause the graft to detach from the ramus.

with OrthoBlast II (The Clinician's Preference, Golden, CO), DBX (Musculoskeletal Transplant Foundation, Edison, NJ) or Grafton (Osteotech, Eatontown, NJ) bone putty. Primary closure of the donor site should be completed after removal and fixation of the bone graft. After the graft is harvested, it may be stored in a suitable medium, such as sterile saline or PRP; however, minimal time should elapse before it is placed in the donor site.

As noted above, it is important to prevent nerve injury when harvesting bone from the ramus. This requires knowledge of where the mandibular canal is located. Although the buccolingual position of the mandibular canal is variable, the distance from the canal to the medial aspect of the buccal cortical plate (ie, the medullary bone thickness) has been found to be greatest at the distal half of the first molar.[15] Damage to the neurovascular bundle can also

Fig 5-4 A bone block is harvested from the ramus.

(a) The space created in the ramus after block removal will heal. However, to completely regenerate without leaving any defect in the area, the space can be filled with one of the commercially available allogeneic bone putties. Alternatively, if desired, it can be filled with freeze-dried bone or reconstituted with platelet-rich plasma (PRP).

(b) The bone block is removed. The last cut (inferior) gives it a hinge-like movement as it is detached.

(c) A 3 × 1–cm block of bone has been harvested and is ready to be contoured and/or divided as needed.

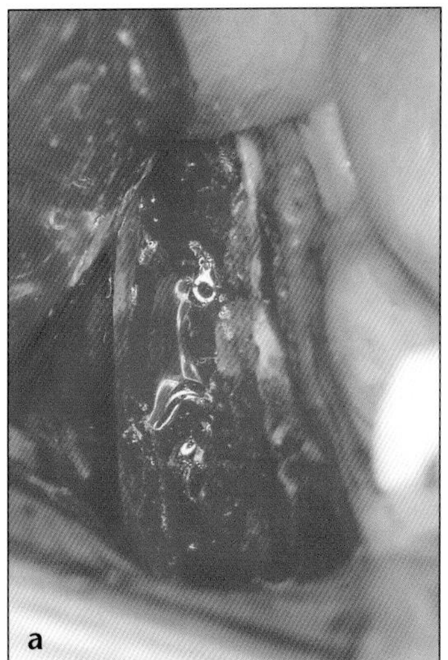

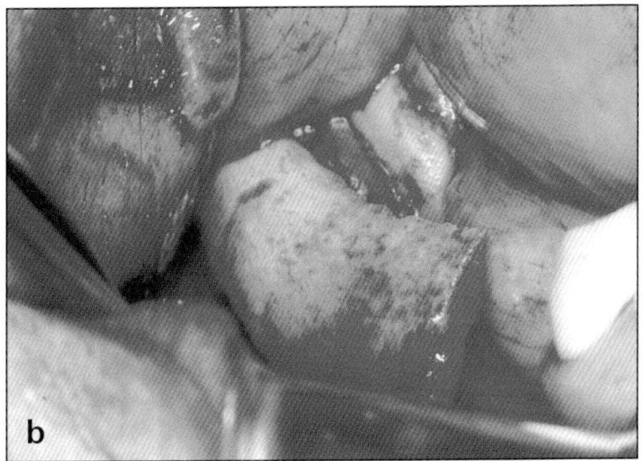

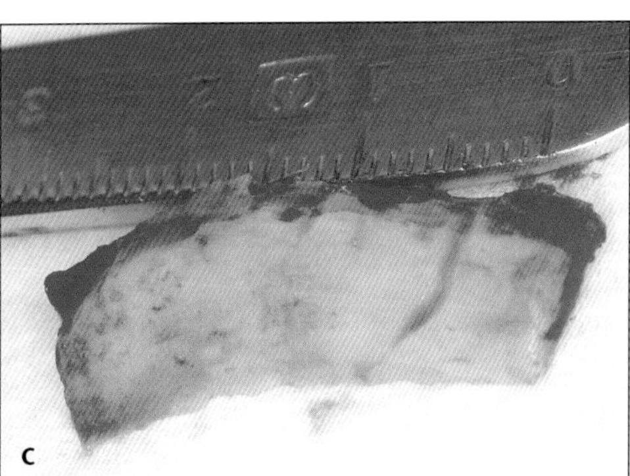

occur during graft removal. To avoid this, bone chisels should parallel the lateral surface of the ramus (Fig 5-5). If the inferior ramus cut is below the level of the inferior alveolar canal, the graft should not be separated from the donor site until the surgeon is certain that the neurovascular bundle is not trapped within it.

Before placing the bone harvested from the ramus graft, the cortex of the recipient site should be perforated to enhance revascularization, and the graft should have intimate contact with the host bone. The graft is mortised in place, and small-diameter screws are typically used for fixation. Tension-free closure is imperative because the main complication risk with onlay bone grafts is wound dehiscence with graft exposure.[1] Although barrier membranes may help minimize autograft resorption, they are not necessary with membranous cortical bone grafts because they typically exhibit minimal volume loss during healing.[7,16] The membranes may also unnecessarily increase the risk of wound dehiscence and graft infection (Fig 5-6).

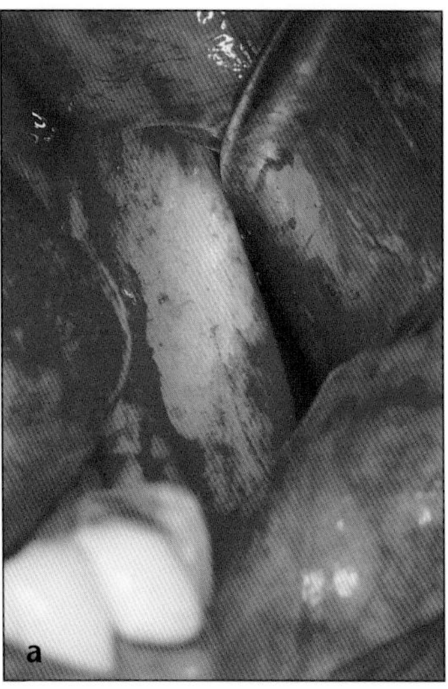
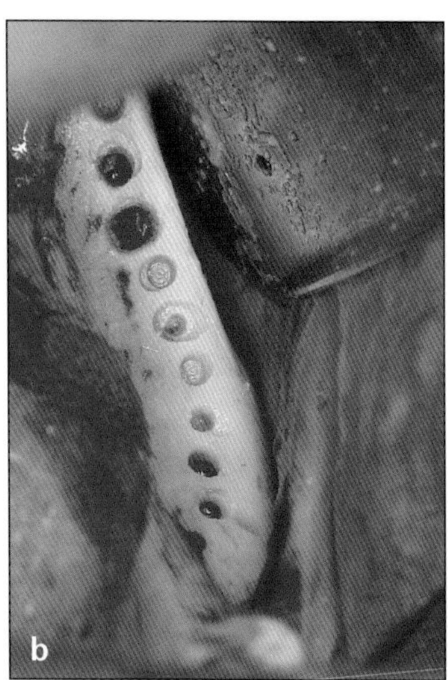
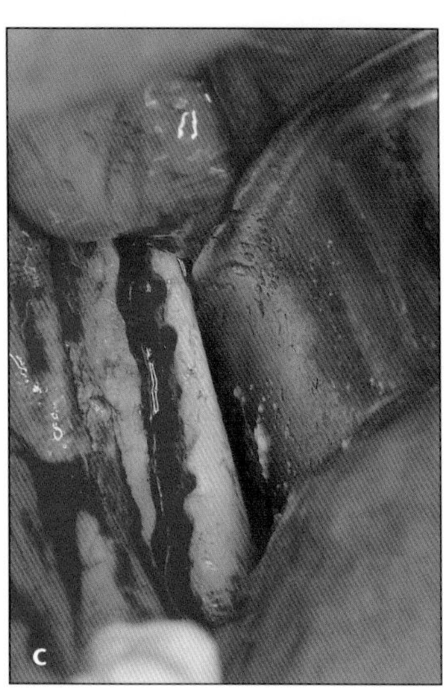
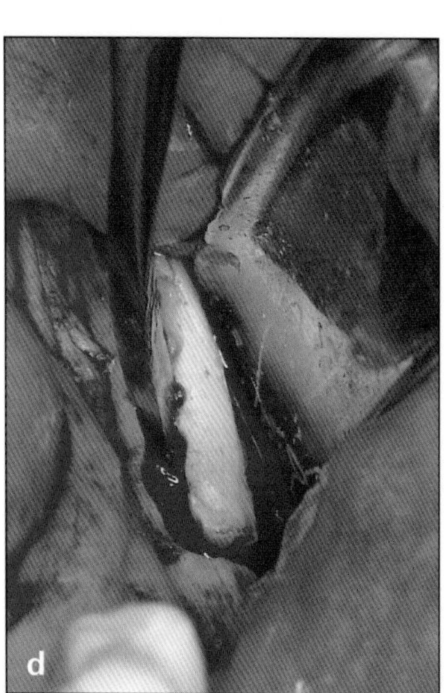
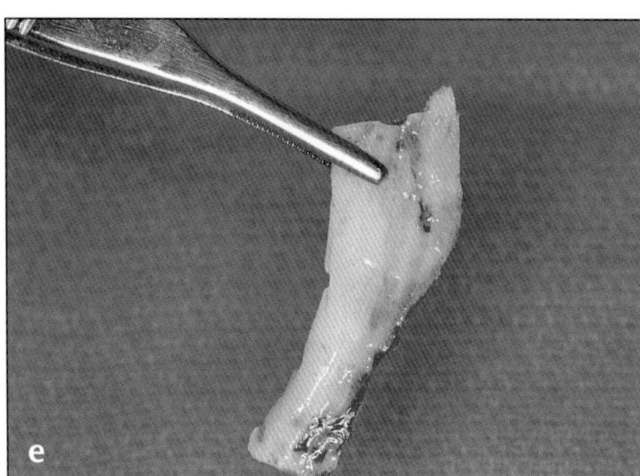
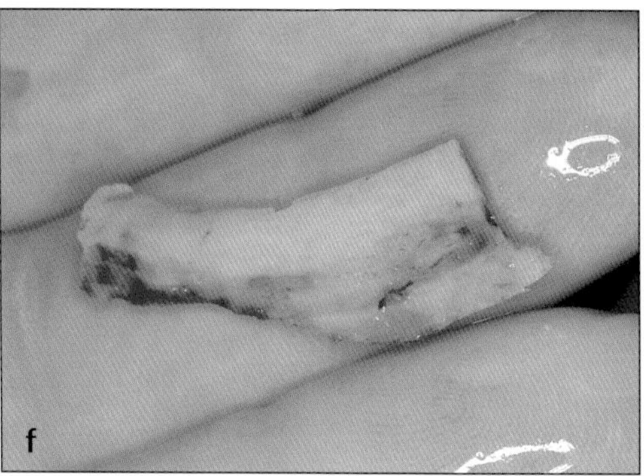

Fig 5-5 A block of bone is harvested from the left ramus (contralateral site), taking care to avoid damaging the neurovascular bundle.

(a) Access to the left ramus was obtained in a manner similar to that used on the right side: The incision was started at the occlusal level of the maxillary posterior molars and brought anteriorly, always touching the bone medial to the external oblique ridge and lateral to the retromolar pad. A wide retractor, such as the Minnesota retractor, is slid between the lateral wall of the ramus and the overlying soft tissues, separating and protecting them. At this level, the lingual tissues are also dissected from the bone just enough to help the clinician visualize the thickness of the bone.

(b) Because a larger section of bone will be harvested on this side, small perforations are made to give the clinician an idea of the potential extension of the cut before the incision is actually made.

(c) The perforations are connected using a no. 1702 Brasseler bur. This bur should cut completely through the cortical bone and into the cancellous bone.

(d) After the four cuts are made, a chisel is again slid through the superior cut. During this part of the procedure, consideration often must be given to the close proximity of the inferior alveolar canal.

(e) Cortical bone block with the inferior alveolar canal imprinted in its internal wall. The inferior alveolar neurovascular bundle was never invaded during this osteotomy procedure, which guarantees that there was no nerve damage. Whenever possible, it is best to harvest the block not only lateral to the inferior alveolar nerve but also superior to it. In this case, it was not possible to harvest superior to the inferior alveolar nerve due to limited bone available in that area.

(f) The block of harvested bone is ready to be cut and shaped to fit the recipient site.

Fig 5-6 Harvested block grafts are placed.

(a) The bone can be divided as needed to fit the recipient site, but each piece must be large enough to hold at least two screws.

(b) The harvested blocks have been cut in segments to fit the curve of the recipient maxilla. The blocks are moved around until the surgeon is satisfied with their position. Sharp edges should be removed from the periphery of the blocks to prevent soft tissue dehiscence.

(c) Once all of the blocks have been placed in their ideal positions, they are affixed one by one with at least two screws apiece to prevent rotation.

(d) The volume of bone that will be obtained from the harvested block is within an acceptable range. Because a certain degree of resorption must be expected, it is best to overestimate rather than underestimate the amount of volume needed since recontouring of the bone to reduce volume is always an option.

(e) A simple resorbable collagen membrane, which resorbs in 2 weeks, is placed over the grafted bone to retard fibrous downgrowth during initial healing. Placement of a longer-lasting resorbable membrane or even a nonresorbable membrane is necessary only if a large amount of particulate bone is placed around the blocks.

(f) The membrane fully covers the grafted area and remains immobilized as the flap is brought down without needing to be tacked down.

(g) Immediate postoperative panoramic radiograph showing the radiolucent donor sites that will gradually fill in with new bone. At the recipient site the metal screws can be observed. These will be removed during the implant placement procedure, just prior to drilling.

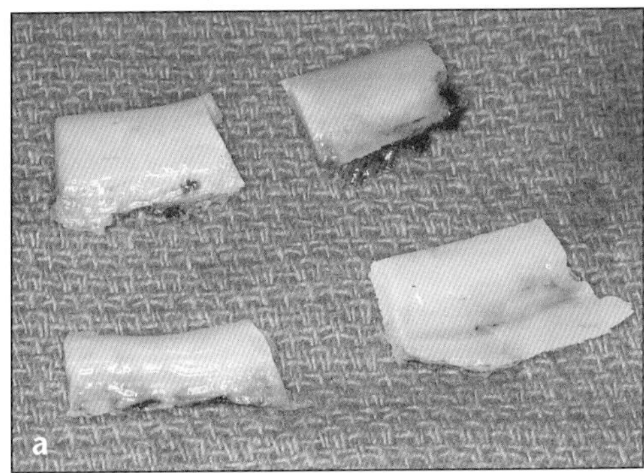
a

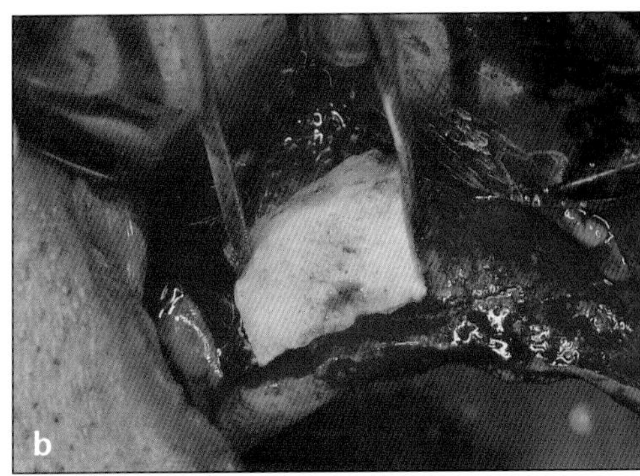
b

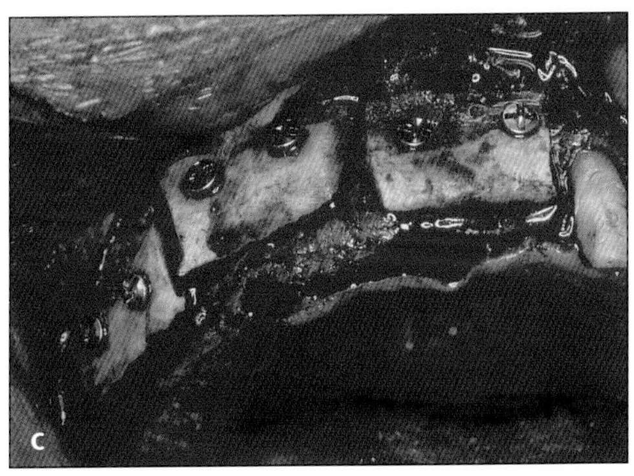
c

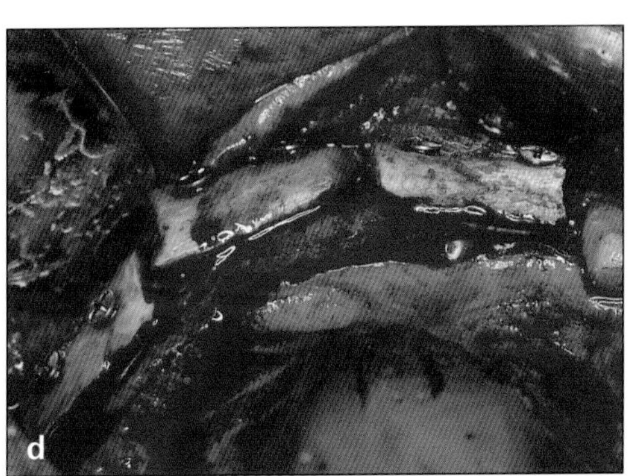
d

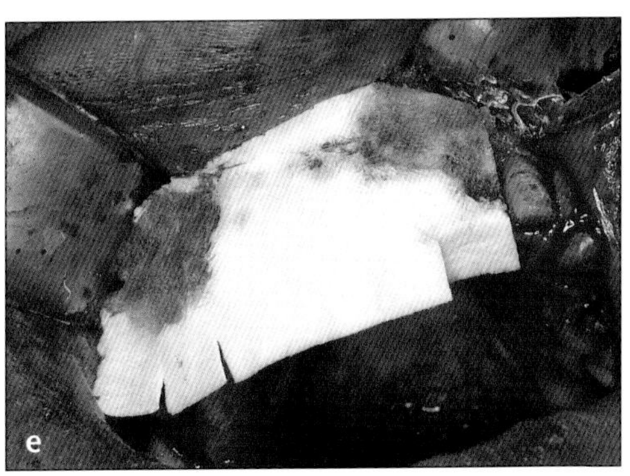
e

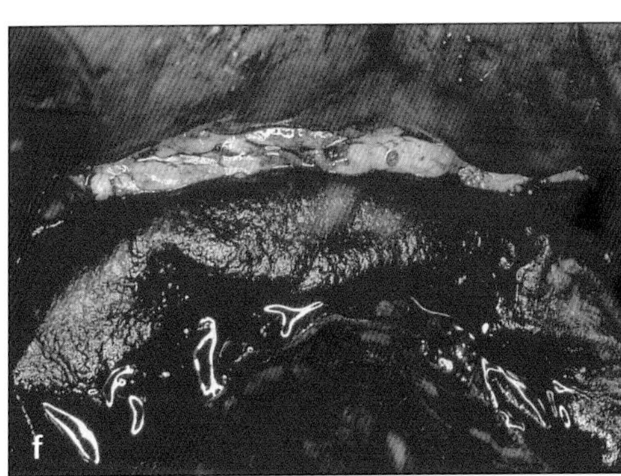
f

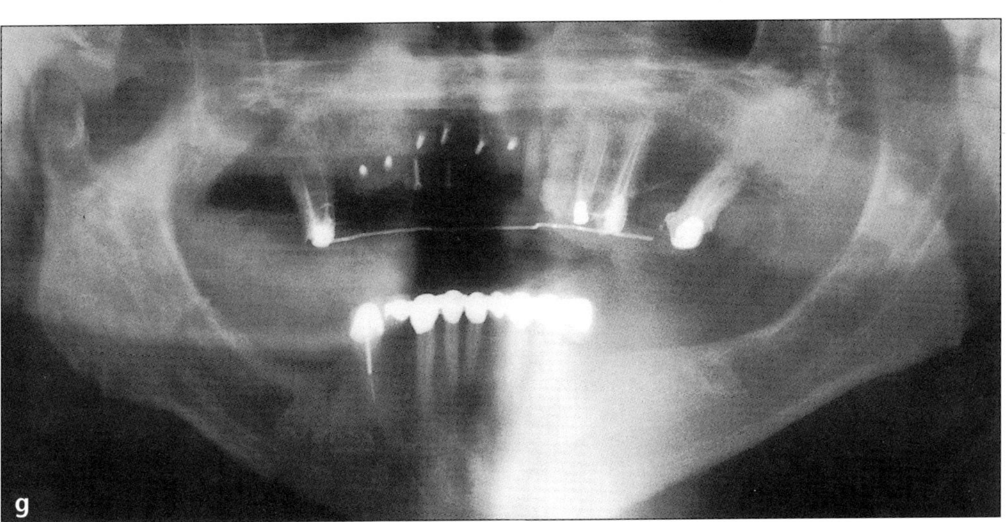
g

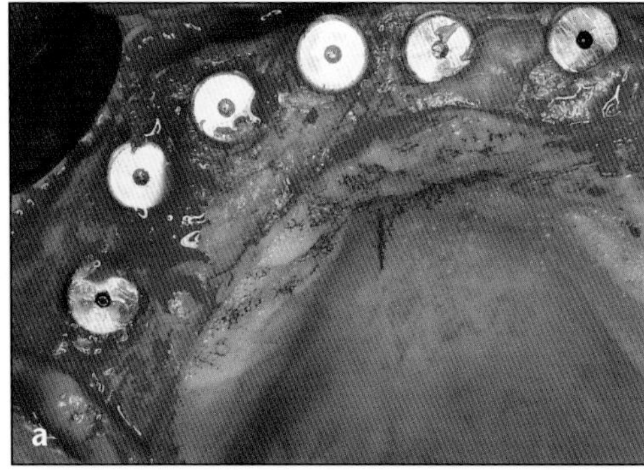
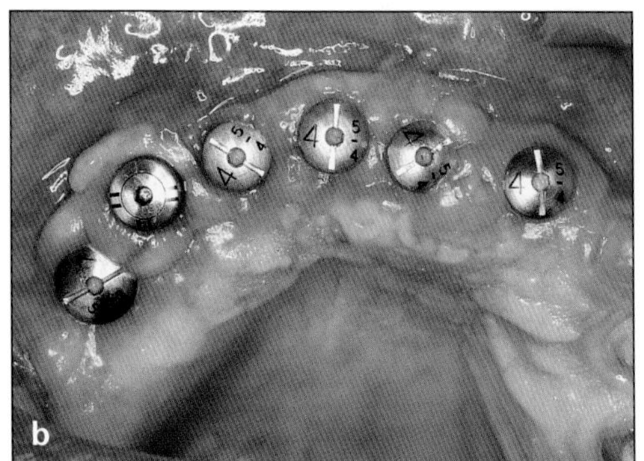
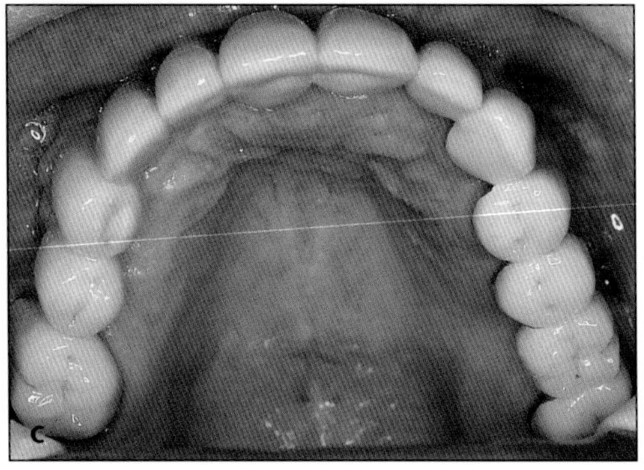

Fig 5-7 Implants are placed in the grafted area. Intraoral block grafts are generally allowed to mature for 4 months in a maxillary recipient site.

(a) The volume of bone obtained enables the implants to be placed in their correct buccopalatal position.

(b) Four months after implant placement and 1 week after stage 2 uncovering surgery, the gingiva is healing around the abutments. An acceptable amount of connective tissue surrounds each healing abutment.

(c) Final restorations supported by the implants and the natural teeth as well as an adequate arch width and height all the way around are possible when a careful treatment plan is followed step-by-step from the beginning of treatment.

Intraoral block grafts like those from the ramus are generally allowed to mature for a minimum of 4 months in a maxillary recipient site and 5 to 6 months in a mandibular site. The longer healing period for mandibular sites ensures an adequate union between the graft and the denser cortex of the host bone. A staged treatment plan in which implant placement is delayed until after graft healing is the preferred method of reconstruction (Fig 5-7).

Potential Complications

Preventing early complications following bone harvesting surgery involves using pressure dressings, topical ice packs, and anti-inflammatory drugs to reduce swelling; prescribing analgesics for pain control; and instructing the patient about the importance of meticulous oral hygiene. Edema is very common following surgery, although its intensity may vary. In most cases, swelling decreases rapidly during the first 2 days postsurgery and complete dissipation occurs within 1 week. Table 5-1 lists other potential complications, along with common reasons for their occurrence and techniques with which to minimize them.

Table 5-1 Potential complications of harvesting bone from the ramus

Complication	Cause	Preventive measures
Potential damage to inferior alveolar nerve	Coronal position of inferior alveolar nerve	Understand the anatomy of the mandibular canal. Limit the harvest to a cortical bone block and keep it coronal to the inferior alveolar nerve.
Limitation of graft size and shape	Generally, harvesting a thin cortical graft to minimize the chances of nerve damage	Take accurate radiographs and preoperative measurements to maximize the graft size while remaining in a safe zone.
Incision dehiscence in donor area	Postoperative edema, hematoma, poor closure of donor site	Use ice packs and anti-inflammatory drugs and consider corticosteroids postoperatively to minimize edema; graft the donor site; and suture the donor site soft tissue carefully.
Postoperative trismus	Excessive trauma during harvesting to muscle fibers attached to the coronoid process	Minimize stripping of the flap superiorly beyond the area required for bone harvest.
Potential damage to lingual nerve during flap incision	Incision placed midcrestally or lingually in area of retromolar pad	Understand the anatomy of the lingual nerve path; make the incision over the retromolar pad area buccal to the midcrestal area.

References

1. Misch C. The use of ramus grafts for ridge augmentation. Dent Implantol Update 1998; 9:41–44.
2. Sindet-Pedersen S, Enemark H. Reconstruction of alveolar clefts with mandibular or iliac crest bone grafts. A comparative study. J Oral Maxillofac Surg 1990;48:554–558.
3. Misch CM. Comparison of intraoral donor sites for onlay grafting prior to implant placement. Int J Oral Maxillofac Implants 1997;12:767–776.
4. Misch CM. Ridge augmentation using mandibular ramus bone grafts for the placement of dental implants: Presentation of a technique. Pract Periodont Aesthet Dent 1996;8: 127–135.
5. Buser D, Dula K, Hirt HP, Schenk RK. Lateral ridge augmentation using autografts and barrier membranes: A clinical study with 40 partially edentulous patients. J Oral Maxillofac Surg 1996;54:420–433.
6. Buser D, Dula K, Belser UC, Hirt HP, Berthold H. Localized ridge augmentation using guided bone regeneration. II. Surgical procedure in the mandible. Int J Periodontics Restorative Dent 1995;15:10–29.
7. Jensen J, Sindet-Pedersen S, Oliver AJ. Varying treatment strategies for reconstruction of maxillary atrophy with implants. Results in 98 patients. J Oral Maxillofac Surg 1994;52: 210–216.
8. Collins TA. Onlay bone grafting in combination with Brånemark implants. Oral Maxillofac Surg Clin North Am 1991;3:893–898.
9. Wheeler SL, Holmes RE, Calhoun CJ. Six-year clinical and histologic study of sinus-lift grafts. Int J Oral Maxillofac Implants 1996;11: 26–34.
10. Lundgren S, Moy P, Johansson C, Nilsson H. Augmentation of the maxillary sinus floor with particulated mandible: A histologic and histomorphometric study. Int J Oral Maxillofac Implants 1996;11:760–766.

11. Heggie AA. The use of mandibular buccal cortical grafts in bimaxillary surgery. J Oral Maxillofac Surg 1993;51:1282–1283.
12. Jensen J, Reiche-Fischel O, Sindet-Pedersen S. Autogenous mandibular bone grafts for malar augmentation. J Oral Maxillofac Surg 1995;53: 88–90.
13. Braun TW, Sotereanos GC. Autogenous regional bone grafting as an adjunct in orthognathic surgery. J Oral Maxillofac Surg 1984;42:43–48.
14. Muto T, Kanazawa M. Mandibular reconstruction using the anterior part of ascending ramus: Report of two cases. J Oral Maxillofac Surg 1997;55:1152–1156.
15. Rajchel J, Ellis E 3rd, Fonseca RJ. The anatomical location of the mandibular canal: Its relationship to the sagittal ramus osteotomy. Int J Adult Orthodont Orthognath Surg 1986;1: 37–47.
16. Marx RE. The science of reconstruction. In: Bell WH (ed). Modern Practice in Orthognathic and Reconstructive Surgery. Philadelphia: Saunders, 1992:1449–1452.

CHAPTER

6 Harvesting Bone from the Mandibular Symphysis

The mandibular symphysis is a good source for procuring smaller grafts, such as those generally used for implant procedures.[1,2] The anterior mandible offers either a block or a particulate configuration of bone. In a block configuration, the symphysis can typically provide a sufficient amount of bone for increasing width deficiencies by 4 to 7 mm, length deficiencies by 15 to 20 mm (about one to three teeth), and height deficiencies by 10 mm. Studies on cadavers suggest this site can yield an average block of 21 × 10 × 7 mm or more.[3,4] Although the ascending ramus may provide more graft material, the mandibular symphysis provides a block graft with more cancellous bone than do other intraoral sites.[5] Unlike the ramus, which studies have shown is a viable source for autogenous bone for ridge augmentation procedures,[6–9] the symphysis yields corticocancellous particulate material in addition to a block graft. As a donor site, the anterior mandible offers moderate to relatively low morbidity[10] and minimal graft resorption following placement.[11–16] This autogenous source has been used successfully to restore many types of defects, including Class III ridge defects (both vertical and buccal bone loss) in the anterior maxilla and other locations (as a block configuration)[17–21] and for sinus elevations (as a particulate configuration).[11,22–29]

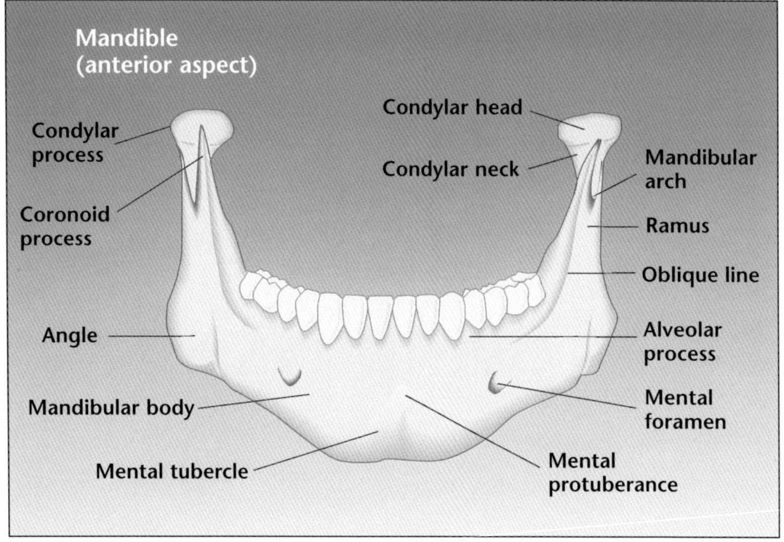

Fig 6-1
Before attempting block graft harvesting from the mandibular symphysis, the clinician should have extensive knowledge of the anatomic landmarks of the mental area (including the inferior alveolar nerve path and anterior loop, mental foramen, incisive nerve, and mandibular width) as well as the probable anatomic variations from case to case.

Biology of the Mandibular Symphysis As a Donor Site

An understanding of the biologic, mechanical, and topographic aspects of the mandible is essential for proper evaluation of the structure as a source of autologous bone grafts (Fig 6-1).[30–33] The most popular graft donor sites are chosen for their cancellous cellular density or for their block configuration to provide structural support. Harvested endosteal osteoblasts and cancellous marrow stem cells must be transferred to the jaw in a viable state and placed into tissue that has sufficient vascularity to diffuse nutrients to the cells before revascularization. New capillaries can then bud into the graft to form a more permanent vascular network. The osteocompetent marrow cells are quite resilient, capable of living outside natural bone for at least 4 hours without losing more than 5% of their viability if stored appropriately.[14]

Cortical membranous grafts revascularize more quickly than endochondral grafts, contain denser cancellous elements,[34] and resorb considerably less.[35–37] This fact may explain why chin grafts, which consist primarily of cortical bone with few osteogenic cells, show good incorporation, less volume loss, and shorter healing times than grafts from the ilium. The biochemical similarity between bone from the mandibular symphysis and the maxillofacial region may partly explain this superior incorporation.[14] Although some research suggests that there is little difference in results when chin or iliac crest grafts are used[38] and that use of the iliac crest results in generally low morbidity,[39] a histologic study comparing maxillary bone grafts with either ilium or chin donor material also revealed a better bone quality result when chin grafts were used.[18]

Using the mandibular symphysis as a donor site allows the clinician to operate in the same field as the recipient site. This ability is often an important benefit to patients, particularly those who are only

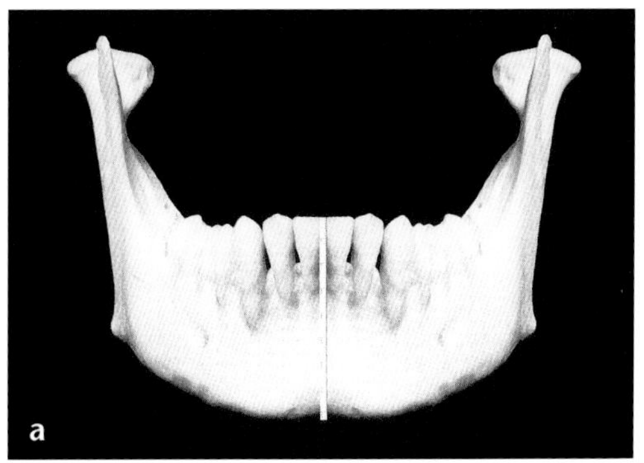

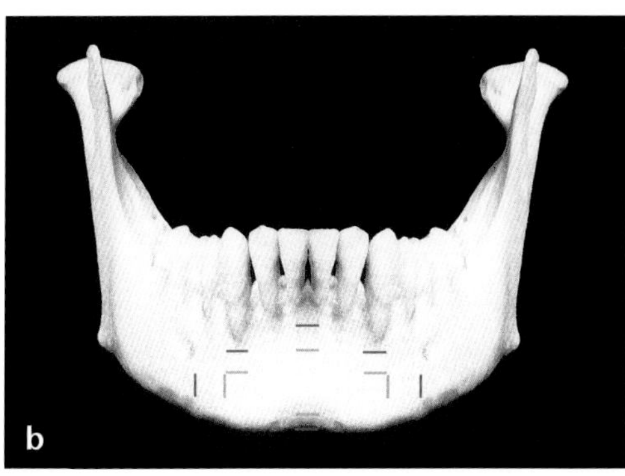

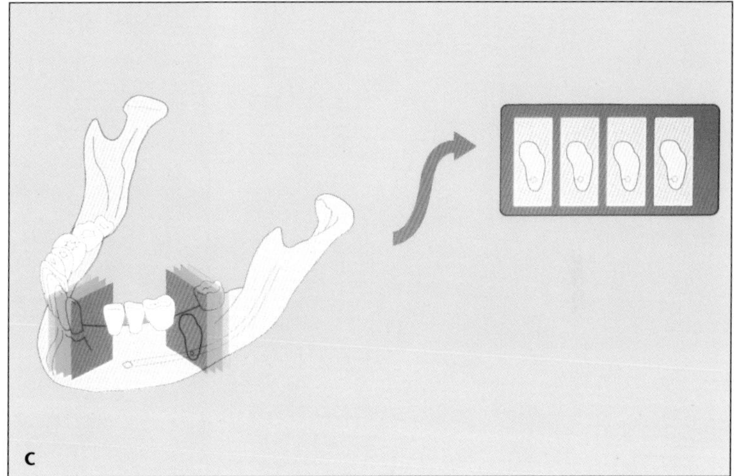

Fig 6-2
(a) Accurate measurements of the apices of the anterior mandibular teeth must be obtained through methods such as periapical radiographs, so that safety markings can be made prior to harvesting bone from the anterior mandible.

(b) Panoramic, periapical, and lateral cephalometric radiographs help establish the working space for bone harvesting, enabling the clinician to avoid tooth apices, the mental foramen, and the mandible's inferior border. Using radiographs, the vital structures to avoid can be measured and marked as indicated in red. The green marks indicate the periphery of the safe zone for harvesting.

(c) Determining the shape and thickness of the anterior mandible at the level where the bone blocks will be taken is essential. A sagittal view with a simple lateral cephalometric radiograph can aid in assessing shape and thickness, along with palpation of the buccal and lingual walls. Computed tomography scans can help determine bone thickness in cases with limited harvesting area.

partially edentulous. Although cutaneous scarring is eliminated with an intraoral donor site, some patients raise concerns about chin deformation. Deformation is not ordinarily a problem with the procedure, but the clinician may take additional steps to prevent it by placing a fill material at the donor site. Chin ptosis can also be avoided if the clinician takes care not to completely deglove the mandible and, most importantly, if he or she sutures the tissues back to their original position.

Many patients do experience reduced sensitivity in the chin or anterior mandibular teeth following procurement from the mandibular symphysis. These effects are typically minimal and eventually disappear, but patients must be informed about this possibility.[40,41] Such sensory changes may be caused by a stretching of the mental nerve or by a disruption of the incisive canal contents, even when an appropriate border depth is maintained below the apices of the anterior tooth roots during chin bone harvesting.[11,18] Proper procurement technique, as described in the next section, minimizes this risk, as does careful patient selection (Fig 6-2).

Patients who are not good candidates for using the mandibular symphysis as a graft donor site include *(1)* those whose mandibles exhibit long anterior tooth roots; *(2)* those who have inadequate mandibular height or width for sufficient graft procurement; and *(3)* those who have a defect exhibiting gross vertical loss or who require width augmentation that spans more than four teeth.

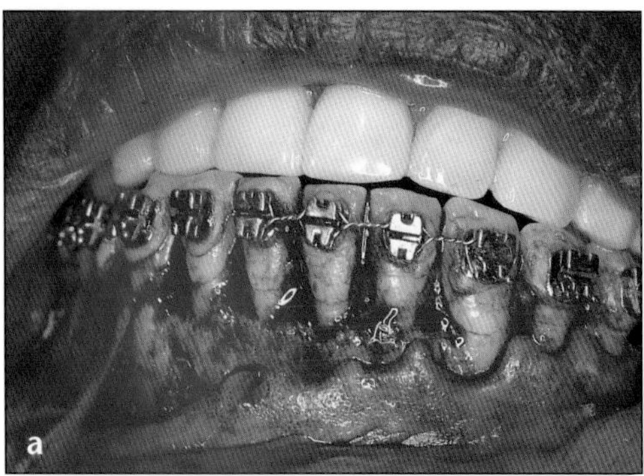

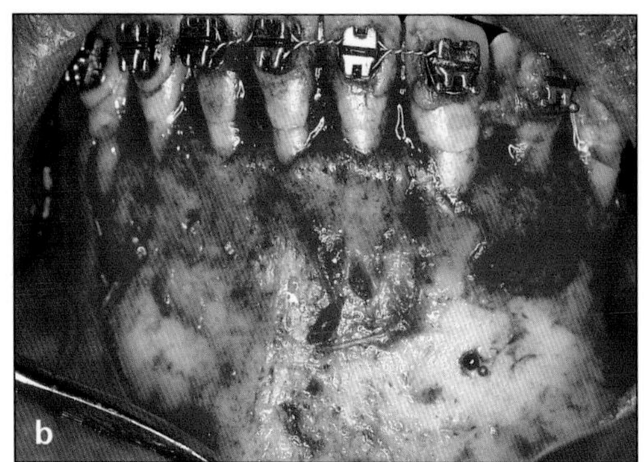

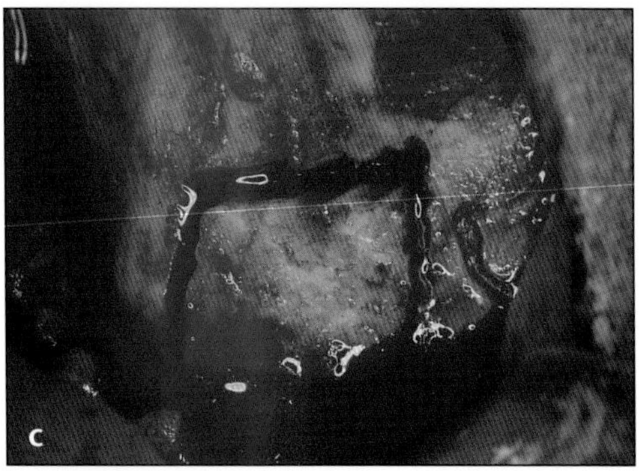

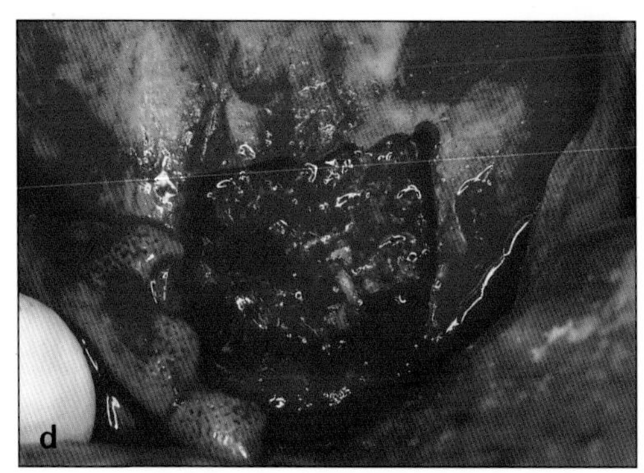

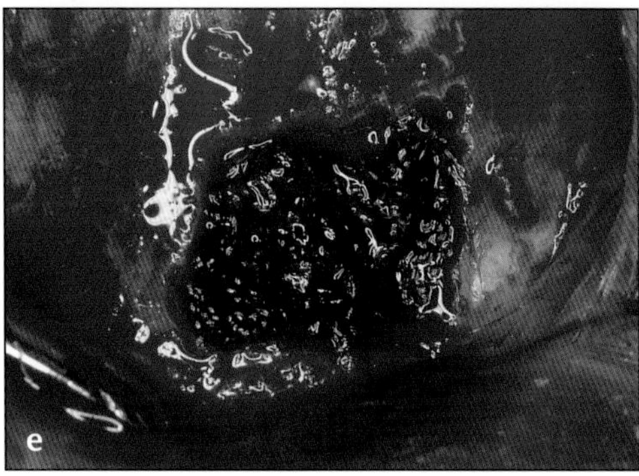

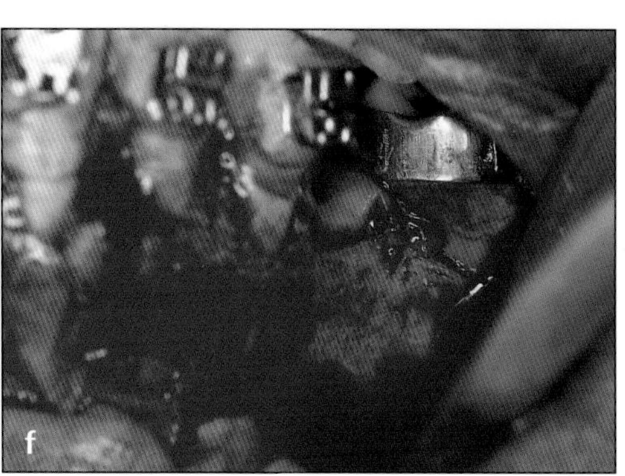

Fig 6-3 The intrasulcular method is indicated for patients with a low vestibule, a tense mentalis posture, and a donor site free of abnormal periodontal circumstances.

(a) An intrasulcular incision is used for this patient, who has thick, flat papillae and broad tooth contacts, requiring a bone graft to an adjacent area (the left posterior mandible). Here, access can be gained to both the donor and recipient sites with one flap. The mental nerve should be protected during flap reflection.

(b) The flap is reflected to expose the donor and recipient sites, to provide adequate visualization of the surgical sites, and to minimize harm to the flap during graft harvesting.

(c) A template created at the recipient site is used to cut an appropriate-sized block at the donor site.

(d) After the block is removed, additional cancellous marrow can be harvested with a no. 2 Molt curette (G. Hartzell & Son, Concord, CA).

(e) After removal of the necessary cancellous marrow, the donor site is packed with Avitene (MedChem Products, Woburn, MA) for hemostasis and then later with a bone putty or allogeneic graft material.

(f) The recipient site is the area of the missing mandibular left first molar. The ridge width is inadequate for implant placement and requires grafting to augment it.

Methods for Harvesting Monocortical Bone Blocks from the Mandibular Symphysis

The clinician obtains the chin bone graft from below the apices of the mandibular incisors and canines. Panoramic and lateral cephalometric radiographs should be taken so that the clinician can evaluate the donor site; he or she must locate the mental foramen as well as determine the form and size of the anterior teeth and the volume of bone available for harvesting. The anteroposterior dimension of the anterior mandible should be determined on a lateral cephalometric radiograph. Additionally, periapical radiographs can be used to

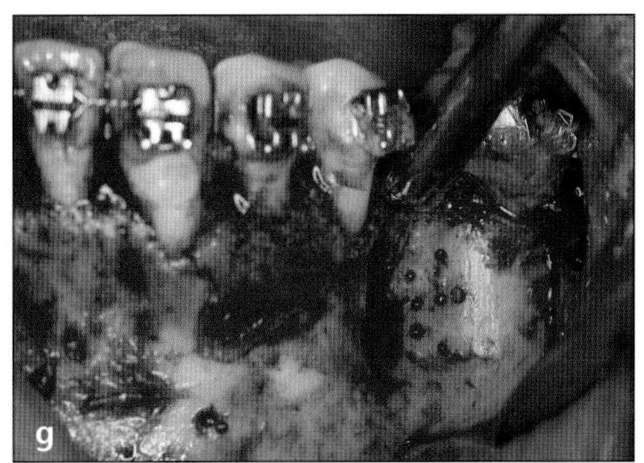

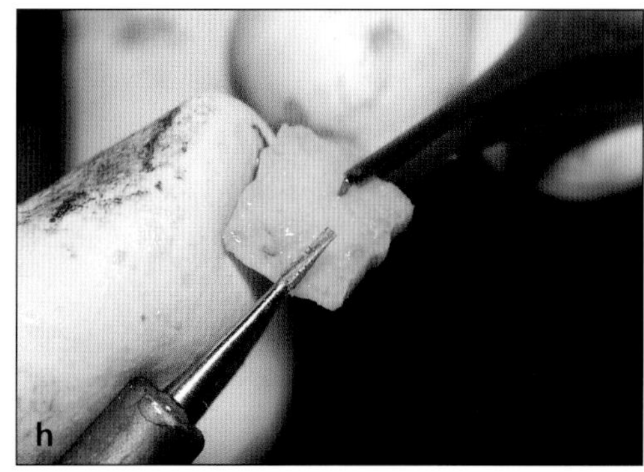

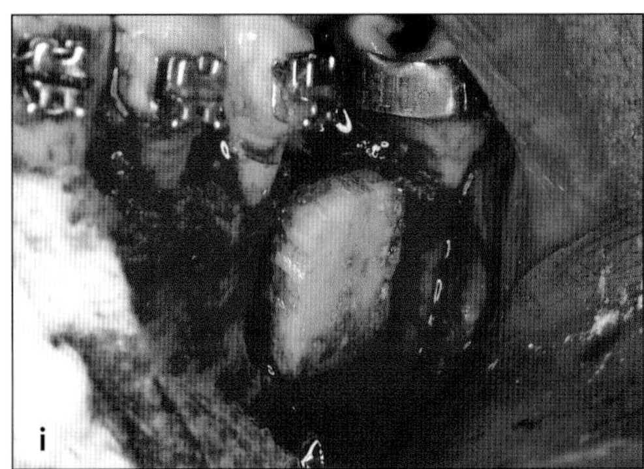

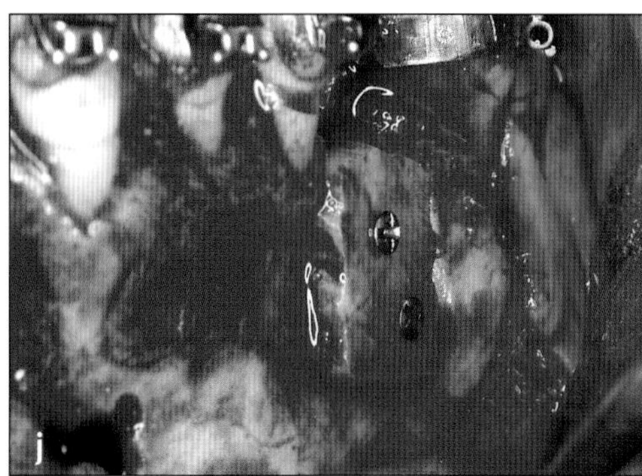

Fig 6-3 *(cont)*
(g) The recipient site is shaped to accommodate the block and perforated with a small drill to add bleeding points for the release of endosteal osteoblasts for optimal bone maturation.

(h) The harvested block is shaped and modified to provide for optimal fit in the defect.

(i) The block graft is set in place to ensure proper fit before stabilization and the creation of fixation screw holes.

(j) The block is fixed in place with screws. The small voids are mortared with particulate graft. Graft material can then be placed in the donor site, and the area is ready for flap replacement and suturing.

determine the measurements of the mandibular tooth roots. It is also important for the clinician to evaluate the recipient site before obtaining the donor material. This evaluation allows the clinician to assess the amount of donor bone needed, to carefully plan the incision and flap reflection design, and to identify any unforeseen complications that preclude harvesting the bone graft. Local anesthesia includes bilateral mandibular blocks of 0.5% bupivacaine with 1:200,000 epinephrine and 2% lidocaine with 1:100,000 epinephrine or articaine with 1:100,000 epinephrine, which are locally infiltrated in the labiobuccal vestibule.

There are three incision options for accessing the donor site, depending on the mandible's musculature and the periodontal status of the mandibular anterior teeth.[42,43] Each has distinct indications, advantages, and disadvantages.

Intrasulcular Method

This straightforward method is indicated for patients with a low vestibule, a tense mentalis posture, and a donor site free of abnormal periodontal circumstances. An intrasulcular incision is made on the facial aspect of the anterior mandibular teeth, as far distal as the canines. A full-thickness flap and the fibrous periosteal layer are then reflected apically to expose the anterior surface of the mentum. The advantages of this incision method include minimized bleeding and trauma and facilitated flap retraction. Disadvantages include suturing difficulty as well as possible recession and loss of bone at the alveolar crest resulting from surgical trauma and loss of periosteal blood supply to part of the facial plate, which can occur if the bone labial to the teeth is thin enough to eliminate marrow space between the cortical bone plates (Fig 6-3).[44]

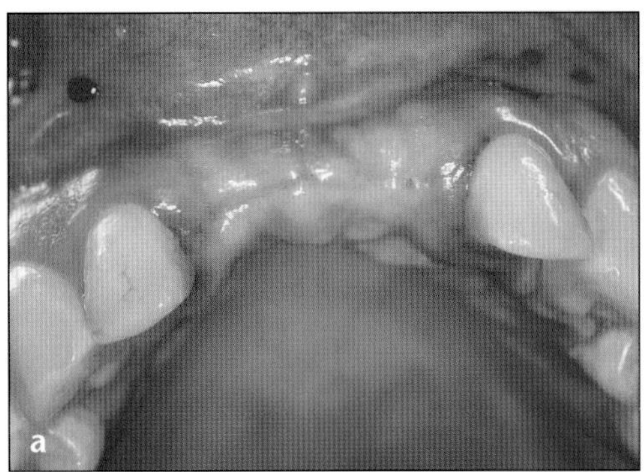

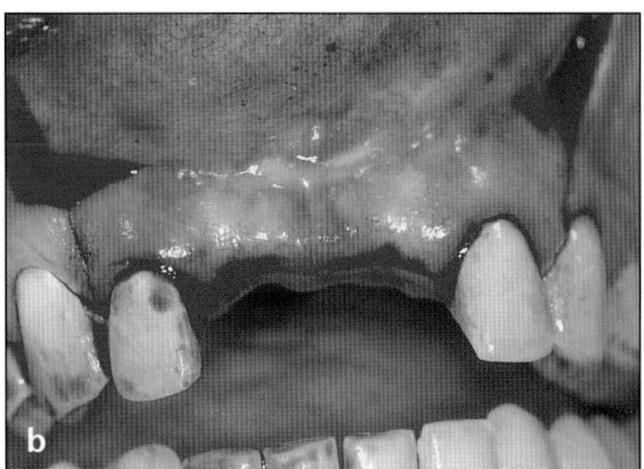

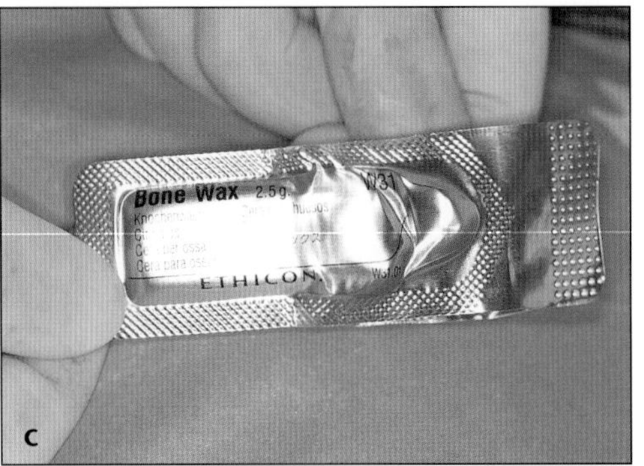

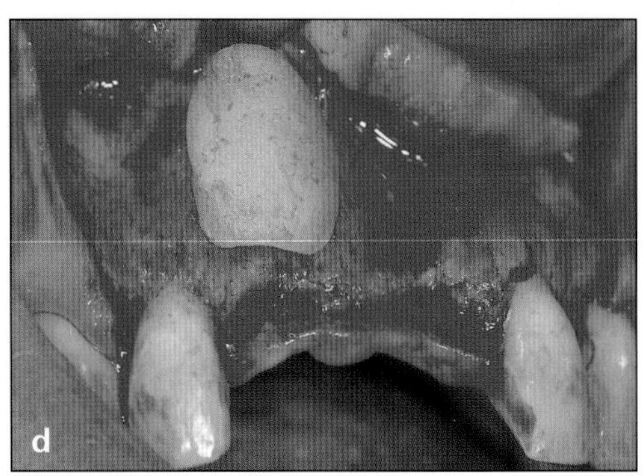

Fig 6-4 The vestibular method is indicated when there is marginal inflammation or existing alveolar bone loss around the incisors.

(a) Two maxillary central incisors and part of the alveolar ridge have been lost as a result of trauma. There is insufficient bone to accommodate dental implants.

(b) A midcrestal incision is made at the edentulous area; vertical incisions to release the flap are made distal to the lateral incisors.

(c) Bone wax, available in sterile packages, is ideal to mold over the bone defect and for hemostasis.

(d) Bone wax can be shaped over the deficient anterior maxilla to help assess the amount of bone volume needed. The bone wax mold can then be used at the donor site as the template for harvesting a bone graft of the correct size and shape.

Vestibular Method

The vestibular method is indicated when there is marginal inflammation or existing alveolar bone loss around the incisors. A vestibular incision is made in the alveolar mucosa 5 mm or more apical to the mucogingival junction between the premolars. Avoiding the mental nerve bundles is crucial to the success of this method; a blunt dissection can be used to uncover the bundles if needed. Limiting the distal extent of the vestibular incision to the canine area can also reduce the incidence of temporary mental nerve paresthesia.[13] Reflection of a full-thickness flap exposes the donor site after the clinician makes an incision apicolingually in the direction of the bone and through the mentalis muscle.[44]

The advantages of this incision method include no interference with the gingiva surrounding the anterior mandibular teeth, no mentalis muscle detachment (thus facilitating accuracy when repositioning it), reduced risk of facial ptosis, closer proximity of the intact part of the periosteum to the donor site, better lateral access, and ability to use a two-step suturing approach (first the muscle, then the mucosal tissues). Disadvantages include greater challenges associated with the initial shallow incision site and the need for subsequent blade redirection,[19] more bleeding and edema, and invisible scarring (Fig 6-4).

Fig 6-4 *(cont)*
(e) The bone wax mold (surgical template) is placed at the ideal position for harvesting bone. It can be moved before perforations are made to mark the size of the bone block needed. Note that a vestibular incision is used in this case.

(f) The initial perforations to guide the final cuts are made with a no. 1701 cylindrical bur (Brasseler, Savannah, GA). Corrections to the size and shape of the block can still be made at this crucial step.

(g) With the same no. 1701 bur, the final perforations in the bone are connected to outline the block. All of the cuts are made with the bur placed perpendicular to the bone, except the anterior vertical one, which should be made with the bur at a 45-degree angle to facilitate the process of sliding in the chisel and lifting up the block.

(h) The bone block is carefully chiseled out and easily extracted if the osteotomy is deep enough (the complete active part of the bur) and the entire outline, even the corners, is cut completely.

(i) Avitene, a hemostatic agent that consists of easily handled collagen fibers, is used to control bleeding.

(j) Once hemostasis has been achieved, the donor site can be sutured.

(k) Bone blocks are placed at the recipient site and fixed with titanium screws. The flap should be properly dissected to separate the mucosa from the periosteum and thus permit tension-free coverage of the grafted area.

(continued)

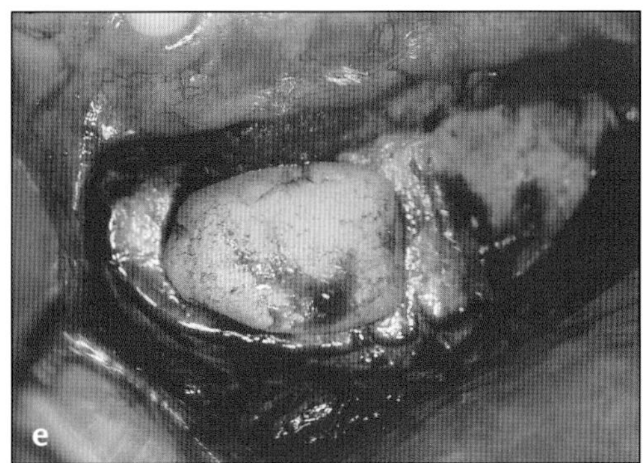

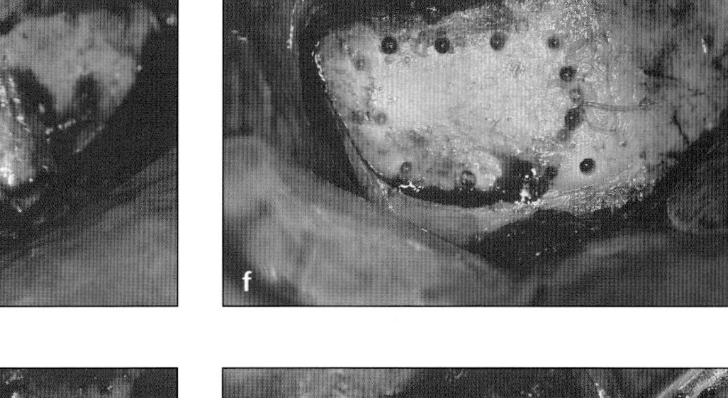

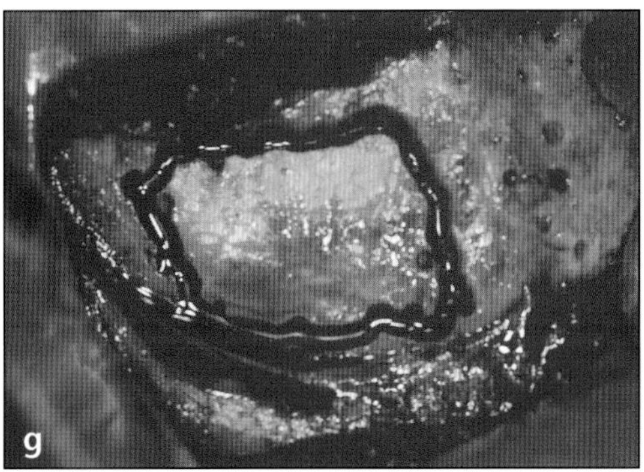

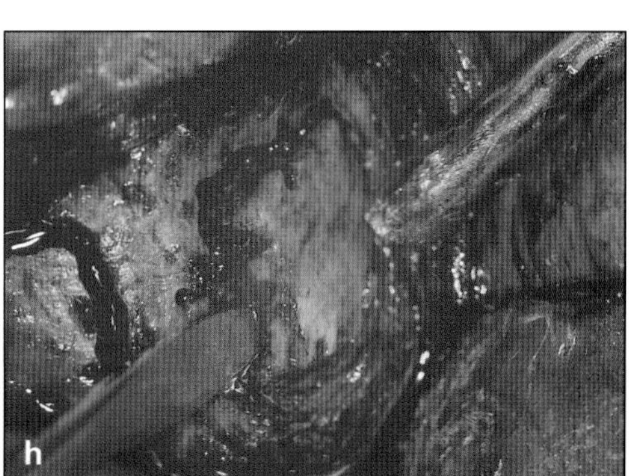

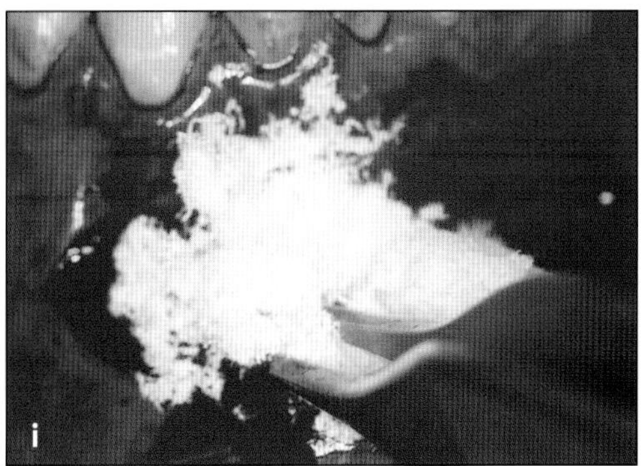

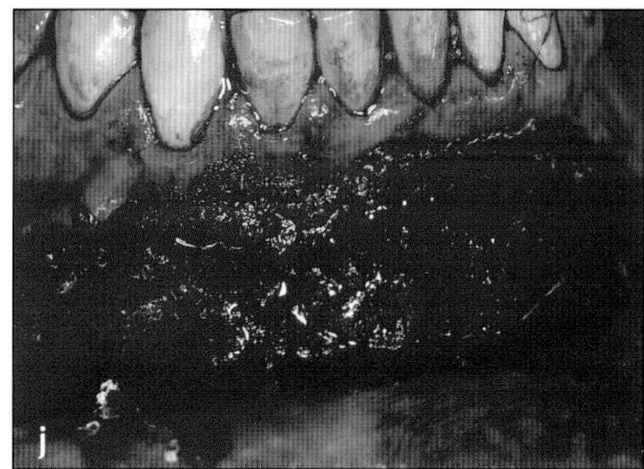

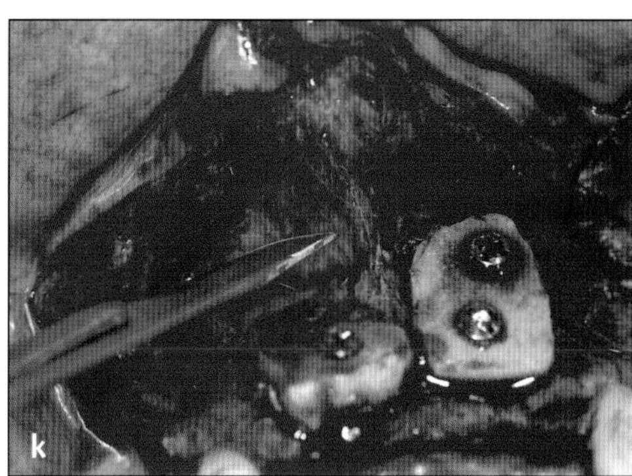

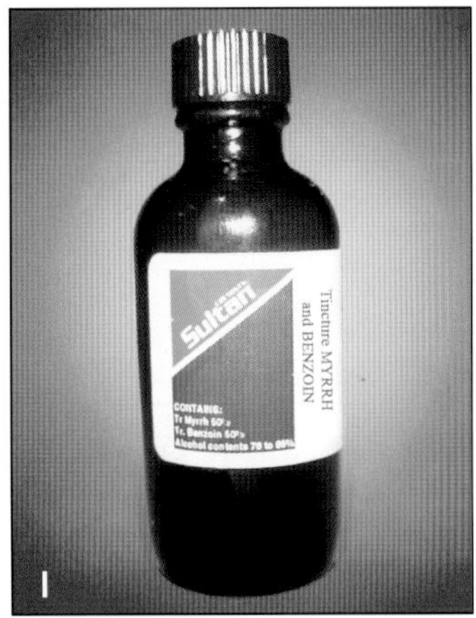

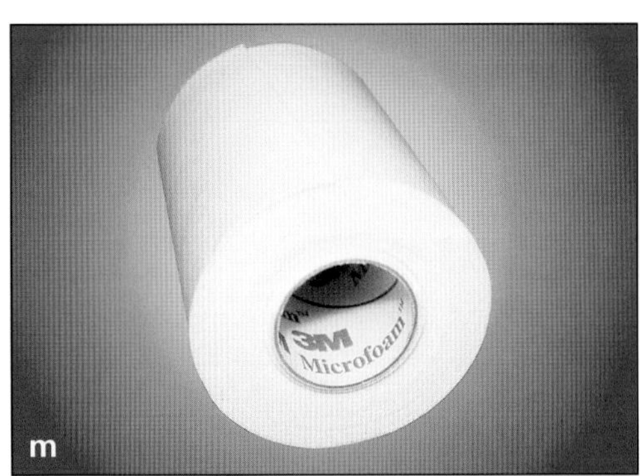

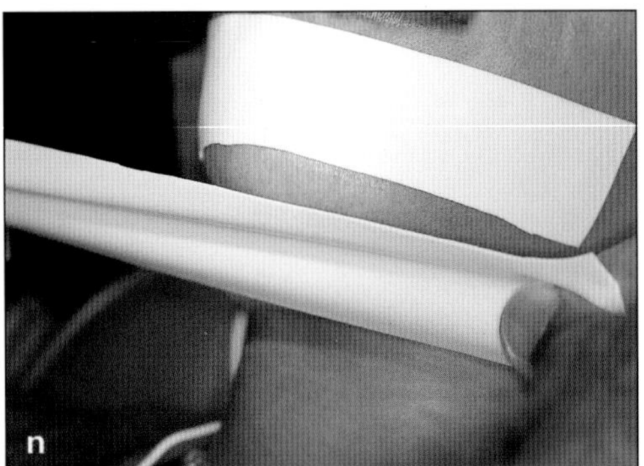

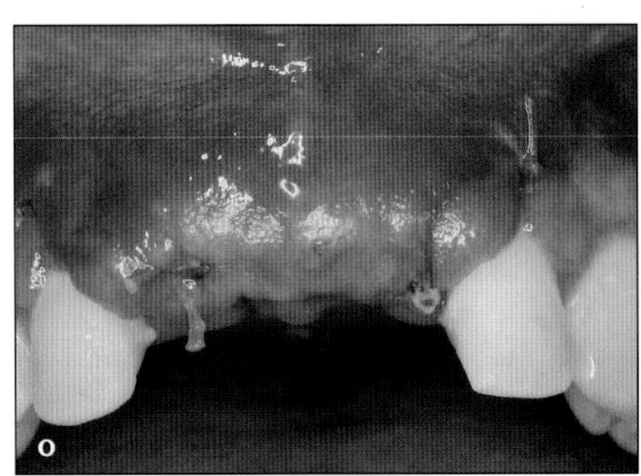

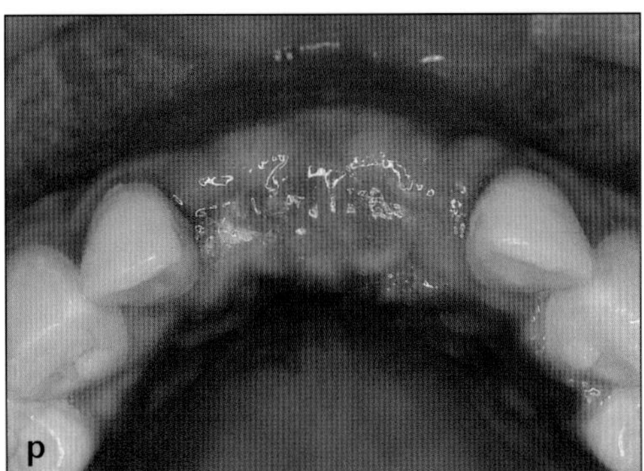

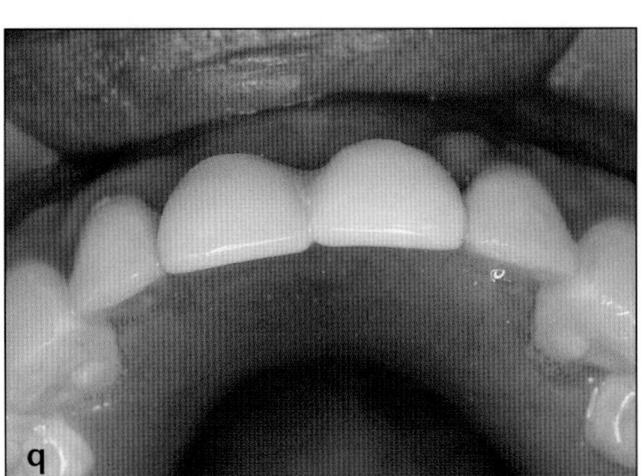

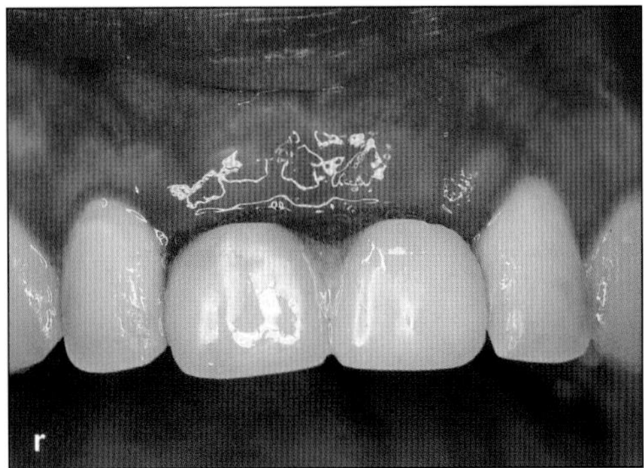

Fig 6-4 *(cont)*
(l) To aid adhesion and minimize irritation from the adhesive, the skin of the mental area is painted with tincture of myrrh and benzoin prior to applying the adhesive surgical dressing.

(m, n) A stretchable microfoam tape is ideal to help keep the soft tissues of the mental area together. The stretchable dressing is placed with one strip pulled back underneath the lower lip and another pulled upward from below the chin.

(o) A 1-week postsurgical view of the grafted site shows that the sutures have not yet been removed and that some swelling persists. The tension-free flap provides perfect coverage with no dehiscence.

(p) A 1-month postsurgical view shows a perfect continuation of ridge contour that will permit the placement of two dental implants.

(q) A provisional acrylic removable partial denture is delivered to the patient as an interim prosthesis.

(r) The provisional partial denture is adjusted so that pressure is exerted over the grafted area, helping ensure integration of the grafts. Ideally, the prosthesis should provide acceptable esthetics and function without compromising graft integration.

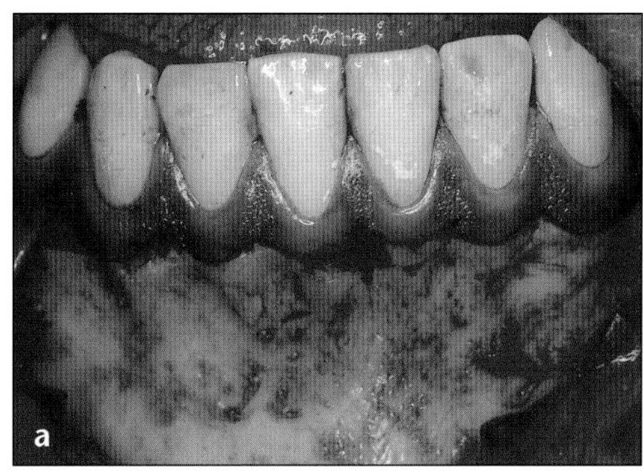

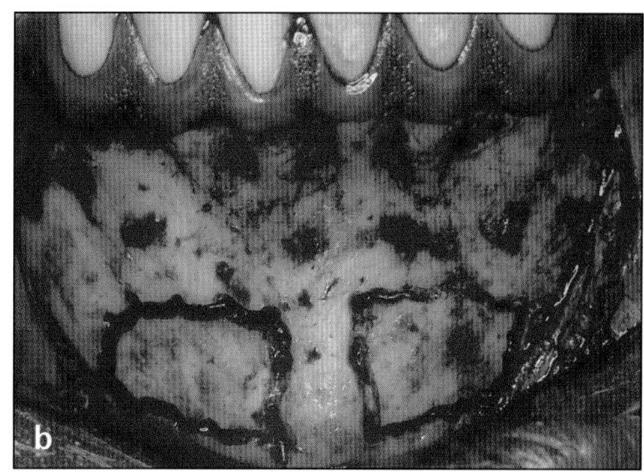

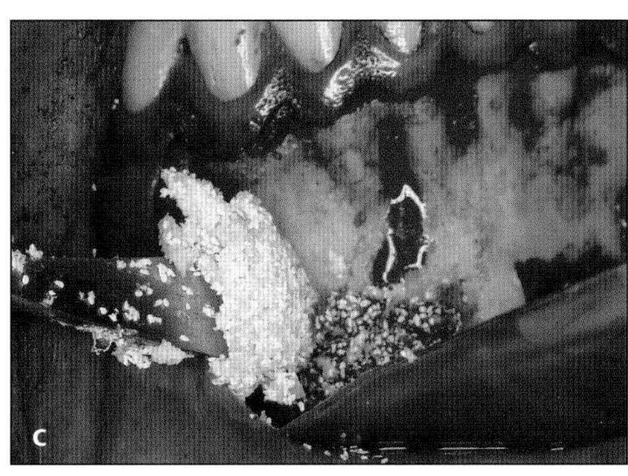

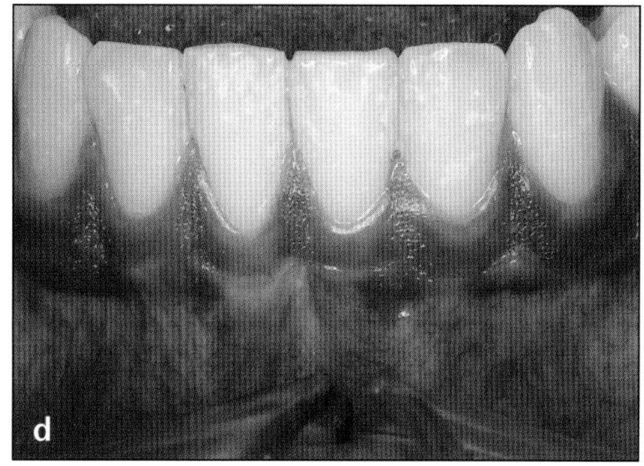

Fig 6-5 The attached gingival method is indicated when at least 3 mm of keratinized gingiva is present and there is some flexibility in the placement of the incision.

(a) The incision can be made within attached gingiva that is more than 3 mm wide. Precise flap reflection with a sharp periosteal elevator totally denudes the bone but does not damage the soft tissues.

(b) The completed osteotomy reveals that the roots of the mandibular incisors can be avoided by using a surgical marker to indicate their location.

(c) The donor sites are filled first with Avitene for hemostasis and then with a graft material (Grafton [Osteotech, Eatontown, NJ] mixed with an alloplast) to facilitate faster and more complete bone regeneration.

(d) Retraction of the lower lip reveals a barely visible scar after 1 month. The incision made at the attached gingiva preserves the original architecture of both gingiva and bone.

Attached Gingival Method

Indications for this method include at least 3 mm of keratinized gingiva and a thin scalloped periodontium, which would potentially have blunting of the papillae with an intrasulcular incision or, in cases with a high frenum, which would be incised with a vestibular incision design. The advantages of the attached gingival incision include prevention of gingival recession or blunting of the papillae, less bleeding and trauma, easier retraction and suturing, and reduced loss of crestal bone as compared to intrasulcular or vestibular incision designs. The main disadvantage of this method is a negligible scar and the requirement for precise postsurgery suturing with fine sutures (Fig 6-5).

Using this method, an incision is carried out in the attached gingiva 3 mm below the gingival margin. It extends from the distal of the first premolar to the distal of the contralateral first premolar with no vertical releasing incisions. The flap is reflected and the mental foramen identified and exposed to prevent damage to the mental nerve from the extension of bone block. The flap should be reflected to 3 mm above the inferior border of the mandible. Once the bone is harvested, and the donor site filled with a bone putty, the flap is replaced, and pressure is applied with gauze soaked in sterile saline. After it is verified to have been repositioned to its original location, the flap is sutured using 5-0 Prolene suture material (Ethicon, Somerville, NJ).

Harvesting for Particulate Grafting

After the symphysis is exposed and the mental foramina are located, a trephine drill should be used to obtain a cylindrical segment of graft material. The depth, of course, is limited by the thickness of the mandible at the harvest sites. The general parameters of the donor site are 5 mm from the inferior border of the chin, 5 mm from the apex of the dentition, and 5 mm anterior to the mental foramen.[19]

The drill is positioned 4 to 5 mm below the apices of the anterior teeth, penetrating the cancellous bone at approximately 50,000 rpm under copious irrigation.

Using continuous drilling with a 4.0-mm-diameter trephine bur, the clinician inserts the drill, being extremely careful during the initial penetration through cortical bone. The bur will tend to jump considerably during this time, and if not properly controlled, it can damage the adjacent soft tissue flap. The core of the bone is broken off at its apex by inserting the drill to its full length and canting it slightly; a small hemostat, cotton pliers, or tissue forceps can then be used to remove the core from the donor site.[15] Alternatively, osteotomes may be used to free the core(s) of bone, and the cancellous bone can be harvested with a no. 2 Molt curette. The bone core harvest includes the facial cortical plate and the attached trabecular bone. A rongeur, an osteocrusher device, or a mini-bone mill can be used to particulate the bone cores as needed.[21] The procured and particulated graft material should be stored in a medium such as sterile saline until placement and should be placed in the recipient site as soon as possible after harvesting.[14]

The inferior border of the mandible should be left intact, and the lingual cortex should not be perforated. Complications such as loss of the airway and excessive bleeding can occur if the clinician perforates the vascular region under the inner cortex.[15] Appropriate allogeneic or alloplastic graft material can be packed into the donor site to restore the defect, and a resorbable collagen membrane can then be placed over the graft material, if desired. Closing the donor-site soft tissue commences once bleeding is under control. Avitene, Surgicel (Johnson & Johnson, New Brunswick, NJ), or platelet-rich plasma (PRP) can be added to the graft material being placed into the donor site if needed for hemostasis. The site should be sutured immediately to reduce possible contamination of mental osseous tissue (Fig 6-6).[12]

Fig 6-6 Bone is harvested from the interior mandible and particulated for immediate use as a graft material.

(a) A patient undergoes intravenous sedation, which is generally required when bone is harvested from the anterior mandible.

(b) Local anesthesia should contain epinephrine for hemostasis, especially when the incision is made through the mentalis muscle.

(c) A 4-mm-diameter trephine bur will provide good-sized cores containing both cortical and cancellous bone when used at the correct depth.

(d) Retraction of the surrounding tissue is essential when drilling with an extremely sharp rotary device such as a trephine bur. A steady grip of the handpiece prevents the bur from jumping when contacting the bone. Copious irrigation with saline solution protects the bone cells from high-temperature friction.

(e) The cores of bone are harvested with the trephine bur. The osteotomies can connect or, as shown, can be made with bone between them. Some trephine burs are designed with markings to control depth. In this case a depth of 8 to 10 mm is generally adequate to ensure a good bone cylinder.

(f) The core of the bone is broken off at its apex by inserting the drill to its full length and canting it slightly; a small hemostat, cotton pliers, or tissue forceps can then be used to remove the core from the donor site.

(g) An assessment of the amount of bone collected should accompany drilling; if more is needed, graft material can also be harvested from the septa between osteotomies with sharp rongeurs.

(h) Removing septal bone from between the trephined osteotomies with the rongeurs will leave a larger defect at the donor site, but harvesting particulate bone this way is safe as long as prescribed anatomic parameters are respected.

(continued)

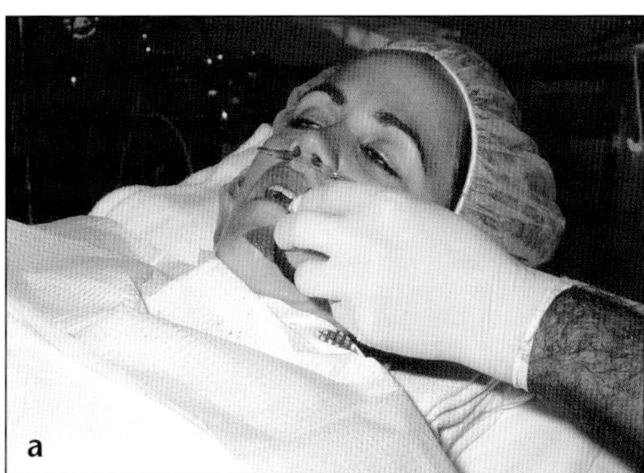
a

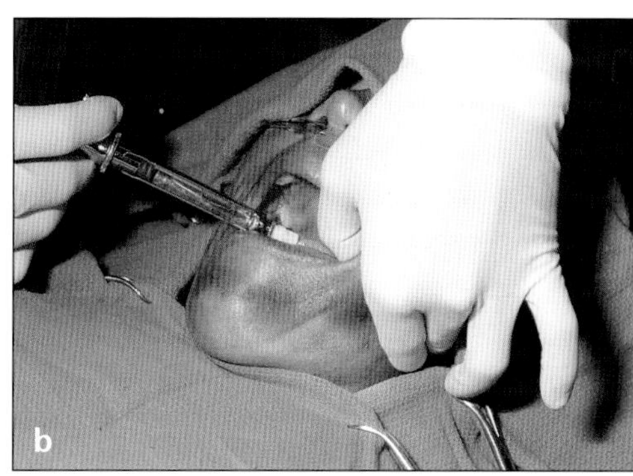
b

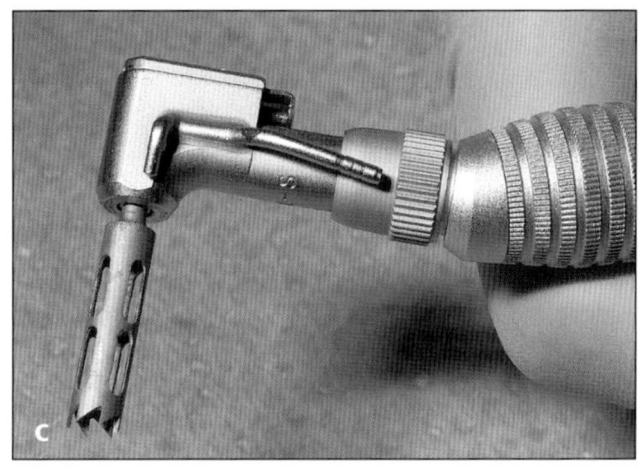
c

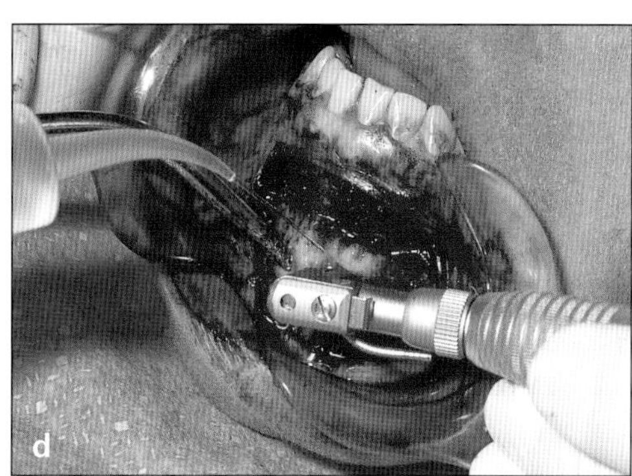
d

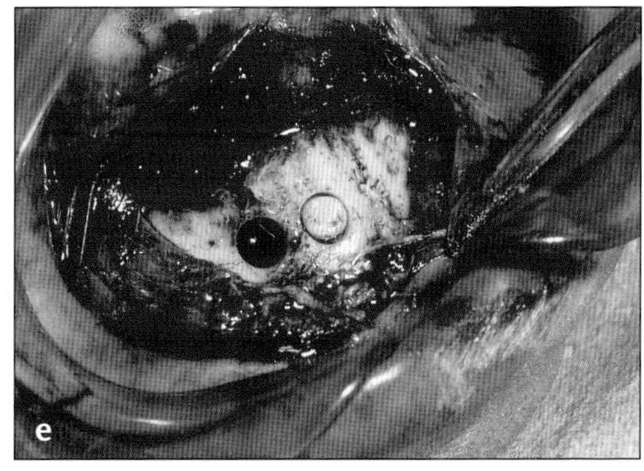
e

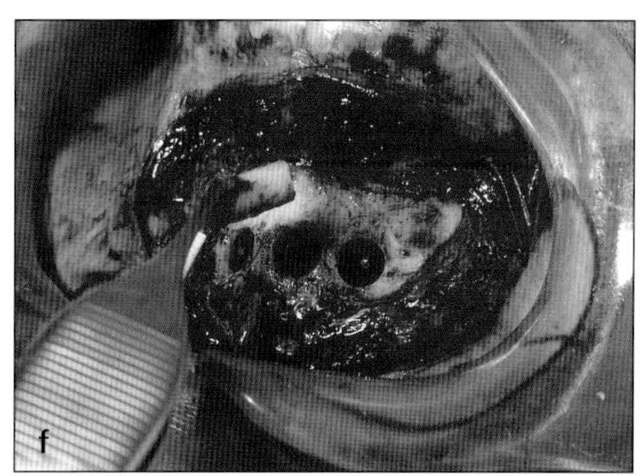
f

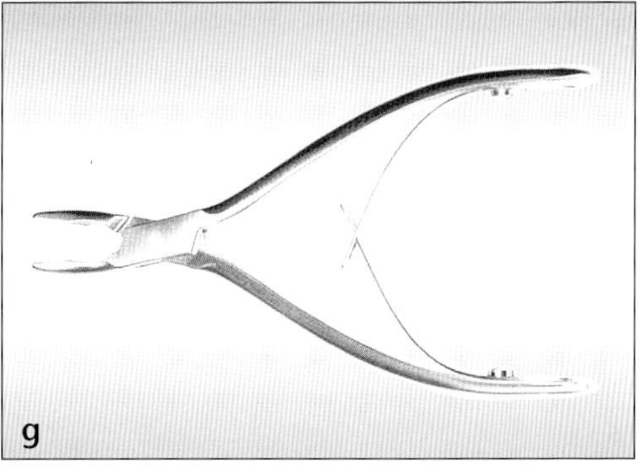
g

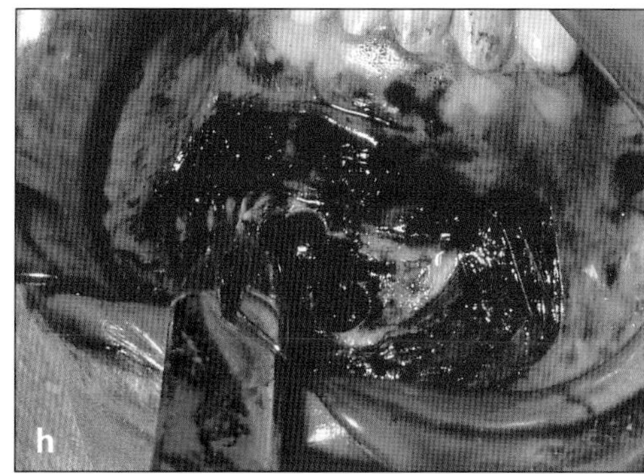
h

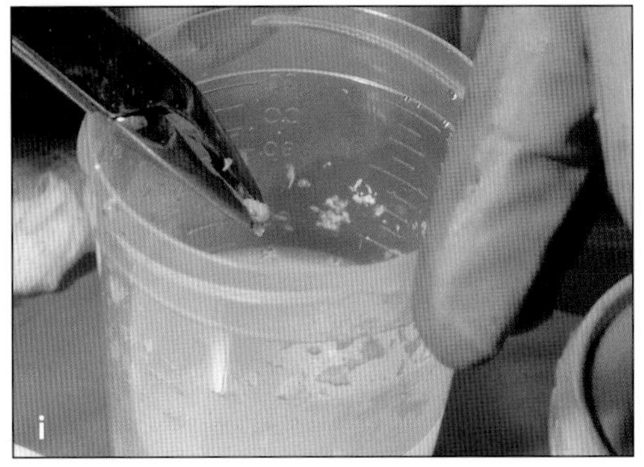

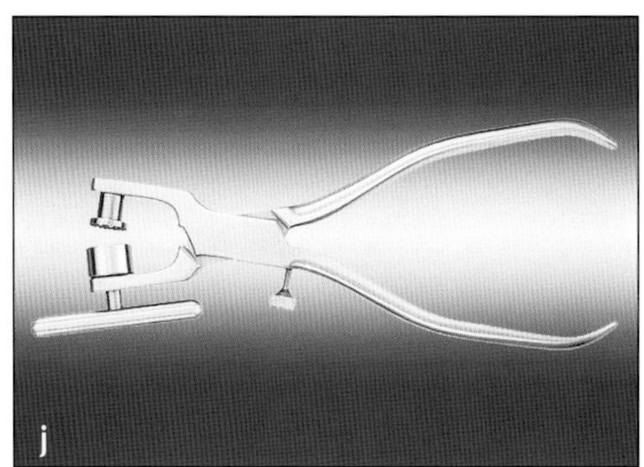

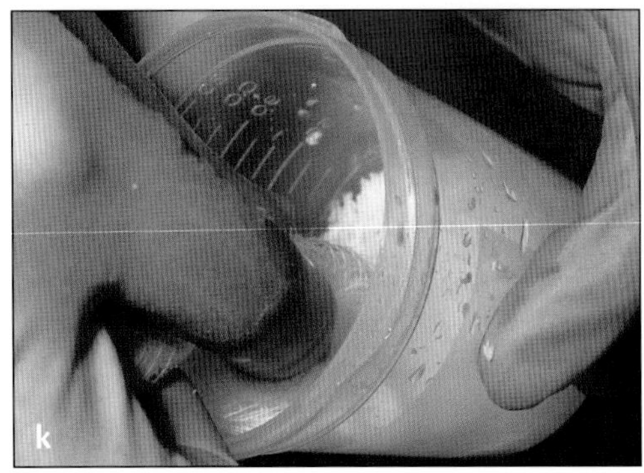

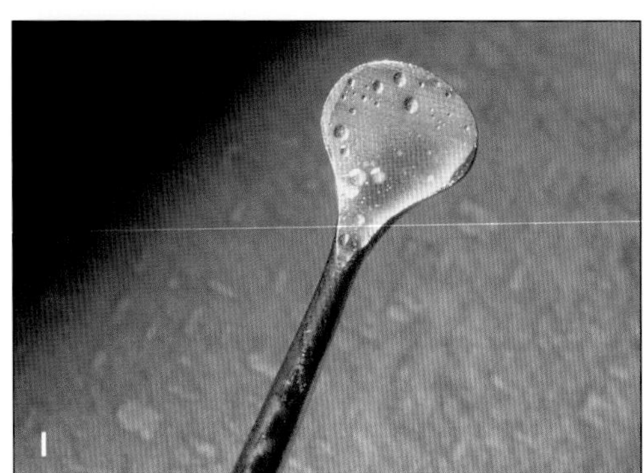

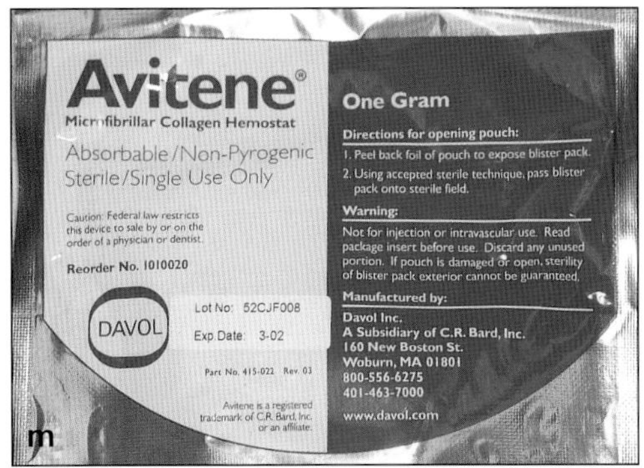

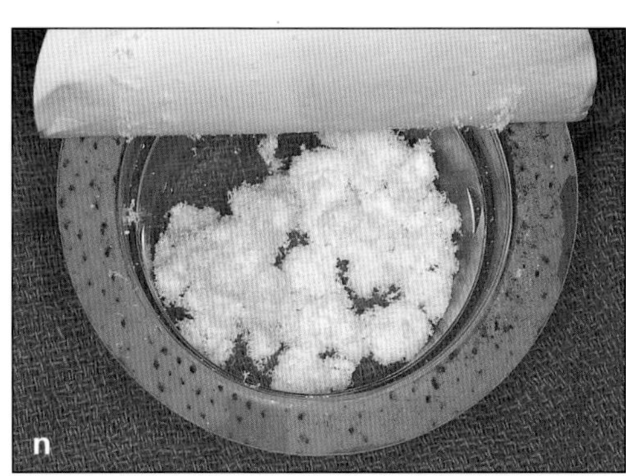

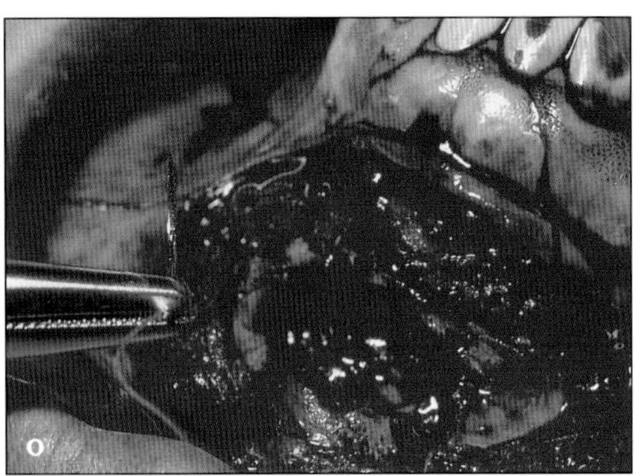

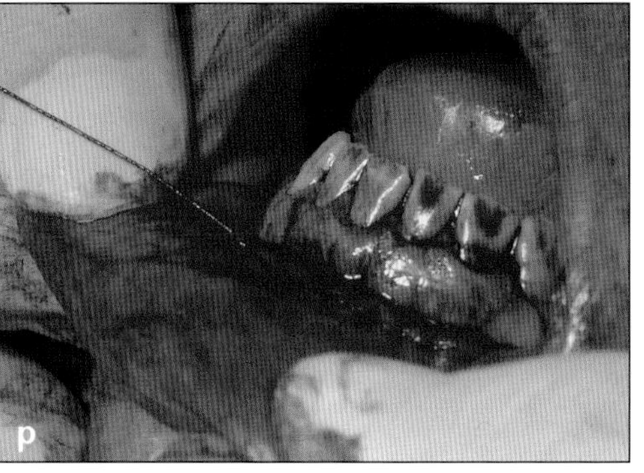

Fig 6-6 *(cont)*

(i) The harvested bone is placed in a sterile saline solution; if it is placed in sterile water, the bone cells will lyse from hypotonicity.

(j) An osteocrusher can reduce bone to particles without waste, which can occur if other instruments, such as rongeurs (airborne particles) or a mini–bone mill (bone waste in the blades) are used. Moreover, the osteocrusher provides a mortised particle size, ideal for handling and for bone growth.

(k) Gauze absorbs excess saline solution from the graft materials before placement.

(l) A no. 2 Molt curette can be used to obtain additional bone marrow from this site if required.

(m) A collagen hemostatic agent such as Avitene can be used to control bleeding.

(n) Avitene's texture and hemostatic efficiency make it ideal for packing this type of defect.

(o) Only after sufficient hemostasis is obtained can the area be packed with graft material and the soft tissues repositioned and sutured. A resorbable suture is used for the periosteum and muscle layer.

(p) A second and final layer of sutures is placed to bind the mucosal layer. The midline and other areas of the flap must be repositioned correctly to return the soft tissue anatomy to its original form.

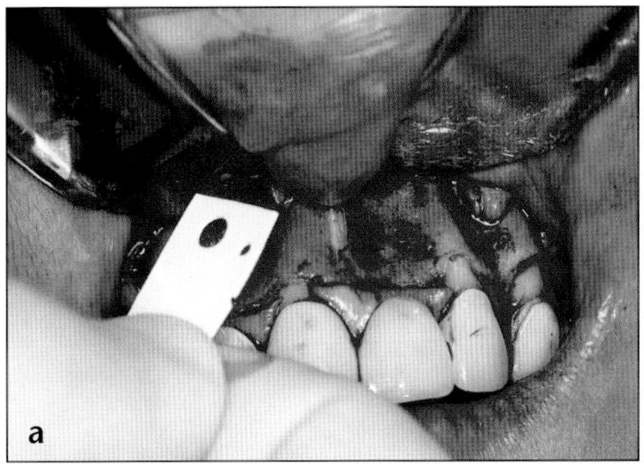
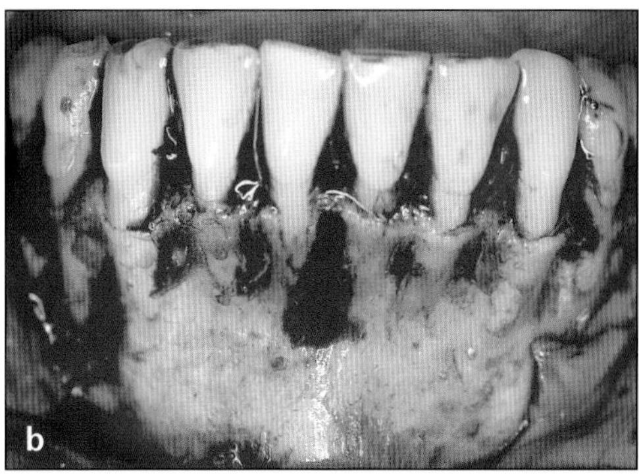
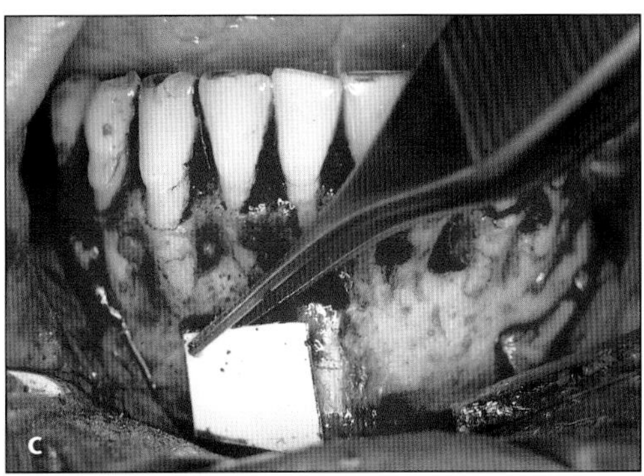
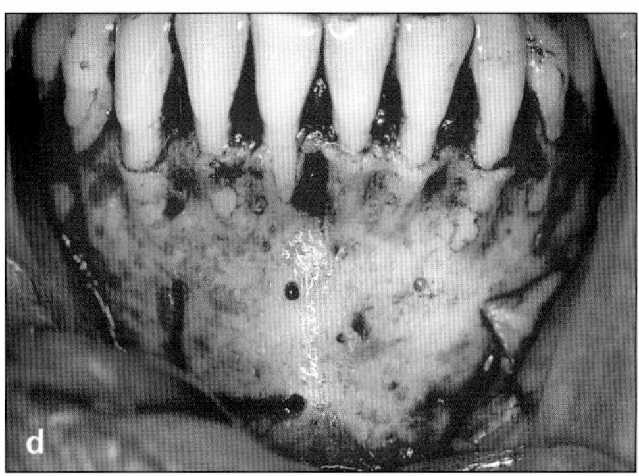
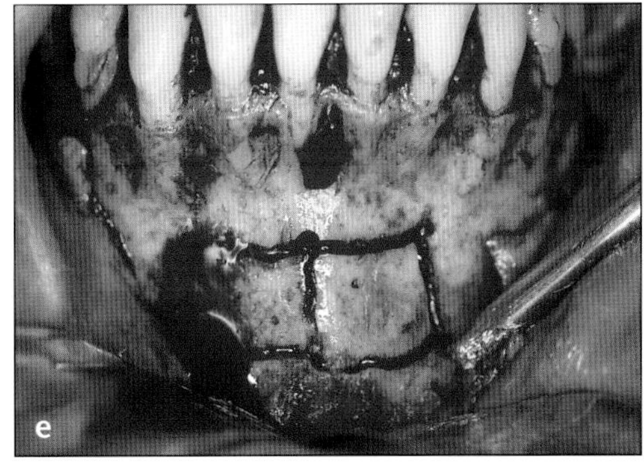
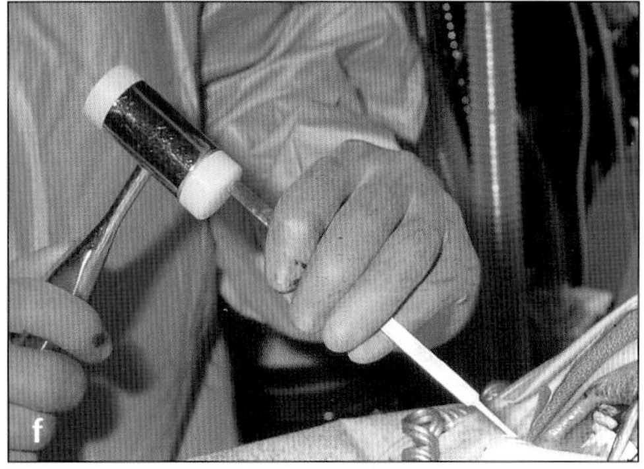

Fig 6-7 Bone blocks are harvested for grafting in a patient who is unhappy with the gingival contour under the pontic areas of a fixed partial denture. The patient wanted dental implants and new restorations. Flap reflection revealed concavities under the pontics.

(a) Volume measurements determine the amount of bone needed for augmentation.

(b) An intrasulcular incision is indicated because of the low vestibule and very tense mentalis muscle.

(c) Readily available sterile plastic sheeting is used as a mold. It is measured at the recipient site and then cut to approximate the graft size required. Here it is shown at the donor site to determine the size of the block required.

(d) Once the flap is well reflected, a no. 1701 bur is used to make cuts at least 5 mm apical to the apices of the mandibular incisors and canines.

(e) Long canine roots make it necessary to remove adjacent blocks.

(f) The chisel is tapped firmly with a mallet as the mandible is held steady to diminish the impact on the condyle area.

(continued)

Harvesting for Block Grafting

After the symphysis has been exposed and the mental foramina are located, the clinician measures the defect to determine the size of bone block(s) required.[45] This measurement can be performed with a simple caliper or templates,[46] or by molding bone wax into the recipient site, lifting the wax, and moving it to the donor site to serve as a guide. The parameters of the donor site are generally 3 mm from the inferior border of the chin, 5 mm from the apex of the dentition, and 5 mm anterior to the mental foramen (Fig 6-7).[19] The outlined graft to be harvested should be approximately 2 to 3 mm larger in each dimension than the size needed for the recipient site. This will allow for some recontouring of the harvested block graft for optimal adaptation

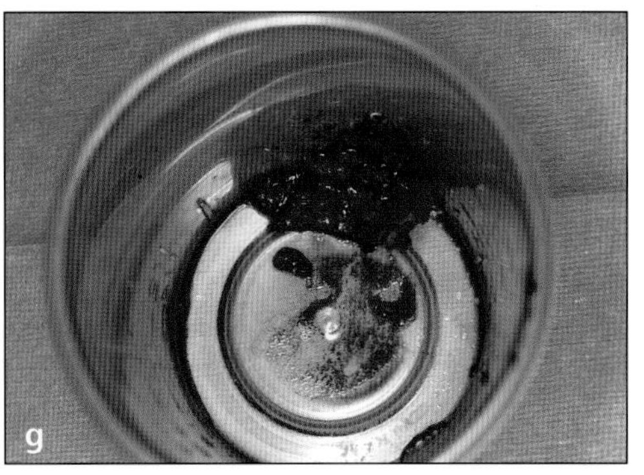

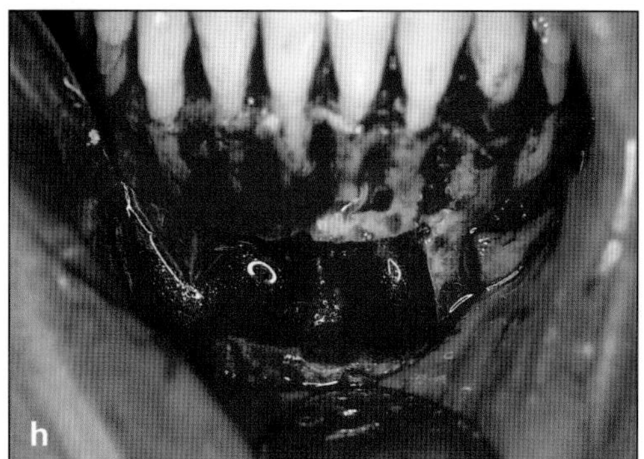

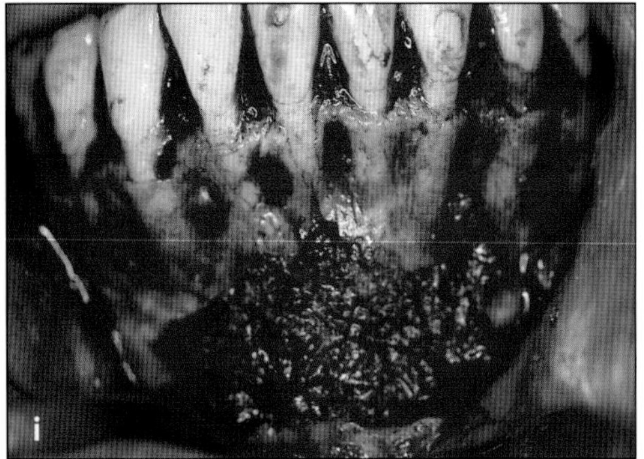

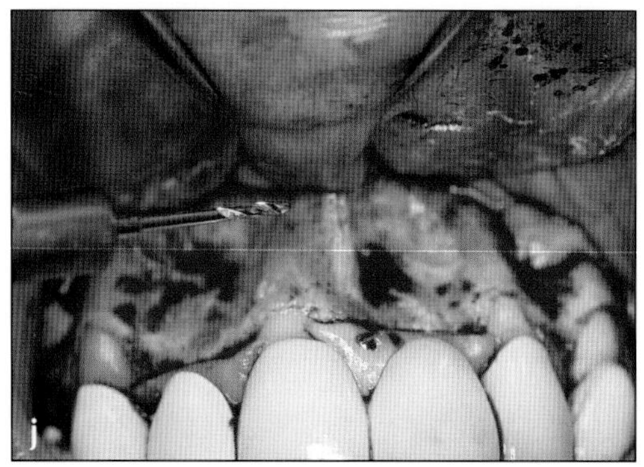

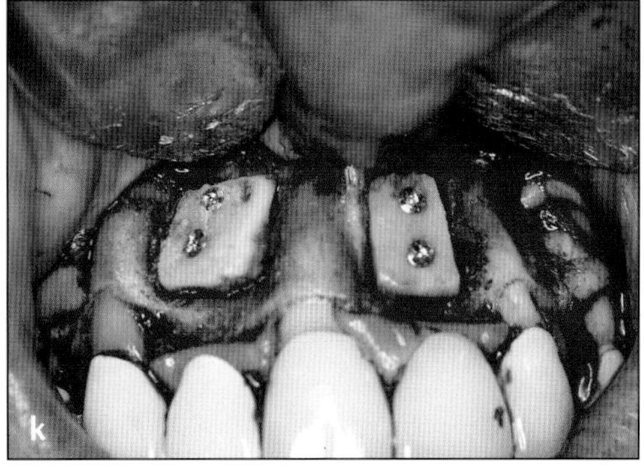

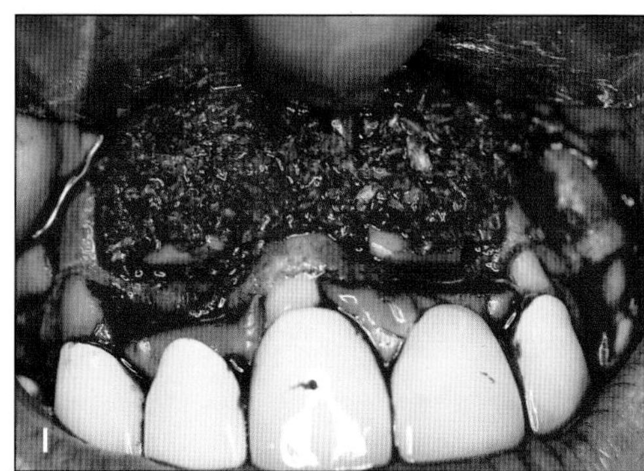

Fig 6-7 *(cont)*
(g) Bone blocks are deposited in a container filled with sterile saline solution while the donor site is prepared for closure.

(h) A large defect in the harvest site is acceptable if maintained within parameters that respect the surrounding anatomy.

(i) The donor site is filled with microfibrillar collagen to provide hemostasis before the graft material is placed and the site is closed.

(j) Perforations are made on the buccal plate of the recipient site to promote bleeding and to help with new vascularization in the bone graft.

(k) The harvested blocks of bone are shaped to fill the defects and screwed into place to ensure proper contact with the underlying bone. Note that any sharp edges on the blocks have been rounded off.

(l) Particulate bone is placed around the blocks and throughout the entire area to provide a smooth contour. Good soft tissue dissection is necessary before the flap—tension free and released from muscle pull—is replaced.

to the defect site. Once the size is determined, a marking pen or surgical bur under copious irrigation at approximately 50,000 rpm can be used at the donor site to outline the external contour of the block graft for the maxillary defect.

Using continuous drilling and a no. 1701 bur, the clinician creates the outline. Alternatively, the Frios MicroSaw (Dentsply, Lakewood, CO), which has a much thinner cut and much less bone waste, can be used for the osteotomy (Fig 6-8). The depth of the osteotomy depends on the thickness of the graft needed. Osteotomes are used to free the block graft and harvest the cancellous bone. The clinician is advised to use caution when the cortical bone is separated from the marrow. An assistant should use an instrument to secure the block so that the specimen is not lost.[19]

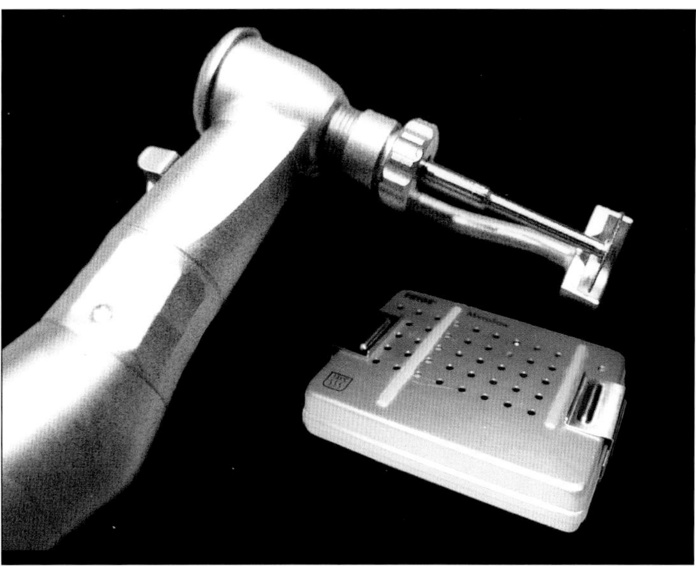

Fig 6-8
A surgical saw such as the Frios MicroSaw can be used to harvest bone from the anterior mandible. A cutting disc with a metal shield can be rotated to a convenient position to protect soft tissues. The disc provides thinner cuts than a bur, preserving more bone but making it more difficult to remove the block from the site.

A rongeur or a chisel can be used to gather additional cancellous bone if needed.[21] The block harvest includes the facial cortical plate and the attached trabecular bone. The procured material should be stored in a medium such as sterile saline until placement, which should be performed as soon as possible following harvesting.[14]

Generally, the inferior border of the mandible should be left intact, and the lingual cortex should not be perforated. Complications such as loss of the airway and excessive bleeding can occur from the perforation of the vascular region under the inner cortex.[15] Appropriate allogeneic or alloplastic material can be packed into the donor site to restore the defect, and a resorbable collagen membrane can be placed over this if desired. The donor-site soft tissues should be closed once bleeding is under control. If needed, Gelfoam (Pharmacia and Upjohn, Kalamazoo, MI) or a synthetic resorbable bone graft can be inserted into the donor site to control bleeding. Because this donor site is considered a five-wall defect, any of the graft materials discussed in chapter 2 can be used. A true barrier membrane is not needed or recommended, although a short-acting collagen, such as CollaTape (Zimmer Dental, Carlsbad, CA), should be used to help hold the graft in place. Avitene, Surgicel, or PRP can be added to the graft material being placed into the donor site if needed for hemostasis. Typically, 1.0- to 1.6-mm titanium alloy screws (KLS Martin, Jacksonville, FL) are used for fixation. Small discrepancies between the graft and host bone can be filled with particulate cancellous bone from the harvest site.

In general, two physical factors—stability of the construct and contact between host bone and the graft—determine the incidence and speed of the union between block bone grafts and the adjacent host bone more than the characteristics of the grafts themselves. In animal models, when the host-graft interfaces were intimately apposed and stably fixed, all interfaces healed.[47] Under stable conditions but without intimate host bone–graft contact, not all interfaces healed, but the biologic characteristics of the graft did not have a discernible effect.[48] When the grafted site was less stable, almost no unions were seen,[49] and a decreasing incidence and maturity of union were noted with decreasing stability of the graft site in that model. The importance of stability of the graft on the parameters of graft incorporation has been noted experimentally[50] and clinically and cannot be overemphasized.[51]

Some research suggests that grafting success in the alveolar ridge can be enhanced by combining autogenous mandibular bone grafts and nonresorbable membranes.[52,53] The author recommends that if greater than half the surface area is particulate rather than block configuration, a membrane barrier with pin fixation should be used. If less than half the surface area of the grafted site is particulate, then a membrane barrier is not critical. Other research suggests that grafting success can be facilitated by early placement of implants after grafting to help prevent resorption[54,55] or by the use of biomaterial instead of autogenous bone.[56–58] However, if an attempt is made to place implants too early into a site with block grafts, there is a strong possibility of the block breaking away from the host bone. For this reason, the author recommends that implants be placed no earlier than 5 months after block grafting. Furthermore, in the author's experience, autogenous bone blocks rather than biomaterials remain the gold standard. However, allogeneic bone blocks with growth factors are showing promising results both clinically and experimentally and can be recommended in less critical cases.

Postsurgery

Amoxicillin or clindamycin should be administered 1 hour prior to the operation and continued for 1 week afterward. Dexamethasone should be prescribed starting the day of surgery and continued for several days postoperatively. Pressure should be applied to the chin for several hours postoperatively to prevent bleeding and to ensure close adaptation of the mentalis muscles. Additionally, ice can be applied to the donor site for the first day following the operation, and chin tape should be used for 48 hours to help control inflammation and minimize bruising at the donor site.[12] After the first week, the patient should use chlorhexidine mouthrinses twice daily for 2 weeks to reduce the risk of infection. Postoperative pain at the donor site is usually minimal to moderate and can be controlled by narcotic analgesics, if necessary.[18] Membrane exposure, infection, and plaque control can be addressed at subsequent appointments. Serious exposure of the membrane may require regrafting or membrane removal; minor exposure may require only the application of a topical antimicrobial (eg, chlorhexidine) as necessary.

Placing block grafts from the mandibular symphysis is discussed in detail in chapter 9. In general, the graft material dimensions are adapted by conservatively trimming the block to achieve a close, customized fit in the recipient site and by smoothing any rough edges that could perforate the overlying flap. These actions help to ensure optimal graft integration and vascularization.

Table 6-1 Potential complications of harvesting bone from the mandibular symphysis

Complication	Cause	Preventive measures
Damaged submental and sublingual arteries	Severely perforated lingual mandibular cortical bone	Understand the buccal-lingual thickness of the mandible from prior to harvesting. The thickness of the block or the length of the bone core should be less than the thickness of the mandible.
Potential damage to mandibular roots	Long anterior tooth roots and/or short anterior mandibular height	Accurately measure the anatomic structures and harvest only from the safe zone.
Mental nerve paresthesia	Extension of incisions for harvesting into the mental foramen area; excessive reflection or retraction of the soft tissue flap	Accurately measure the anatomic structures and harvest only from the safe zone. Guard the mental nerve during flap reflection and retraction.
Incision dehiscence in donor area	Postoperative edema, vigorous chin musculature, hematoma, inappropriate or poor closure of soft tissues	Use a pressure dressing for 3 days postsurgery. Perform a layered closure when possible. Caution the patient to minimize stretching the tissues to look at the area for 5 days after surgery.
Temporary altered sensation of lower teeth	Extension of cut for harvesting too close to tooth apices; frequently occurs postsurgery as a normal sequelae	Explain this common postoperative sequelae to the patient before surgery; monitor closely if it occurs.
Chin ptosis	Failure to preserve the mentalis muscle attachment; suturing the soft tissue flap into an incorrect position	Carefully reposition the flap to its original position and suture in layers

Potential Complications

Preventing early complications following bone harvesting surgery involves using pressure dressings, topical ice packs, and anti-inflammatory drugs to reduce swelling; prescribing analgesics for pain control; and instructing the patient about the importance of meticulous oral hygiene.

Edema is very common following surgery, although its intensity may vary. In most cases, swelling decreases rapidly during the first 2 days postsurgery and complete dissipation occurs within 1 week. Table 6-1 lists other potential complications, along with common reasons for their occurrence and techniques with which to minimize them.

References

1. Cotter CJ, Maher A, Gallagher C, Sleeman D. Mandibular lower border: Donor site of choice for alveolar grafting. Br J Oral Maxillofac Surg 2002;40:429–432.
2. McCarthy C, Patel RR, Wragg PF, Brook IM. Dental implants and onlay bone grafts in the anterior maxilla: Analysis of clinical outcome. Int J Oral Maxillofac Implants 2003;18: 238–241.
3. Montazem A, Valauri DV, St-Hilaire H, Buchbinder D. The mandibular symphysis as a donor site in maxillofacial bone grafting: A quantitative anatomic study. J Oral Maxillofac Surg 2000;58:1368–1371.
4. Gungormus M, Yilmaz AB, Ertas U, Akgul HM, Yavuz MS, Harorli A. Evaluation of the mandible as an alternative autogenous bone source for oral and maxillofacial reconstruction. J Int Med Res 2002;30:260–264.
5. Pikos MA. Facilitating implant placement with chin grafts as donor sites for maxillary bone augmentation—Part I. Dent Implantol Update 1995;6:89–92.
6. Proussaefs P, Lozada J, Kleinman A, Rohrer MD. The use of ramus autogenous block grafts for vertical alveolar ridge augmentation and implant placement: A pilot study. Int J Oral Maxillofac Implants 2002;17:238–248.
7. Sauvigne T, Fusari JP, Monnier A, Breton P, Freidel M. The retromolar area, an alternative for the mandibular symphysis graft in implant surgery: Quantitative and qualitative analysis of 52 samples [in French]. Rev Stomatol Chir Maxillofac 2002;103:264–268.
8. Gungormus M, Yavuz MS. The ascending ramus of the mandible as a donor site in maxillofacial bone grafting. J Oral Maxillofac Surg 2002;60:1316–1318.
9. Capelli M. Autogenous bone graft from the mandibular ramus: A technique for bone augmentation. Int J Periodontics Restorative Dent 2003;23:277–285.
10. Herford AS, King BJ, Audia F, Becktor J. Medial approach for tibial bone graft: Anatomic study and clinical technique. J Oral Maxillofac Surg 2003;61:358–363.
11. Jensen J, Sindet-Pedersen S. Autogenous mandibular bone grafts and osseointegrated implants for reconstruction of the severely atrophied maxilla: A preliminary report. J Oral Maxillofac Surg 1991;49:1277–1287.
12. Jensen J, Sindet-Pedersen S, Oliver AJ. Varying treatment strategies for reconstruction of maxillary atrophy with implants: Results in 98 patients. J Oral Maxillofac Surg 1994;52: 210–216.
13. Jensen J, Reiche-Fischel O, Sindet-Pedersen S. Autogenous mandibular bone grafts for malar augmentation. J Oral Maxillofac Surg 1995;53:88–90.
14. Misch CM, Misch CE. The repair of localized severe ridge defects for implant placement using mandibular bone grafts. Implant Dent 1995;4:261–267.
15. Smiler DG. Small-segment symphysis graft: Augmentation of the maxillary anterior ridge. Pract Periodontics Aesthet Dent 1996;8: 479–483.
16. Schwartz-Arad D, Dori S. Intraoral autogenous onlay block bone grafting for implant dentistry [in Hebrew]. Refuat Hapeh Vehashinayim 2002;19:35–39, 77.
17. Misch CM, Misch CE, Resnik RR, Ismail YH. Reconstruction of maxillary alveolar defects with mandibular symphysis grafts for dental implants: A preliminary procedural report. Int J Oral Maxillofac Implants 1992;7: 360–366.
18. Garg AK, Morales MJ, Navarro I, Duarte F. Autogenous mandibular bone grafts in the treatment of the resorbed maxillary anterior alveolar ridge: Rationale and approach. Implant Dent 1998;7:169–176.
19. Hunt DR, Jovanovic SA. Autogenous bone harvesting: A chin graft technique for particulate and monocortical bone blocks. Int J Periodontics Restorative Dent 1999;19:165–173.
20. Cordaro L, Amade DS, Cordaro M. Clinical results of alveolar ridge augmentation with mandibular block bone grafts in partially edentulous patients prior to implant placement. Clin Oral Implants Res 2002;13:103–111.
21. John V, Gossweiler M. Implant treatment planning and rehabilitation of the anterior maxilla, part 2: The role of autogenous grafts. J Indiana Dent Assoc 2002;81:33–38.
22. Khoury F. Augmentation of the sinus floor with mandibular bone block and simultaneous implantation: A 6-year clinical investigation. Int J Oral Maxillofac Implants 1999; 14:557–564.
23. De Andrade E, Otomo-Corgel J, Pucher J, Ranganath KA, St George N Jr. The intraosseous course of the mandibular incisive nerve in the mandibular symphysis. Int J Periodontics Restorative Dent 2001;21:591–597.

24. Armand S, Kirsch A, Sergent C, Kemoun P, Brunel G. Radiographic and histologic evaluation of a sinus augmentation with composite bone graft: A clinical case report. J Periodontol 2002;73:1082–1088.
25. Wang PD, Klein S, Kaufman E. One-stage maxillary sinus elevation using a bone core containing a preosseointegrated implant from the mandibular symphysis. Int J Periodontics Restorative Dent 2002;22:435–439.
26. Schwartz-Dabney CL, Dechow PC. Variations in cortical material properties throughout the human dentate mandible. Am J Phys Anthropol 2003;120:252–277.
27. Chuenchompoonut V, Ida M, Honda E, Kurabayashi T, Sasaki T. Accuracy of panoramic radiography in assessing the dimensions of radiolucent jaw lesions with distinct or indistinct borders. Dentomaxillofac Radiol 2003;32:80–86.
28. Cordaro L. Bilateral simultaneous augmentation of the maxillary sinus floor with particulated mandible. Report of a technique and preliminary results. Clin Oral Implants Res 2003;14:201–206.
29. McCarthy C, Patel RR, Wragg PF, Brook IM. Sinus augmentation bone grafts for the provision of dental implants: Report of clinical outcome. Int J Oral Maxillofac Implants 2003;18:377–382.
30. Jin H, Kim BG. Mandibular osteotomies after drawing out the inferior alveolar nerve along the canal. Aesthetic Plast Surg 2003;27:126–129.
31. da Fontoura RA, Vasconcellos HA, Campos AE. Morphologic basis for the intraoral vertical ramus osteotomy: Anatomic and radiographic localization of the mandibular foramen. J Oral Maxillofac Surg 2002;60:660–665.
32. Cutright B, Quillopa N, Schubert W. An anthropometric analysis of the key foramina for maxillofacial surgery. J Oral Maxillofac Surg 2003;61:354–357.
33. Nomura T, Gold E, Powers MP, Shingaki S, Katz JL. Micromechanics/structure relationships in the human mandible. Dent Mater 2003;19:167–173.
34. Fukuda M, Takahashi T, Yamaguchi T, Kochi S. Placement of endosteal implants combined with chin bone onlay graft for dental reconstruction in patients with grafted alveolar clefts. Int J Oral Maxillofac Surg 1998;27:440–444.
35. Alonso N, Machado de Almeida O, Jorgetti V, Amarante MT. Cranial versus iliac onlay bone grafts in the facial skeleton: A macroscopic and histomorphometric study. J Craniofac Surg 1995;6:113–118.
36. Bahr W, Coulon JP. Limits of the mandibular symphysis as a donor site for bone grafts in early secondary cleft palate osteoplasty. Int J Oral Maxillofac Surg 1996;25:389–393.
37. Misch CM. Comparison of intraoral donor sites for onlay grafting prior to implant placement. Int J Oral Maxillofac Implants 1997;12:767–776.
38. Matsumoto MA, Filho HN, Francischone E, Consolaro A. Microscopic analysis of reconstructed maxillary alveolar ridges using autogenous bone grafts from the chin and iliac crest. Int J Oral Maxillofac Implants 2002;17:507–516.
39. Kalk WW, Raghoebar GM, Jansma J, Boering G. Morbidity from iliac crest bone harvesting. J Oral Maxillofac Surg 1996;54:1424–1429.
40. Marx RE, Morales MJ. Morbidity from bone harvest in major jaw reconstruction: A randomized trial comparing the lateral anterior and posterior approaches to the ilium. J Oral Maxillofac Surg 1988;46:196–203.
41. Matsumoto MA, Filho HN, Francischone E, Consolaro A. Microscopic analysis of reconstructed maxillary alveolar ridges using autogenous bone grafts from the chin and iliac crest. Int J Oral Maxillofac Implants 2002;17:507–516.
42. Nkenke E, Schultze-Mosgau S, Radespiel-Troger M, Kloss F, Neukam FW. Morbidity of harvesting of chin grafts: A prospective study. Clin Oral Implants Res 2001;12:495–502.
43. Gapski R, Wang HL, Misch CE. Management of incision design in symphysis graft procedures: A review of the literature. J Oral Implantol 2001;27:134–142.
44. Raghoebar GM, Louwerse C, Kalk WW, Vissink A. Morbidity of chin bone harvesting. Clin Oral Implants Res 2001;12:503–507.
45. Zeiter DJ, Ries WL, Sanders JJ. The use of a bone block graft from the chin for alveolar ridge augmentation. Int J Periodontics Restorative Dent 2000;20:618–627.
46. Scher E, Holmes S. Simplified transfer of intraoral bone grafts in ridge-augmentation procedures. Implant Dent 2003;12:113–115.

47. Stevenson S, Li XQ, Martin B. The fate of cancellous and cortical bone after transplantation of fresh and frozen tissue-antigen-matched and mismatched osteochondral allografts in dogs. J Bone Joint Surg Am 1991;73:1143–1156.
48. Stevenson S, Li XQ, Davy DT, Klein L, Goldberg VM. Critical biological determinants of incorporation of non-vascularized cortical bone grafts. Quantification of a complex process and structure. J Bone Joint Surg Am 1997;79:1–16.
49. Feighan JE, Davy D, Prewett AB, Stevenson S. Induction of bone by a demineralized bone matrix gel: A study in a rat femoral defect model. J Orthop Res 1995;13:881–891.
50. Lin KY, Bartlett SP, Yaremchuk MJ, Fallon M, Grossman RF, Whitaker LA. The effect of rigid fixation on the survival of onlay bone grafts: An experimental study. Plast Reconstr Surg 1990;86:449–456.
51. Vander Griend RA. The effect of internal fixation on the healing of large allografts. J Bone Joint Surg Am 1994;76:657–663.
52. Donos N, Kostopoulos L, Karring T. Alveolar ridge augmentation by combining autogenous mandibular bone grafts and non-resorbable membranes. Clin Oral Implants Res 2002;13:185–191.
53. Kaufman E, Wang PD. Localized vertical maxillary ridge augmentation using symphyseal bone cores: A technique and case report. Int J Oral Maxillofac Implants 2003;18:293–298.
54. Dortbudak O, Haas R, Bernhart T, Mailath-Pokorny G. Inlay autograft of intra-membranous bone for lateral alveolar ridge augmentation: A new surgical technique. J Oral Rehabil 2002;29:835–841.
55. Bell RB, Blakey GH, White RP, Hillebrand DG, Molina A. Staged reconstruction of the severely atrophic mandible with autogenous bone graft and endosteal implants. J Oral Maxillofac Surg 2002;60:1135–1141.
56. Araujo MG, Sonohara M, Hayacibara R, Cardaropoli G, Lindhe J. Lateral ridge augmentation by the use of grafts comprised of autologous bone or a biomaterial. An experiment in the dog. J Clin Periodontol 2002;29:1122–1131.
57. Feuille F, Knapp CI, Brunsvold MA, Mellonig JT. Clinical and histologic evaluation of bone-replacement grafts in the treatment of localized alveolar ridge defects. Part 1: Mineralized freeze-dried bone allograft. Int J Periodontics Restorative Dent 2003;23:29–35.
58. Knapp CI, Feuille F, Cochran DL, Mellonig JT. Clinical and histologic evaluation of bone-replacement grafts in the treatment of localized alveolar ridge defects. Part 2: Bioactive glass particulate. Int J Periodontics Restorative Dent 2003;23:129–137.

CHAPTER

7 Harvesting Bone from the Tibia

The tibia offers the surgeon access to a large quantity of quality autogenous bone that can be harvested either in the office setting under local anesthesia and intravenous sedation or in the operating room under general anesthesia.[1] Licensure varies by state and country regarding the degree and/or specialty required to perform this procedure. It is imperative for the clinician to research and confirm that he or she is permitted to perform the procedure in his or her locale prior to undertaking it without supervision.

A tibial bone harvest is generally an excellent graft choice when approximately 20 to 40 cm^3 of cancellous particulate bone is needed.[2] Bone obtained from a donor site such as the tibial plateau contains osteocompetent cells, an island of mineralized cancellous bone, fibrin from blood clotting, and platelets from within the clot. Within hours of graft placement, the clot's platelets degranulate, releasing platelet-derived growth factor (PDGF), transforming growth factors-beta$_1$ and -beta$_2$ (TGF-β_1 and TGF-β_2), and other growth factors to initiate the process of bone regeneration.[3] However, knowledge of the patient's history is always essential for determining which donor site to use in each case.[4,5] Other important considerations regarding the donor site include understanding aging and metabolic disease states[6] and using caution regarding tibial harvesting in children.[7,8]

Advantages and Contraindications

The proximal lateral tibial graft harvest has a number of advantages over other donor sites and techniques:

1. From 20 to 40 cm^3 of noncompressed cancellous bone can be harvested from the marrow space.

2. The procedure is straightforward and can be performed using in-office conscious sedation or general anesthesia.
3. The total procedure time averages only 20 to 40 minutes.
4. Blood loss is minimal, and drainage is not required.
5. Patients report minimal postoperative pain and dysfunction.
6. The procedure allows immediate postoperative weight bearing.
7. Studies show relatively fewer complications and less morbidity is found than with other techniques, such as the iliac crest graft.[9,10] The incidence of complications for tibial grafts ranges from 1.3% to 3.8%, which compares favorably with the 8.6% to 9.2% incidence of complications for iliac crest harvesting.[11]
8. Studies reveal that postoperative bruising is minimal, healing is generally uneventful, and postoperative scarring is unremarkable.

Contraindications for the procedure include:

1. The need for block bone (This procedure provides only cancellous marrow [particulate] bone.)
2. Patients 18 years of age or younger
3. Patients with a history of knee injury or knee surgery
4. Patients with advanced rheumatoid or degenerative arthritis
5. Patients with metabolic bone disease

Anatomy

The tibia is the larger of the two lower leg bones in the tibia-fibula complex and the main structural support of this portion of the leg. Whether a medial or a lateral approach is used to obtain bone graft material, it is important for the clinician to note preoperatively the key anatomic landmarks associated with the tibia.[12–13]

The tibial condyles should be palpated immediately below the knee and marked. On the anterior surface of the proximal end of the tibia between the condyles is an oval protuberance called the *tibial tuberosity* or *Gerdy tubercle*; this should be located, palpated, and marked. The Gerdy tubercle is a ridge on the lateral anterior aspect of the tibia, approximately 1.5 to 2.0 cm below the articulating surface. The iliotibial tract attaches to the top portion of the Gerdy tubercle, and the tendon of the tensor fascia lata muscle attaches to the bottom of the tubercle (Fig 7-1). The iliotibial tract is the tensor fascia lata and the tensor fascia lata muscle, which originates from the external tip of the anterior ilium, crosses the hip joint and the knee joint at the lateral band of the leg, and enters the Gerdy tubercle. Inferior to the ridge of the Gerdy tubercle is the anterior tibialis muscle. This ridge is located on the lateral side of the tibia, two-thirds of the way between the head of the fibula and the midline of the tibial shaft, both of which are readily palpable.

Properly locating the Gerdy tubercle prior to making the incision is essential to avoid violating the articular surface of the tibial plateau and damaging the articulation of the knee (Fig 7-2). Maintaining this anatomic position also prevents involvement of the head of the fibula, which is subcutaneous at this level and should be located, palpated, and marked, as should the patella, the iliotibial tract, and the anterior tibialis muscle.

The small blood vessels in the immediate vicinity of the lateral proximal tibia include:

- Branches of the medial superior and inferior genicular arteries, which pass under the cover of the patellar ligament

Fig 7-1 It is important for the clinician to note the key anatomic landmarks associated with the tibia prior to tibial harvesting.

(a) Anterior and lateral view of the tibia. The red circle indicates the access area for bone harvesting at the Gerdy tubercle.

(b) Tibiofemoral and tibiofibular joints in a cadaver specimen. The head of the fibula, the Gerdy tubercle (the protuberance just below the tibial condyle), and the tibial condyle vary in protuberance and should be clearly identified by palpation before the procedure begins.

(c) Anterior radiographic view of the area showing the exact location of the Gerdy tubercle and the volume of the medullary space within the head of the tibia.

(d) Muscles and attachments in the area of bone harvest.

(e) Vascular network in the area of bone harvest.

(f) Muscles and attachments, vascular network, harvest site, and angulation. Harvesting at this site and angulation can prevent damage to the vascular network and muscles.

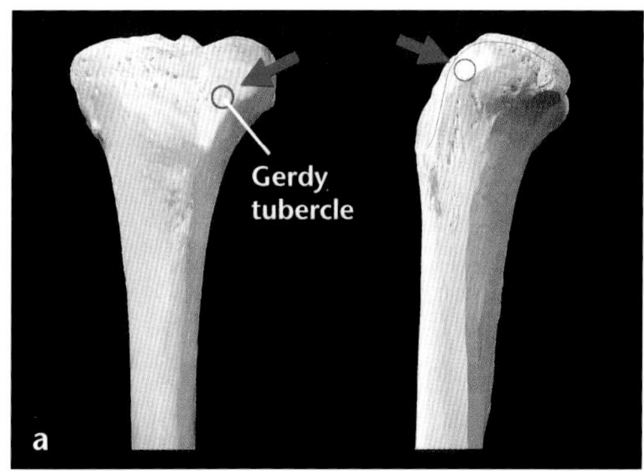

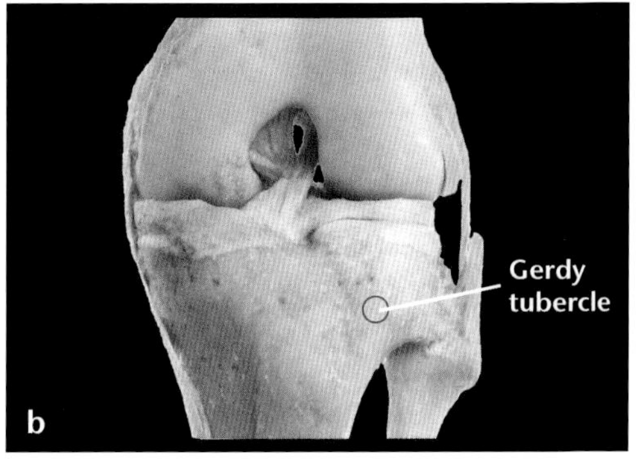

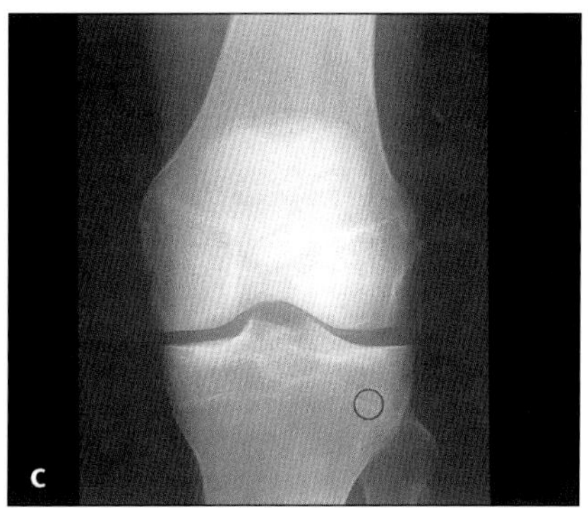

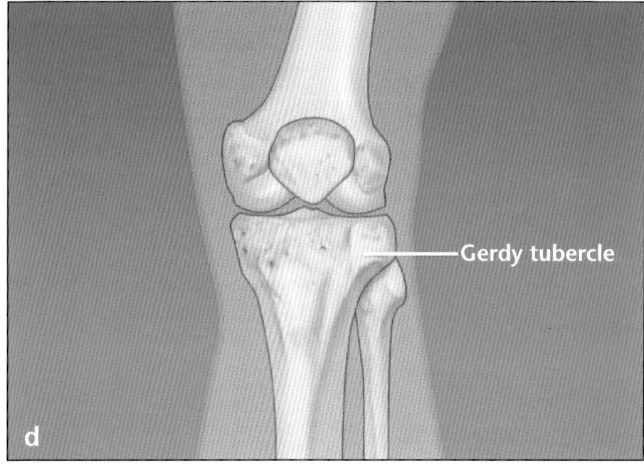

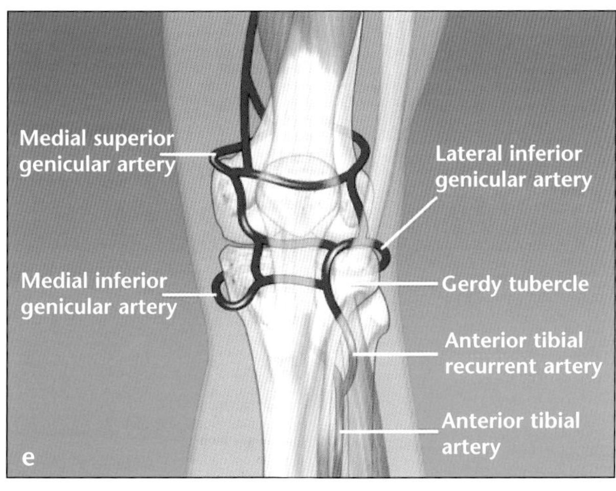

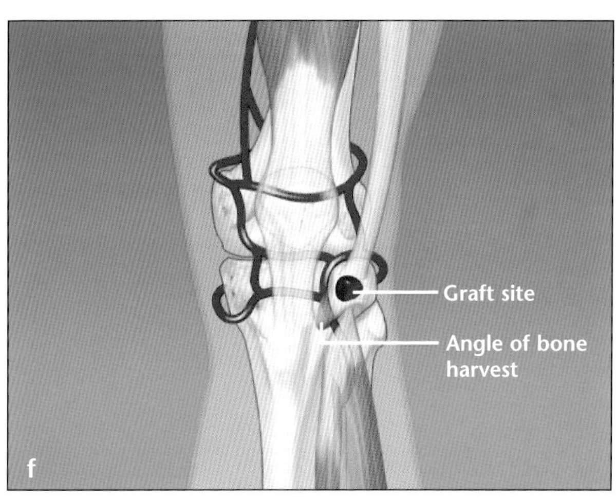

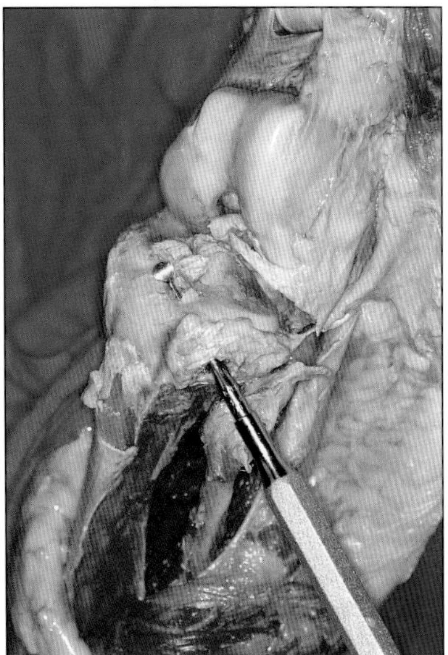

Fig 7-2
The Gerdy tubercle owes its protuberance to the "pull" of the muscles attached to it. The instrument used for harvesting bone from the site should always be directed medially and downward. In this figure, an opening is made over the Gerdy tubercle of a dissected cadaver tibia. The curette has been intentionally directed upward to illustrate how far off-angle the surgeon would have to be in order to enter the articulation of the knee. The surgeon should also keep in mind that extreme force must be exerted to perforate the flat articular surface of the tibia.

- Branches of the lateral inferior genicular, fibular, and anterior recurrent tibial arteries
- Branches of the anterior tibial arteries

Bleeding from these vessels is minimal and easily controlled with the use of electrocautery. The two vessels most at risk in the immediate surgical area are the anterior tibial recurrent and lateral inferior genicular arteries. Appropriate placement of the incision is essential to avoid injury to these vessels.

The primary muscle in this surgical area is the anterior tibialis, located on the lateral surface of the tibia. Its fibers course vertically, overlapping the anterior tibial vessels and the deep peroneal nerve in the proximal tibial region. This nerve rises from the bifurcation of the common peroneal nerve between the fibula and the peroneus longus muscle and continues deep to the extensor digitorum longus muscle and on to the anterior surface of the interosseous membrane. Injury to this nerve is easily avoided by the proper placement of the initial incision.

Surgical Approach and Technique

First, the patient is placed in a supine position. A roll should not be placed under the ipsilateral hip and beneath the knee to help flex the knee and to elevate the anterolateral tibia. However, a Crescent Knee Support (Crescent Products, North Minneapolis, MN) can be used to elevate and comfortably flex the knee (Fig 7-3a). Covered in medical-grade vinyl for easy disinfection, this support is 16 inches wide and covers almost the entire width of a standard dental chair. A gripping material on the bottom of the support prevents shifting.

The donor site is shaved and prepared with iodine or a povidone-iodine solution and appropriate sterile draping (Fig 7-3b). A sterile Betadine (Purdue Pharma, Stamford, CT) or similar preparation and sterile drapes, gloves, and gowns are required. Draping should be relatively wide so that the surgeon can see all adjacent and relevant landmarks clearly and thus ensure proper graft site orientation (Figs 7-3c to 7-3e).

Fig 7-3 Surgical approach and technique for harvesting bone from the tibia.

(a) A Crescent Knee Support pillow, designed specifically for knee surgery, can be used under the knee during the tibia harvest.

(b) The skin is disinfected with Betadine applicators to remove surface bacteria.

(c) A sterile surgical marker will be needed after the skin is disinfected.

(d) Anatomic landmarks are drawn on the skin to help maintain proper orientation.

(e) The location of the patella, the head of the tibia, and the Gerdy tubercle are marked on the skin. Other landmarks (eg, fibula, muscles) can also be marked for greater accuracy.

(continued)

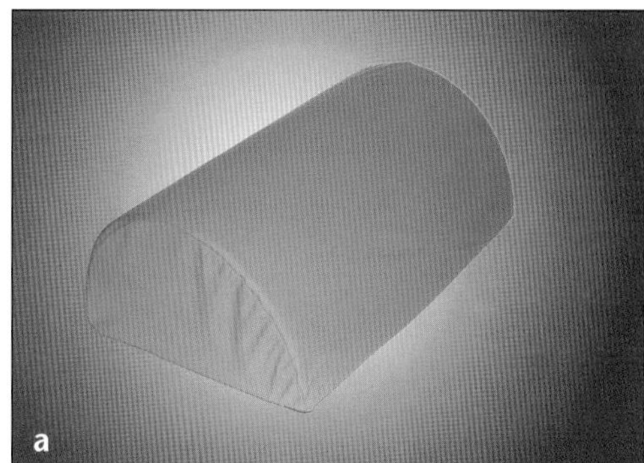

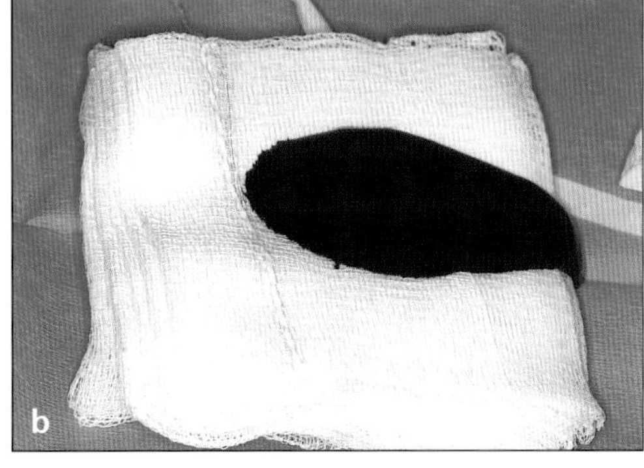

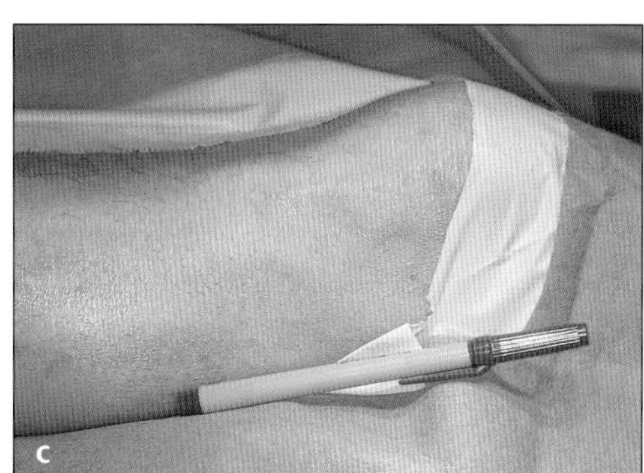

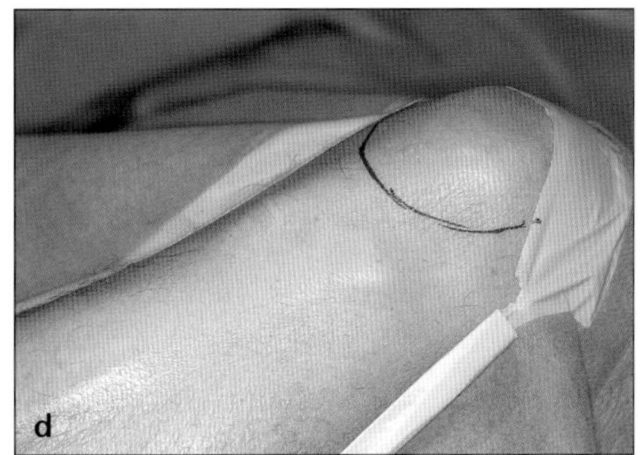

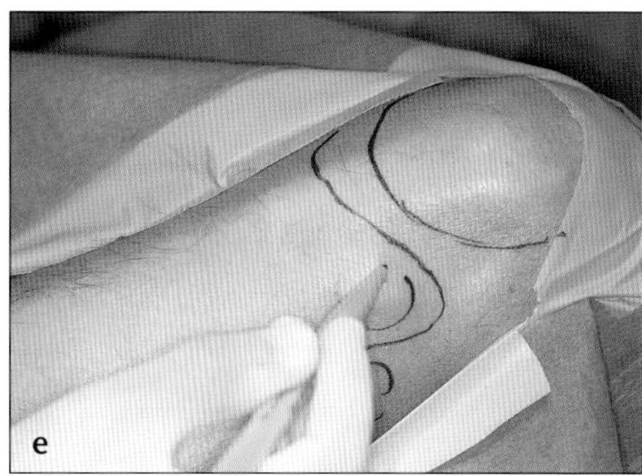

Typically, the left tibia is used, allowing one surgeon to harvest bone on the patient's left side and another surgeon to stand near the right side of the patient's head to place the bone graft. Taking bone from the left tibia provides a natural angle for a right-handed surgeon; for a left-handed surgeon, the right tibia provides a more natural angle for harvesting (Fig 7-3f).

Following sterile preparation and draping, 1 to 2 mL of 2% lidocaine with 1:1,000,000 epinephrine is placed subcutaneously (Fig 7-3g). After allowing 1 to 2 minutes to anesthetize the superficial skin, another 1 to 2 mL is deposited on the periosteum (Fig 7-3h). There are almost no nerve fibers in the bone marrow, so this area will not require local anesthesia; however, there are nerve fibers in the periosteum and the skin, so good filtration to the skin and then to the periosteum layer is required.

A 2- to 3-cm incision is made directly over the Gerdy tubercle through skin and subcutaneous tissues in layers with a no. 15 scalpel blade (Fig 7-3i). The incision should be angled with its cephalad limit just above and medial to the origin of the tibialis anterior muscle and its caudal extent lateral to the patellar ligament. The incision is made through the skin, subcutaneous tissue, and fascia of the iliotibial tract of the fascia lata, as well as through the periosteum (Fig 7-3j).

The periosteum is reflected, which may require some effort because it is bound rather tenaciously to the underlying bone (Fig 7-3k). A bony window, approximately 1 to 1.5 cm in diameter, is delineated with a surgical handpiece and straight fissure no. 702 bur (Brasseler, Savannah, GA). A series of bur holes is created circumferentially (Fig 7-3l) and then connected. The diameter of the opening is slightly larger than the diameter of the tip of a no. 4 Molt curette (G. Hartzell & Son, Concord, CA).

The surgeon then removes the small cortical bone plug with a no. 4 Molt curette and introduces the curette to begin harvesting bone (Fig 7-3m). To remove the cancellous marrow from the tibia, the surgeon should stand at or above knee level so that the natural direction of entry is downward and across the tibia. This approach will automatically direct the instrument away from the knee joint. Although the subchondral bone is dense and is therefore unlikely to be perforated, thus allowing entrance to the knee joint, it is unnecessary to harvest from this area and to accept even the remote risk of a knee joint entrance.

The use of the no. 4 Molt curette is followed by the use of straight (Lorenz no. 152 and no. 153 [W. Lorenz Surgical, Dayton, OH]) and curved (Lorenz no. 157) orthopedic curettes to harvest the desired quantity of cancellous bone (Fig 7-3n). To obtain bone further in the shaft, the surgeon can use the curved orthopedic curettes. In addition to obtaining bone from the center of the tibial head, it is also desirable to curette along the inner aspect of the cortex, where the greatest concentration of mesenchymal cells is located.

Generally, 20 to 40 mL of cancellous bone can be procured from each tibia. Because this procedure removes minimal amounts of cortical bone and does not disrupt the continuity of the cortex, which provides strength to the bone and enables it to resist fractures, the tibia is not weakened by this surgery (Figs 7-3o and 7-3p). The use of hand instruments is recommended, and the curette should be oriented inferiorly and medially to avoid the subchondral bone just beneath the tibial plateau. Using trephines or other power instruments in this area is not recommended, although Sandor et al report favorable patient and clinical results using a minimally invasive power-driven trephine for harvesting bone from the anterior iliac crest.[14]

Graft Handling

The methods used to store and handle the graft in the period between harvest and implantation can considerably alter its viability. The bone cells in this cancellous graft are relatively hardy and able to survive for several hours without losing any significant viability.[15] A graft with this cancellous cellular density is best transferred to the recipient site within 30 to 180 minutes so that the cells have optimum viability and activity. The recipient site should have optimum vascularity so as to allow nutrients to diffuse into these cells and begin the formation of capillary ingrowth.

The graft material should be stored in a very small amount of sterile saline. Any bone substitutes for graft expansion can be added at this time. Platelet-rich plasma (PRP), if indicated, should be added imme-

Fig 7-3 *(cont)*
(f) For the right-handed surgeon, the left tibia offers a more favorable donor site, providing a more comfortable angle and helping to keep instruments away from the articular site.

(g) The same local anesthetic with vasoconstrictor is used for the tibia site and for the oral recipient site. The agent is first placed subcutaneously, following the direction of the subsequent incision.

(h) The needle is then directed perpendicular to the site, penetrating the periosteum.

(i) A no. 15 blade is used to make a 2- to 3-cm incision in layers—through the skin, subcutaneous tissue, muscle fibers, and periosteum.

(j) As the incision progresses, continuous palpation verifies that the cuts are made directly over the tubercle.

(k) A sharp periosteal elevator must be used to reflect the periosteum, which is firmly attached to bone, and uncover the bony surface.

(l) The osteotomy begins as a series of holes made with a no. 701 bur (Brasseler) at the 12, 3, 6, and 9 o'clock positions, forming a circle with a circumference no larger than 1 cm; these perforations are later connected with the same bur, and the central cortical plug is removed with the aid of a no. 4 Molt curette.

(continued)

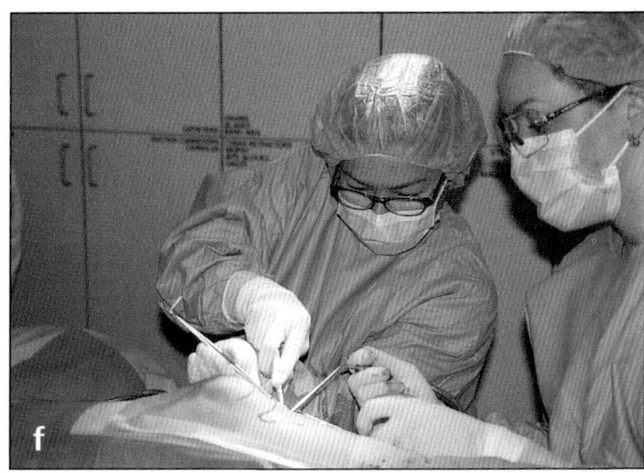
f

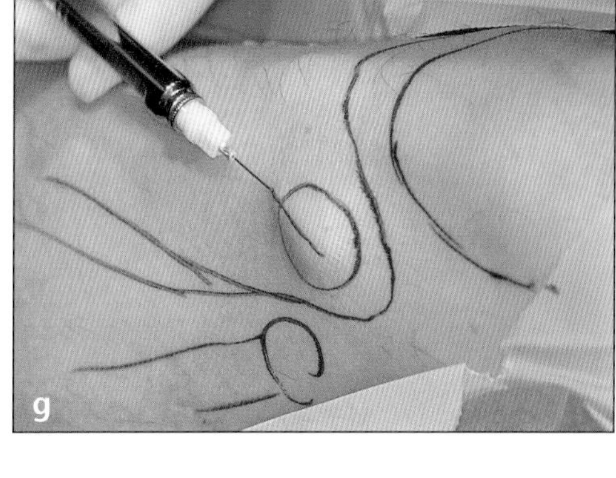
g

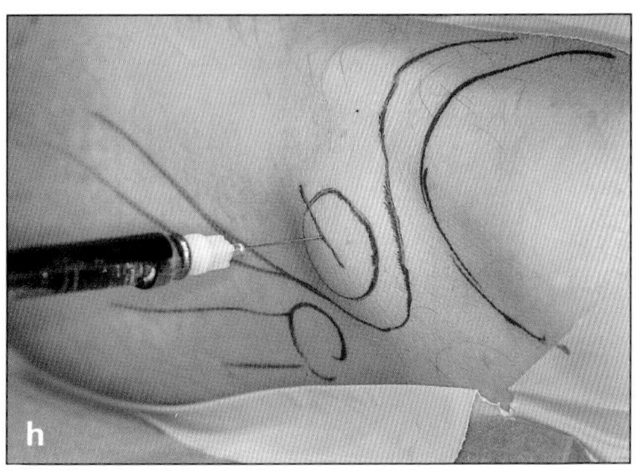
h

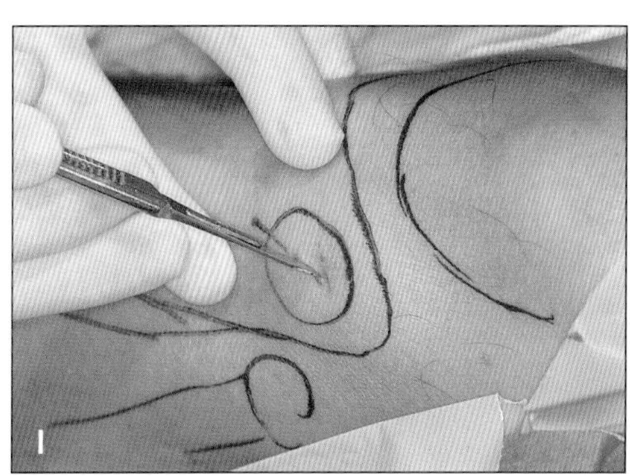
i

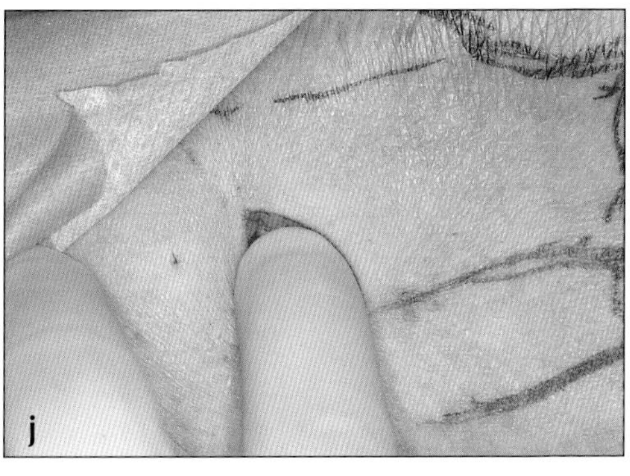
j

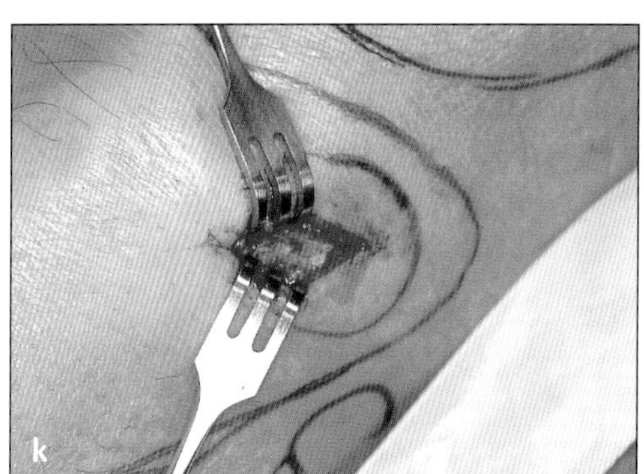
k

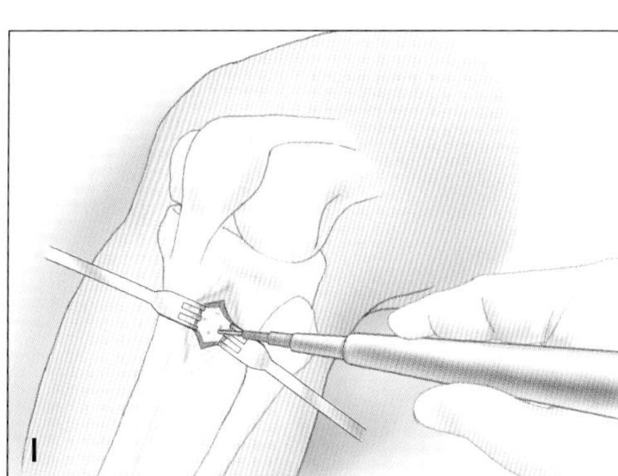
l

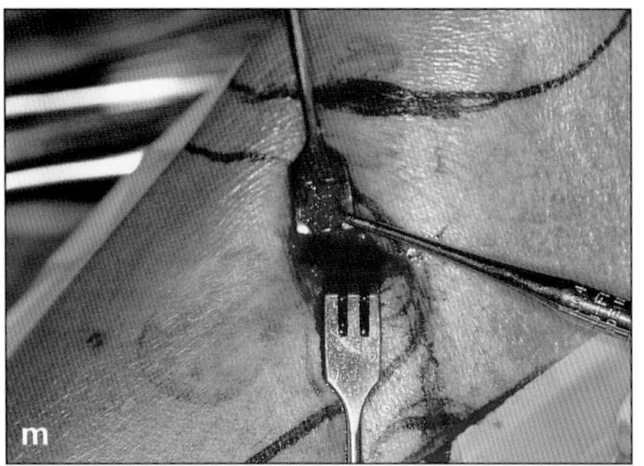

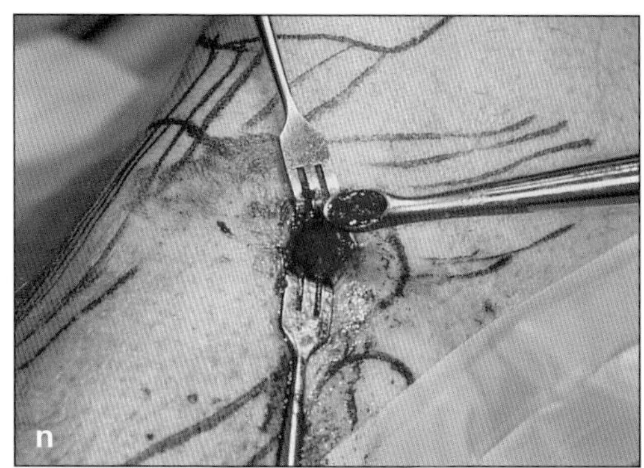

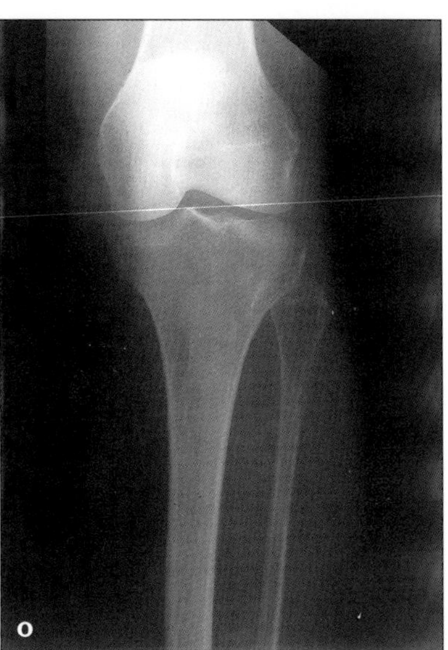

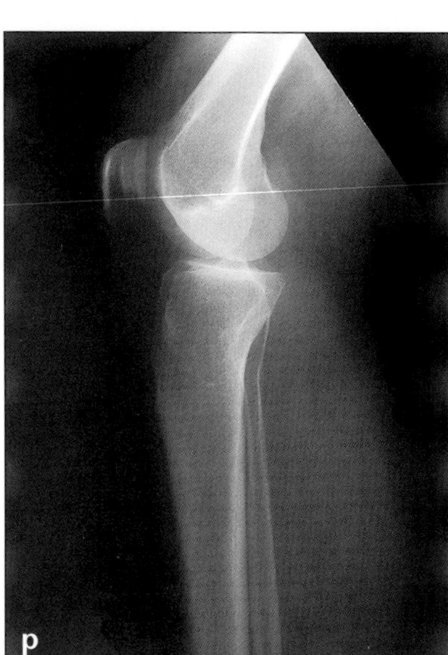

Fig 7-3 *(cont)*
(m) Cancellous bone is scooped out of the tibia through the osteotomy using the sharp edges and spoon-like shape of a no. 4 Molt curette.

(n) In some cases, orthopedic curettes, which provide different reaching angles, can be used to harvest cancellous bone; however, caution is advised because such curettes tend to exert more force during the scraping action because of their rigidity.

(o) Four-month postoperative radiographic view of the anterior tibia shows good bone density throughout the tibial head.

(p) Four-month postoperative view of the lateral tibia reveals no radiolucent spaces.

diately preceding delivery of the graft to the recipient site. Of the many temporary storage solutions that have been tested, simple room-temperature saline or tissue culture media have been found to maintain the best viability.[6] Cooling the storage media can extend cell viability, whereas heating it will shorten viability times sustainable at room temperatures.[15] Sterile water and other hypotonic solutions are highly lytic to cell membranes and should be avoided.[6]

Postoperative Wound Management

There is no need to fill the metaphyseal dead space with an alloplastic material; however, a hemostatic agent should be placed into the harvested cavity at this point. Hemostatic agents, such as Avitene (MedChem Products, Woburn, MA), Surgicel (Johnson & Johnson, New Brunswick, NJ), or autologous PRP or platelet-poor

Fig 7-4 Postoperative wound management includes hemostatic agents, suturing, and antibacterial ointment. The wound does not need to be drained nor the metaphyseal dead space filled with alloplastic material.

(a) Before closure of the tibial donor site, a hemostatic agent (Avitene, Surgicel, PRP, or PPP) should be placed in the cavity.

(b) PPP, delivered to the cavity with a plastic syringe, is very effective. It is a cost-effective hemostatic agent with a gel-like consistency that fills the cavity and stays in place.

(c) Closure of the soft tissues with a resorbable suture (eg, 3-0 Vicryl) is performed in layers, starting with the periosteum.

(d) The muscle is sutured with 4-0 chromic gut, which resorbs slightly more quickly than Vicryl suture material.

(e) For the skin, a 5-0 Prolene suture is ideal. Different suture techniques can be used with good results. The continuous subcuticular technique, shown here, provides optimal esthetic results.

(continued)

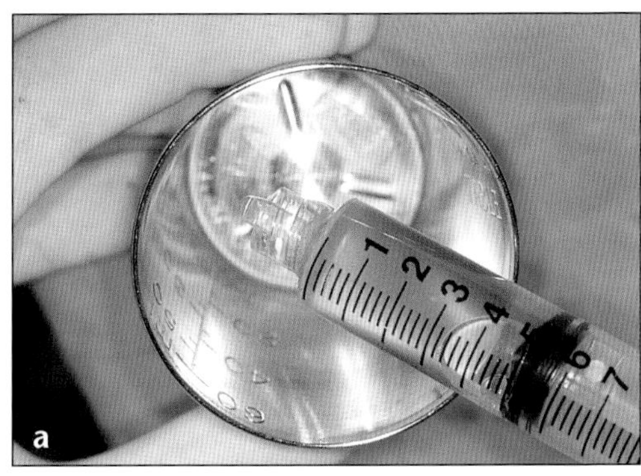
a

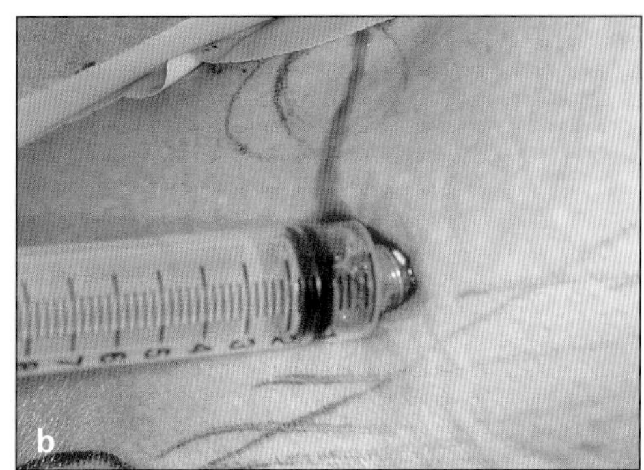
b

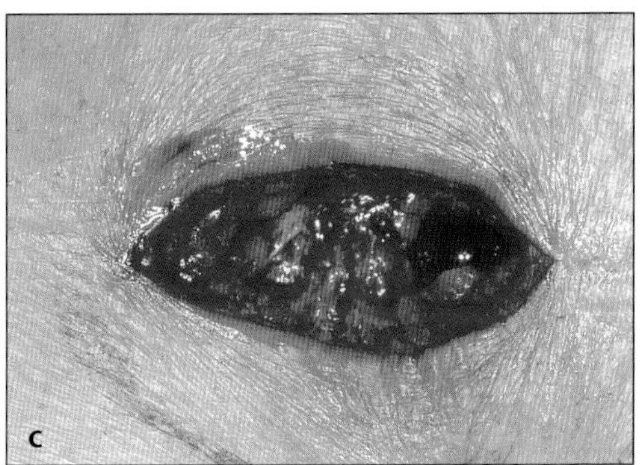
c

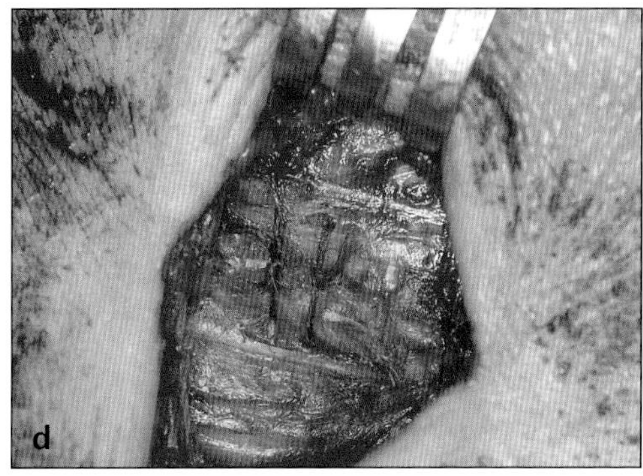
d

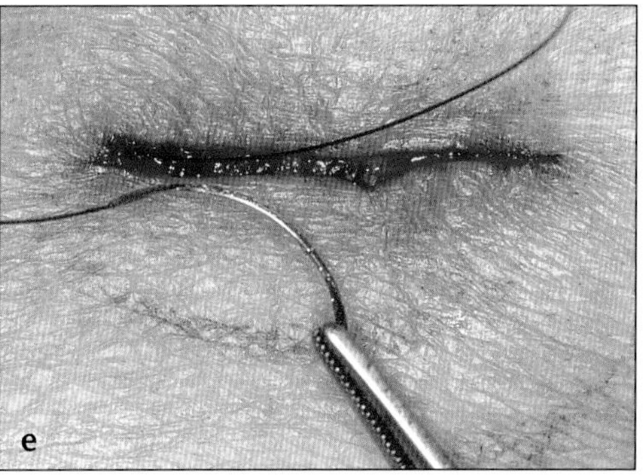
e

plasma (PPP), have all been used successfully in this wound. PRP is generally recommended for the donor sites if an adequate amount remains after using it for the recipient site. If not, the PPP can be used for the donor site for purely hemostatic purposes (Figs 7-4a and 7-4b).

The wound does not require placement of a surgical drain and can be closed in layers. The periosteum should be approximated with 3-0 Vicryl sutures (Ethicon, Somerville, NJ) and the muscle layer with 4-0 chromic gut sutures. For the skin layer, either a continuous subcuticular or an interdermal suture may be used for optimal esthetic results with a 5-0 Prolene suture (Ethicon). An antibacterial ointment is placed over the incision, and then Steri-Strips (3M, St Paul, MN) are placed and a nonstick dressing (eg, a large adhesive bandage) is applied (Figs 7-4c to 7-4h). A pressure dressing is not required for this procedure.

All patients should receive a course of intravenous or oral antibiotics for the donor site procedure if antibiotics were

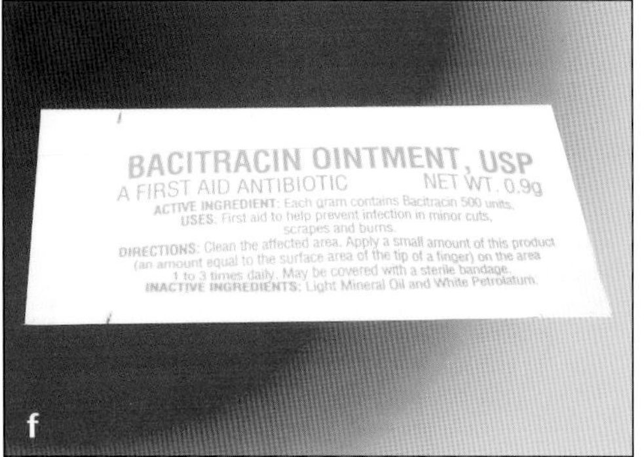

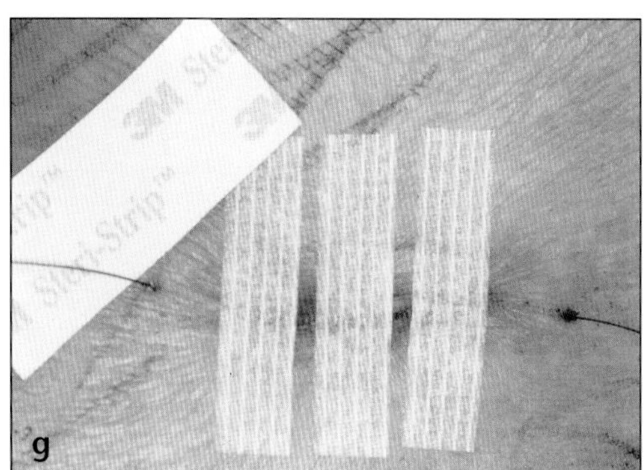

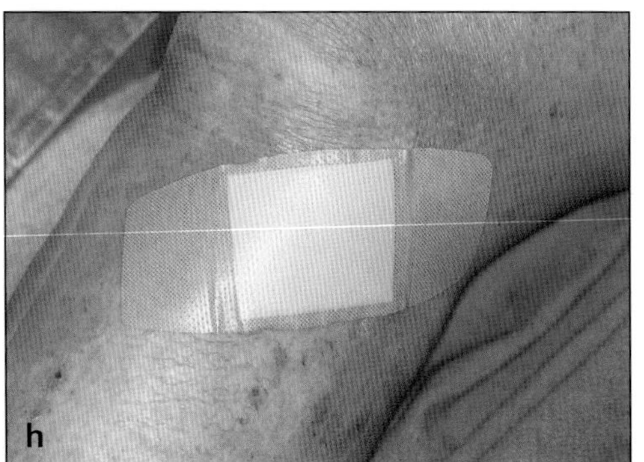

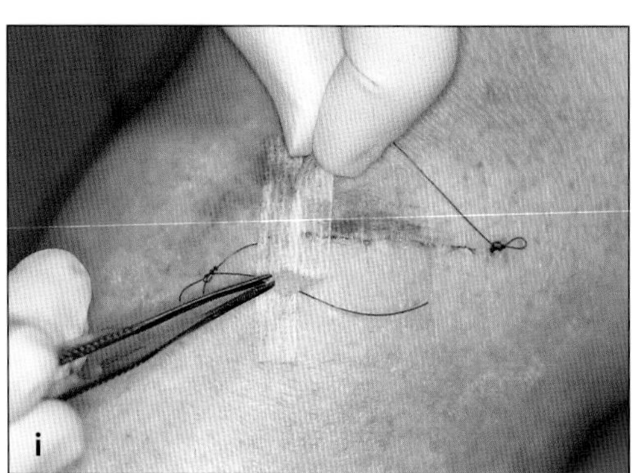

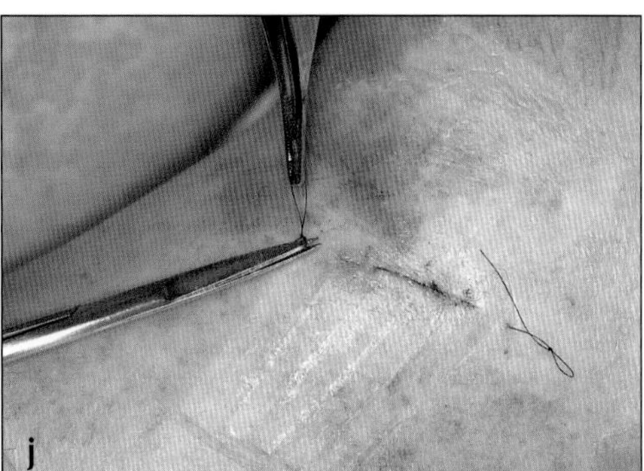

Fig 7-4 *(cont)*
(f) An antibacterial ointment (eg, bacitracin) is applied over the wound after closure. The ointment should be limited to the incision line so that the subsequent dressings can adhere to the skin.

(g) Steri-Strips are placed across the incision line, helping to approximate the wound.

(h) A large bandage can protect the site during the postoperative phase.

(i) When sutures are removed (at approximately 7 days), the area should be cleaned with hydrogen peroxide, and bacteria-accumulating scabs should be removed. No local anesthesia is necessary.

(j) An antibacterial ointment is used for several days after suture removal.

not prescribed for the primary surgical procedure. Postoperative instructions to the patient are relatively straightforward.[5,9] The patient should get bed rest the first two postoperative days, with only minimal walking (eg, to the bathroom). The patient can return to work on the third day but with limited walking and standing. Walking should be limited to short distances for 1 week. No sports or strenuous activity should be undertaken for 6 weeks. Patients should attempt to keep the donor area as dry as possible when showering or bathing. Skin sutures are removed 5 to 7 days after surgery (Figs 7-4i and 7-4j). Swelling and ecchymosis can extend up to the thigh and down to the ankle. Since this is the most common postoperative finding, patients should be specifically forewarned and reassured that such swelling and bruising are entirely expected and normal.

Table 7-1 Potential complications of harvesting bone from the tibia

Complication	Cause	Preventive measures
Potential entrance into joint space	Losing track of landmarks, directing instruments at an incorrect angle, using trephine burs or rotary instruments to harvest (which may accidentally and quickly slip to inappropriate areas or angles)	Understand the anatomy of the Gerdy tubercle and adjacent areas. Limit the harvest to particulate cancellous bone marrow and keep instruments directed downward at a 45-degree angle.
Limited size and shape of graft	Hesitation to harvest due to inexperience with the procedure or inadequate sedation; patient with poor quality or quantity of bone available for harvest	Provide adequate sedation for the procedure. Gain experience with the procedure under supervision. If an inadequate quantity of bone is obtained from a particular patient, add volume expanders to harvested bone.
Entrance into fibula head instead of tibia	Inadvertently marking the tibial head as the Gerdy tubercle	Understand the anatomy of the Gerdy tubercle and adjacent areas. Determine and, using a surgical marker, accurately mark all adjacent surgical landmarks.
Postoperative edema or ecchymosis	Excessive trauma during harvesting to muscle fibers attached to the Gerdy tubercle. Most often this is normal and will subside in 2 weeks.	Minimize stripping of the flap superiorly beyond the area required for bone harvest. Use ice packs and anti-inflammatory drugs and consider the use of corticosteroids postoperatively to minimize edema.
Large and/or unsightly scar	Incision other than a straight line (eg, U-shaped incision); inappropriate surgical closure.	Place the incision in a natural skin crease, use an intradermal suture and Steri-Strips, and use PRP on the incision line if available.

Potential Complications

Preventing early complications following bone harvesting surgery involves using pressure dressings, topical ice packs, and anti-inflammatory drugs to reduce swelling; prescribing analgesics for pain control; and instructing the patient about the importance of meticulous oral hygiene. Edema is very common following surgery, although its intensity may vary. In most cases, swelling decreases rapidly during the first 2 days postsurgery and complete dissipation occurs within 1 week. Table 7-1 lists other potential complications, along with common reasons for their occurrence and techniques with which to minimize them.

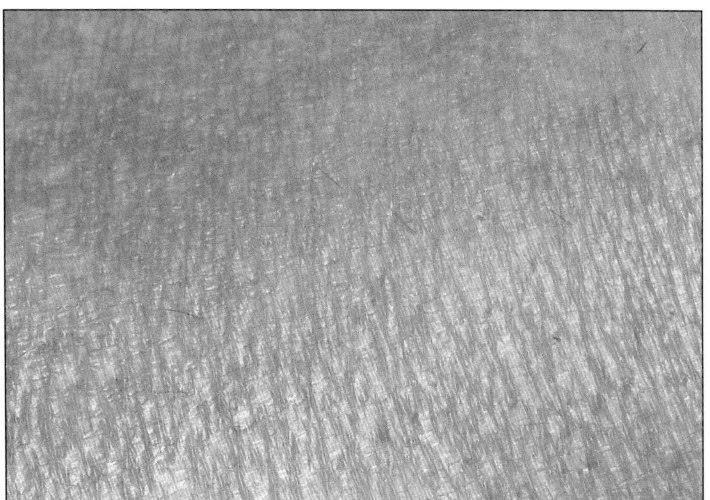

Fig 7-5
The scar left by the tibial bone harvest varies from patient to patient, but a careful technique will help reduce scarring. Successful 4-month postoperative results are seen in this patient.

Conclusion

A low complication rate, minimal patient discomfort, minor bruising, and limited postoperative scarring make the lateral proximal tibia a practical and viable bone source for implant-related bone grafting procedures (Fig 7-5). While the use of allografts, synthetic graft composites, and recombinant grafts may one day offer viable and cost-effective alternatives to autogenous bone grafts,[16–20] the tibial cancellous autograft should remain high on the clinician's list of grafting choices. In fact, improved methods for harvesting autogenous bone not only from the tibia[21] but also from the iliac crest[12,22] will keep these clinical options attractive for some time to come.

The lateral proximal tibial metaphysis offers a practicable alternative source of moderate amounts of cancellous bone with minimal morbidity. Harvesting bone from the lateral proximal tibia is a straightforward procedure when the surgeon is familiar with the anatomy of the lower extremity. Keeping the graft in a saline solution and minimizing the amount of time between harvesting and implantation will ensure bone graft viability. This in-office procedure has the added advantage of being relatively quick, with the patient under conscious sedation.

The cases shown in Figs 7-6 and 7-7 demonstrate the procedures described in this chapter.

Fig 7-6 Tibial harvesting for a bilateral sinus graft case.

(a) After being shaved, the skin above the lateral side of the tibia is disinfected via a Betadine-soaked gauze applied in a circular motion starting from the center and advancing to the periphery. The Betadine is left to dry.

(b) As sedation begins, local anesthesia is injected first in the subcutaneous tissue, which swells as the anesthetic solution seeps in.

(c) The needle is then directed perpendicular to the site, depositing the solution within the periosteum.

(d) An oblique incision is made over the Gerdy tubercle. The skin is stretched and kept in place with the free hand.

(e) The incision should be approximately 2 to 3 cm long to allow for good visualization once bone is reached; however, because the skin over this area can be moved up and down freely, to ensure the correct location, the area must be palpated frequently as the incision progresses into deeper layers.

(f) After the bony surface is denuded, the osteotomy begins with a no. 701 cylindrical bur. Perforations forming a circle are made and later connected.

(g) The bony cortical plug is removed using a no. 4 Molt curette for leverage. This curette, or other orthopedic curettes in different sizes, are used to scrape and scoop out the bone marrow until the amount required for the grafting procedure has been harvested.

(h) This bilateral sinus graft case requires approximately 18 mL of bone; PRP is added to enhance bone regeneration.

(continued)

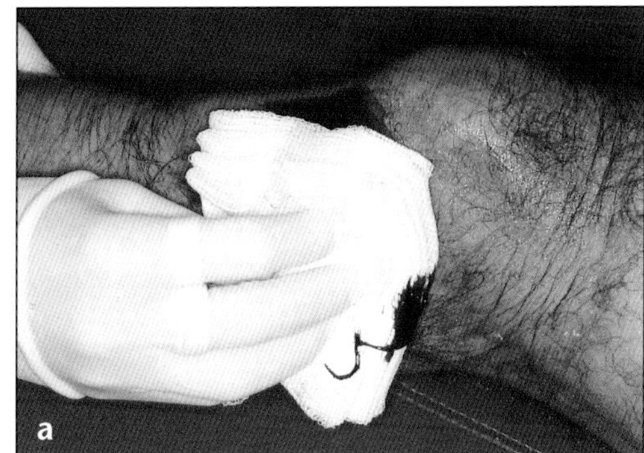

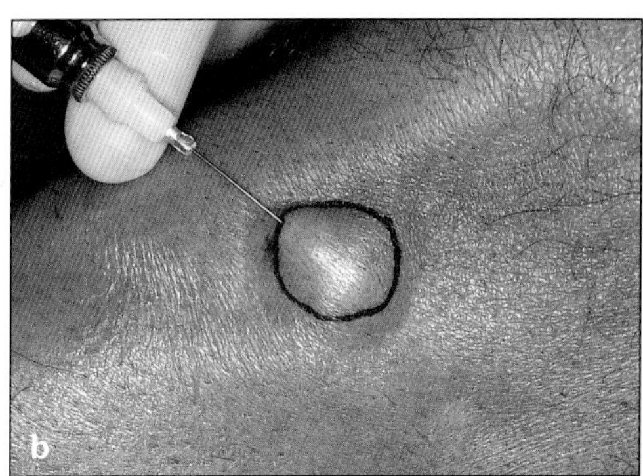

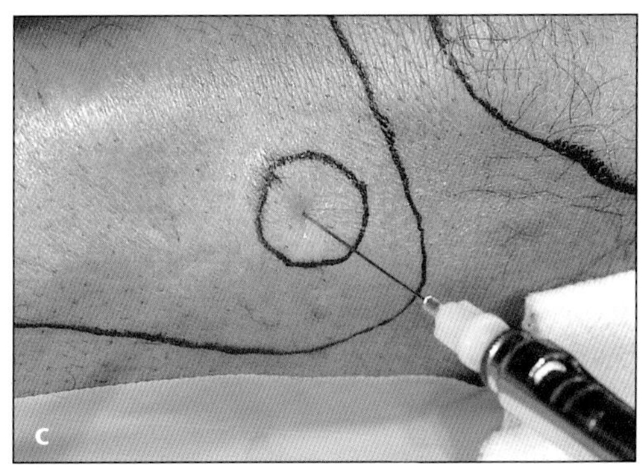

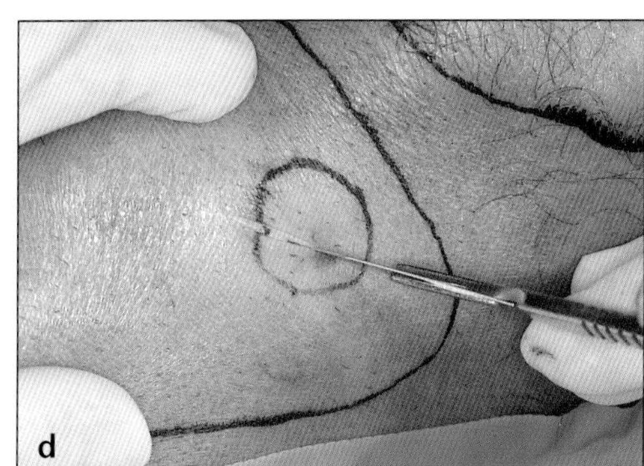

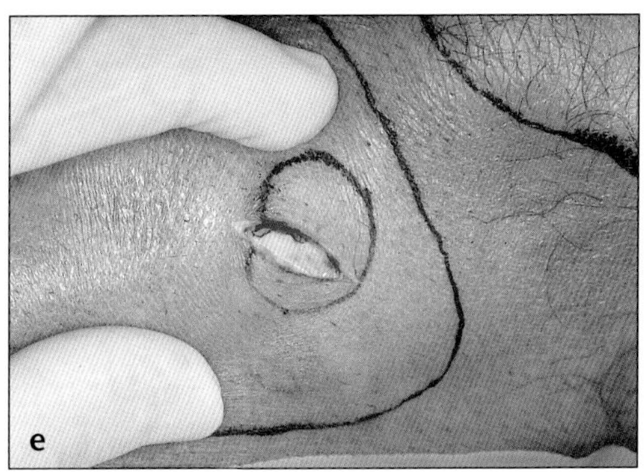

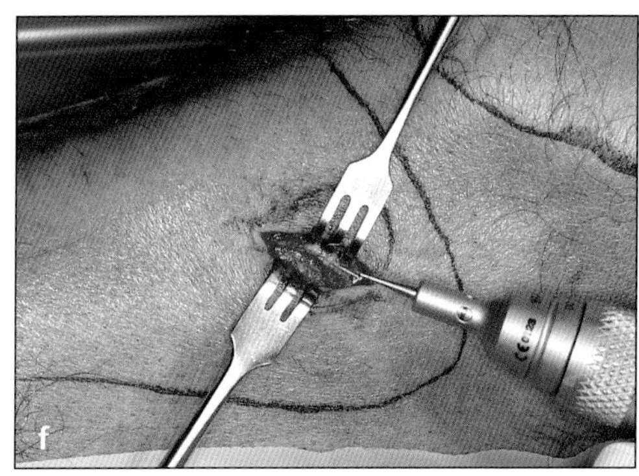

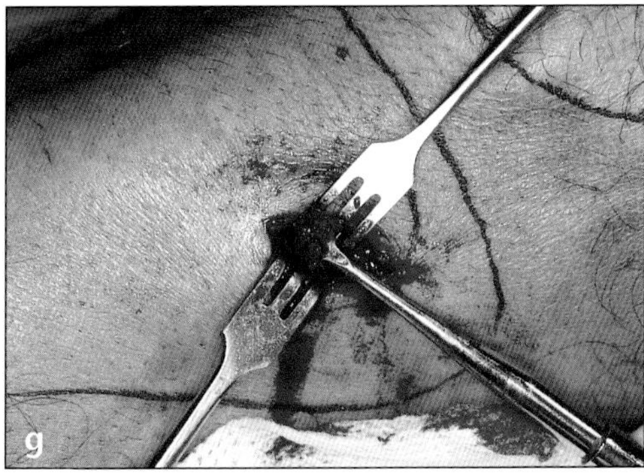

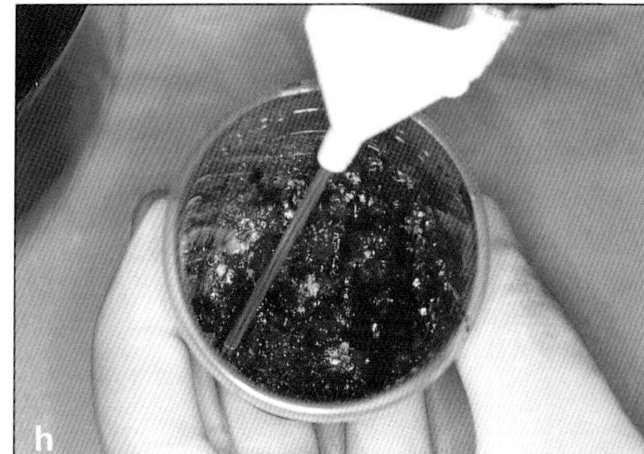

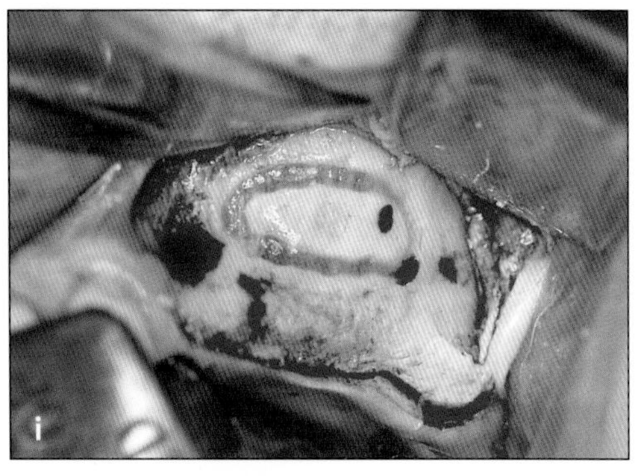

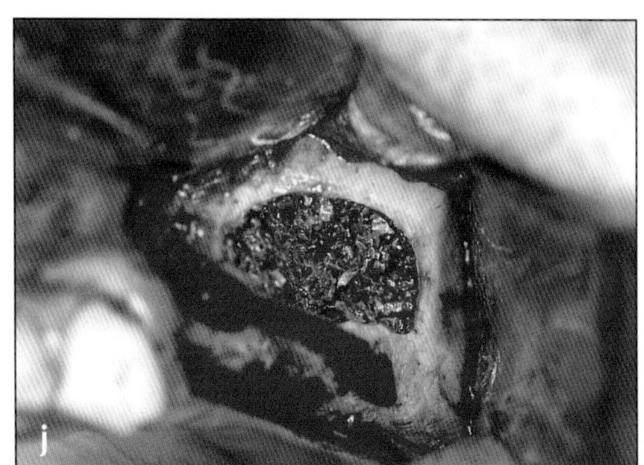

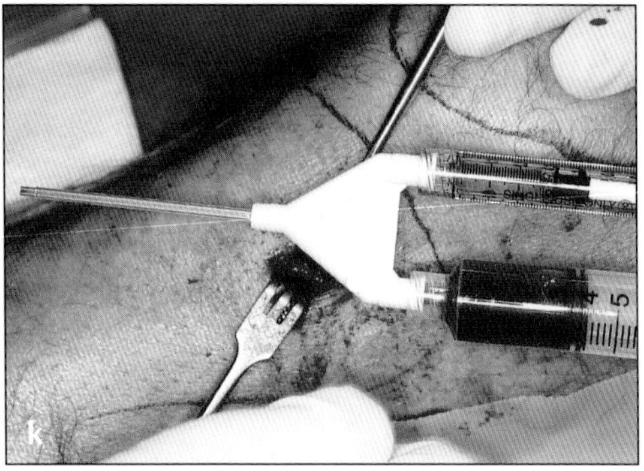

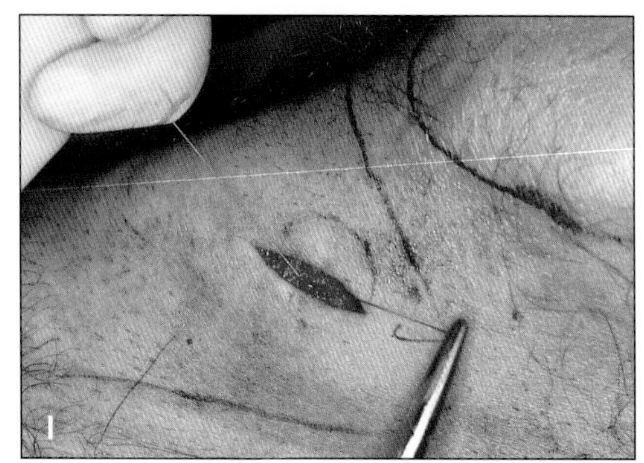

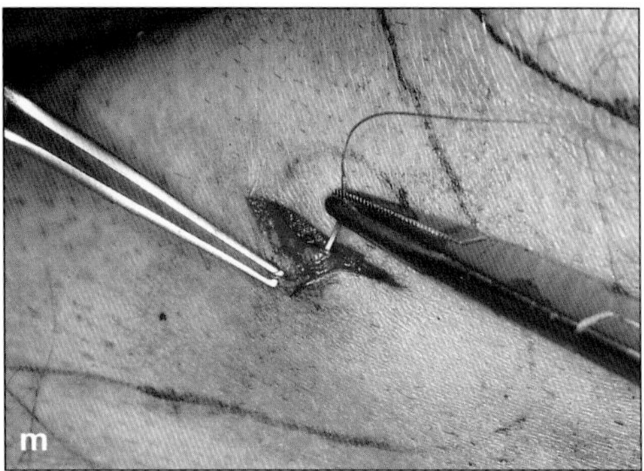

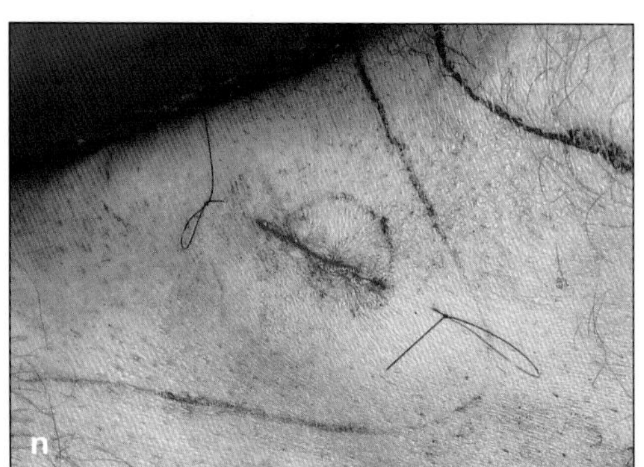

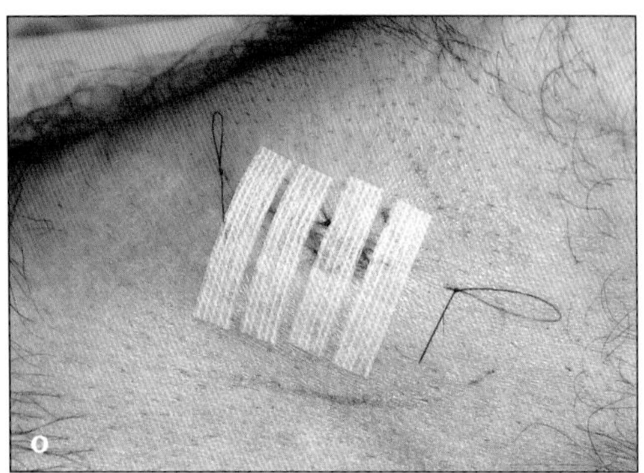

Fig 7-6 *(cont)*
(i) Sinus lift procedure at the time of osteotomy for antral access.

(j) Once both cavities are completely filled, closure of the tibia site can begin.

(k) In this case, there was enough PRP to use within the graft and in the cavity left in the tibia. PRP promotes hemostasis better than PPP and improves healing.

(l) Suturing is done in layers. The muscle is brought together with 3-0 Vicryl suture.

(m) The subcutaneous tissue is sutured with 4-0 chromic gut in an interrupted fashion.

(n) The skin is sutured with 5-0 Prolene with a continuous subcuticular technique.

(o) Steri-Strips are placed across the incision line to reinforce the sutures.

Fig 7-6 *(cont)*
(p) Four months after sinus elevation, 10 implants were placed. Six months after placement, the implants have osseointegrated. One week after uncovering, healing abutments have been removed in order to take impressions for Atlantis (Atlantis Components, Cambridge, MA) abutment fabrication.

(q) Atlantis abutments in perfect angulations and positions, as received in the cast.

(r) Panoramic radiograph of bilateral sinus grafts, including 10 posterior maxillary implants with Atlantis abutments.

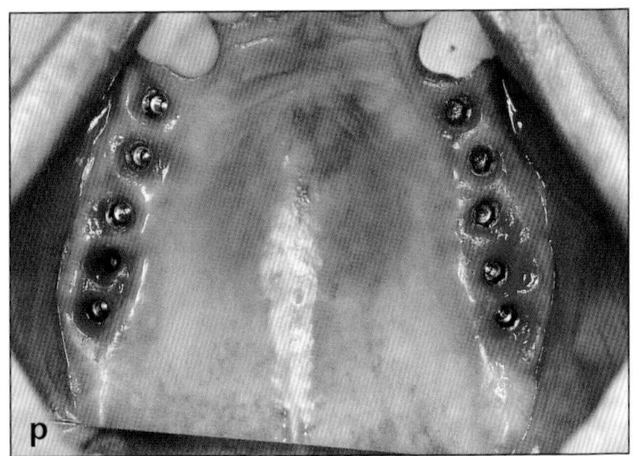

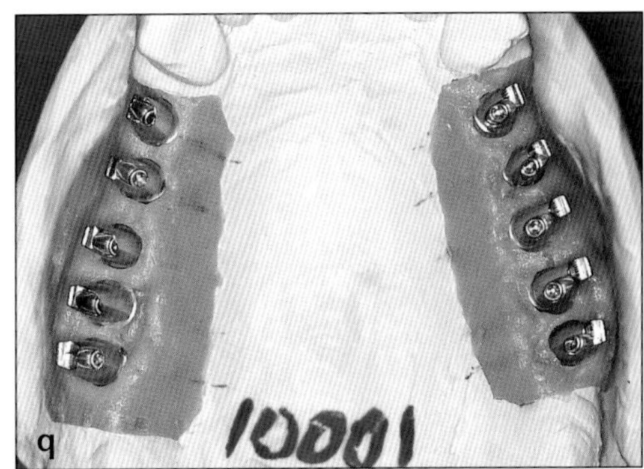

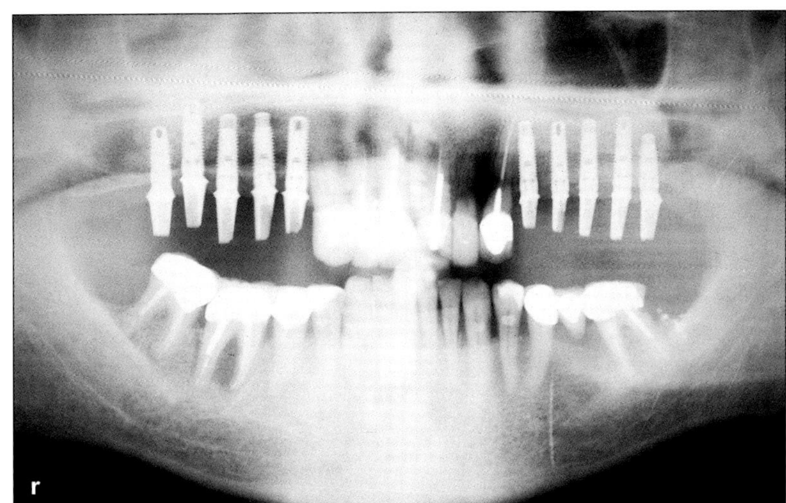

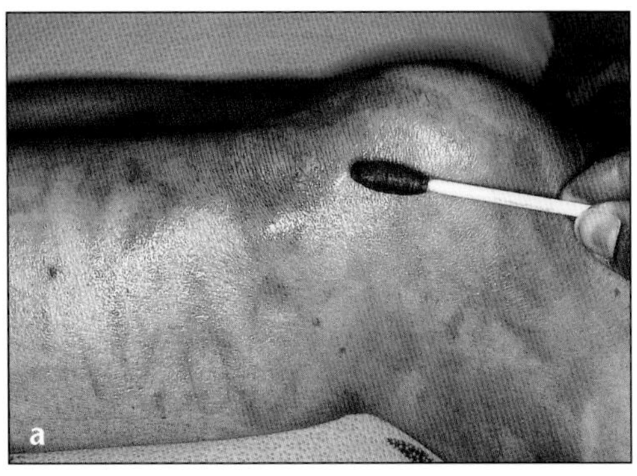

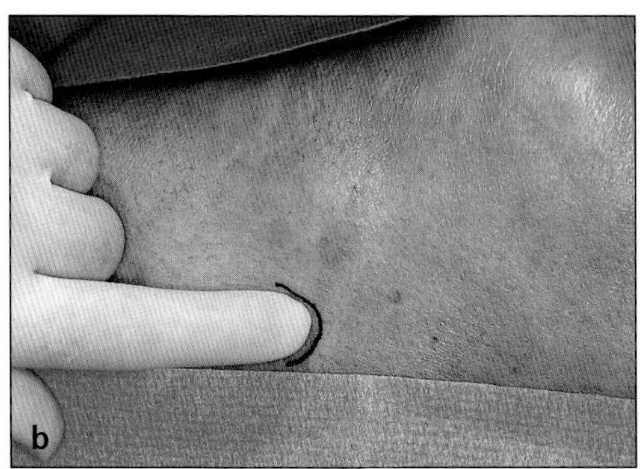

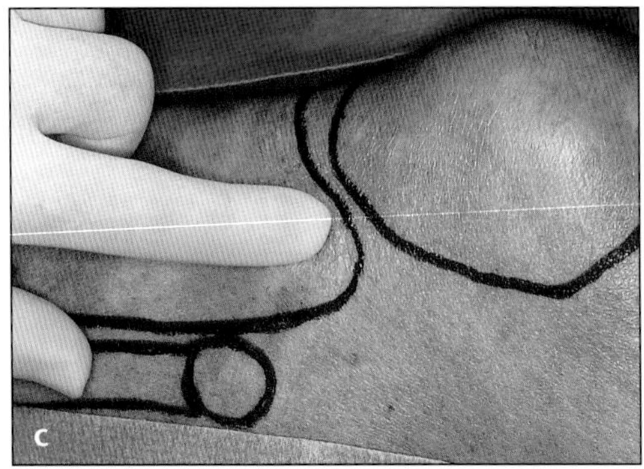

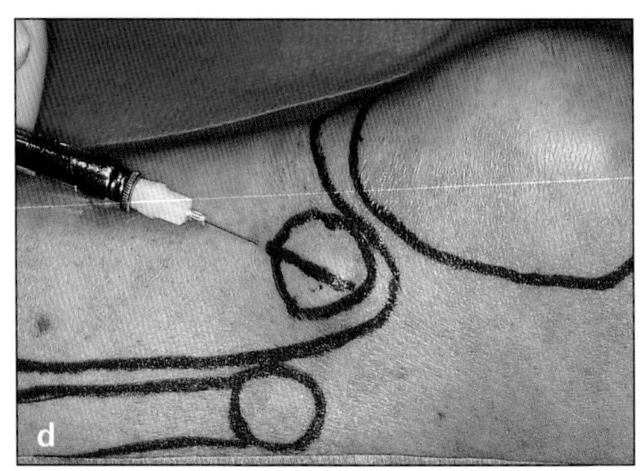

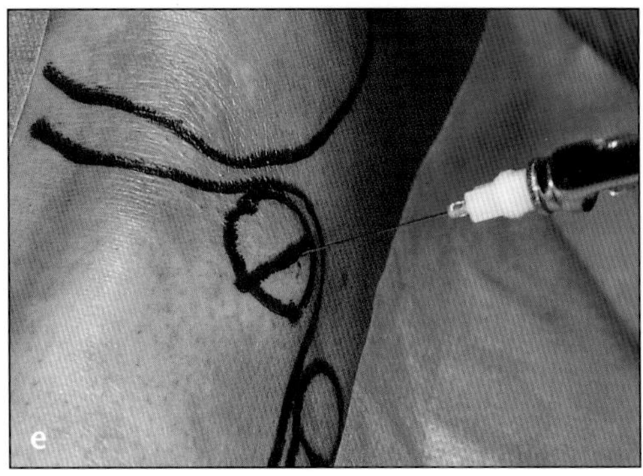

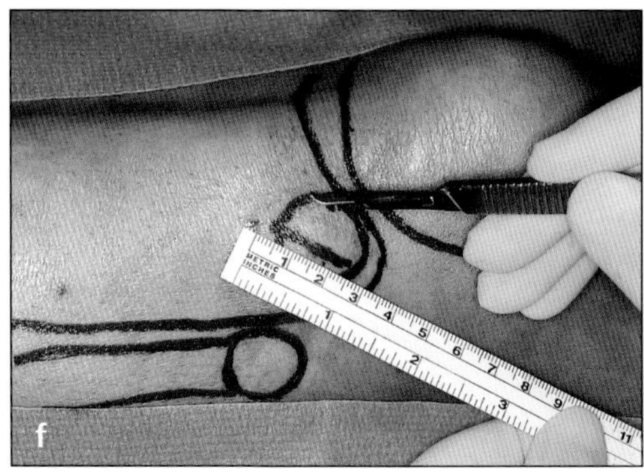

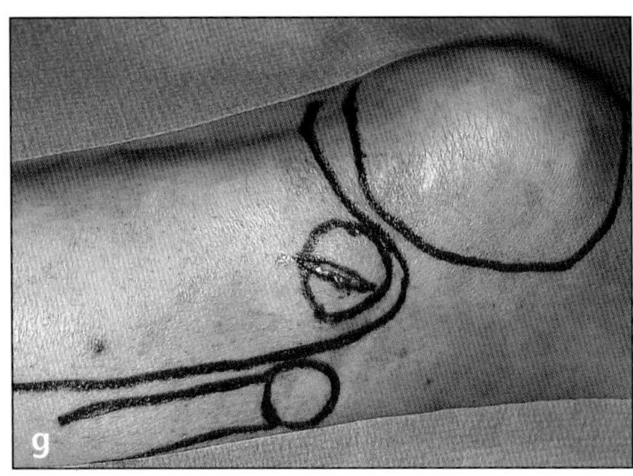

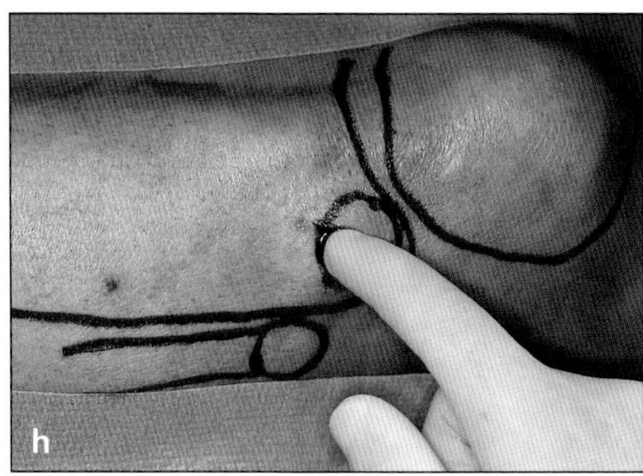

Fig 7-7 Cancellous bone is harvested from the tibia in preparation for a grafting procedure.

(a) The disinfected area should extend well beyond the incision site to provide a sterile surgical field.

(b) Several important anatomic landmarks should be carefully identified before the incision is started. Here, the clinician palpates and marks the head of the fibula.

(c) The head of the tibia is marked, followed by the Gerdy tubercle, the most important landmark for this procedure.

(d) After the incision location is marked, local anesthesia is deposited in the subcutaneous tissue. The needle is inserted all the way, and the solution is slowly applied as the needle is extracted.

(e) The last step in delivering local anesthesia at the tibial site is to deposit the solution at the level of the periosteum, placing the needle perpendicular to the skin's surface.

(f) The oblique incision, made directly over the protuberance (Gerdy tubercle), should measure 2 to 3 cm.

(g) The incision is made with a no. 15 scalpel blade and progresses in layers. If needed, cauterization can be used to control bleeding.

(h) The position of the incision is continually confirmed by palpation.

Fig 7-7 *(cont)*
(i) Rakes are ideal for retracting the skin and exposing the subcutaneous tissues. The thick, white periosteum is easy to identify. The blade should be pressed firmly over this tissue for a clean cut straight down to the bone.

(j) Once the bone is reached, a no. 701 surgical bur is used for the osteotomy, accompanied by good irrigation and suction.

(k) Perforations in the shape of a circle are made in the bone and then connected to form a 1- to 2-cm window. The cortical bone plug is then removed.

(l) Cancellous bone is scooped out of the bony window with a no. 4 Molt curette.

(m) The bone graft can be simultaneously placed into the recipient site. PRP was required for this case, mixed with the autogenous graft before delivery to the recipient site.

(n) Before closure, more PRP is applied for hemostasis and for delivery of growth factors to the donor site. Note how the entire cannula can be used to deliver the PRP, allowing the clinician to gain a sense of the volume and orientation of the cavity from which the bone marrow was taken.

(o) The sutures are placed in layers starting with periosteum and bone and followed by the subcutaneous layer.

(p) Bacitracin ointment is placed over the wound for added antibacterial protection. Placement of Steri-Strips helps reinforce the sutures and protect the incision line.

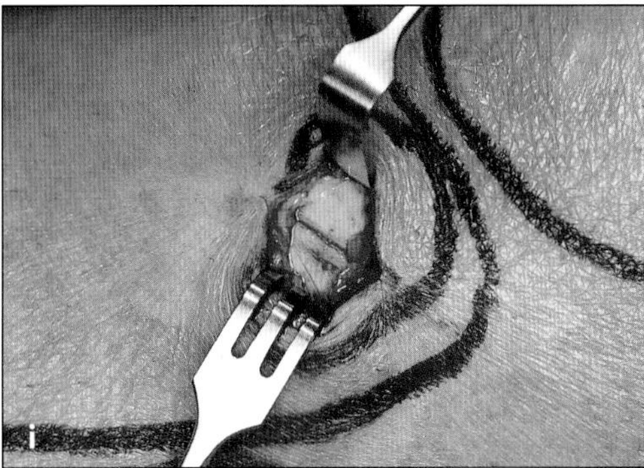

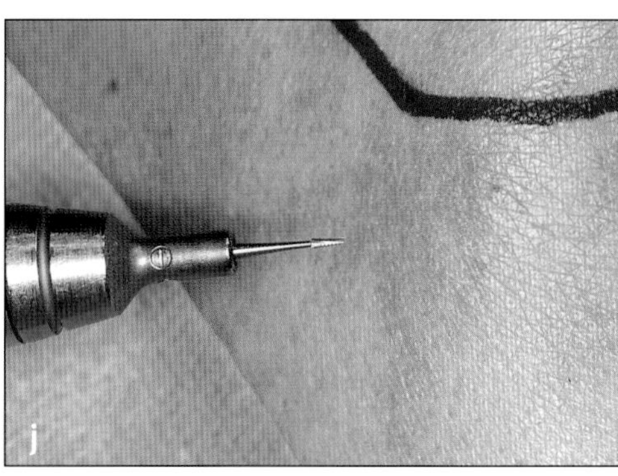

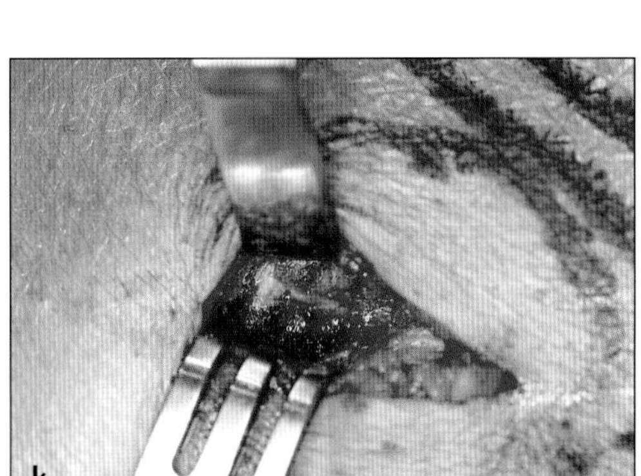

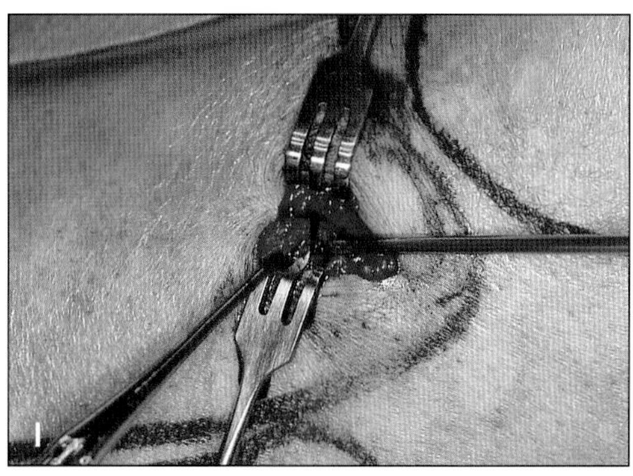

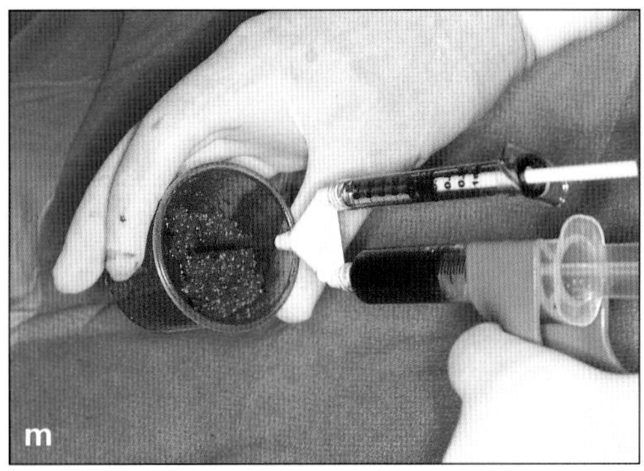

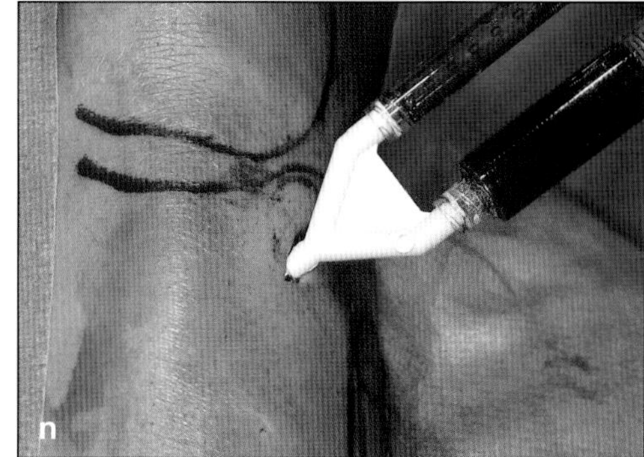

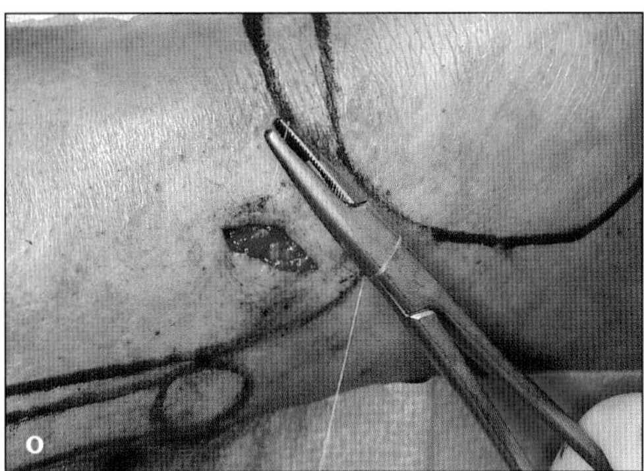

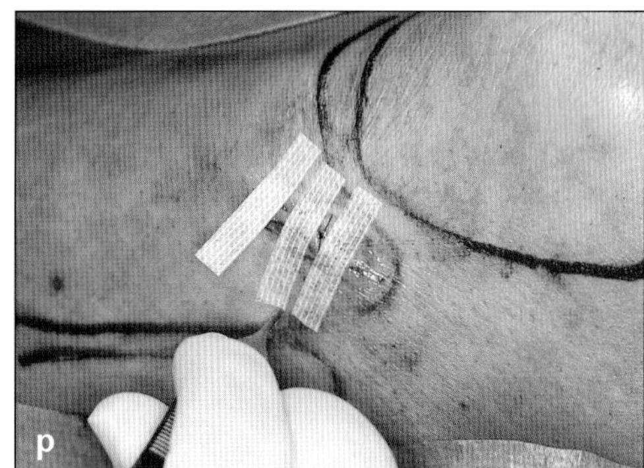

References

1. Huizinga PJ, Kushner GM, Alpert B. Tibial Bone Graft Technique. Louisville, KY: University of Louisville, 2000:7–8.
2. Garg AK. Lateral proximal tibia bone harvest for use in augmentation procedures. Dent Implantol Update 2001;12:33–37.
3. Garg AK. The use of platelet-rich plasma to enhance the success of bone grafts around dental implants. Dent Implantol Update 2000; 11:17–21.
4. Daffner RH. Case report 592: Bone graft donor site of tibia. Skeletal Radiol 1990;19:73–75.
5. Catone GA, Reimer BL, McNeir D, Ray R. Tibial autogenous cancellous bone as an alternative donor site in maxillofacial surgery: A preliminary report. J Oral Maxillofac Surg 1992; 50:1258–1263.
6. Marx RE, Garg AK. Bone structure, metabolism, and physiology: Its impact on dental implantology. Implant Dent 1998;7:267–276.
7. Besly W, Ward Booth P. Technique for harvesting tibial cancellous bone modified for use in children. Br J Oral Maxillofac Surg 1999; 37:129–133.
8. van Damme PA, Merkx MA. A modification of the tibial bone-graft-harvesting technique. Int J Oral Maxillofac Surg 1996;25:346–348.
9. Alt V, Nawab A, Seligson D. Bone grafting from the proximal tibia. J Trauma 1999;47: 555–557.
10. Ilankovan V, Stronczek M, Telfer M, Peterson LJ, Stassen LF, Ward-Booth P. A prospective study of trephined bone grafts of the tibial shaft and iliac crest. Br J Oral Maxillofac Surg 1998;36:434–439.
11. O'Keeffe RM Jr, Riemer BL, Butterfield SL. Harvesting of autogenous cancellous bone graft from the proximal tibial metaphysis. A review of 230 cases. J Orthop Trauma 1991; 5:469–474.
12. Herford AS, King BJ, Audia F, Becktor J. Medial approach for tibial bone graft: Anatomic study and clinical technique. J Oral Maxillofac Surg 2003;61:358–363.
13. Jakse N, Seibert FJ, Lorenzoni M, Eskici A, Pertl C. A modified technique of harvesting tibial cancellous bone and its use for sinus grafting. Clin Oral Implants Res 2001;12: 488–494.
14. Sandor GK, Rittenberg BN, Clokie CM, Caminiti MF. Clinical success in harvesting autogenous bone using a minimally invasive trephine. J Oral Maxillofac Surg 2003;61:164–168.
15. Marx RE, Snyder RM, Kline SN. Cellular survival of human marrow during placement of marrow-cancellous bone grafts. J Oral Surg 1979;37:712–718.
16. Boeck-Neto RJ, Gabrielli M, Lia R, Marcantonio E, Shibli JA, Marcantonio E Jr. Histomorphometrical analysis of bone formed after maxillary sinus floor augmentation by grafting with a combination of autogenous bone and demineralized freeze-dried bone allograft or hydroxyapatite. J Periodontol 2002;73: 266–270.
17. Valen M, Ganz SD. A synthetic bioactive resorbable graft for predictable implant reconstruction: Part one. J Oral Implantol 2002;28: 167–177.
18. Ganz SD, Valen M. Predictable synthetic bone grafting procedures for implant reconstruction: Part two. J Oral Implantol 2002;28: 178–183.
19. St John TA, Vaccaro AR, Sah AP, et al. Physical and monetary costs associated with autogenous bone graft harvesting. Am J Orthop 2003; 32:18–23.
20. Turner TM, Urban RM, Hall DJ, Cheema N, Lim TH. Restoration of large bone defects using a hard-setting, injectable putty containing demineralized bone particles compared to cancellous autograft bone. Orthopedics 2003;26(5 suppl):561–565.
21. Marchena JM, Block MS, Stover JD. Tibial bone harvesting under intravenous sedation: Morbidity and patient experiences. J Oral Maxillofac Surg 2002;60:1151–1154.
22. Cowan N, Young J, Murphy D, Bladen C. Double-blind, randomized, controlled trial of local anesthetic use for iliac crest donor site pain. J Neurosci Nurs 2002;34:205–210.

PART

III

Bone Grafting

CHAPTER

8 Augmentation Grafting of the Maxillary Sinus for Placement of Dental Implants

Dental implant placement in patients who are edentulous in the posterior maxilla can be difficult for a variety of reasons, including increased pneumatization of the maxillary sinus (and thus close approximation of the maxillary sinus floor to the alveolar crestal bone) or inadequate ridge width.[1] Sinus pneumatization, which typically occurs with aging, often minimizes or completely eliminates the vertical bone available for endosteal implant placement in the maxillary sinus. Often, the bone partition between the alveolar mucosa and the maxillary sinus is as thin as 1 mm (Fig 8-1).[2]

Since the mid-1990s, bone grafting the sinus floor to increase vertical height and improve bone quality for implant placement has become increasingly successful. It is an excellent and predictable procedure for treating patients who have a severely atrophic posterior maxilla.[3] Using a pull-out test of dental implants in various types of bone, one study found that bone-grafted areas tend to have an even higher bone-to-implant contact and greater pull-out resistance than normal bone. Thus, bone grafting around implants is recommended in sites that are deficient in bone volume or density or in sites such as the maxilla that have a history of implant failure.[4]

Grafting of the antral floor was originally developed and described by Tatum in the early 1970s (Fig 8-2).[5-7] Initially, he used an alveolar crestal access to the maxillary sinus. Subsequently, a modified Caldwell-Luc procedure was developed in which he approached the sinus by infracturing the lateral wall of the maxilla and using the wall to elevate the maxillary sinus membrane (Fig 8-3). An autogenous bone graft was then placed in the area previously

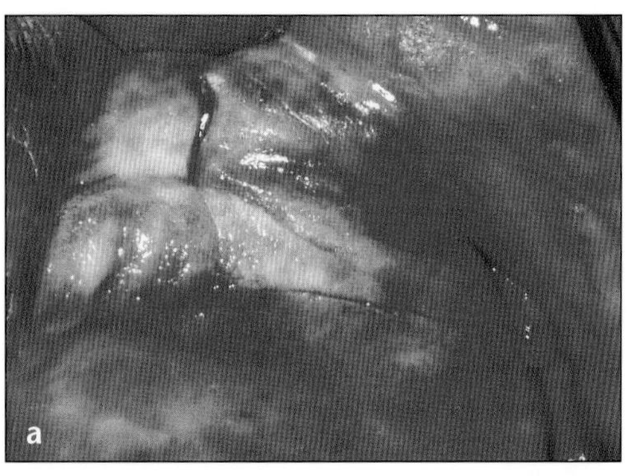

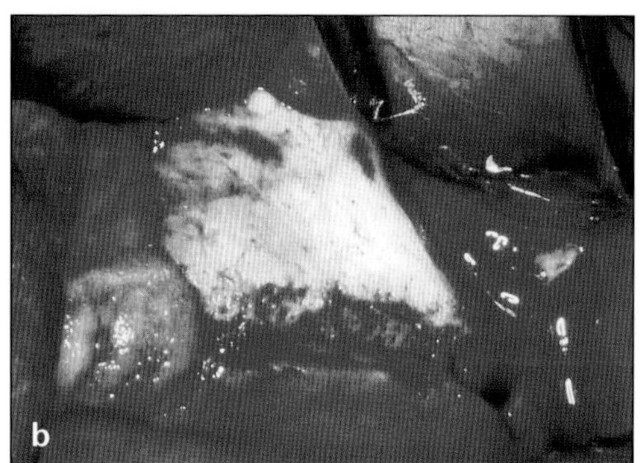

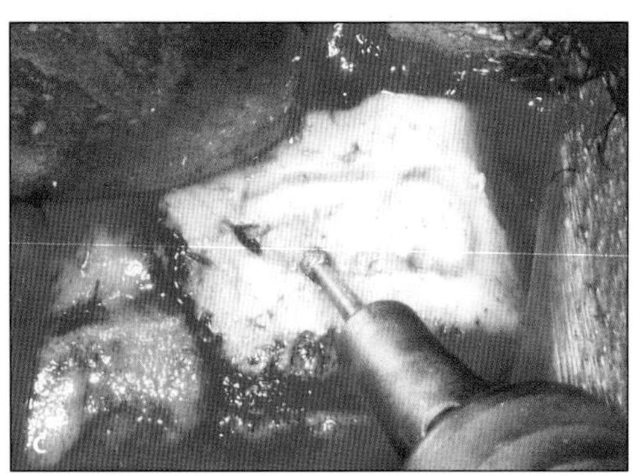

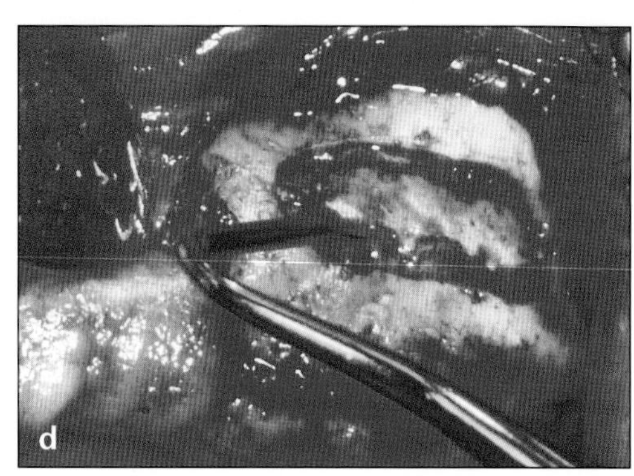

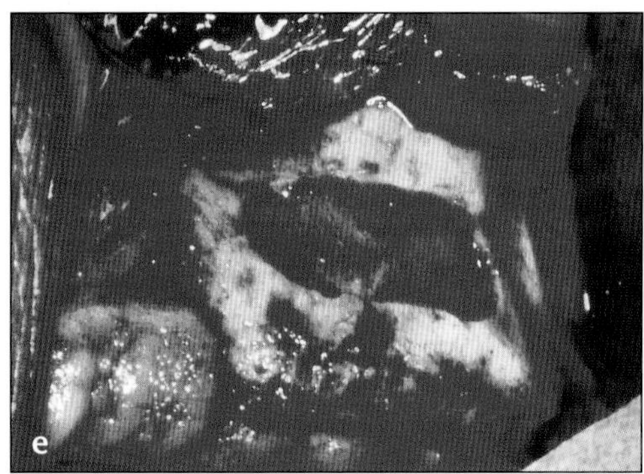

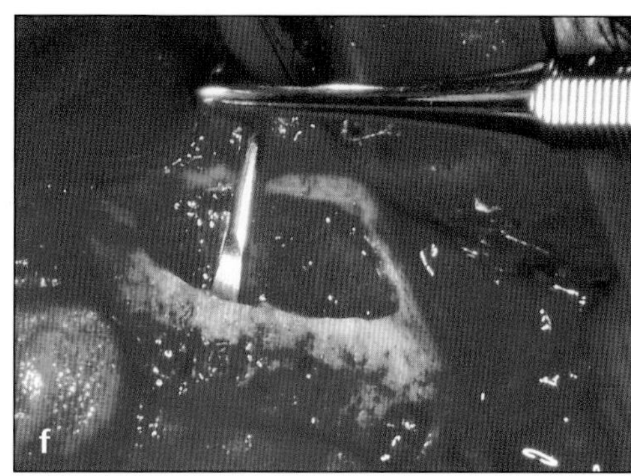

Fig 8-1 Sinus pneumatization often minimizes or eliminates the vertical bone available for implant placement in the maxillary sinus, necessitating bone grafting of the sinus floor to increase vertical height and improve bone quality.

(a) Maxillary ridges showing sufficient width for implant placement but inadequate height because of sinus cavity hyperpneumatization. The maxillary sinus lateral wall and floor are approximately 1 to 2 mm thick. An incision is made with a sharp no. 15 blade down to the bone, resulting in a clean cut through the tissues.

(b) A mucoperiosteal flap is reflected with a sharp periosteal elevator to avoid shredding of mucosa or periosteum. Vertical incisions permit adequate elevation of this flap for good visibility of the lateral wall of the maxilla.

(c) The osteotomy is shaped according to the sinus cavity. This step should be performed carefully, as the thickness of bone varies greatly from one patient to another.

(d) The island of bone that remains after the osteotomy is carefully elevated. The resistance of residual bone is variable, so this should be done slowly to prevent or minimize tears. Note the minimal thickness of the bone.

(e) The maxillary sinus membrane is exposed and ready to be reflected. Smooth edges facilitate the next step.

(f) The sinus membrane is reflected with specially designed curettes. Note that there are areas of the residual alveolar crest that are 0 mm thick.

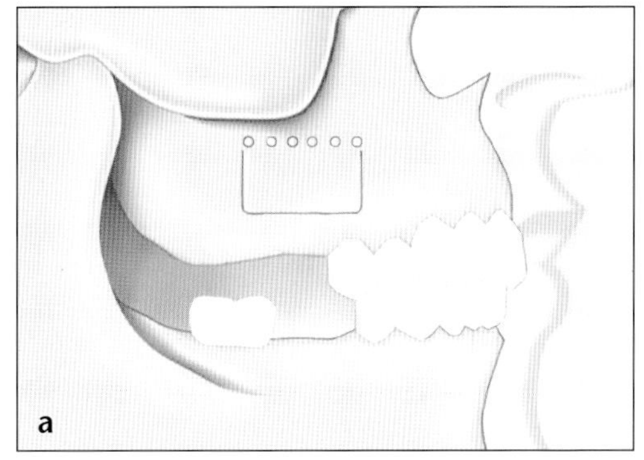

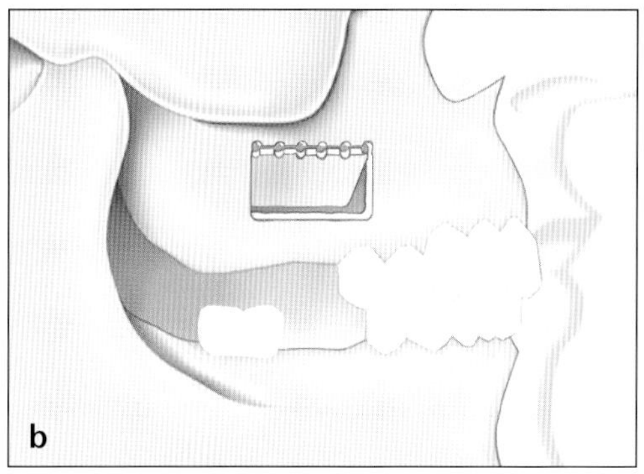

Fig 8-2
(a) The classic window design for augmentation grafting of the maxillary sinus. A rectangular or trapezoidal osteotomy is created and the superior portion is not contiguous. The underlying schneiderian membrane is left intact. A modified and recommended technique is presented later in this chapter.

(b) The bony island is fractured with an osteotome and mallet and elevated superiorly while simultaneously elevating the underlying schneiderian membrane.

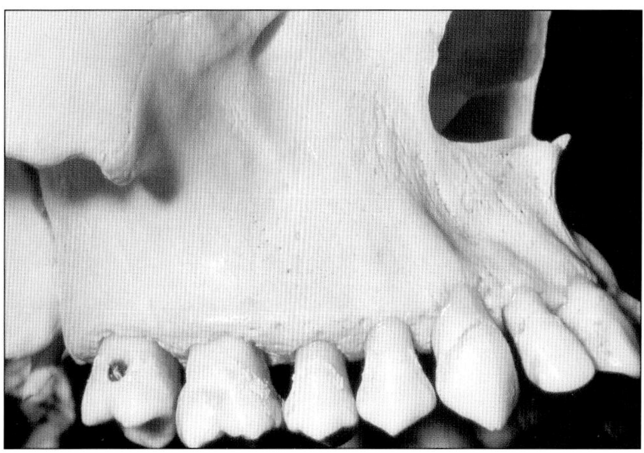

Fig 8-3
Lateral wall of the maxilla. Note the relationship of the infraorbital foramen and the sinus area. Also note the position of the zygoma in relation to the area for the osteotomy; this will be a landmark to use when designing the osteotomy. It is important to maintain the window inferior to the zygoma to minimize the chances of damaging the infraorbital nerve with the bur or the retractor.

occupied by the inferior third of the sinus. This technique provided adequate bone in the posterior maxilla, permitting various implant placement options.

In 1980, Boyne and James described a similar clinical procedure and demonstrated bone formation in the maxillary antrum following placement of autogenous marrow and cancellous bone in the maxillary sinus.[8] In 1984, Misch modified the technique, combining sinus augmentation and blade-vent implant placement in the same procedure.[9] In 1997, a further modified technique was published by Garg and Quinones in which sinus augmentation and rough-surface implants were combined and the window shape and design were modified along with recommended instrumentation[10] (Fig 8-4). These procedures differ in the initial surgical approach, the type or donor site of grafting material, and the type of implant used.

Sinus lift grafting and implant placement can be accomplished as either a one- or two-step procedure. Many authors have reported good initial results with both approaches.[1,11–25] If there is sufficient alveolar bone width and only partial pneumatization of the sinus, bone grafting and implant placement can be performed at the same time. This one-step approach offers the advantages of minimizing total treatment

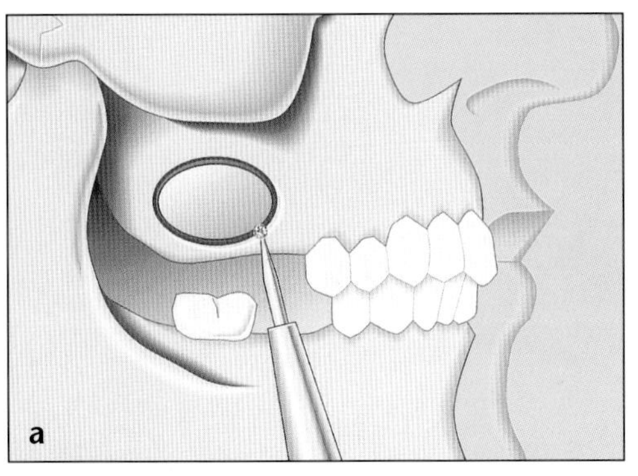

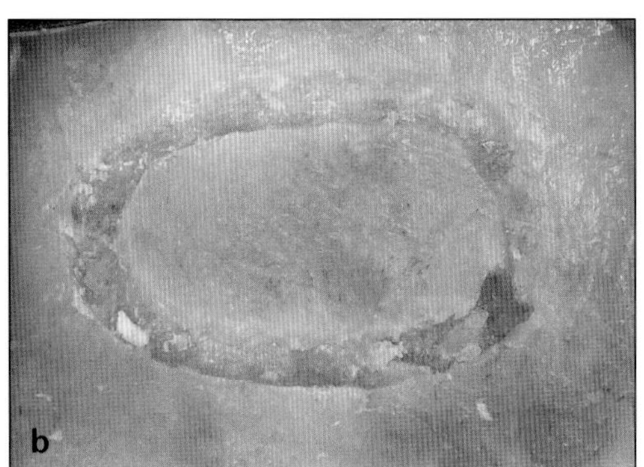

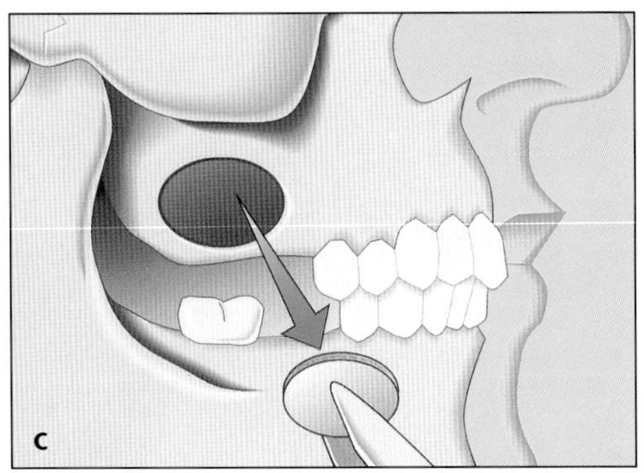

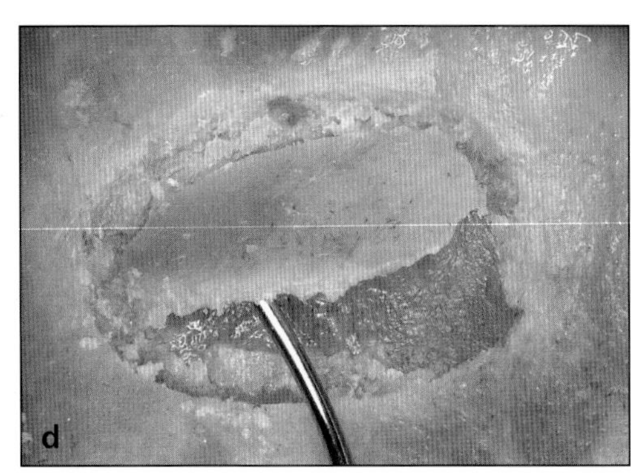

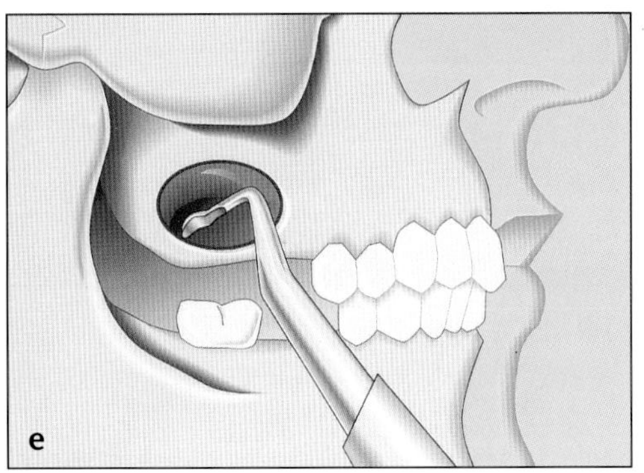

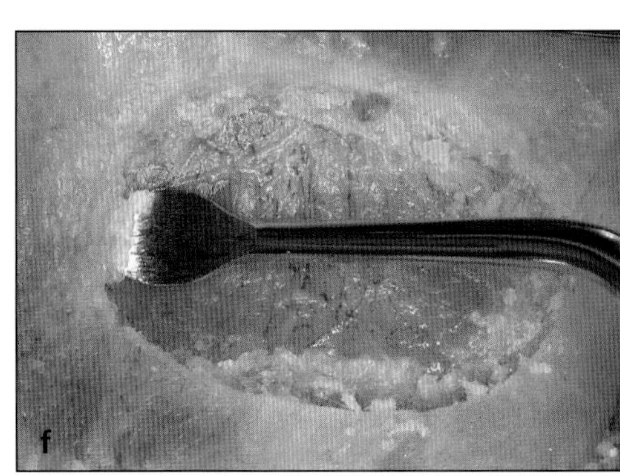

Fig 8-4 Sinus augmentation grafting technique using rough-surface implants and a modified window shape and design.

(a) The ideal shape of the osteotomy should be ovoid and contiguous. In this manner, the chances of schneiderian membrane perforation with sharp corners from a rectangular or trapezoidal osteotomy are minimized. This also minimizes membrane perforations due to sharp edges arising from a greenstick-fractured area superiorly.

(b) Osteotomy perfomed on a cadaver specimen. The size and shape of the osteotomy should follow the contours of the maxillary sinus.

(c) Removal of the island of bone. This should be performed gently to minimize the chances of perforating the underlying membrane.

(d) Elevation of the island of bone in a cadaver specimen.

(e) Sinus membrane elevation using a specially designed curette. Sharp curettes should be used and the membrane should be reflected off the bone as opposed to attempting to simply push it off the bone.

(f) Sinus membrane elevation with a curette in a cadaver specimen.

Fig 8-4 *(cont)*
(g) Coronal view of sinus membrane elevation. Note that the inferior portion of the window is approximately 3 mm above the sinus floor. This allows the surgeon to avoid some 1 to 2 mm sinus septa during elevation of the sinus window and allows for a small lip of bone to help contain the graft material. The superior portion of the window depends on the size of the implant that will be placed. The superior portion of the window should be measured from the ridge crest and should be at least the same height as the implant that is planned for the area.

(h) Membrane elevation in a cadaver specimen.

(i) Sinus cavity grafted with the amount of material needed for future implant placement. Note that this does not obliterate the entire sinus cavity.

(j) Grafting the sinus cavity returns the original contour of the lateral wall of the maxilla on this cadaver specimen.

(k) Coronal view of the grafted sinus cavity after some maturation of the graft has occurred.

(l) Coronal view of the implant site after the implant is placed and surrounded by sufficient bone.

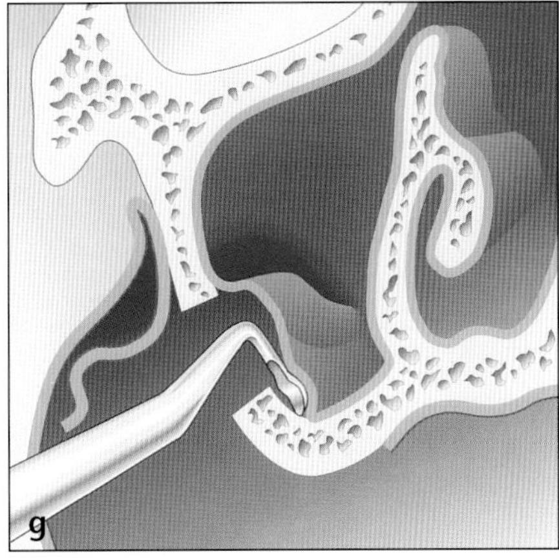

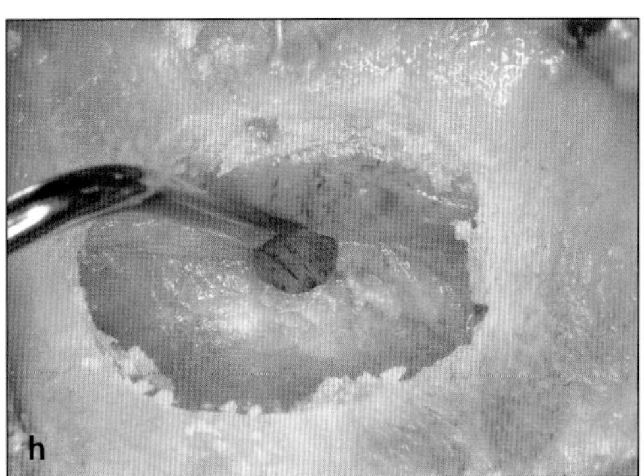

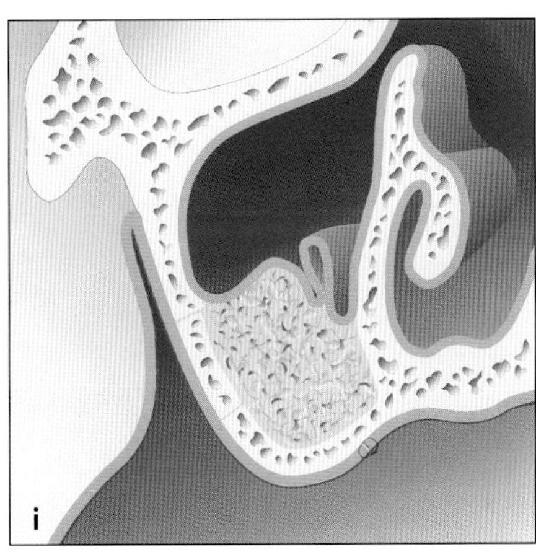

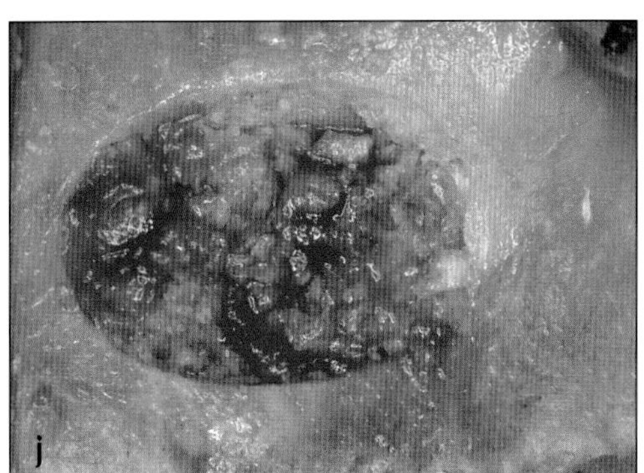

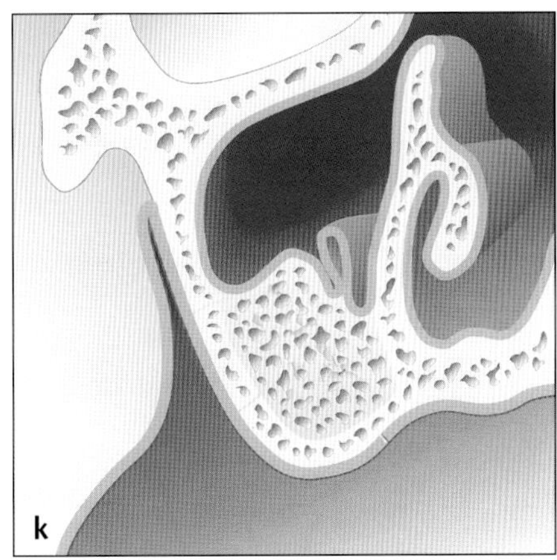

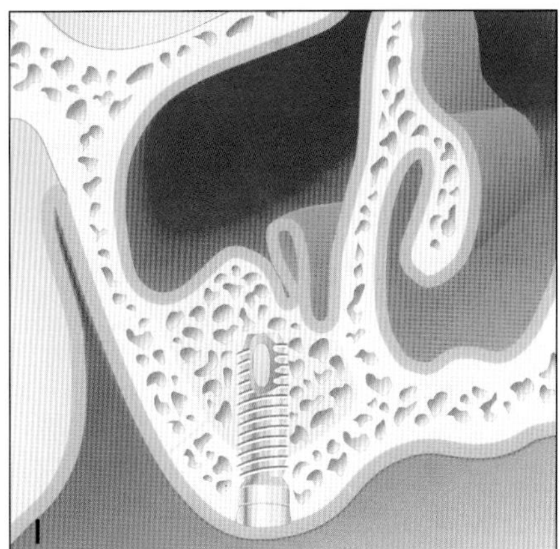

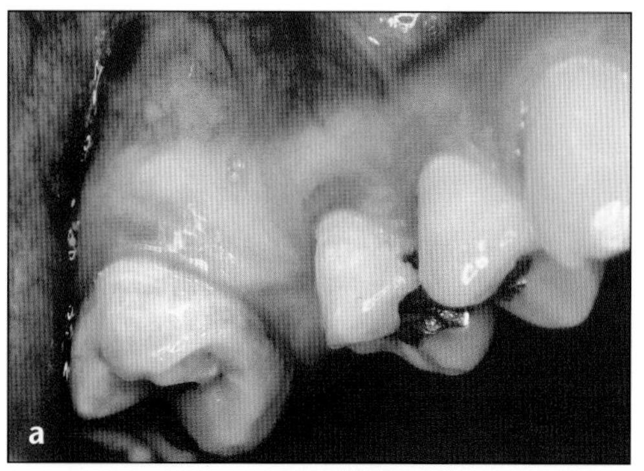

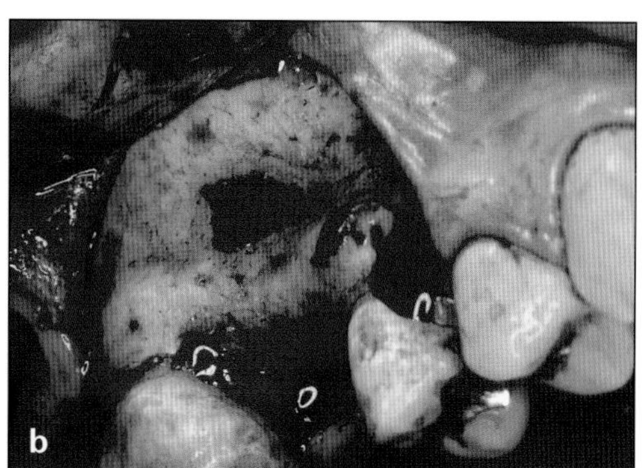

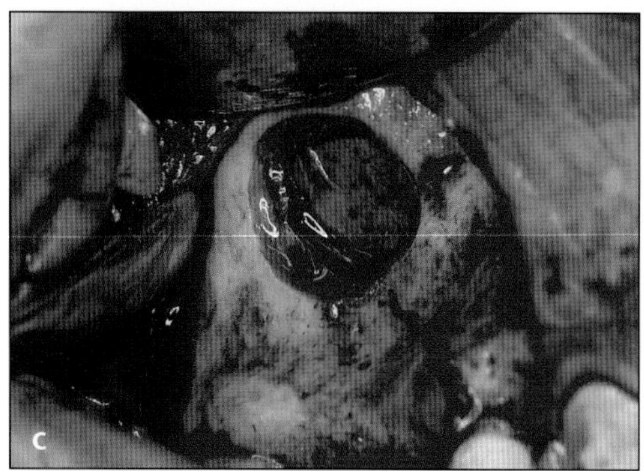

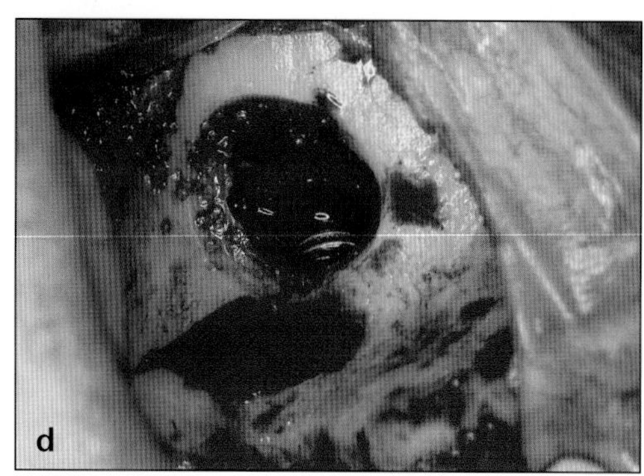

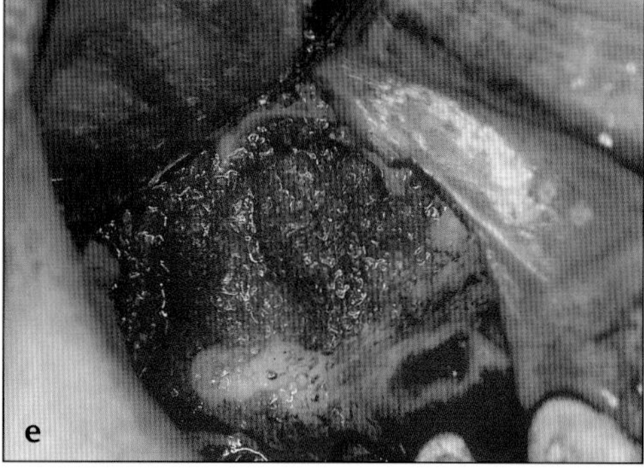

Fig 8-5 If there is sufficient alveolar bone width and only partial pneumatization of the sinus, bone grafting and implant placement can be performed at the same time.

(a) Sites with just one missing tooth can have enough pneumatization that the area requires sinus grafting. Bone grafting and placement can be performed simultaneously. The vertical release should be extended to the depth of the vestibule.

(b) The size of the flap is determined according to the site, but achieving good visualization always should be a consideration.

(c) In this case, a small osteotomy can be performed, thus avoiding any damage to adjacent teeth. Smooth edges are recommended to facilitate reflection.

(d) Integrity of the sinus membrane can be assessed by asking the patient to take a few deep breaths through the nose. At this point the implant osteotomy is performed, the medial half of the sinus is grafted, and the implant is placed.

(e) The sinus is then filled flush with the existing contours. A resorbable membrane extending beyond the borders of the window 3 mm circumferentially will be placed and the flap closed primarily.

time by eliminating a second surgical procedure and of allowing a coordinated consolidation of the graft around the implant[1] (Fig 8-5).

In the past, available host bone measuring less than 5 mm in height was deemed inadequate to mechanically maintain an endosteal implant. Thus, in these cases simultaneous bone grafting and implant placement were contraindicated in favor of the two-step approach, in which implant placement is delayed until 4 to 6 months after graft placement.[12,13] In recent years, this concept has been challenged, with success reported using the one-step approach for posterior maxillary ridges measuring as little as 1 mm in height.[2,26–29] The critical factor appears to be adequate ridge width for placement of the intended implant (Fig 8-6).

Because few vital anatomic structures encroach upon the surgical site, the risks with sinus lift grafting are negligible, morbidity is low, and postoperative complications can be treated relatively easily with medical or surgical intervention. Bone re-

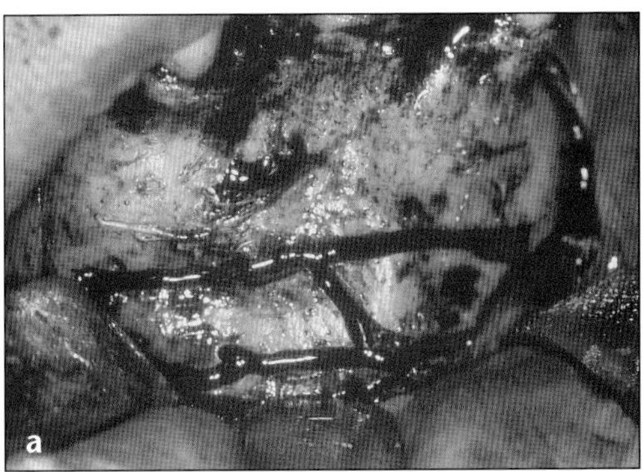

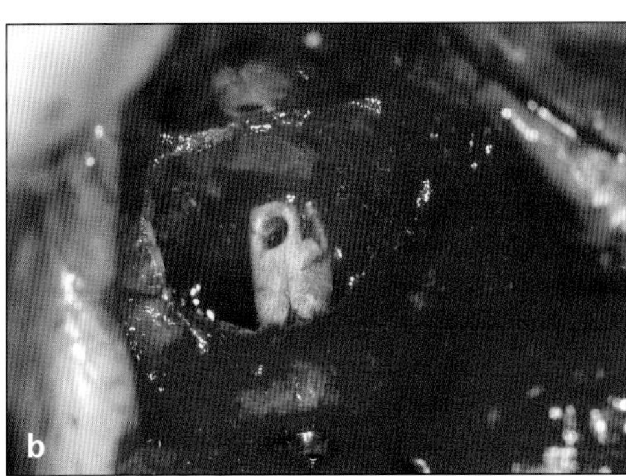

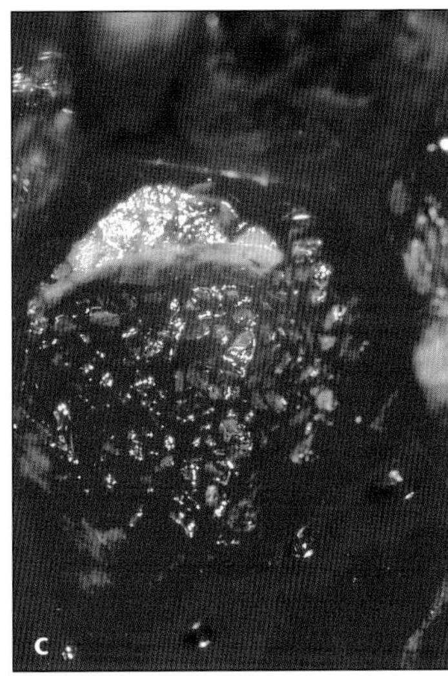

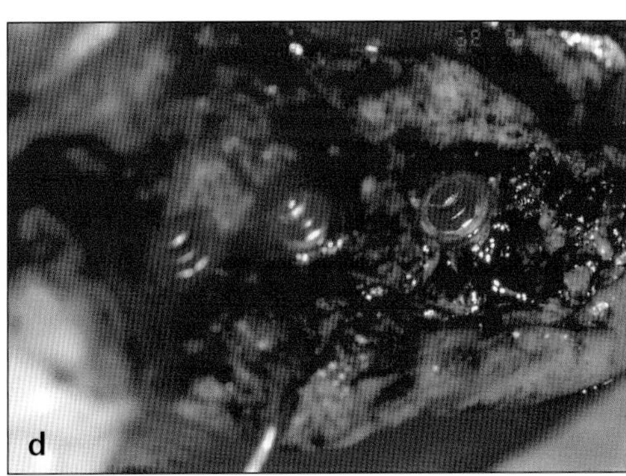

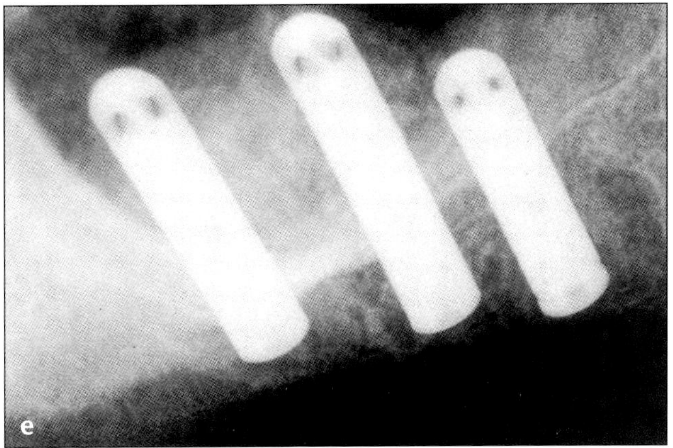

Fig 8-6 Recent studies show high success rates following simultaneous implant placement with sinus grafting, even in cases with as little as 1 mm of crestal bone height.

(a) Harvest of autogenous bone from anterior mandible to use for the graft. When performing grafting for hyperpneumatized sinuses, use of autogenous bone is recommended.

(b) Simultaneous implant placement with sinus grafting in cases with as little as 1 mm of crestal bone height must be performed by an experienced clinician, and a minimum of 8 mm of bone width is required. The lateral aspect will then be grafted.

(c) Multiple implants were placed simultaneously in the graft with good initial stabilization of the implants in spite of the minimal residual height of bone. Packing the bone in a careful, meticulous manner—densely in the sinus and around the implants—ensures that the implants remain in the same position.

(d) After 5 months of maturation, excellent results can be seen without any complications for stage 2 surgery.

(e) Radiographically, the bone is still mineralizing, and the position of the implants has been maintained as expected.

sponse is excellent, and different graft materials produce bone that is demonstrable on histologic examination.[26] The graft and new bone appear to remodel in response to functional loading. The prosthetic alternatives are also predictable; fixed, fixed removable, or removable prosthetic reconstructions can be placed over implants within the sinus graft.[1]

Maxillary Sinus Anatomy

Maxillary bone is primarily medullary (ie, spongy) (Fig 8-7) and finely trabecular. The quantity and osseous density of bone in this area is lower than that of premaxillary or mandibular bone. The adjacent cortices consist of compact bone; however, they are generally very thin, providing minimal strength compared with the cortices surrounding the mandible. Because of its spongy nature, medullary bone must establish a stress-bearing surface next to an endosteal implant in order for the functioning implant to remain stable and be able to transmit physiologic load to the supporting bone.[5,30]

The maxillary sinus is an approximately 15-mL-volume air space, although the actual size depends on the amount of resorption that has occurred. It resembles a sloped paperweight, with its largest and only flat side composing the medial wall (which is also the lateral wall of the nasal cavity).[31-33] Septa may divide the sinus into two or more cavities that may communicate. The sinus begins to form in the second to third year of life, and its formation is nearly complete by 8 years of age. It has a nonphysiologic drainage port high on the medial wall (maxillary ostium) that drains into the middle meatus of the nose. The ostium is considered nonphysiologic because it serves as an overflow drain rather than as a dependent complete drainage system.

The bony walls of the sinus are thin, except for the anterior wall and the alveolar ridge in the dentate individual. In the edentulous person, the alveolar bone is frequently atrophied and may be only 1 to 2 mm thick, making it unsuitable as an implant site without appropriate grafting. Thus, the purpose of sinus lift surgery is to restore a sufficient amount of alveolar bone so that implants can be successfully placed.

The maxillary sinus is lined with a pseudostratified columnar epithelium, which is also called the *schneiderian membrane.* Beneath the surface epithelium is a loosely cellular but highly vascular thin tissue. Beneath this, in all areas, is a periosteum. The delicate mucosa of the sinus attaches to the periosteum on its osseous surface. However, this feature is not an important source of bone formation in sinus lift surgery. A thin layer of respiratory epithelium, which lines the schneiderian membrane, cannot be differentiated from the periosteum of the bones to which it is firmly affixed.

The blood supply to the maxilla normally emanates from three parent arteries—the superior labial, anterior ethmoidal, and, primarily, the internal maxillary arteries. The area of sinus lift surgery is mainly supplied by branches from the internal maxillary artery. The sinus floor derives some of its blood flow from the greater and lesser palatine vessels as well as the incisal artery, a terminal branch of the sphenopalatine artery (which is yet another portion of the internal maxillary artery). These vessels penetrate the bony palate and ramify within the sinus floor and its medial and lateral walls. Another vascular contributor is the posterosuperior alveolar artery, which enters the maxilla in the superior tuberosity area to supply most of the posterior and lateral walls. The infraorbital branch of the internal maxillary artery helps to supply blood to the superolateral sinus area. The anterior ethmoidal artery, which is a terminal branch of the internal carotid system (via the ophthalmic artery), supplies the superomedial sinus area (Fig 8-8).

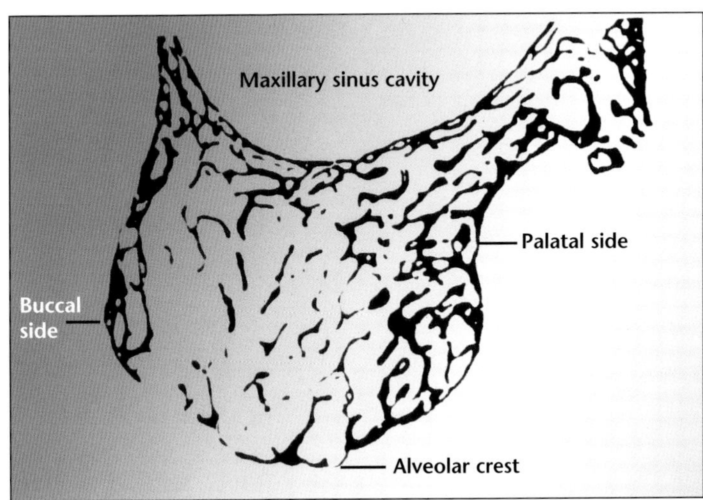

Fig 8-7
Coronal aspect of a decalcified histologic section of a maxillary ridge and its relationship to the sinus cavity. Note the spongy nature of the bone in this area.

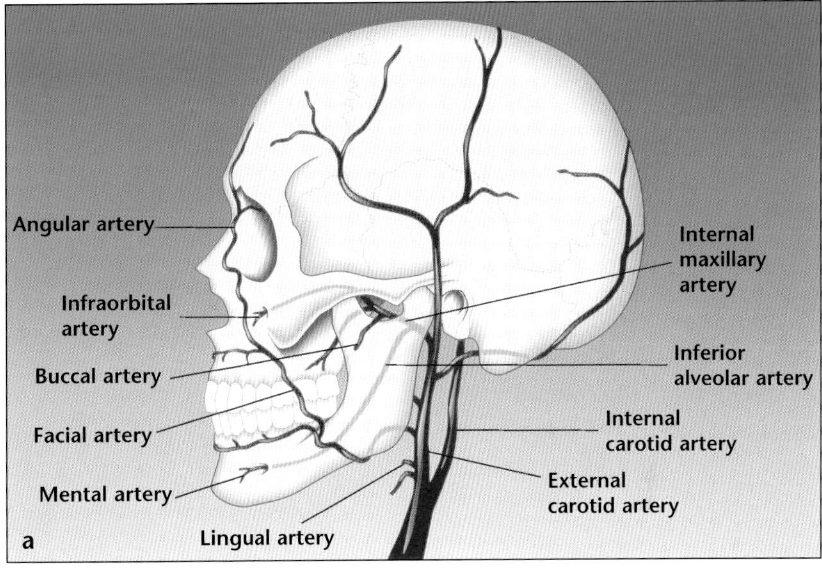

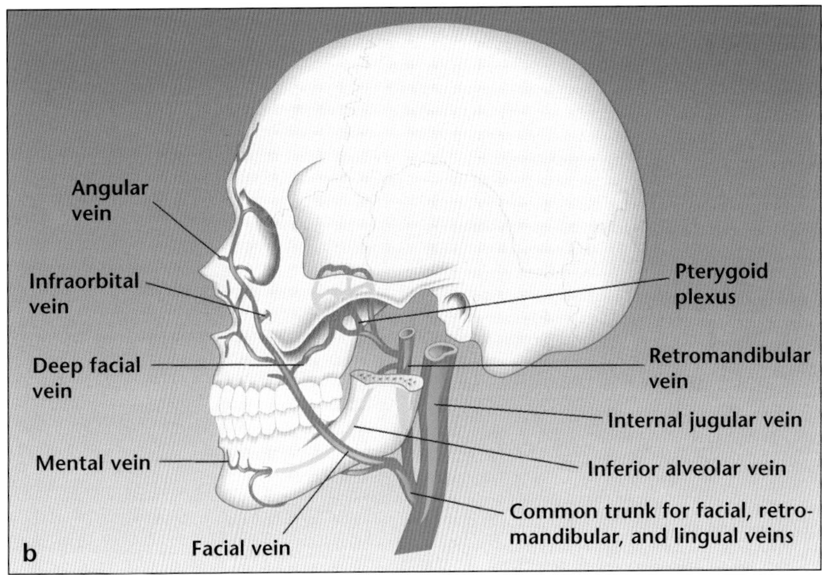

Fig 8-8
(a) Blood supply to the sinus starting at the common carotid artery.

(b) Venous drainage from the facial area.

Maxillary Sinus Physiology

The function of the maxillary sinus is purportedly to warm air and to provide resonance to the voice. The sinus is probably also the product of an evolutionary natural selection to assist the scalp veins and intracranial venous sinuses in dissipating the intense heat produced by the metabolically active human brain. Similarly, it also lightens the weight of the craniofacial complex.

The healthy maxillary sinus is self-maintained by postural drainage and actions of the ciliated epithelial lining, which propels bacteria toward the ostium. The sinus also produces mucus-containing lysosomes and immunoglobulins. The rich vascularity of the sinus membrane also helps to maintain its healthy state by allowing lymphocytic and immunoglobulin access to the membrane and sinus cavity. The healthy sinus contains its own normal flora, of which *Haemophilus* species are the most common. Other common flora may include streptococci, anaerobic gram-positive cocci, and aerobic gram-negative rods.

Mechanisms of Bone Grafting

Transplanted osteogenesis is another term for bone grafting; the phrase emphasizes that bone is dynamic and forms by cellular regeneration, which produces osteoid that becomes mineralized. A graft is not a solid bone block that heals into place.[34] Bone grafting is accomplished through osteogenesis, osteoinduction, and/or osteoconduction.[35-38] *Osteogenesis* refers to the formation and development of bone by osteocompetent cells. Osteogenic graft material, which is derived from or composed of tissue involved in the natural growth and repair of bone, can encourage bone formation in soft tissues and can stimulate faster bone growth in bone implant sites. *Osteoinduction* is the process of activating osteogenesis by recruiting cells from the surrounding natural bone that then differentiate into bone-forming cells. Osteoinductive grafts can enhance bone regeneration, sometimes even resulting in the extension or growth of bone where it is not normally found. *Osteoconduction* is the process by which the graft material acts as a nonviable scaffold onto and within which the patient's own natural bone grows. Osteoconductive grafts are conducive to bone growth and allow apposition from existing bone, but they do not produce or trigger bone formation themselves when placed in soft tissue.

Bone-Grafting Materials

Many materials have been used for sinus lift procedures, including autogenous bone,[11-16] bone allografts,[17,35,38-43] and alloplasts such as tricalcium phosphate (TCP), resorbable and nonresorbable hydroxyapatite,[1,38,44-46] bovine-derived bone mineral,[47] and bioactive glasses. An ideal graft is nontoxic, nonantigenic, noncarcinogenic, strong, resilient, easily fabricated, able to permit tissue attachment, resistant to infection, readily available, and inexpensive.[48]

Autogenous Bone

To date, there is no official consensus as to which graft material or combination of materials is best for augmenting the sinus antral void created by the sinus lift operation.[1,49-51] Autogenous bone has long been considered the gold standard among grafting materials because of its highly osteogenic, osteoinductive, and osteoconductive properties, a combination not found in the alternatives.[52] These properties allow bone to form more rapidly and in conditions where significant bone augmentation or repair is required. In a 1993 histomorphometric study of patients who underwent maxillary sinus augmentation, Moy et al assessed the bone composition of four different graft materials using biopsies taken from graft sites at the time of implant placement.[49] Particulated autogenous chin grafts contained 59.4% bone; composite grafts of hydroxyapatite and chin bone contained 44.4% bone; grafts of hydroxyapatite alone contained 20.3% bone; and grafts of demineralized freeze-dried bone alone contained 4.6% bone. Lorenzetti et al performed a similar study, which revealed that autogenous chin grafts contained 66% bone; autogenous iliac bone grafts contained 53% bone; and 50-50 composite grafts of autogenous chin bone and hydroxyapatite granules contained 44% bone.[53]

Cancellous particulated bone from the iliac crest continues to be an excellent source of autogenous graft material,[54] as is that from the tibial plateau (the procedure is described in greater detail in chapter 7). Intraoral sites such as the mandibular symphysis, maxillary tuberosity, ramus, and exostoses and debris from an implant osteotomy have also been used with success.[13,17,18,38,55] Mandibular bone grafts reportedly resorb less than do iliac crest grafts,[13,18] and the procedure can be easily accomplished in an office setting with the patient under parenteral sedation and local anesthesia (the procedure is described in greater detail in chapters 2, 5, and 6). Thus, there is no postoperative hospitalization, which results in lower costs and better patient acceptance.

A disadvantage of intraorally obtained bone grafts is that donor sites provide a smaller volume of bone than what can be obtained from the iliac crest or tibial plateau. A typical sinus requires approximately 4 to 5 mL of bone volume for grafting for dental implants. The total graft volume required is naturally dependent on the amount of bone resorption (sinus pneumatization and ridge resorption) that has occurred at the time the patient presents for surgery. Typically, 5 mL of bone can be harvested from the anterior mandible, 5 to 10 mL from the ascending ramus, 20 to 40 mL from the tibial head, 70 mL from the anterior ilium, and approximately 140 mL from the posterior iliac crest.

The use of cortical and corticocancellous blocks adapted to the sinus floor has also been reported, although healing time is longer compared with that associated with particulated graft material.[56] In a 6-year follow-up investigation of 216 sinus lift procedures with immediate placement of 467 implants into bone measuring 1 to 5 mm in height, Khoury observed the best bone regeneration in patients grafted completely with autogenous material comprising a percentage of cortical bone.[2]

The choice of donor site usually depends on the volume and type of bone desired. In extremely healthy patients, patients with minimal sinus resorption, and patients who refuse to undergo an extraoral bone graft harvest, it may be appropriate to expand the volume of autogenous bone harvested intraorally by combining it with other graft materials, such as allografts or alloplasts. However, some recent studies indicate that bone formed in autogenous bone–grafted sinuses is retained signficantly longer than in sites grafted with a combination of autogenous and demineralized freeze-dried bone allografts (DFDBA).[57] Lorenzetti et al showed that in maxillary sinuses grafted with a combination of autogenous bone and hydroxyapatite granules, soft tissue prevailed over bone, and a year after placement the hydroxyapatite granules were clearly distinguishable and surrounded by only a very thin layer of bone.[53]

Allografts

Bone allografts such as freeze-dried bone allografts (FDBA) or DFDBA may be cortical or trabecular. They are obtained from cadavers or living donors other than the patient, processed under complete sterility, and stored in bone banks. Fresh allografts are the most antigenic; however, this antigenicity can be reduced considerably by freezing or freeze-drying the bone, as is customary.[39]

Whether these grafts form bone by osteoinduction, osteoconduction, or some combination of both is the subject of continued debate. In the 1960s, Urist suggested that allografts form bone by osteoinduction because they contain osteoinductive proteins called *bone morphogenetic proteins* (BMPs).[58] FDBA can be used in either a mineralized or demineralized form. Both FDBA and DFDBA contain BMPs; however, in the quantities used clinically, the amount of BMPs is generally inadequate to account for osteoconduction. Demineralization removes the mineral phase and purportedly exposes the underlying bone collagen and growth factors, particularly BMPs.[35,40,41] Although the demineralization process exposes growth factors, it also destroys approximately half of the growth factors contained in FDBA. Additionally, the demineralization process removes the mineral portion of the graft (hydroxyapatite), which is critical for maintaining the matrix of the grafted site and providing for osteoconduction. Several authors have since challenged this theory based on unpredictable results with DFDBA, suggesting that these allografts may contain inconsistent and often inadequate levels of BMPs because of factors such as handling and processing technique.[59-62] One study suggested that using DFDBA in combination with hydroxyapatite may somewhat improve its effectiveness.[54] These concerns are valid; hence, the author recommends FDBA rather than DFDBA for bone grafting. This is discussed in more detail in chapter 2.

Irradiated cancellous bone has also been used as a substitute graft material for autogenous bone.[42,43] However, by using mineralized FDBA, a local substrate of mineral is provided for the graft and no BMPs are destroyed in the demineralizing process. Jensen and Greer found that radiated mineralized allografts used in conjunction with maxillary antroplasty, a screw-form implant, and an expanded polytetrafluoroethylene (e-PTFE) membrane barrier provided more predictable ossification than demineralized cancellous allograft.[50] They concluded that this graft material was the best option other than autogenous bone.

Advantages of allografts include ready availability, minimization of the amount of autogenous bone harvested from the patient, reduced anesthesia and surgical time, decreased blood loss, and fewer complications.[38] The disadvantages are primarily their dimished capacity to produce bone as compared to autogenous bone, and perhaps the theoretical disadvantages associated with tissues transplanted from another individual[35,38,46] (cadaver bone can be rejected like other transplanted tissues or organs). Technical problems include the precision required to insert bulk allografts, the necessity for rigid fixation to the host bone to obtain successful union, and the high rates of infection, nonunion, and graft fracture.[35,39] Because allografts are not osteogenic, adding this material to autogenous bone means that bone formation will proceed more slowly and result in less volume than with purely autogenous grafts.[38] Studies have shown that DFDBA for the maxillary sinus is often not completely remodeled by the host and does not always produce a sufficient amount or quality of new bone, even when a protective membrane is used.[1,50,51]

Alloplasts

Alloplasts, which may be natural or synthetic materials, heal only through osteoconduction. The most commonly used alloplasts are bioactive ceramics, which include synthetic calcium phosphate materials (eg, hydroxyapatite) and those derived from natural sources (eg, deorganified bovine bone). Ceramics such as hydroxyapatite are safe and well tolerated but have little ability to encourage new attachments.[44] Nonresorbable hydroxyapatite has also been criticized as being of modest value for grafting the maxillary sinus for implant placement.[63,64] Calcium phosphate ceramics act primarily as filler materials, with new bone formation taking place along their surface.[45,46] The objective in using them is to help provide a scaffold for enhanced bone tissue repair and growth.

Combining allograft or alloplastic grafting material with autogenous bone can decrease the amount of harvested bone necessary for the sinus lift procedure,[3] but as noted earlier, bone formation may be less complete or proceed more slowly than when autogenous bone is used alone.

Biologic growth factors and bone grafts

The application of BMPs and other growth factors is the subject of increased research today as a way to enhance bone regeneration and possibly even to replace bone grafting altogether for inducing osteogenesis. For instance, Boyne et al studied the efficacy, safety, and technical feasibility of delivering human recombinant BMP-2 via an absorbable collagen sponge implant in various cases.[65–67] In animal studies involving maxillary sinus augmentation,[65,68] the authors reported that this technique resulted in significant new bone formation in the floor of the maxillary sinus and that the delivery system did not induce any significant immune or other adverse response.

Preoperative Evaluation

Before undertaking sinus lift and grafting procedures, a thorough medical history must be obtained. In particular, the patient should be evaluated for seasonal allergies, allergic rhinitis, or sinus congestion upon waking, all of which may indicate potential sinus pathosis. A patient with sinusitis, sinus disease, or invasive lesions should be referred to an appropriate medical therapist for treatment before surgery proceeds.

The patient should also be asked about tobacco use and the ability to refrain from use before and after surgery, as this can severely impact the success of bone grafting. Nicotine impairs bone healing, diminishes osteoblast function, causes autogenous bone graft morbidity, and decreases graft biomechanical properties.[69]

Panoramic radiographs (Fig 8-9) are necessary and can be supplemented with sinus radiographs and computed tomography (CT) scans (Fig 8-10) to help the clinician determine the available maxillary alveolar bone height, the location of sinus floor convolutions (septa), and the surgical entry site. An anesthesia light wand may also help to illuminate the sinus and to guide placement of the sinus wall osteotomy.[70] The wand is placed transnasally or in the palatal region intraoperatively. It can also be used postoperatively to evaluate the density of graft material in the sinus prior to closure, since it illuminates any voids or uneven placement of the graft material.

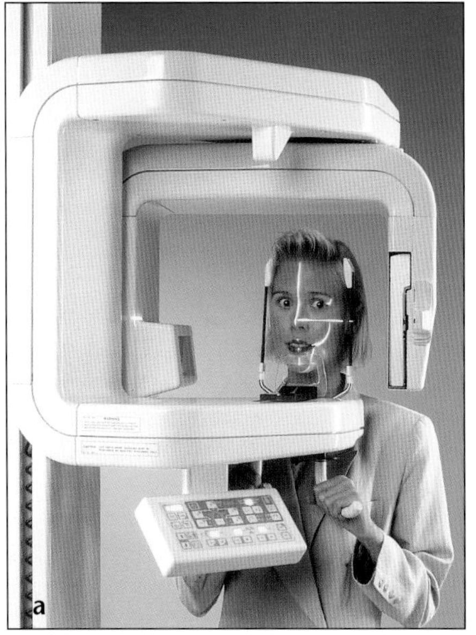

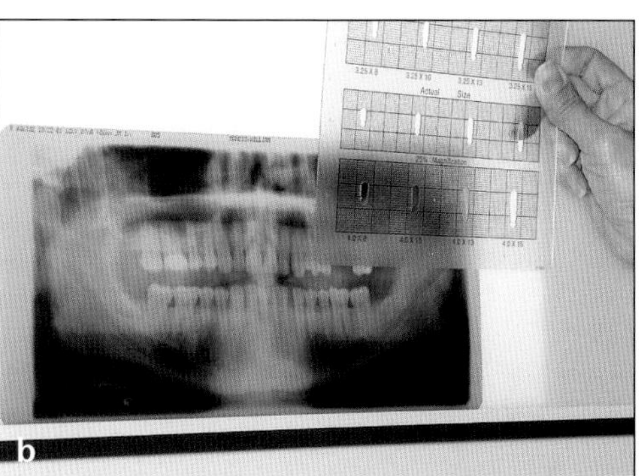

Fig 8-9

(a) The panoramic radiograph is the main radiographic tool for initial assessment of the maxillary sinus.

(b) Grids showing the average percentage of magnification that is expected from the panoramic radiographs are available from various manufacturers. They provide a quick, relatively accurate way to measure dimension height and mesiodistal spacing.

The interdental space is evaluated for the available space between the gingiva and the proper plane of occlusion, which should be greater than 5 mm. If there is less than 5 mm of vertical space present for prosthetic reconstruction, a gingivectomy, vertical osteotomy of the maxillary posterior alveolar process, and/or correlation of the mandibular plane is indicated.[5,9] If more than 20 mm of vertical space is available for prosthetic reconstruction, ridge augmentation in addition to sinus grafting should be considered. It is also important to determine if any active disease or disorders (eg, acute sinusitis, retained root tips, polyps, tumors, cysts in the antral cavity) exist in the sinus. It has been shown that patients with periodontal disease have an increased incidence of maxillary sinus disease, which may have an impact on implantation.[71] All remaining maxillary teeth should be evaluated to ensure that there is no periodontal disease extending from the tooth into the maxillary sinus. The presence of any of these entities contraindicates performing the procedure until they are corrected. After the relevant patient workup has been accomplished, the surgical procedure can be performed.

Fig 8-10
(a) In some cases, the panoramic radiograph can be supplemented with CT scans to help determine the presence of anatomic variations such as septa and polyps.

(b, c, d) The scanner takes images in a coronal, a sagittal, and an axial plane. This information can then be reformatted by the computer to provide images in a variety of formats.

(e) A tomographic image in which specialized software was used to provide slices perpendicular to the facial aspect of the maxilla. The anterior maxillary ridge, posterior maxillary ridge, and maxillary sinus can be seen in the various images.

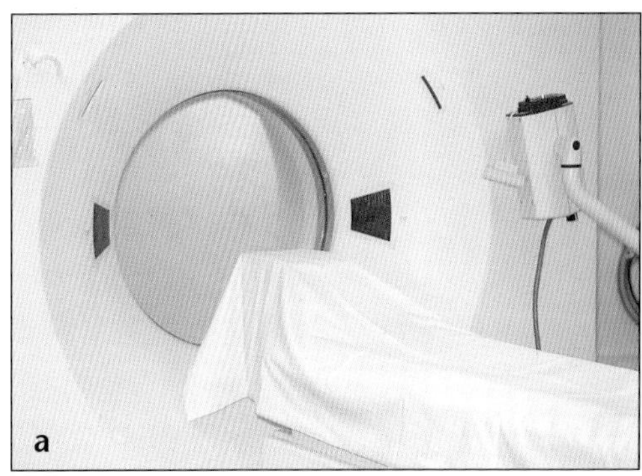

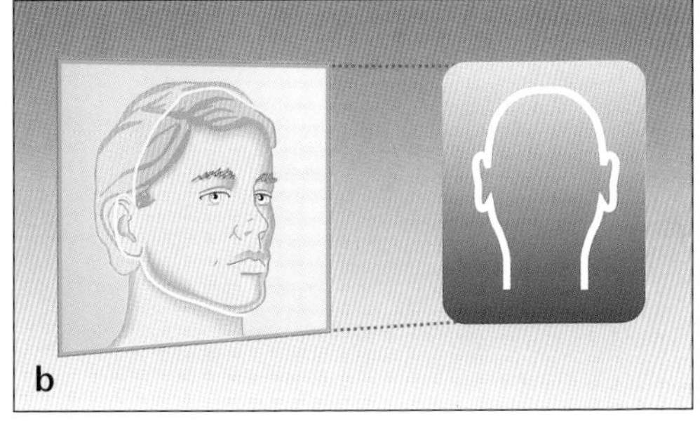

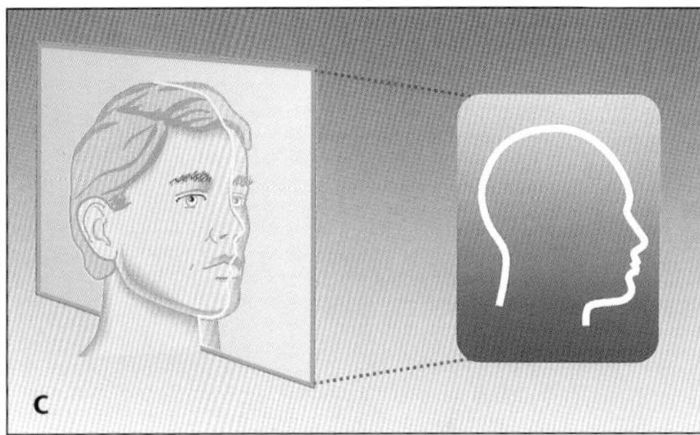

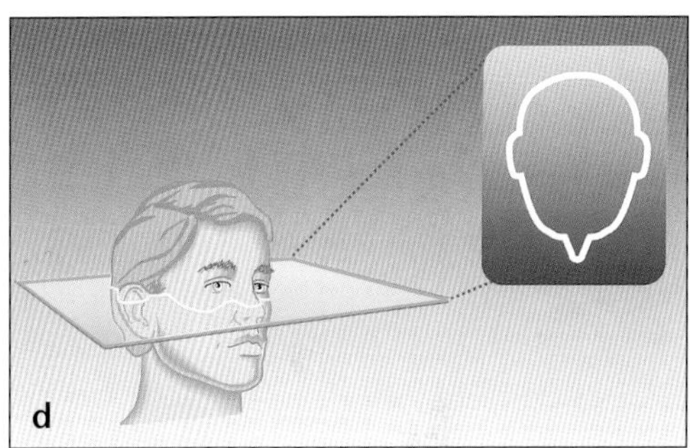

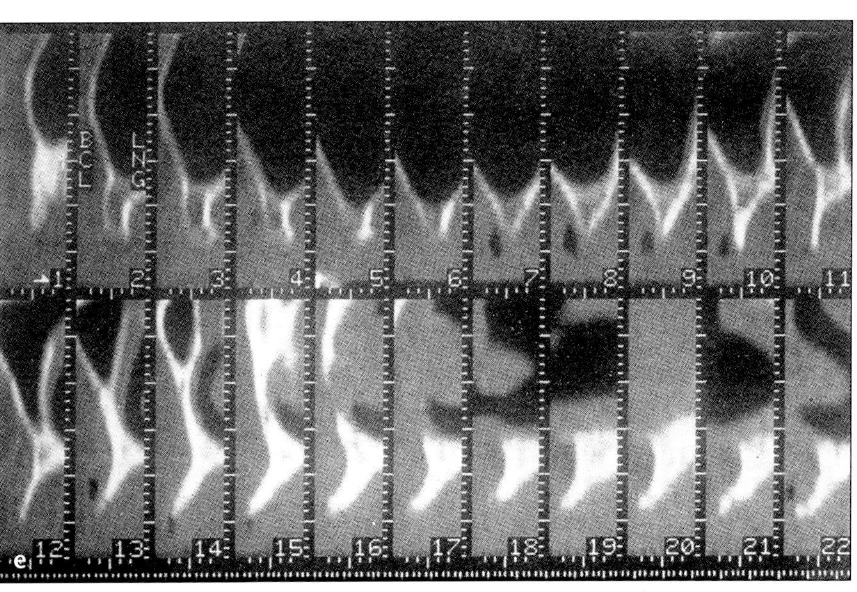

Surgical Technique

Appropriate antibiotics that are effective against both aerobic and anaerobic bacteria should be administered preoperatively and continued for 7 to 10 days postoperatively.[72,73] The surgery can be performed with the patient sedated with intravenous medication unless the graft material is procured from the iliac crest, in which case general anesthesia should be used. A local anesthetic with a vasoconstrictor for hemostasis is infiltrated into the maxillary surgical site and any intraoral graft donor site. The surgery can also be performed with local anesthesia, posterosuperior alveolar, and greater palatine nerve blocks combined with infiltration. A second-division nerve block, entered from the greater palatine canal, can also be used.

A horizontal incision is made on the crest or palatal aspect of the edentulous ridge, with extensions beyond the areas of the osteotomy and with consideration of the amount of attached gingiva on the alveolar crest. The incision is carried forward beyond the anterior border of the sinus (Fig 8-11). A vertical releasing incision to the depth of the vestibule in the canine fossa area helps to reflect the flap and expose the bone and also ensures good soft tissue closure over the bone. The lateral wall of the maxilla is exposed by reflecting the mucoperiosteal flap superiorly to the level of the malar buttress. Elevation of the periosteum adjacent to the implant site should be minimized to preserve the blood supply to the alveolar crest. The periosteum should be reflected superiorly just beyond the height of the superior aspect of the anticipated opening into the maxillary sinus (approximately at the level of the zygoma).

After the lateral maxillary wall has been completely exposed, a no. 8 round diamond bur should be used in an oval configuration at low speed and high torque to make an oval osteotomy in the lateral wall of the maxillary sinus (Fig 8-12). If the maxillary wall is thick, a no. 8 round carbide bur can be used to initiate the osteotomy to cut more quickly and then exchanged for a diamond bur of the same size and shape when approaching the schneiderian membrane in order to minimize the risk of perforating the membrane with the bur. Slight variations in osteotomy technique have been described; some authors[11] create a U-shaped osteotomy with the vertical arms of the osteotomy parallel to facilitate infracturing, and others[1] make a trapezoid-shaped osteotomy with a no. 1701 fissure cut bur. An oval-shaped osteotomy is recommended to avoid sharp edges that may tear the schneiderian membrane.[10] Similarly, the round diamond bur is recommended to minimize perforations of the schneiderian membrane. A brush-stroke type of touch is used to penetrate through the bone while avoiding the schneiderian membrane. To ensure that the bone has been penetrated all the way around the oval osteotomy, it should be tapped gently, and any movement should be noted. This bone can be either pushed in to serve as the roof of the graft or removed to create a window for better visualization and access. In cases in which a septum is attached to the bone window, the window can be drilled down and obliterated so the sinus is separated into two or more smaller chambers by the septum (Fig 8-13).

At this point, the underlying schneiderian membrane is exposed. Meticulous care should be taken to reflect the membrane superiorly without perforating it. A curette is gently introduced along the margin of the created access window, with the curved portion placed against the schneiderian membrane and the sharp edges placed against the bone (Fig 8-14). The curette is slid along the bone, 360 degrees around the margin of the access window.

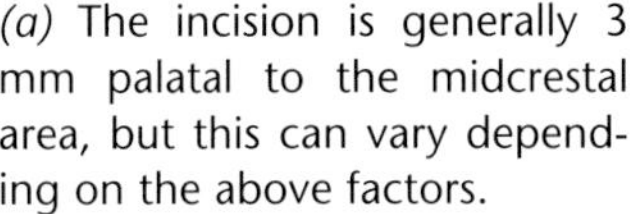

Fig 8-11 The anatomy of the ridge, the ridge width, and the amount of attached gingiva are some of the factors to consider before starting the incision.

(a) The incision is generally 3 mm palatal to the midcrestal area, but this can vary depending on the above factors.

(b) A vertical releasing incision is made mesial to the site where the osteotomy will be performed. The incision should be made in such a fashion that the base is wider than the tip. The extension of this incision superiorly will depend on the area where the osteotomy will be performed but generally is to the depth of the vestibule. A small posterior vertical release is usually helpful in achieving adequate reflection of the flap.

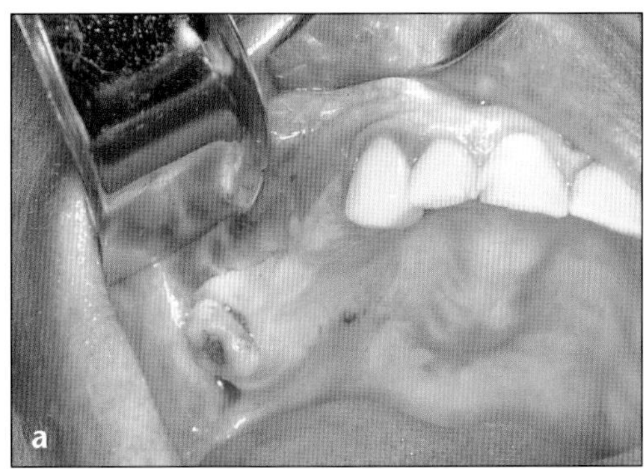

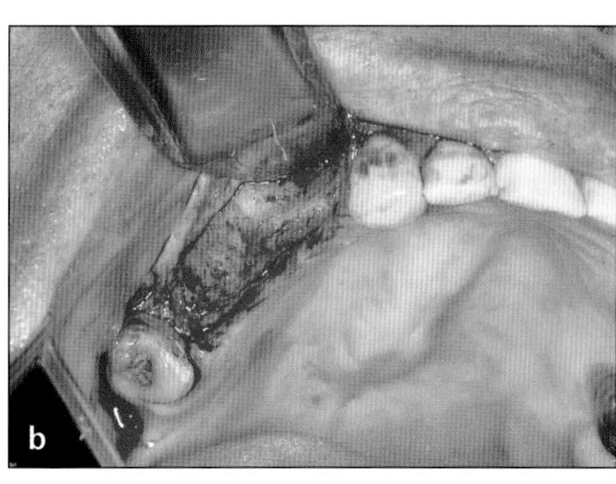

Fig 8-12 The thickness of the maxillary wall and the surgeon's preference and experience will determine the type of bur used to make the osteotomy in the lateral wall of the maxillary sinus.

(a) A no. 8 round diamond bur is a good choice for surgeons who are learning this procedure or for thin walls and relatively small windows.

(b) The 4.0 oval bur (Brasseler, Savannah, GA) shown is a good option for thick walls and large windows and in experienced hands.

(c) The shape of the osteotomy is generally oval; this will depend on the contours of the maxillary sinus. As the osteotomy progresses, the membrane will start to show as the bone thins in the area of drilling. It is a good idea to stop occasionally and assess the proximity of the membrane to avoid perforations.

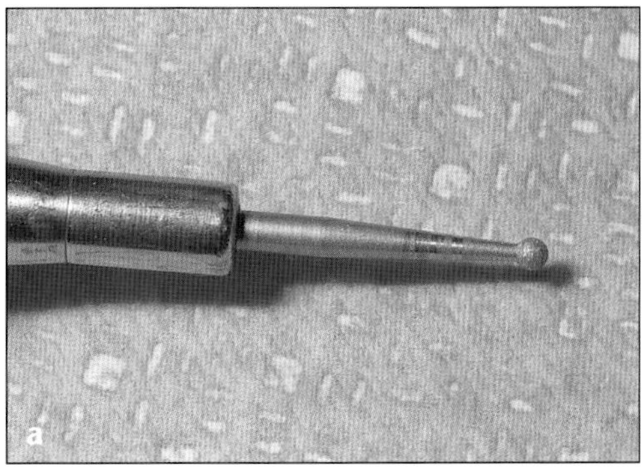

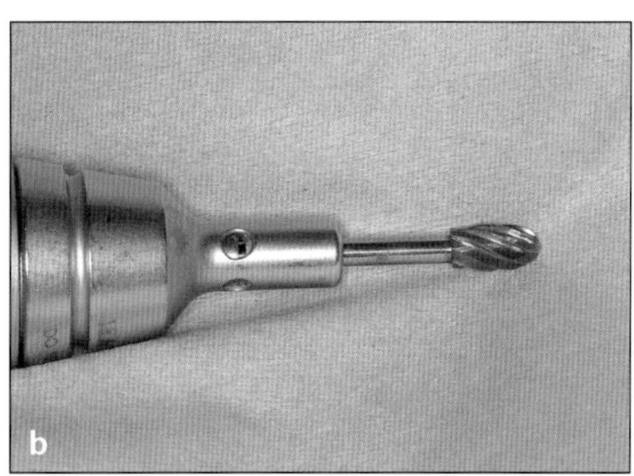

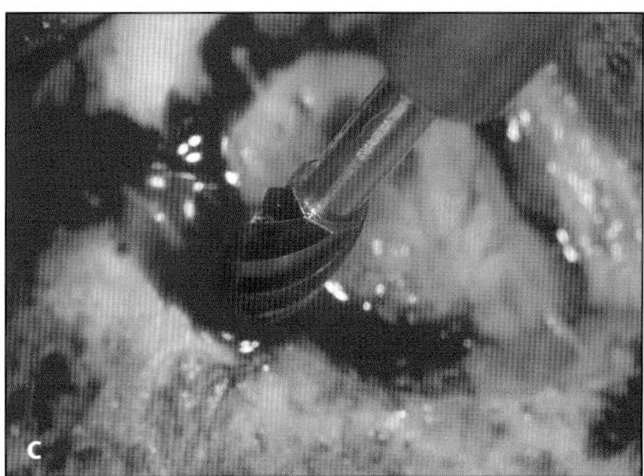

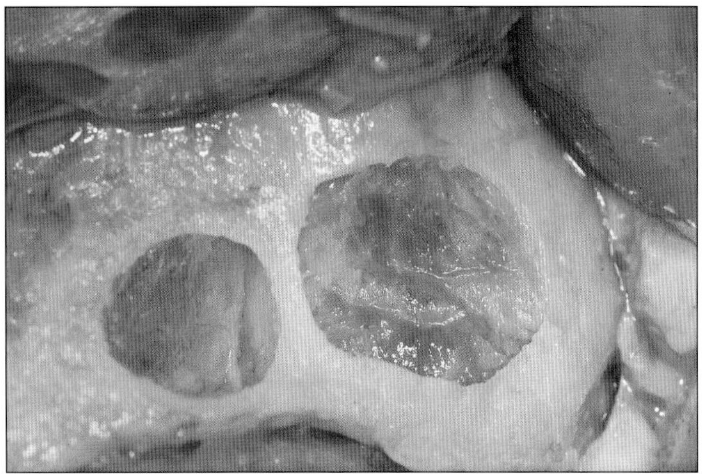

Fig 8-13
In some patients, septa may be encountered. If a septum is not very high, it may be possible to go around it with just one window. If a septum is too high, as shown, two separate windows may be made to facilitate the reflection of the membrane, both anterior and posterior to the large septum.

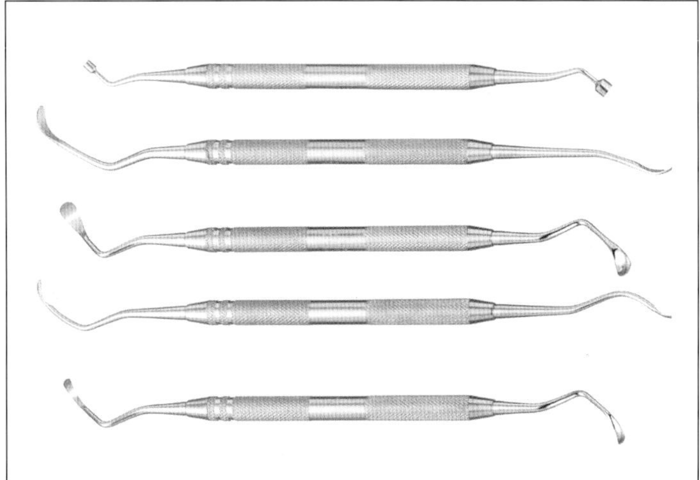

Fig 8-14
The curettes used for membrane reflection should provide different angles and sizes so they can be easily used in anatomically varied sinuses. The edges of the curettes should be sharp and should always be placed against the bone. The movement for reflection could be described as a "scrape-push." The instrument kit should include a wide surface condenser/plugger for moving the graft into the correct position and compacting it.

The schneiderian membrane is then carefully elevated from the floor inferiorly, anteriorly, and posteriorly through the osteotomy sites. If it is an extremely small window, then the process should be performed with a sufficiently small curette. For the usual sinus window, the largest possible curette should be used to minimize the chances of perforating the schneiderian membrane and to maximize the efficiency of the membrane-reflection process.

Perforation of the schneiderian membrane during surgery most often occurs if the lateral wall is being infractured, but it can also happen when the membrane is being elevated off the inferior and anterior bony aspects of the sinus. The most common areas of perforation are at the level of the inferior osteotomy, the level of the greenstick fracture if used, and the inferomedial portion of the sinus window.[1] For small perforations in the membrane, a small piece of a collagen membrane can be placed in the area to adapt to the perforation, occlude it, and allow it time to heal and repair itself.[1] For larger perforations, a longer-lasting, stiff, collagen-based membrane should be shaped into a dome and placed in the sinus to occlude the perforation and contain the graft. It is important to ensure that all of the schneiderian membrane has been reflected off the sinus floor so that the bone graft is lying not on the epithelium but rather on raw bone.

The sinus floor septa (convolutions) are not necessarily altered. A variable number of septa (also referred to as the *Underwood septa*) divide the floor of the maxillary sinus into several recesses and may complicate sinus lift procedures.[74,75] Most of the septa are located in the region between the second premolar and the first molar. Septal formation may be caused by the different phases of maxillary sinus pneumatization of the empty alveolar process following tooth extraction. To minimize the chance of complications from a septum, it is advisable to create the inferior portion of the osteotomy at least 3 mm above the sinus floor and thereby avoid it. If a septum is present and is higher than 3 mm from the floor (something that should be noted preoperatively, because it will affect the surgery), the oval-shaped osteotomy should be split into three by making vertical cuts through the bony window just anterior and just posterior to the septum. This will create bony windows over the left and right compartments that are lifted off and a bony window over the septum that is not lifted off but rather is ground down with the drill and diamond bur.

Intraoperative Bleeding

Because there are no major vascular structures in the surgical area, any intraoperative bleeding that does occur usually is from capillary soft tissue or bony ooze. The interconnecting vascular contributions to the maxilla and maxillary sinus likely account for the forgiving nature and rapid healing of maxillary sinus surgery; however, the vascular system can produce a brisk intraoperative oozing that is usually related to the patient's systemic blood pressure or the presence of local inflammation and only rarely to a bleeding disorder or coagulopathy. Most hemostatic disorders have already been diagnosed by the time a patient reaches the age when a sinus lift would be required, or else they are noted while obtaining a thorough preoperative history. For patients who claim to be "bleeders" or who have a suspicious history of bleeding problems, a simple battery of screening blood tests will identify 98.5% of bleeding disorders. This series of tests includes a complete blood count (CBC) with a platelet count and differential, a bleeding time test, a prothrombin time, and a partial thromboplastin time.

If brisk intraoperative oozing develops, the patient's systemic blood pressure should be checked. Hypertension control is usually established by reinforcing the local anesthesia, verbally reassuring the patient, and using additional sedation if necessary. It is rare but possible that a procedure may have to be stopped because of uncontrollable hypertension. Locally, brisk oozing is best controlled by temporarily packing the wound (Fig 8-15). Saturating the packing with 2% lidocaine with 1:100,000 epinephrine or 4% liquid cocaine will sometimes assist hemostasis, particularly if the oozing is coming from soft tissue. If the oozing is coming from bone and cannot be controlled with temporary packing, pressing bone wax into the area is usually effective. In addition, microfibrillar bovine collagen (Avitene, MedChem Products, Woburn, MA) is an excellent resorbable and compatible agent that initiates clot formation. Two additional "leave-in" agents, Gelfoam (Pharmacia and Upjohn, Kalamazoo, MI) and Surgicel (Johnson & Johnson, New Brunswick, NJ), also assist in clot formation and hemostasis. However, the most effective means of control that permits completion of the sinus lift procedure is to use Avitene for slower-paced bony oozing and bone wax for more rapid oozing. Chapter 11

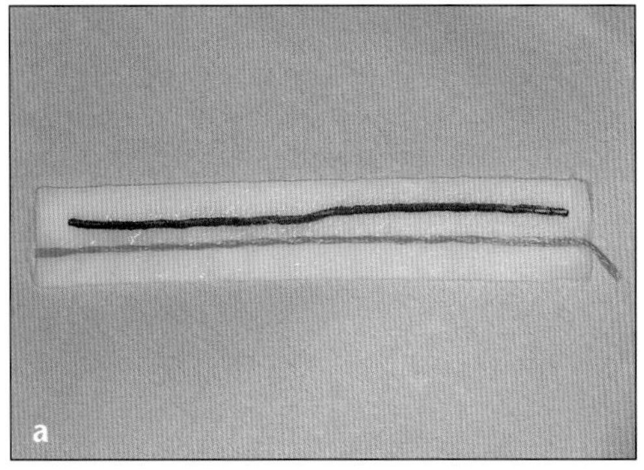

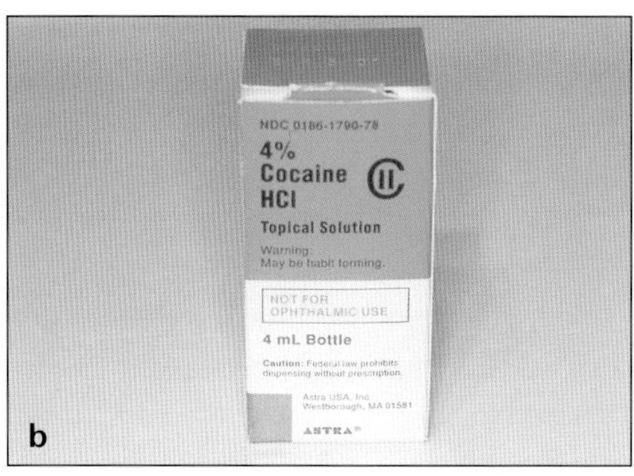

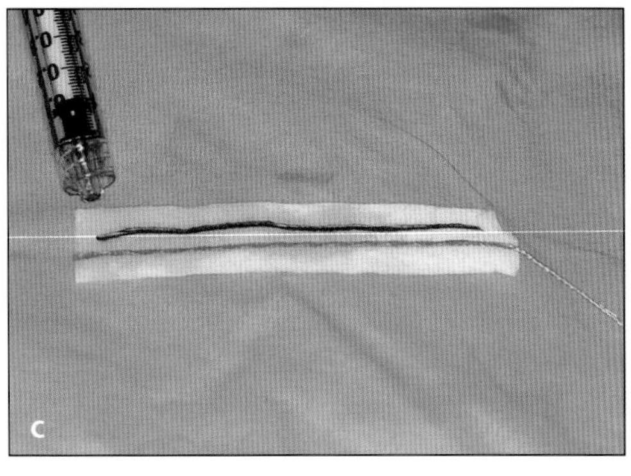

Fig 8-15 Brisk introperative oozing is best controlled by temporarily packing the wound.

(a) Hemostasis inside the sinus cavity can be achieved with the use of a Cottonoid strip (Codman, Raynham, MA), a thin $\frac{1}{2} \times 3$-inch strip of highly absorbent gauze with a long strip of green thread to help identify it once it becomes soaked with blood and a darker radiopaque strip for radiographic detection if necessary.

(b) Before the Cottonoid strip is placed in the sinus, it should first be impregnated with a liquid hemostatic agent such as 4% cocaine solution.

(c) The Cottonoid strip is saturated. An alternative to 4% cocaine solution is to use lidocaine with 1:50,000 epinephrine; the epinephrine acts as the hemostatic agent.

discusses the hemostatic properties of PRP that make it the hemostatic agent of choice when available.

Grafting Procedure

During the sinus lift grafting procedure, autogenous bone is harvested from the preselected site and, if appropriate, mixed with other graft materials. This mixture is then packed and compacted into 1- or 3-mL syringes and set aside.

As described earlier, a one-step procedure can be performed in which the graft and implant are placed simultaneously. When this approach is selected, essential surgical modifications will be necessary, including a wide lateral window opening, the use of a bone mill to homogenize the graft material, meticulous condensation of the graft, and clinical measurements to ensure implant parallelism.[26] The implant sites should be drilled using a surgical stent as a guide. It is important to protect the sinus membrane during this procedure. After preparing the implant sites, the top of the syringes should be cut off with scissors and the graft mixture injected into the maxillary sinus and packed against the intact medial wall.

After grafting the medial portion of the sinus, the implants are placed. Bone is then packed against the anterior and posterior maxillary walls, molding the bone against and over the implant to a height of 10 to 12 mm. During this part of the procedure, it is important to maintain the implant in the proper position to avoid compromising subsequent prosthetic restoration. Next, the lateral portion of the surgical site should be firmly packed with the bone graft. If the diameter of the implant is greater than the width of the alveolar crest, bone should be placed and secured outside the sinus against the lateral surface of the implants. The area of the access window should then be covered with a membrane barrier to prevent soft tissue ingrowth, the mucoperiosteal flap should be repositioned, and the incisions should be closed with interrupted sutures. The graft can mature while the implant is integrating.

If a two-step surgical approach (ie, separate grafting and implant placement surgeries) is used, adequate graft material is placed in the maxillary sinus to accommodate the length of the implant. Once adequate graft material has been placed, the window is then covered with a resorbable membrane barrier, as with the one-step procedure. The mucoperiosteal flap is repositioned, and the incisions are closed with interrupted resorbable sutures. After the bone has matured (approximately 4 to 12 months depending on the graft materials used, the graft size, and the patient's systemic health), it is evaluated to ensure that there is sufficient bone height for implant placement. The implants can then be placed in the mature graft material following the surgical protocol prescribed for that system and allowed to integrate.

Postoperative Considerations

Postoperative considerations for the maxillary sinus grafting procedure are similar to those for most oral surgery and sinus manipulation procedures. After the first week, a chlorhexidine mouthrinse should be used twice daily for 2 weeks to reduce the chance of infection. Blowing the nose, sucking liquid through a straw, and smoking cigarettes, all of which create negative pressure, should be avoided for at least 2 weeks after surgery. Coughing or sneezing should be done with an open mouth to relieve pressure. Pressure at the surgical site, ice, elevation of the head, and rest are also recommended. Analgesics should be used to control postoperative pain and discomfort. An anti-inflammatory medication and an antihistamine can also be used. Preoperative prophylactic antibiotic therapy, such as 500 mg Augmentin (GlaxoSmithKline, Research Triangle Park, NC) or a similar suitable antibiotic, should be used and continued postoperatively three times a day for 7 to 10 days. A nasal decongestant such as Sudafed (Warner Lambert, Morris Plains, NJ), 30 to 60 mg per day, should be prescribed, and Afrin (Schering-Plough, Kenilworth, NJ) nasal spray should be used on an as-needed basis for nasal congestion.

Depending on the graft materials and the host osteogenic potential, 3 to 12 months should be allowed for the bone graft and implants to integrate before the prosthodontic phase begins. During this period, the patient can wear a conventional prosthesis that has been relined with a soft material. If an intraoral donor site has been used, it is usually well tolerated and recuperation normally takes 1 to 2 weeks.

Potential Postoperative Complications

Possible complications that can occur after this procedure include sinus congestion, infection of the graft, poor wound healing, and the formation of insufficient quality or quantity of bone in the grafted site.[76] Sinus congestion and pain should be treated with decongestants and analgesics. If the graft becomes infected (which is relatively uncommon), the graft material should be completely removed, the sinus membrane should be removed in a radical sinus antrectomy procedure, the area should be well irrigated, and antibiotic

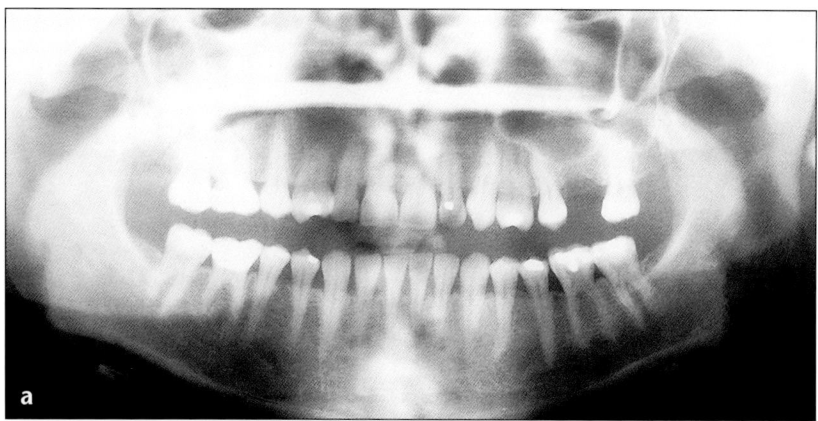

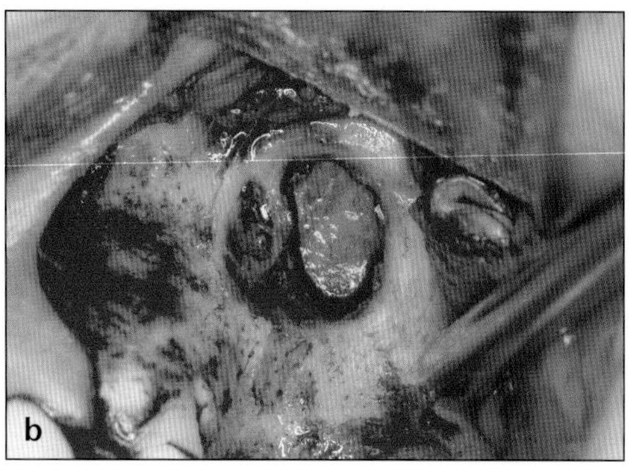

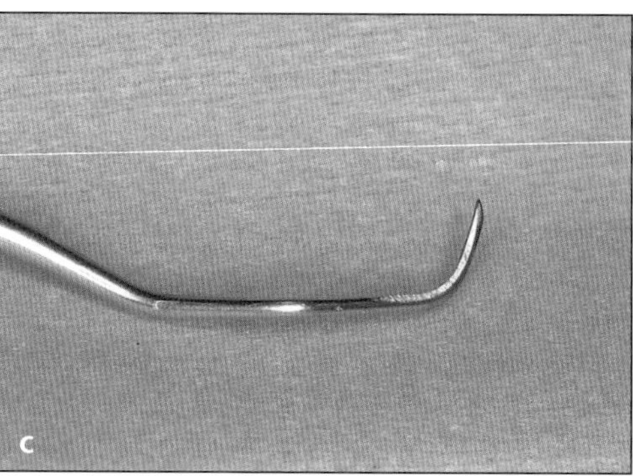

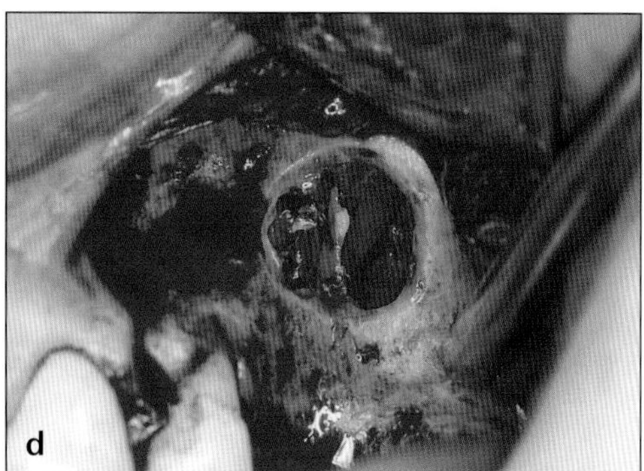

Fig 8-16 Cases involving an individual tooth are frequently encountered and are ideal for sinus grafting and implant placement if the patient wants to maintain the integrity of adjacent teeth and avoid preparation for a partial denture.

(a) In this patient there is approximately 4 mm of crestal bone height.

(b) Bony septa are frequently encountered in sinus cavities. These can usually be visualized radiographically, allowing the clinician to plan ahead and have the right instruments available, which is particularly important in small osteotomies such as this.

(c) In small osteotomies and especially in those with septa, very small instruments, such as a Gracey periodontal scaler (Hu-Friedy, Chicago, IL), can be used.

(d) Reflection of the membrane above and around the septum reveals that the area is contiguous.

therapy should be prescribed. A nasal antrostomy procedure is generally not required. The sinus can be regrafted after the crestal soft tissue has healed and radiographs show the sinus to be clear.

If the blood supply to the tissue is interrupted or impeded, there may be poor wound healing and an early loss of the bone graft or implant. If the incision does not close properly, the remaining graft should be removed, the membrane inspected for perforations, and the sinus void irrigated. Appropriate antibiotics should be prescribed, and the wound should be allowed to heal by secondary intention.

If the graft fails to produce sufficient quality or quantity of new bone to sustain implants, the sinus void can be regrafted. After the lateral aspect of the sinus has been exposed, the graft material is removed, the surgical defect inspected, and the sinus regrafted with a different combination of materials.[1] Trauma to an implant

Fig 8-16 *(cont)*
(e) Graft material, in this case allogeneic bone, is reconstituted in nonactivated PRP.

(f) Once reconstituted, the graft material is mixed with activated PRP. It will now be easier to manipulate because the particles will clump together.

(g) In this case of immediate graft and implant placement, the sinus is grafted medially, the implant is placed, and the area is grafted laterally. In some cases, as shown here, it is necessary to overcontour the lateral wall of the maxilla in order to compensate for any concavity in that area.

(h) The implant and bone graft were placed simultaneously. Notice the bone around the apex of the implant. Performing simultaneous graft and implant placement allows the clinician to place the bone exactly where it is needed for the implant.

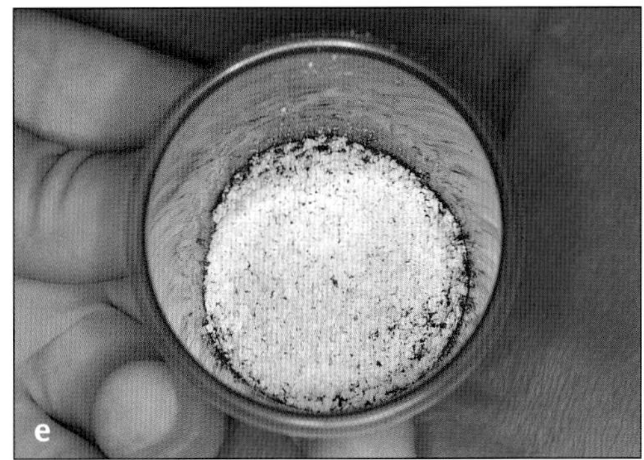

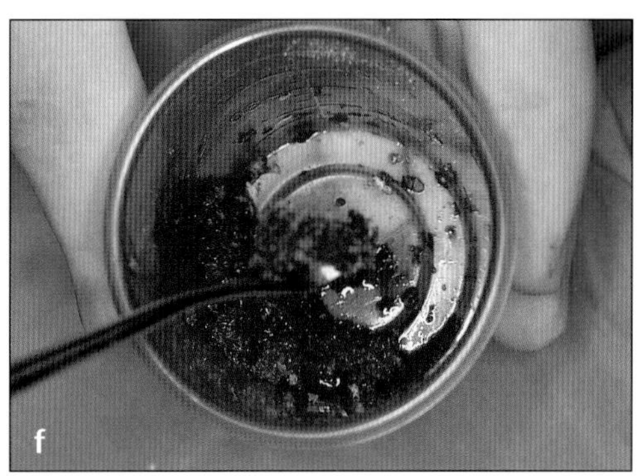

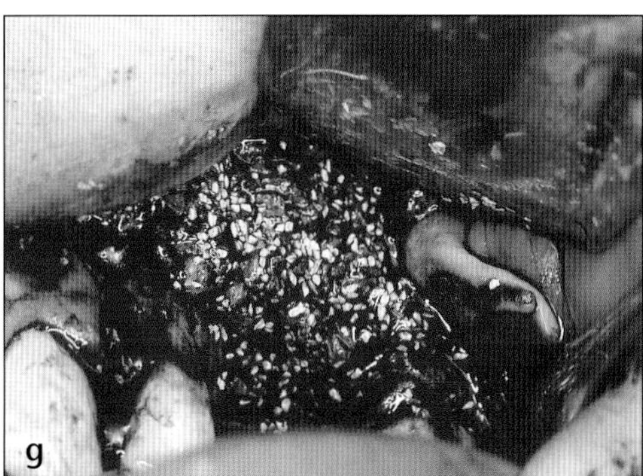

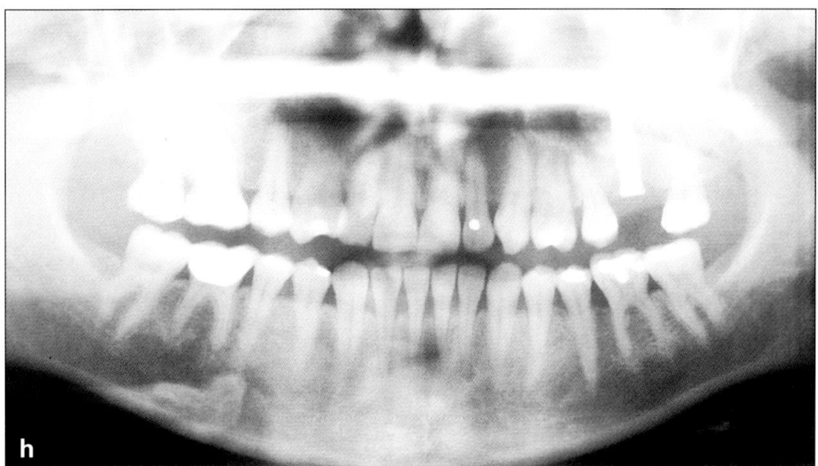

during the healing process or pathologic loading from the restoration can also cause premature loss of implants. The loss of maxillary implants can create oro-antral openings that may require surgery for closure.[17]

Clinical Cases

Figures 8-16 to 8-23 present several cases demonstrating the procedures described in this chapter.

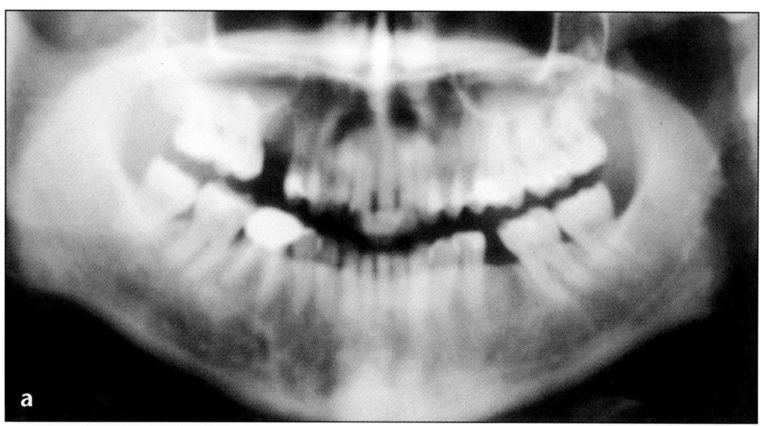

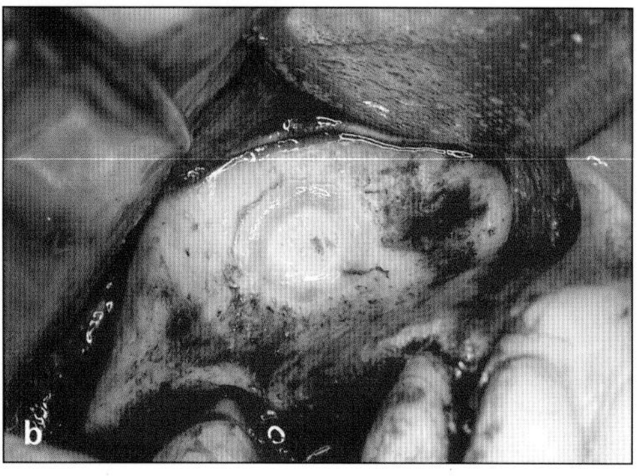

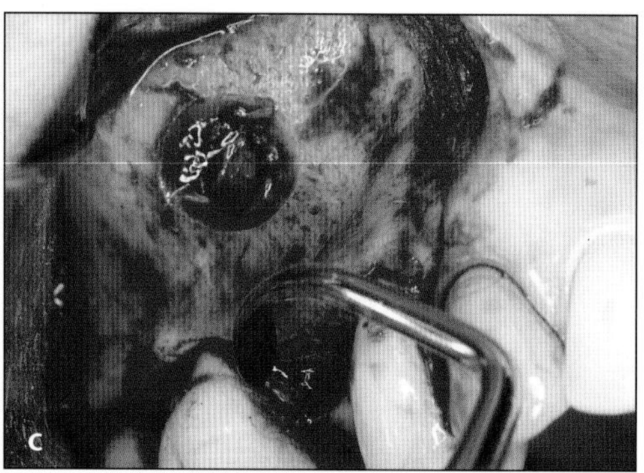

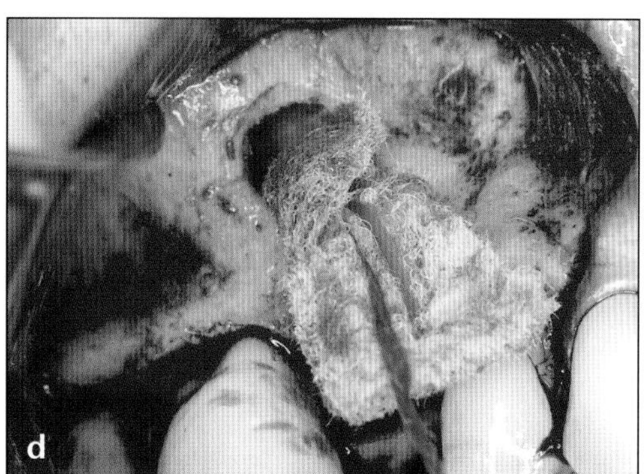

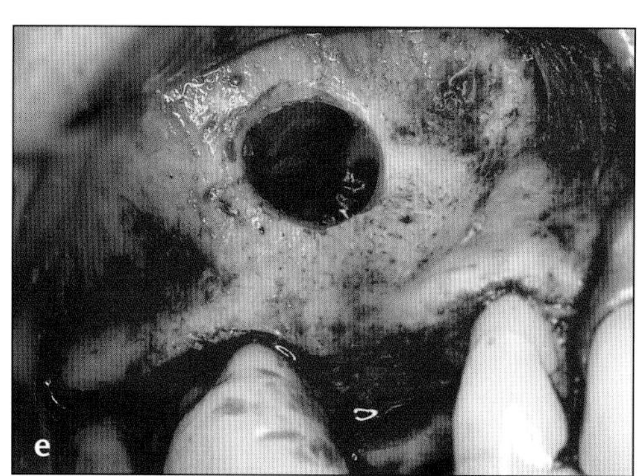

Fig 8-17 Maxillary sinus augmentation for single implant placement.

(a) This panoramic radiograph shows a missing first molar and inadequate bone height for implant placement.

(b) For this single implant patient, a very small osteotomy is created. Note the size and configuration of the flap, which allows for good visualization of the osteotomy site and adjacent areas.

(c) A small curette with several angles allows for access to the different areas of the sinus.

(d) After being impregnated with a hemostatic agent, the Cottonoid strip is carefully packed in, which assists in reflecting the membrane. In addition, the strip keeps the schneiderian membrane elevated temporarily after its removal.

(e) After removal of the Cottonoid, it is easier to assess the volume and whether the amount of reflection is adequate.

Fig 8-17 *(cont)*
(f) The graft material is sprayed with activated PRP at the time it will be placed into the recipient site. The special dual lumen syringe tip mixes the PRP with the calcium chloride and thrombin.

(g) After filling the sinus cavity, placing a resorbable membrane, and suturing the crestal and the distal release of the flap, more graft material is added. Not suturing the vertical incision leaves a pouch that can easily be filled with more graft material to augment the thickness of the lateral wall of the maxilla in the areas needed.

(h) The graft material is carefully packed with the plugger. A fine pickup pliers is used to separate the flap and resorbable membrane from the residual alveolar bone and to hold the pouch open.

(i) When a sufficient amount of graft material is placed, the vertical releasing incision of the pouch is sutured.

(j) When suturing is complete, a gentle finger massage of the area can help disperse the graft material and mold it to the desired ridge shape.

(k) In this patient, the implant was placed after graft maturation in a staged fashion because of lack of adequate crestal width at the time of grafting. An ideal position, length, and diameter of the implant was achieved because of the gain in height from the sinus graft and the gain in width achieved with the pouch technique.

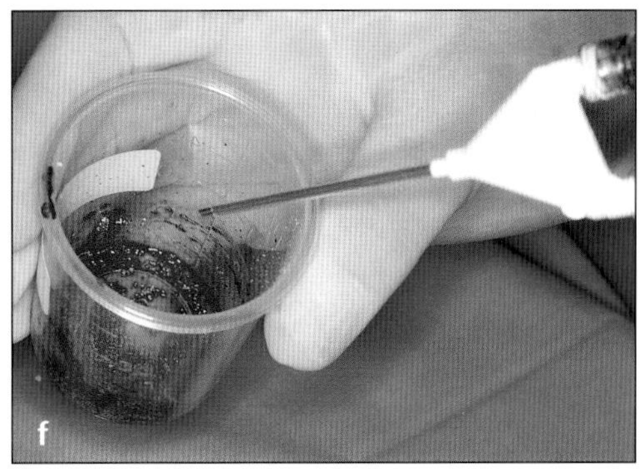
f

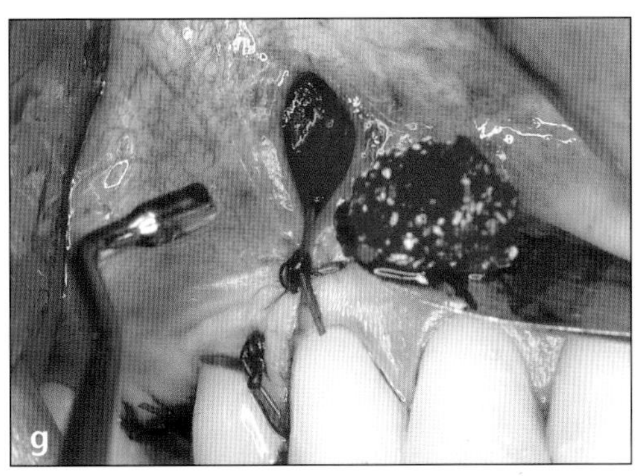
g

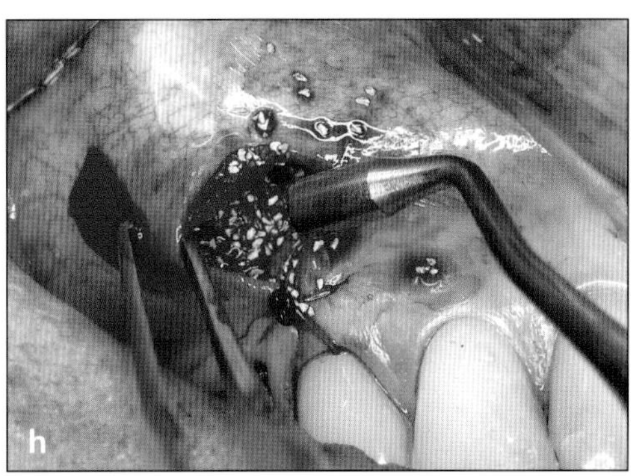
h

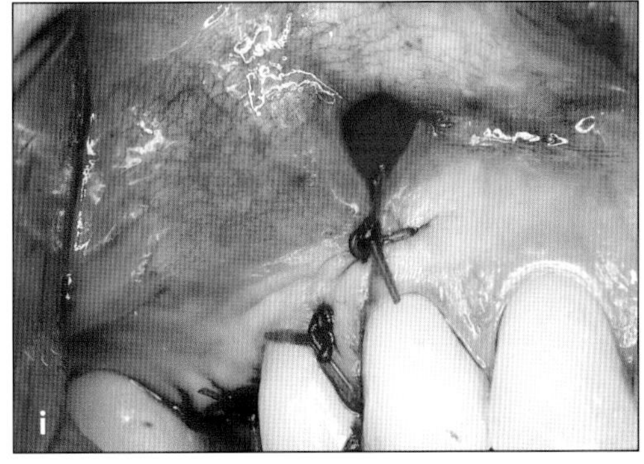
i

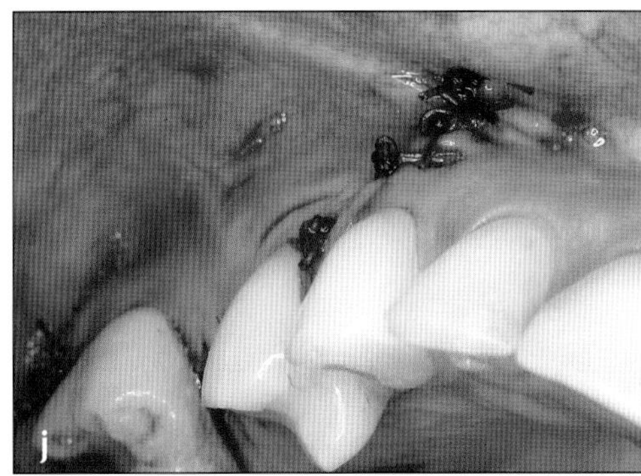
j

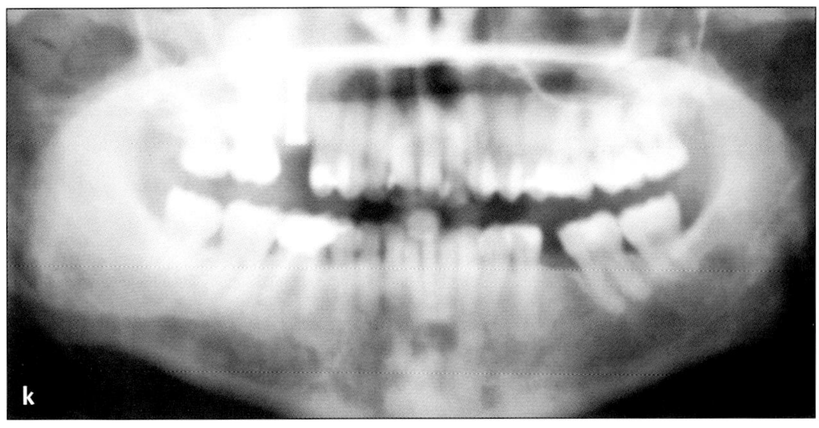
k

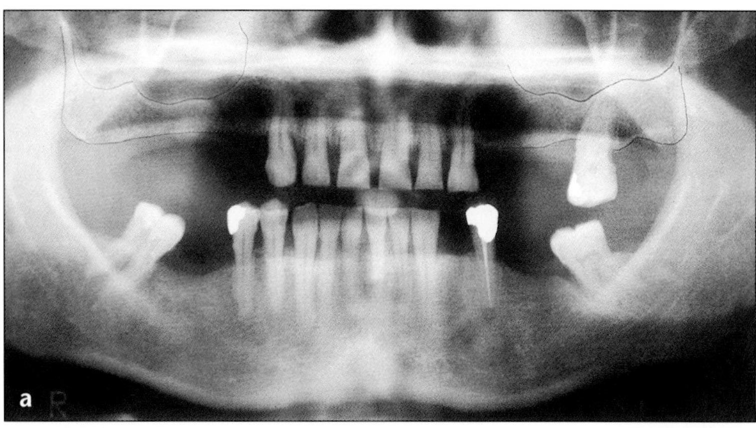

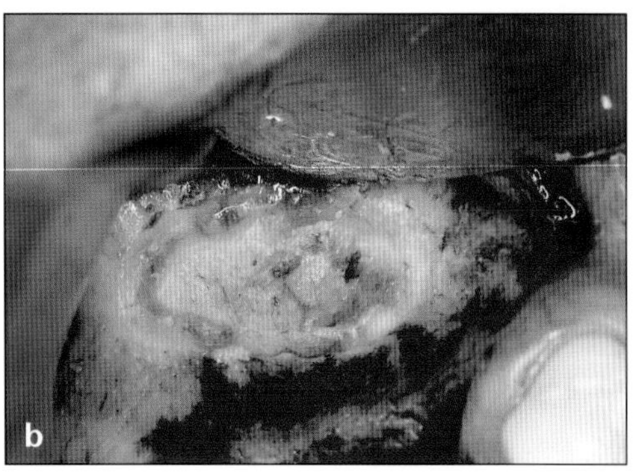

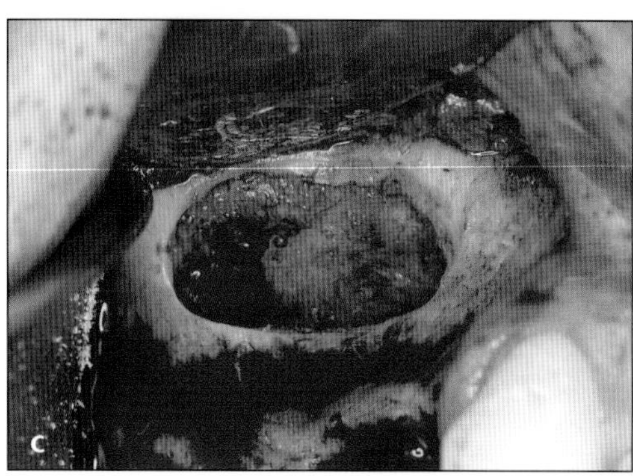

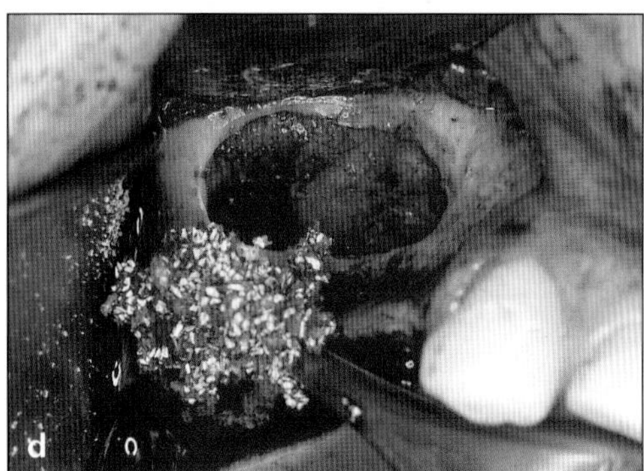

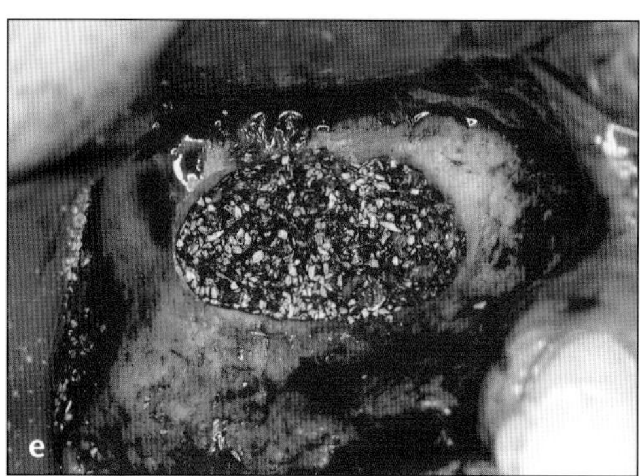

Fig 8-18 Bilateral sinus grafting of hyperpneumatized sinuses for implant placement.

(a) Panoramic radiograph showing bilaterally pneumatized maxillary sinuses.

(b) The size and shape of the osteotomy depends on the sinus being grafted and the number and positioning of implants that will be placed. It is important to plan ahead and know the exact area that the implants will occupy in height as well as mesiodistally and mediolaterally.

(c) After the island of bone is removed, the membrane can be reflected.

(d) Following adequate reflection and the placement and removal of the Cottonoid, the graft material is placed in the recipient site, where it is manipulated with the condenser to the correct position and then compacted appropriately.

(e) Complete filling of the sinus cavity restores the intial contour of the lateral wall of the maxilla.

Fig 8-18 *(cont)*
(f) The amount of bone gain can be appreciated in the sinus cavities. The dome shape in this radiograph shows that the integrity of the membrane was maintained and the elevated area was filled completely.

(g) Implants placed in the grafted sites have been allowed to integrate and were uncovered at stage 2 surgery. Note the healthy mucosa surrounding the healing abutments.

(h) The successful result of a process that began with bilateral sinus grafts of hyperpneumatized sinuses.

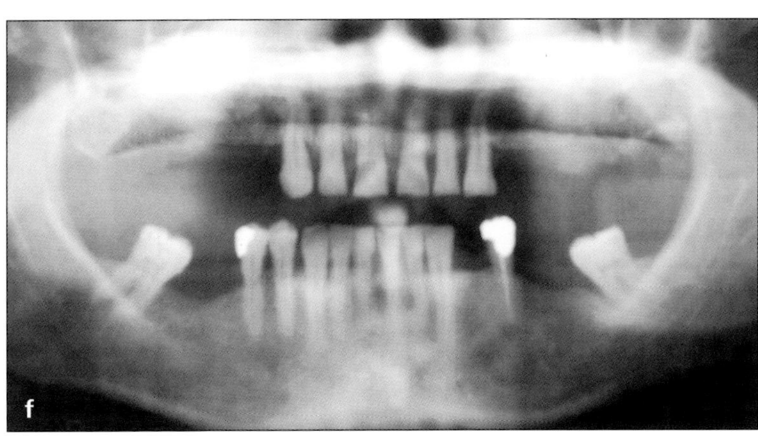

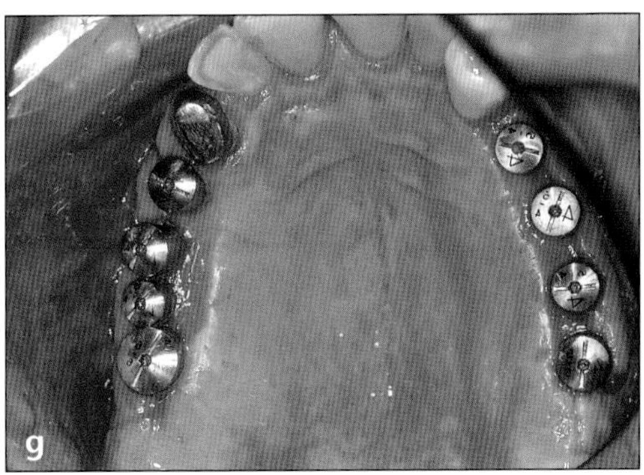

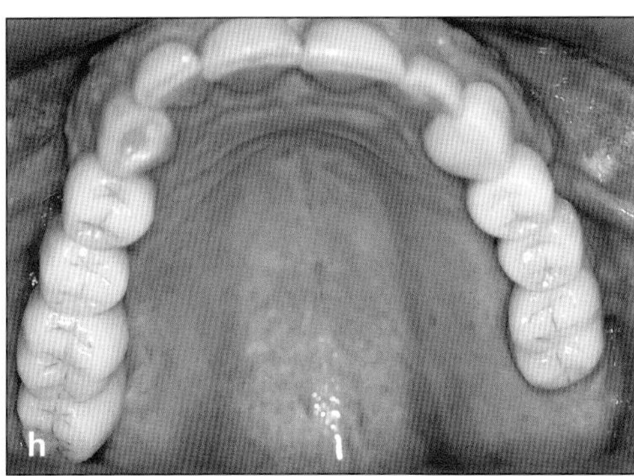

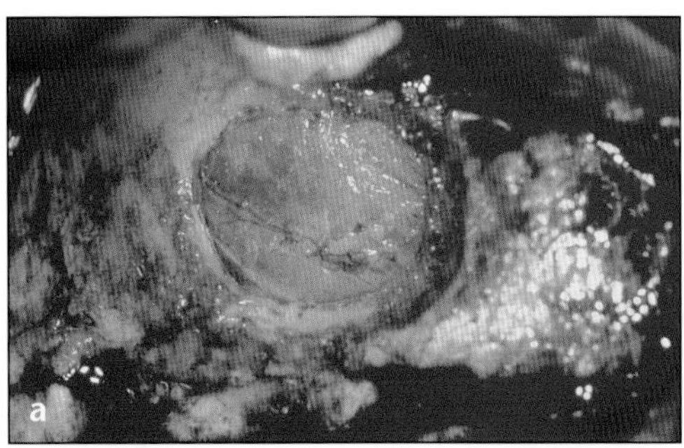

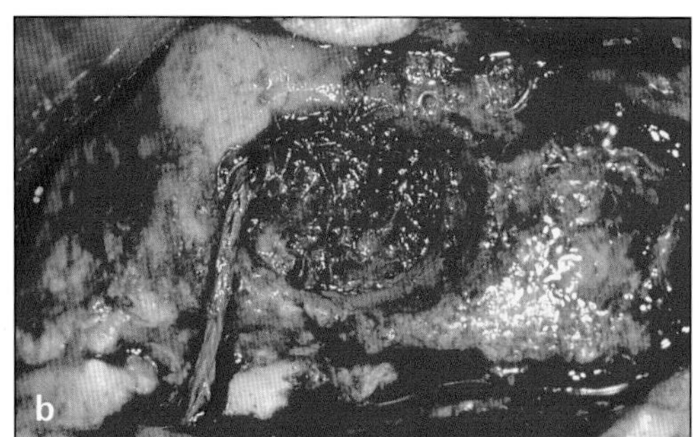

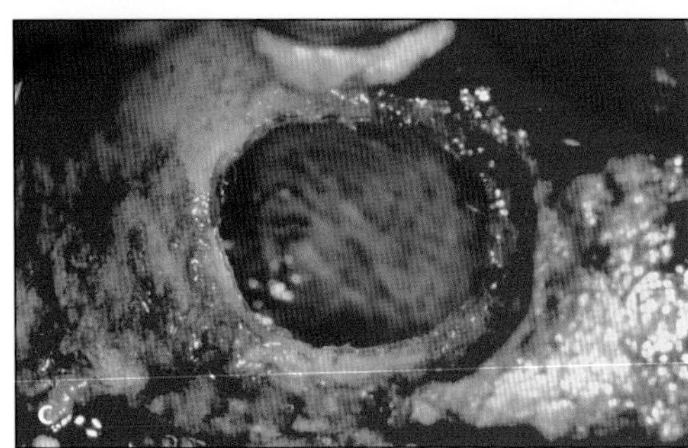

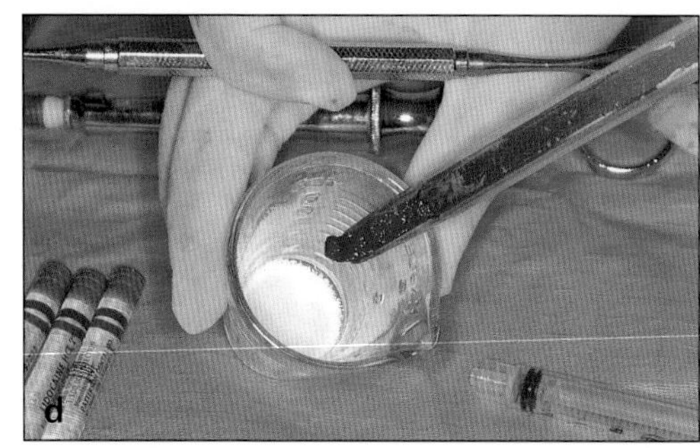

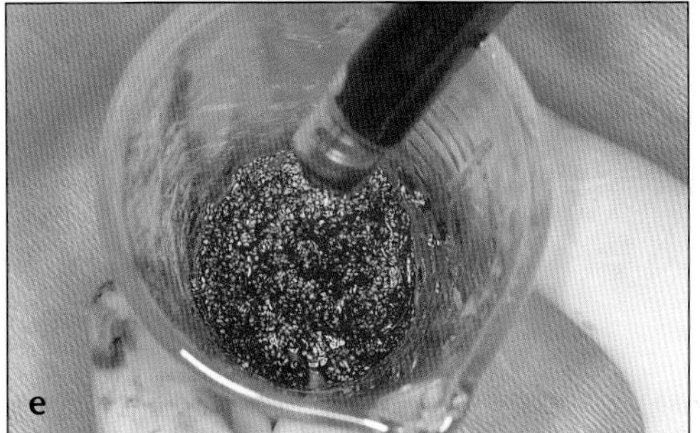

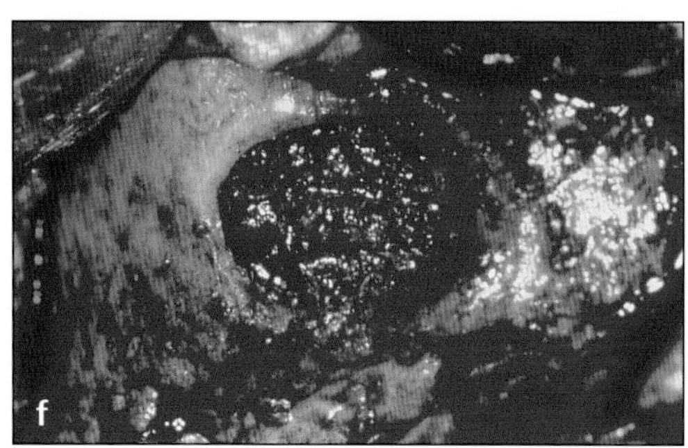

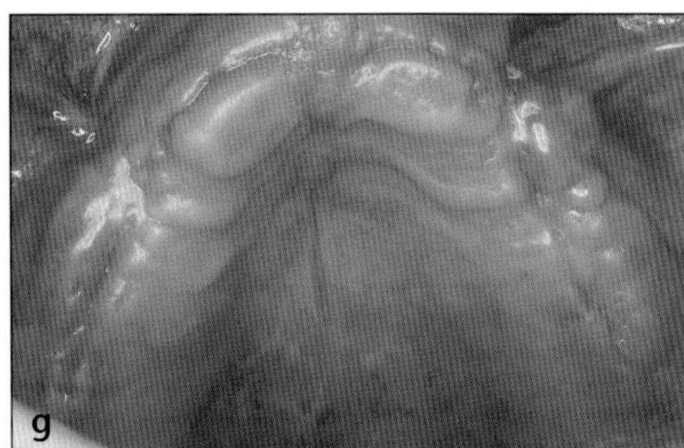

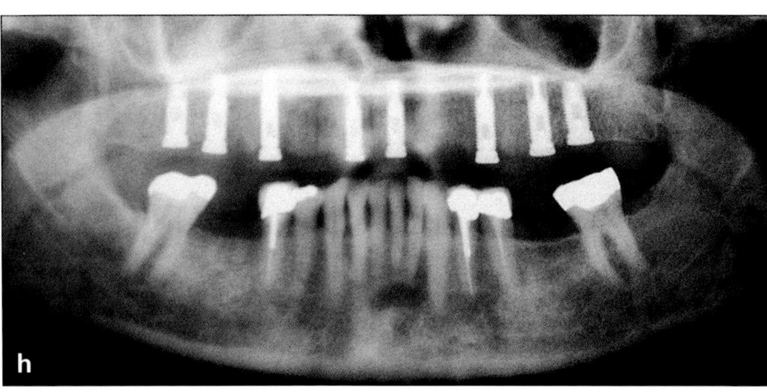

Fig 8-19 Two-step sinus grafting and implant placement procedure.

(a) In this case, a more rounded osteotomy was required to fit the anatomy and to provide access to the areas that required membrane reflection and subsequent grafting and implant placement.

(b) The hemostatic agent–soaked Cottonoid in place with the green string hanging out to permit its identification even if if becomes soaked with blood. This provides excellent hemostasis and visualization of the area upon removal.

(c) After the Cottonoid is removed, the volume of the cavity achieved by membrane reflection can be evaluated to determine if more reflection is necessary.

(d) Bone is harvested from the adjacent area using a commercially available bone shaver. These bone shavings can be mixed with other graft materials according to the patient's needs.

(e) Nonactivated PRP is added to this composite graft to reconstitute the allogeneic bone. Once saturated, activated PRP is added to allow for release of growth factors and to allow it to gel. The gelling action of the PRP will simplify the surgical manipulation of the material and its placement into the sinus.

(f) Complete filling of the maxillary sinus. A resorbable membrane will be placed and the area primarily closed.

(g) Well-healed ridges 2 weeks after sinus grafting. The patient continued to wear her denture immediately after surgery, so the contours of the ridges have not changed. A small amount of scarring can be seen in the areas of the vertical releases.

(h) Posterior implants placed in the bone-grafted areas. Note the ideal length and positioning of the implants because of the graft.

Fig 8-20 Bilateral sinus grafts to provide needed height for implant placement in a completely edentulous maxilla.

(a) Panoramic radiograph showing a completely edentulous maxilla with moderate ridge resorption. The patient's teeth have recently been extracted. Immediate implant placement will be performed in this case.

(b) Venipuncture is performed to draw blood for development of the PRP. This is a procedure that most patients easily accept once they learn of the benefits of PRP.

(c) Instrumentation for the graft, including a specialized retractor.

(d) Autogenous bone shavings harvested with the bone shaver.

(e) Allogeneic bone is mixed with the autogenous bone.

(continued)

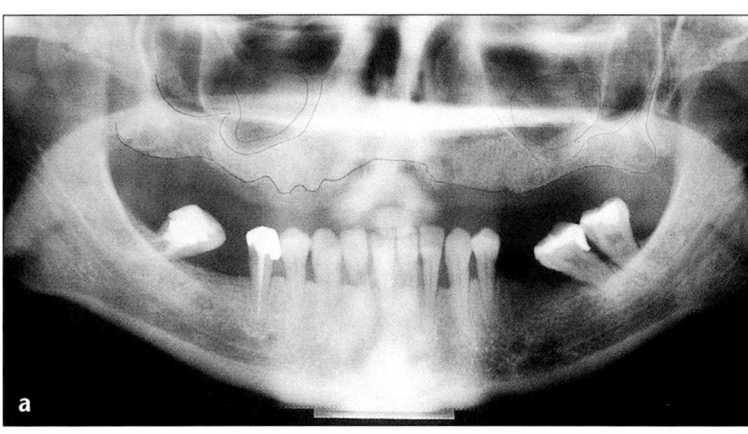

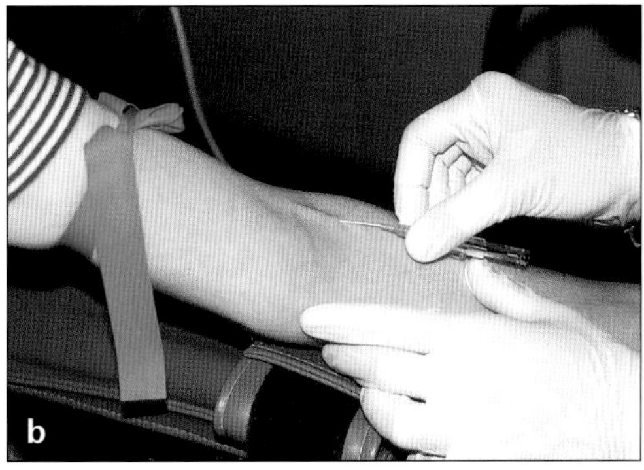

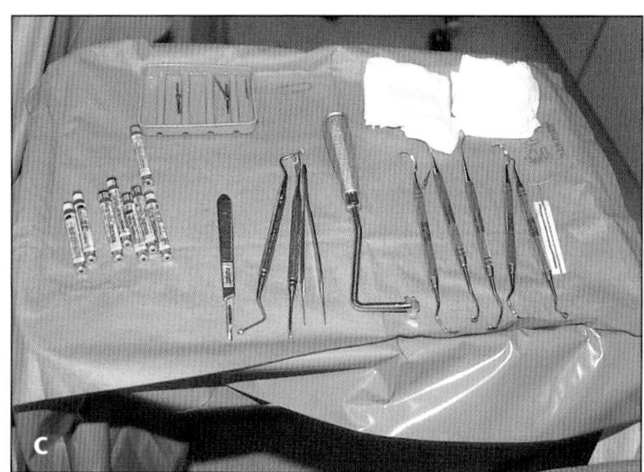

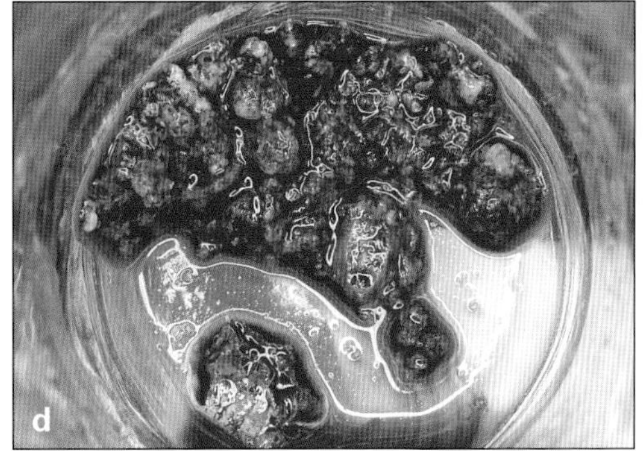

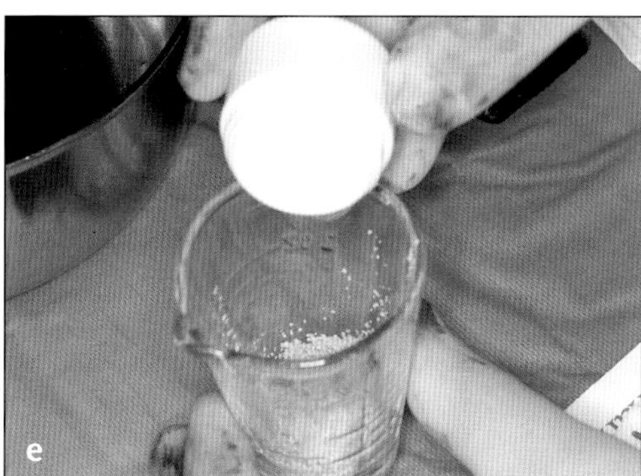

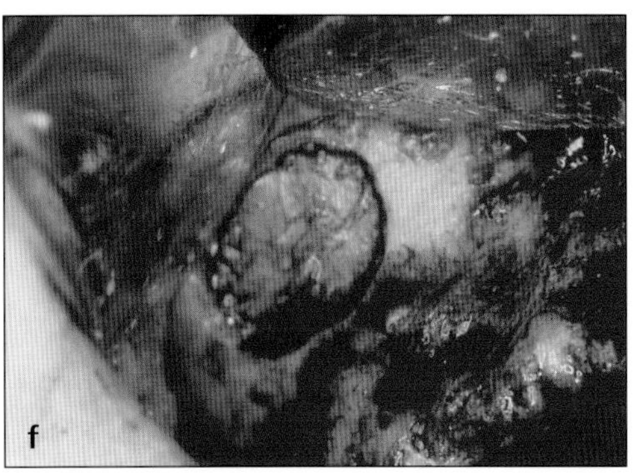

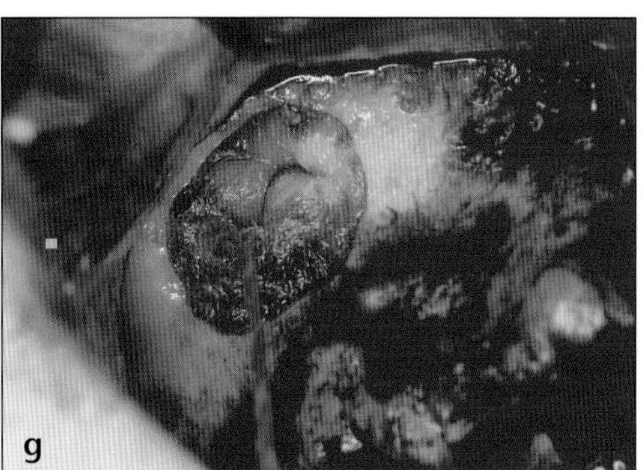

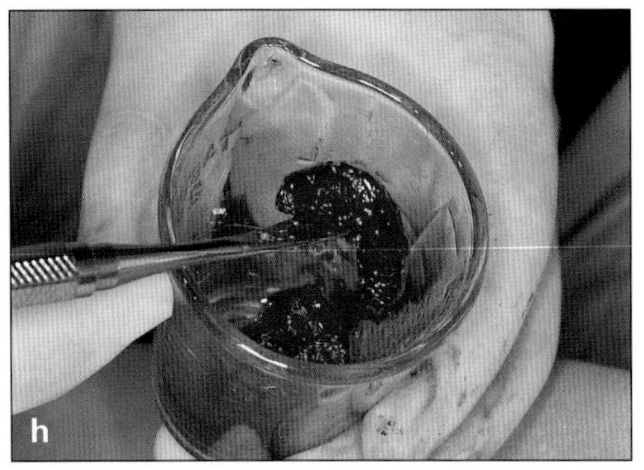

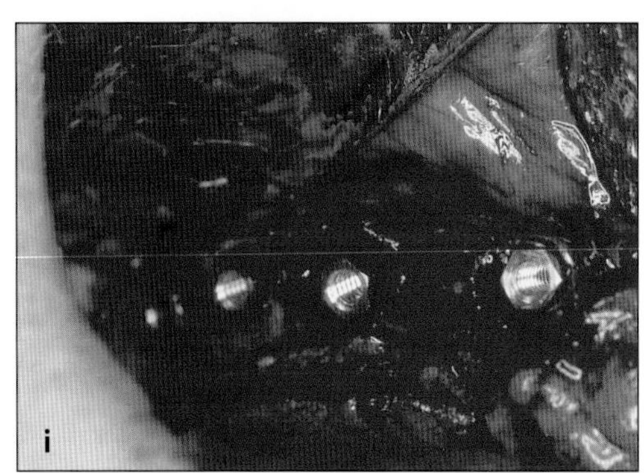

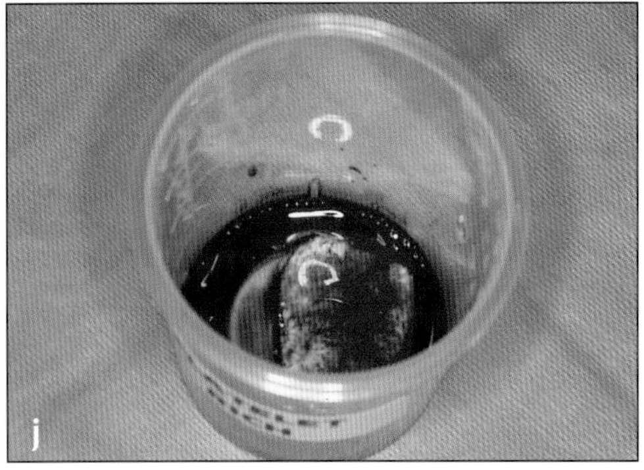

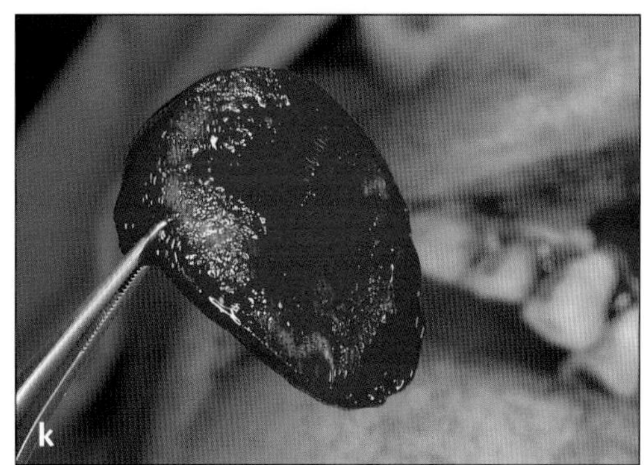

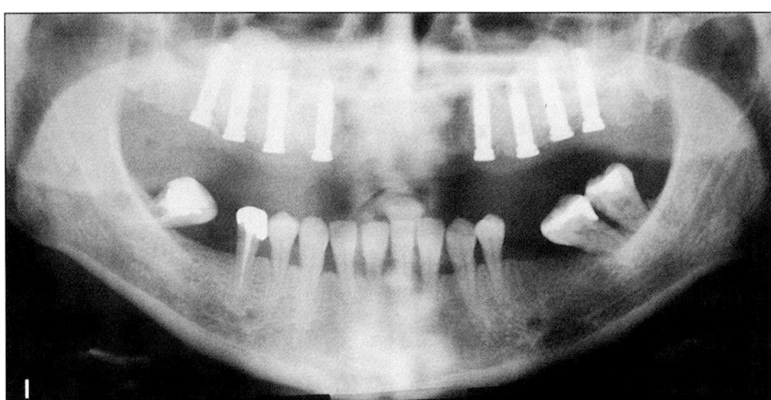

Fig 8-20 *(cont)*
(f) Some sinus membranes are very thin and translucent, while others are thicker and more dense. The level of difficulty involved in reflecting a membrane depends mostly on the strength of its attachment to the bone.

(g) When performing a bilateral sinus graft, it is ideal to leave one side packed with the Cottonoid strip while working on the contralateral side.

(h) Graft material saturated with PRP is picked up to carry to the recipient site.

(i) Implants were placed simultaneously with the sinus grafts bilaterally.

(j) A resorbable membrane saturated with activated PRP will be used over the osteotomy window. The membrane should cover the window and extend beyond the edges at least 3 mm circumferentially.

(k) The collagen membrane is carried toward the lateral aspect of the maxilla. It is important that this membrane does not slide from its correct position covering the window when the flap is sutured. It can be tacked in position if necessary.

(l) An immediate postoperative panoramic radiograph shows the implants in place with a length that could not have been achieved without grafting.

Fig 8-21 Bilateral sinus grafts to provide needed height for implant placement in a moderately resorbed, fully edentulous maxilla.

(a) After the osteotomy has been completed, the island of bone can be carefully separated and lifted from the underlying membrane. In cases where it is extremely adherent, it may be left attached and the membrane and bone reflected together. When the island of bone is not removed, the procedure is more difficult and visualization of the extent of the sinus is decreased. If removed carefully and gently, the residual bone detaches from the membrane easily and without any risk of tearing.

(b) The piece of bone should be removed slowly and carefully; a quick or aggressive pull before it is completely separated may cause a tear.

(c) The buccal plate can be crushed and used as a small portion of the graft.

(d) The Cottonoid strip is saturated with lidocaine with 1:50,000 epinephrine for hemostasis.

(e) The Cottonoid strip is removed gently and carefully to avoid tearing the schneiderian membrane.

(f) Some autogenous bone shavings are mixed with the allogeneic bone graft material to create a composite graft.

(g) Before starting to pack the graft material, it is important to take the time to assess the volume of the cavity and ensure that the implant site is adequately reflected for grafting.

(h) The graft material should be packed in a careful, orderly manner to avoid leaving any gaps in the area of the graft and to ensure that the graft is in good contact with host bone.

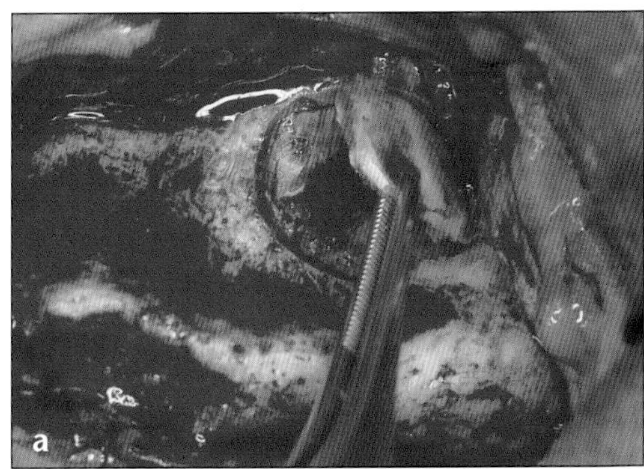
a

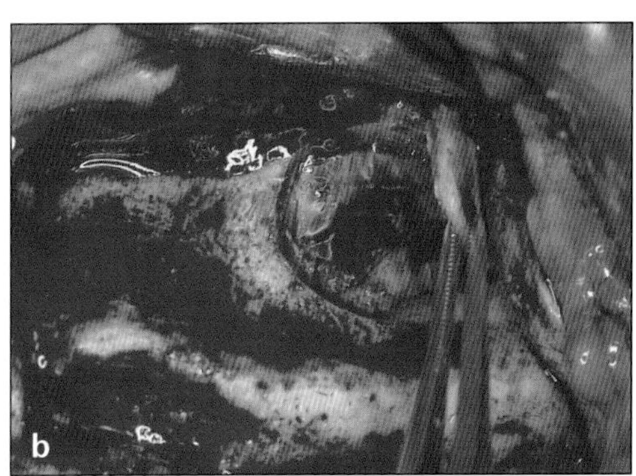
b

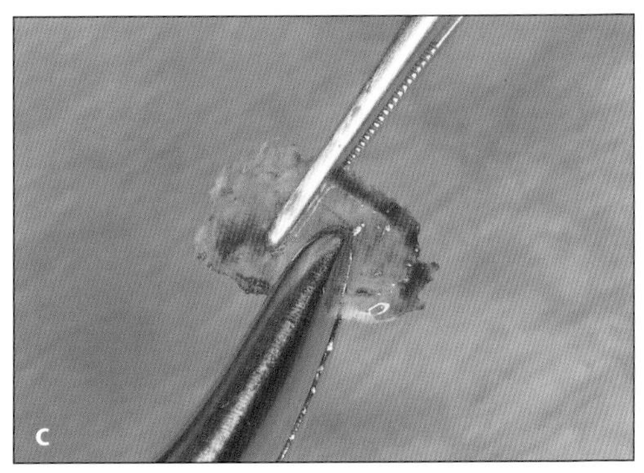
c

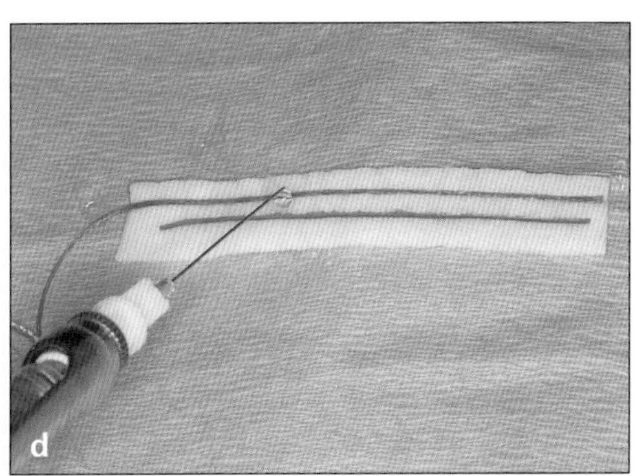
d

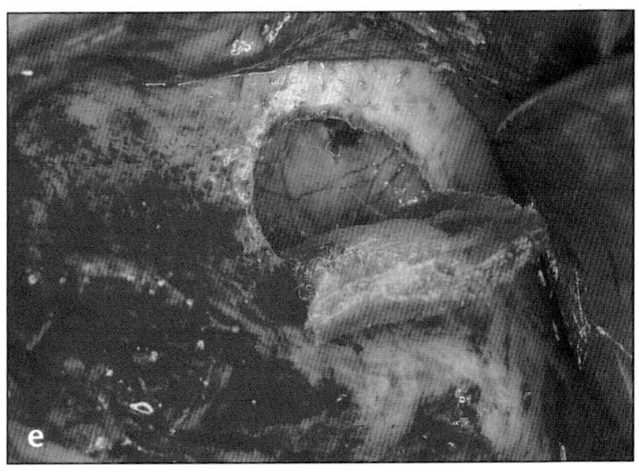
e

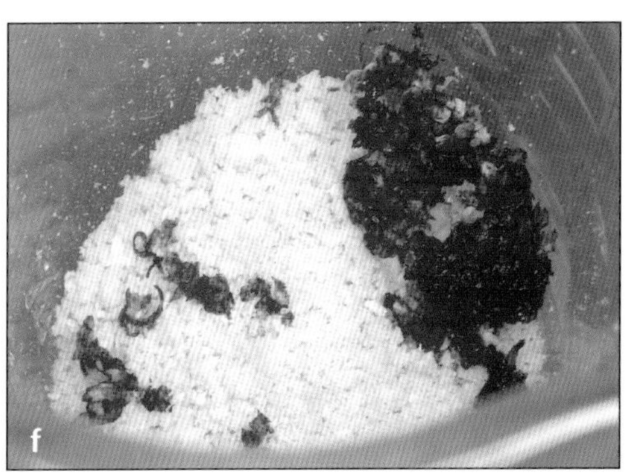
f

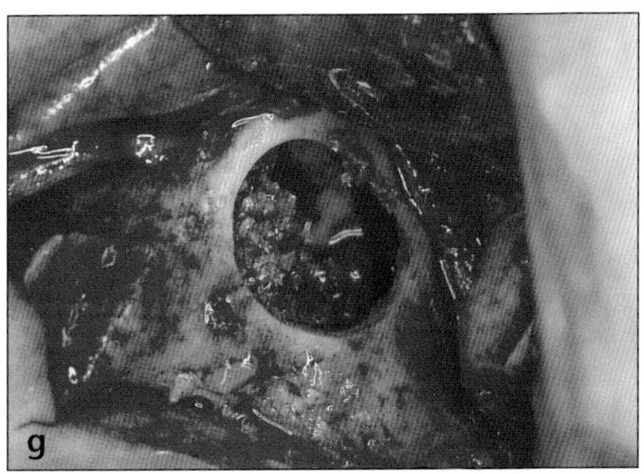
g

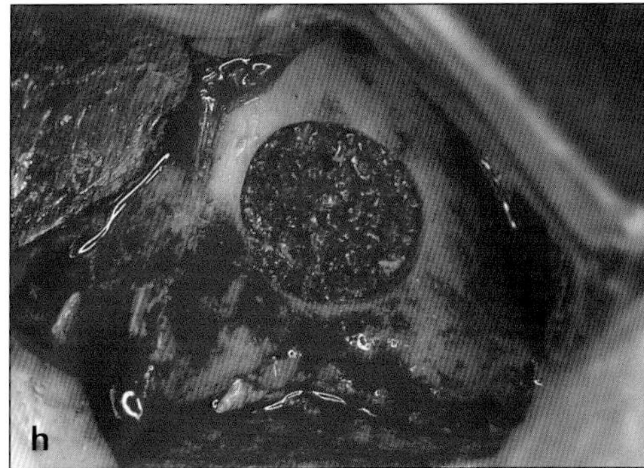
h

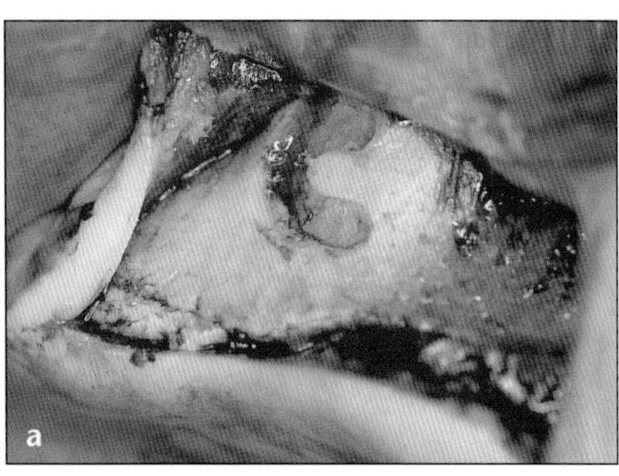

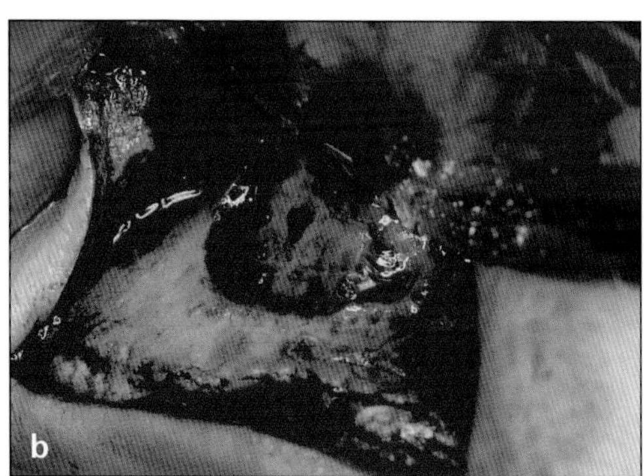

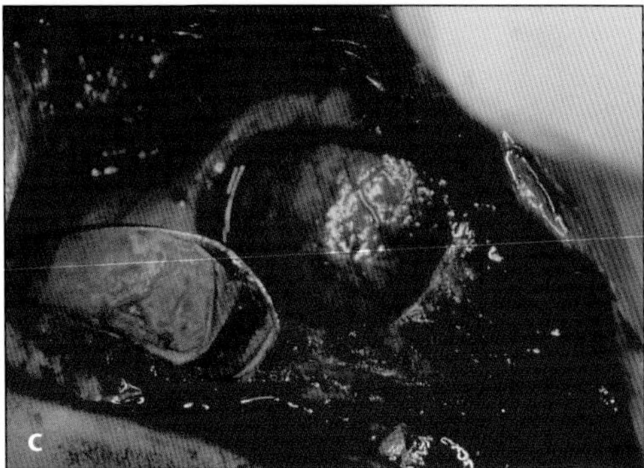

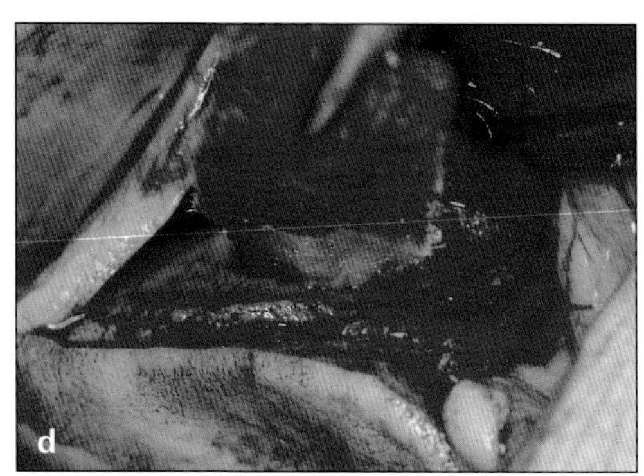

Fig 8-22 Sinus augmentation grafting in a patient with hyperpneumatized maxillary sinuses.

(a) The osteotomy is started in a C shape in order to locate and localize a sinus septum. After its position is well established, the osteotomy is continued.

(b) Good reflection, suction, and irrigation are important during osteotomy and membrane reflection.

(c) Asking the patient to take a few deep breaths through the nose and to hold them for a few seconds helps during reflection of the membrane. It is also helpful in determining if the membrane is torn—a torn membrane will not lift when the patient inhales.

(d) The Cottonoid is removed after approximately 5 minutes.

Fig 8-22 *(cont)*
(e) The schneiderian membrane is appropriately elevated, and the sinus cavity is now ready to be packed with graft material. Note how the area can be visualized due to the hemostasis achieved with the Cottonoid strip.

(f) The graft material should be positioned close to the oral cavity to facilitate taking it from the container to the sinus cavity. Contamination with saliva should be avoided.

(g) The force applied while packing the graft with the condenser should be applied carefully and downward toward the bony floor. Force that is excessive and/or directed toward the schneiderian membrane could cause the membrane to tear and the graft to be pushed beyond it.

(h) Graft material placed level with the buccal wall.

(i) A PRP membrane is placed over the window. It has a consistency that permits this type of manipulation.

(j) Postoperative healing at 2 weeks.

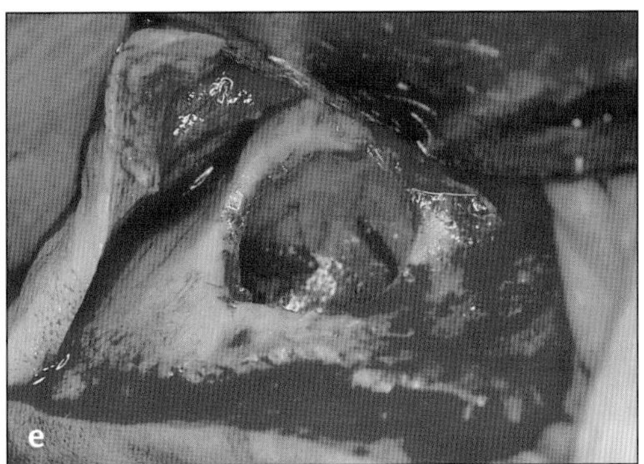

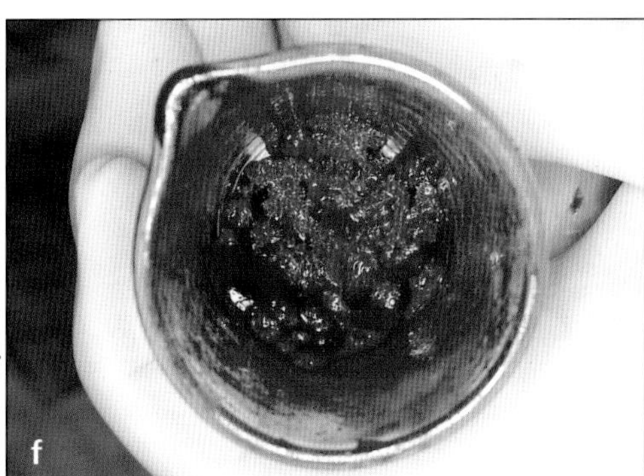

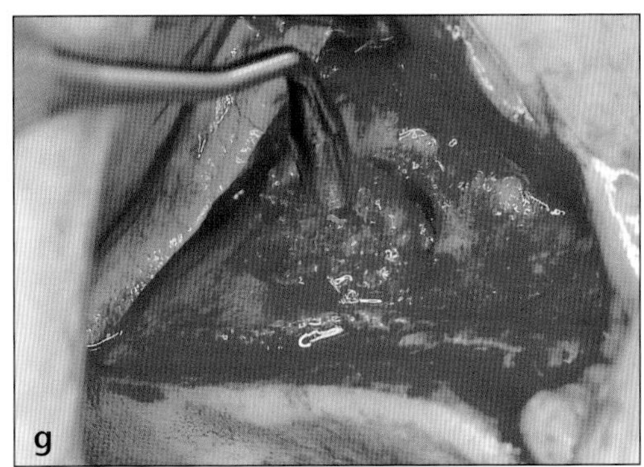

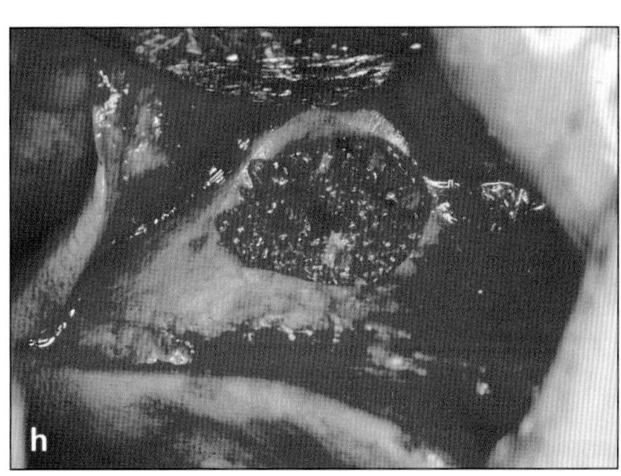

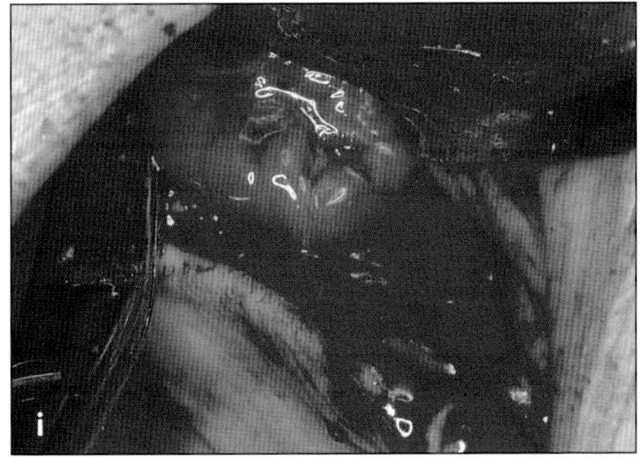

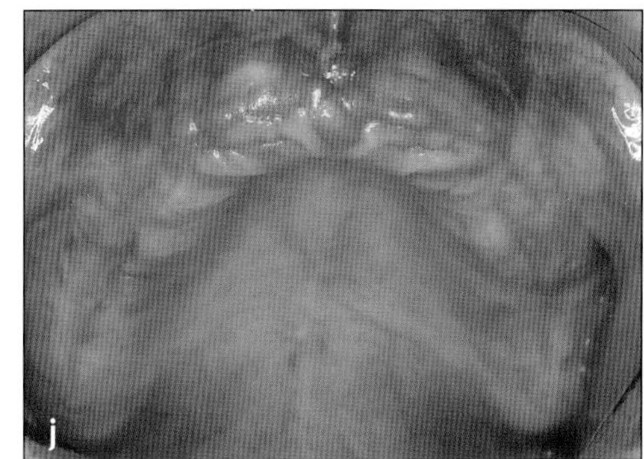

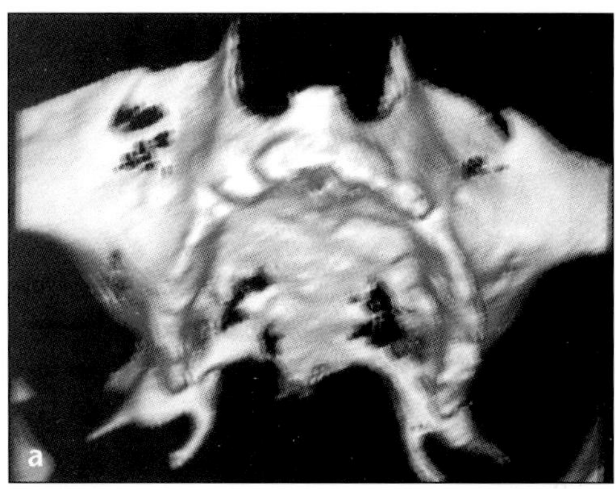

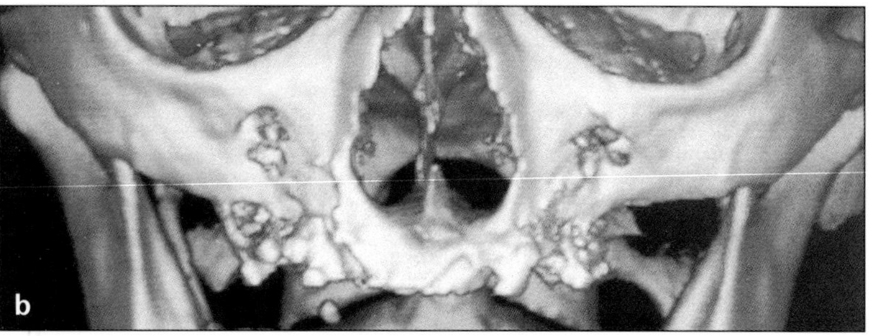

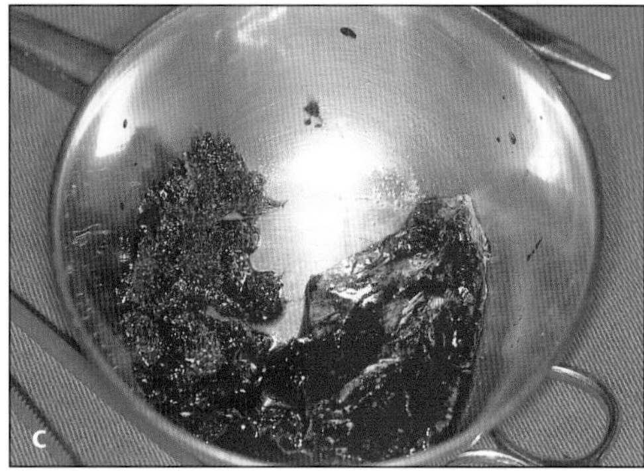

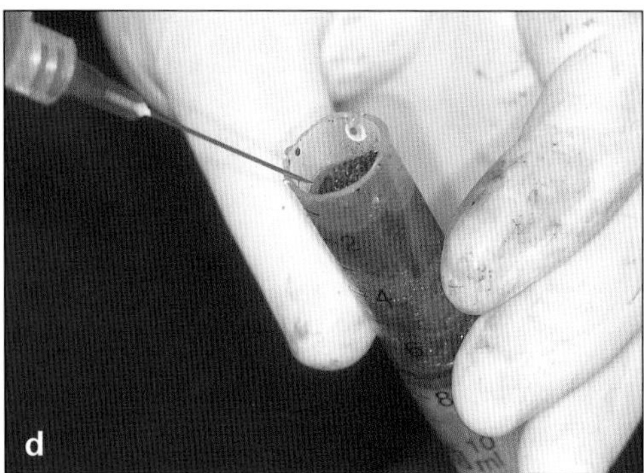

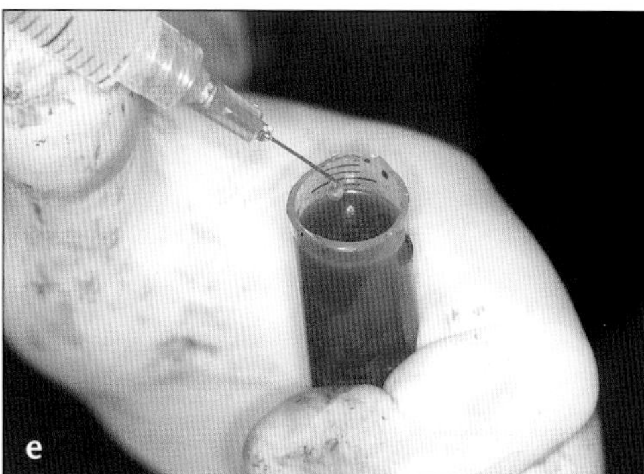

Fig 8-23 Particulate and block grafting for implant placement in a patient with severe alveolar ridge resorption.

(a) Digital three-dimensional tomograph of the maxilla shows an average crestal bone width of 2 mm.

(b) The anterior and posterior maxillary alveolar ridges have resorbed almost to the floor of the nose. There is approximately 2 to 3 mm of crestal bone height.

(c) The amount of bone loss in this patient requires not only particulate bone but also bone blocks. Because of the volume and configurations required, bone was harvested from the iliac crest in an operating room under general anesthesia.

(d) The particulate bone is placed in a 5-mL syringe with the tip cut off. This is an inexpensive, readily available, sterile way to carry bone to the recipient sites. Moreover, it allows the clinician to measure the bone volume and condense the bone with the plunger. Nonactivated PRP is added to saturate the particulate bone.

(e) Once the nonactivated PRP has saturated the graft material, the activating agent is injected. This step is performed immediately prior to placement of the graft in the recipient site.

Fig 8-23 *(cont)*
(f) The graft material is injected out of the syringe.

(g) For demonstration purposes, the graft material is pushed out onto a sterile towel. Clinically, it is dispensed directly to the recipient site in this manner.

(h) The graft material holds together even when fully released from the syringe because of the gelatinous consistency of the PRP.

(i) The sinus cavities are filled first and, using a condenser, the bone is pressed into all necessary areas of the sinus and condensed well.

(j) The harvested bone blocks are cut into smaller blocks and carefully measured to fit deficient areas on the ridge.

(k) Both the blocks and the ridge are contoured and shaped for excellent adaptation and stabilization. They should be positioned to create an ideal ridge width for dental implants as well as an ideal maxillomandibular relationship.

(l) The screws for affixing the bone blocks should be high quality and of appropriate length and diameter with a well-fitting driver.

(m) At least two screws should generally be used for each block to prevent rotation or movement.

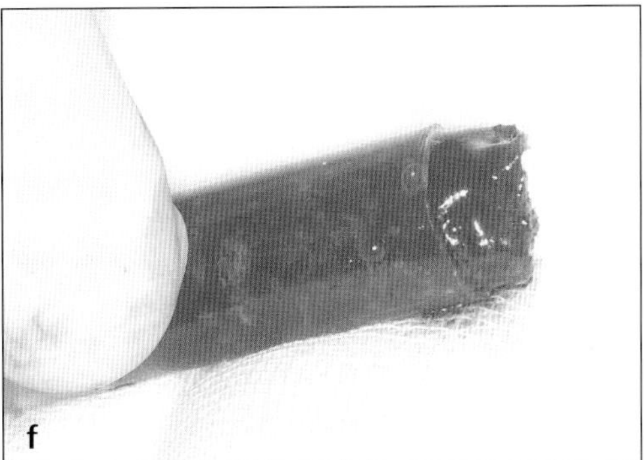
f

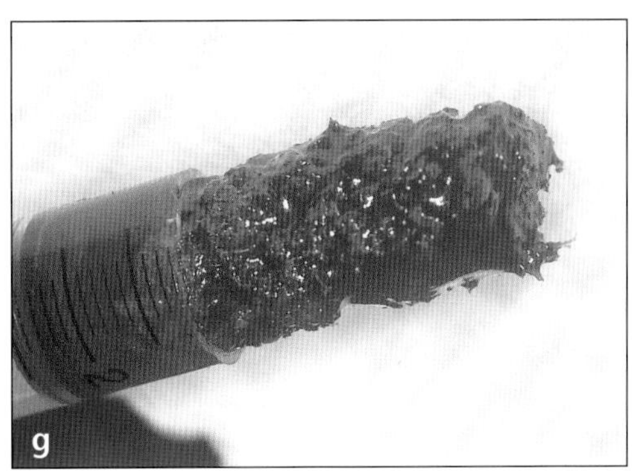
g

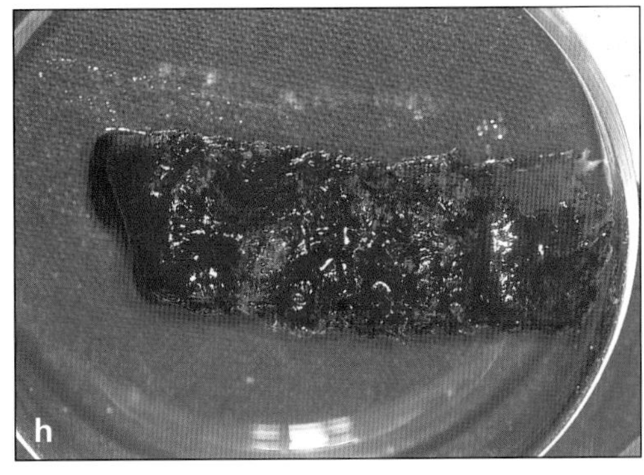
h

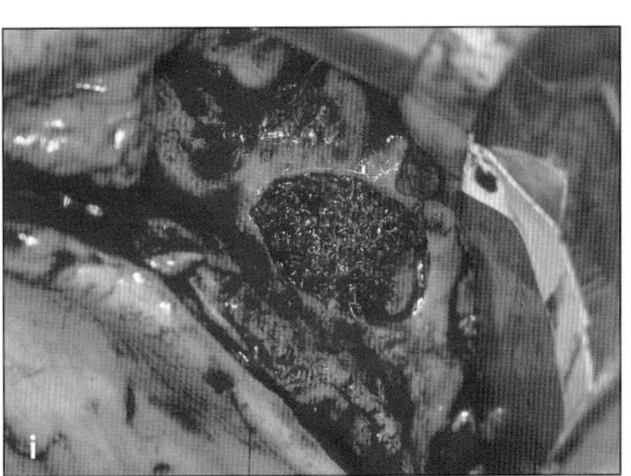
i

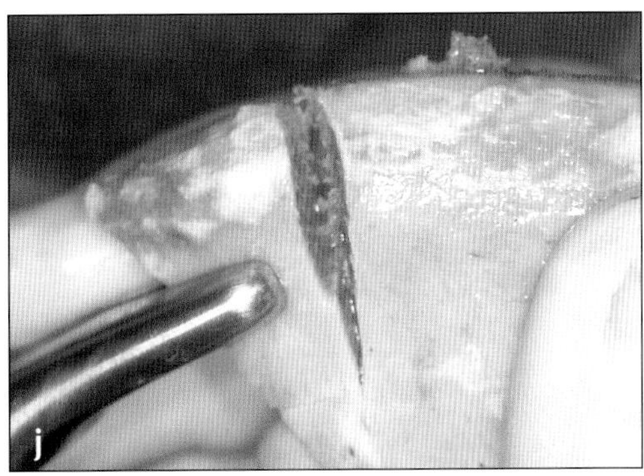
j

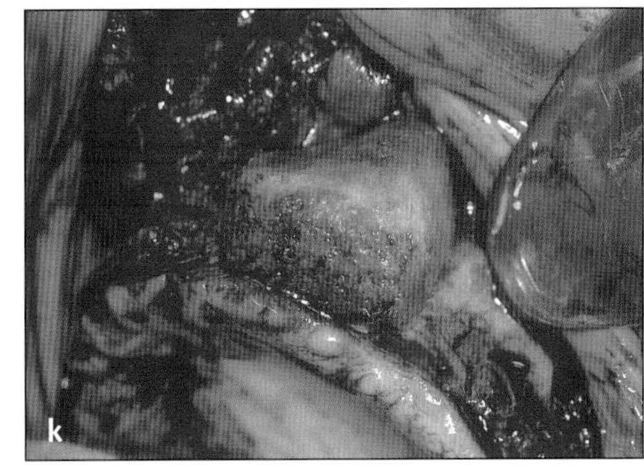
k

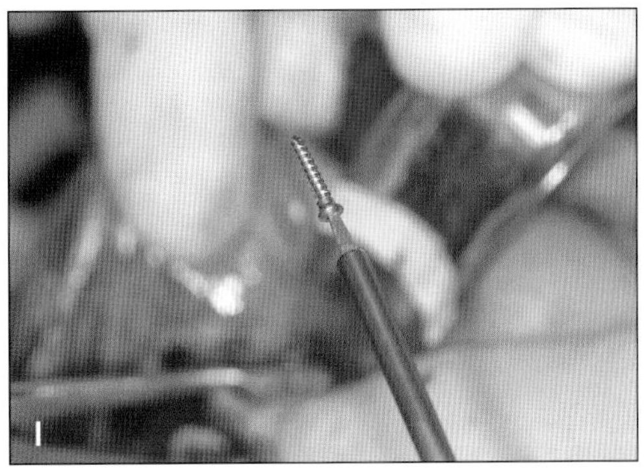
l

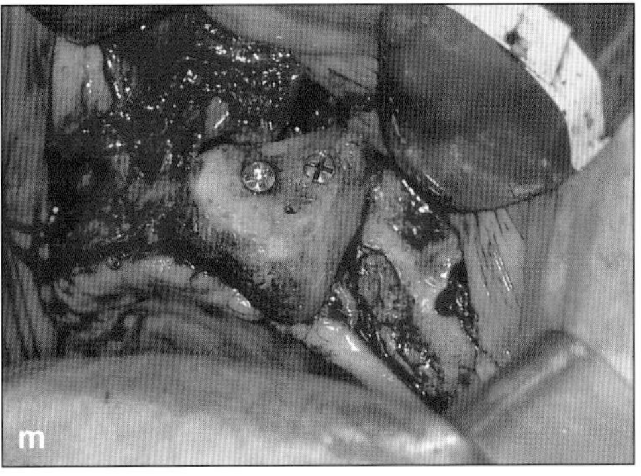
m

(continued)

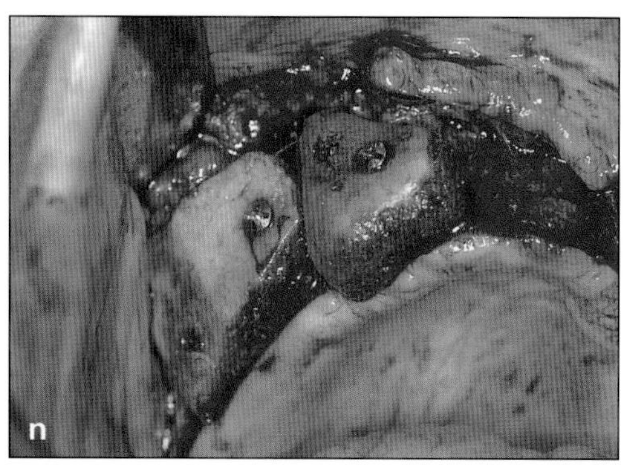
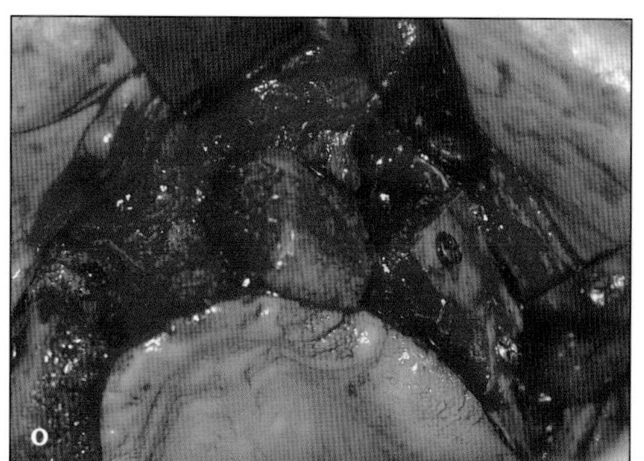
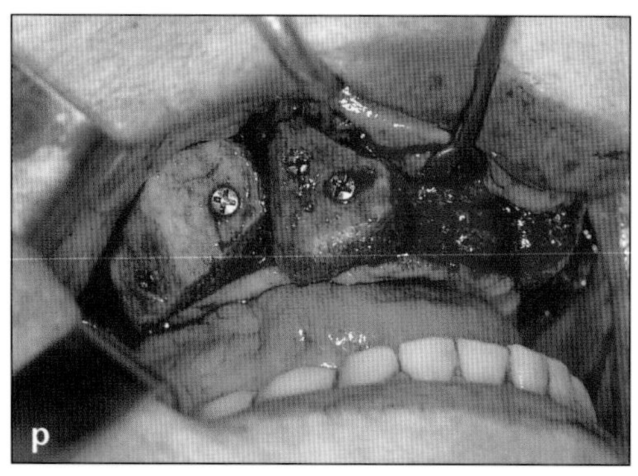
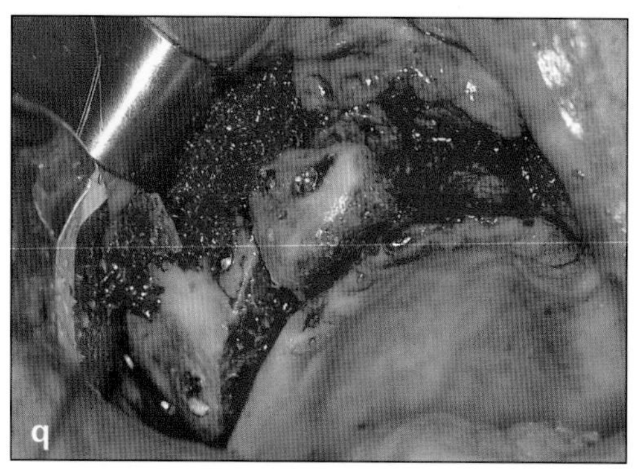
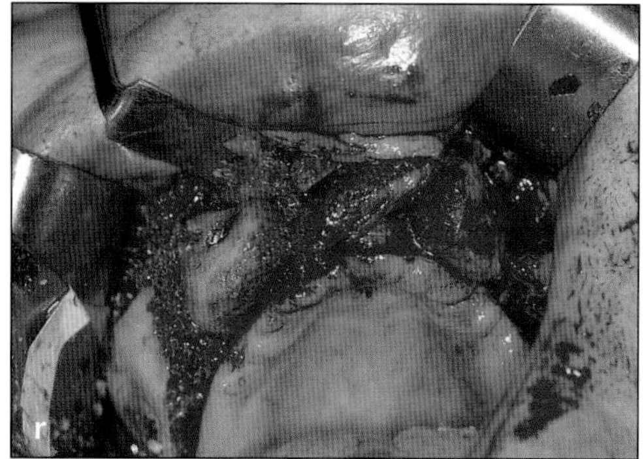
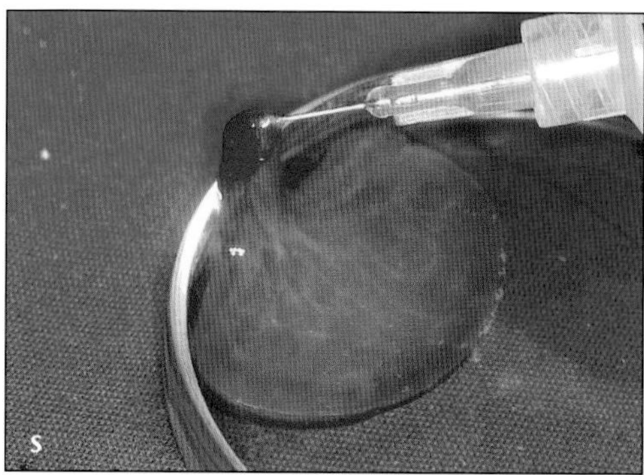
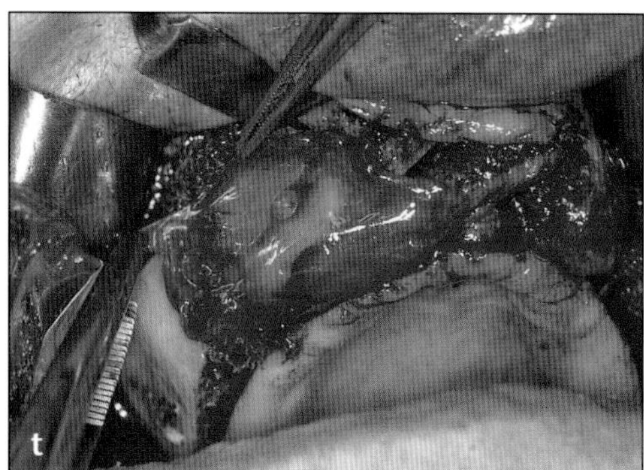
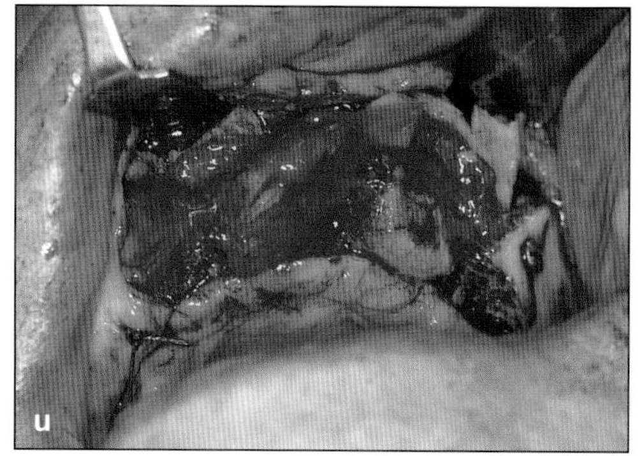

Fig 8-23 *(cont)*
(n) Reshaping of the blocks continues as they are placed to fill the spaces.

(o) The edges of the blocks can be contoured once they have been screwed into position.

(p) It is important to check the intermaxillary relationship during block placement to ensure that an appropriately dimensioned ridge is being created.

(q) Particulate bone is used to fill the space between the blocks and create a smoother and denser contour.

(r) A PRP membrane is formed and will be used. Since most of the surface of the graft is cortical block bone and not particulate bone, a true guided bone regeneration–type membrane is not necessary.

(s) A PRP membrane is created by placing a small pool of activated PRP onto a smooth sterile surface.

(t) This membrane is placed over the blocks of bone.

(u) The entire grafted area should be covered with a membrane.

Fig 8-23 *(cont)*
(v) A thorough dissection of the buccal flap should be performed to permit a wide stretch of the mucosa and ensure a complete and tension-free primary closure. It is important that the flap be mucosal only and not contain buccinator or obicularis oris muscle fibers. This strategy will minimize tension and movement to the flap during smiling and chewing. If necessary, a vestibuloplasty can be performed at a later time.

(w) Twelve dental implants of adequate length, diameter, and position have been successfully placed in a patient with 2 to 3 mm of ridge height and width prior to grafting.

(x) Clinical view of the 12 healing abutments after stage 2 surgery, surrounded by healthy attached gingiva.

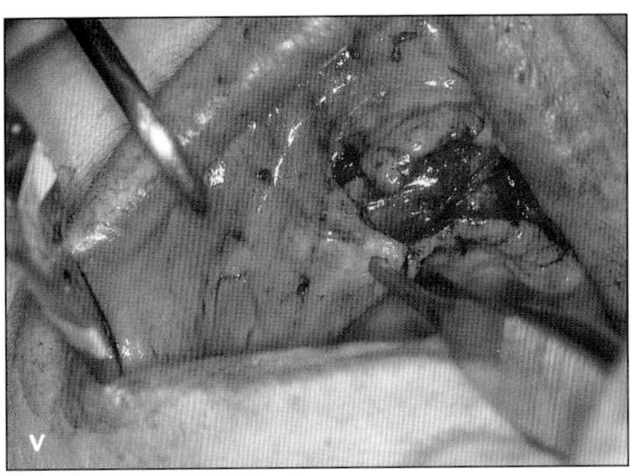

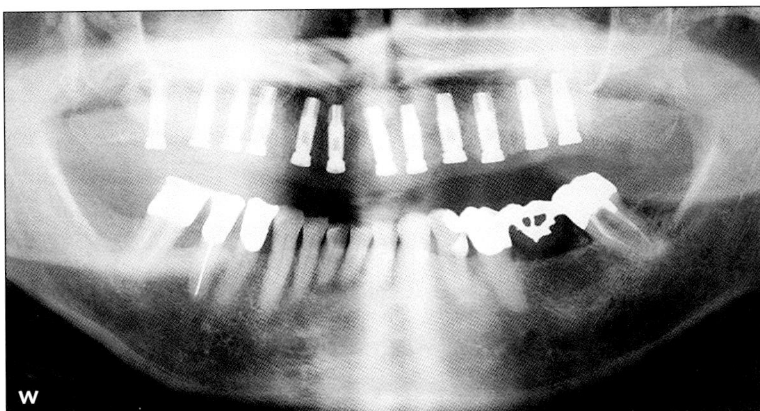

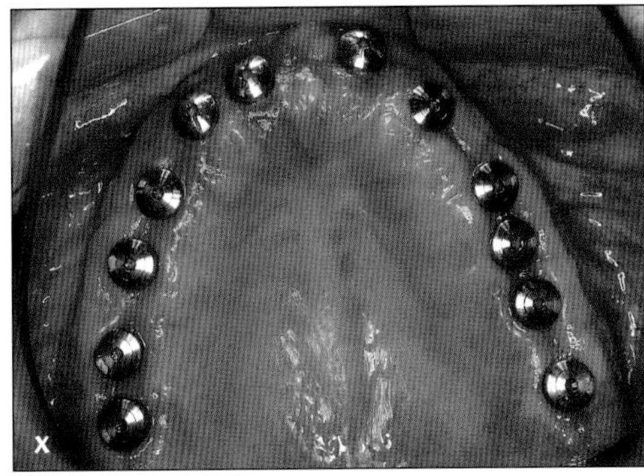

References

1. Smiler DG, Johnson PW, Lozada JL, et al. Sinus lift grafts and endosseous implants. Treatment of the atrophic posterior maxilla. Dent Clin North Am 1992;36:151–186.
2. Khoury F. Augmentation of the sinus floor with mandibular bone block and simultaneous implantation: A 6-year clinical investigation. Int J Oral Maxillofac Implants 1999;14:557–564.
3. Chanavaz M. Sinus grafting related to implantology. Statistical analysis of 15 years of surgical experience (1979–1994). J Oral Implantol 1996;22:119–130.
4. Marx RE. Clinical application of bone biology to mandibular and maxillary reconstruction. Clin Plast Surg 1994;21:377–392.
5. Tatum H Jr. Maxillary and sinus implant reconstructions. Dent Clin North Am 1986;30: 207–229.
6. Tatum H Jr. Endosteal implants. CDA J 1988;16:71–76.
7. Tatum H. Maxillary implants. Florida Dent J 1989;60:23–27.
8. Boyne PJ, James RA. Grafting of the maxillary sinus floor with autogenous marrow and bone. J Oral Surg 1980;38:613–616.
9. Misch CE. Maxillary sinus augmentation for endosteal implants: Organized alternative treatment plans. Int J Oral Implant 1987;4: 49–58.
10. Garg AK, Quinones CR. Augmentation of the maxillary sinus: A surgical technique. Pract Periodontics Aesthet Dent 1997;9:211–219.
11. Kent JN, Block MS. Simultaneous maxillary sinus floor bone grafting and placement of hydroxylapatite-coated implants. J Oral Maxillofac Surg 1989;47:238–242.
12. Jensen J, Simonsen EK, Sindet-Pedersen S. Reconstruction of the severely resorbed maxilla with bone grafting and osseointegrated implants: A preliminary report. J Oral Maxillofac Surg 1990;48:27–32.
13. Raghoebar GM, Brouwer TJ, Reintsema H, Van Oort RP. Augmentation of the maxillary sinus floor with autogenous bone for the placement of endosseous implants: A preliminary report. J Oral Maxillofac Surg 1993;51: 1198–1203.
14. Adell R Lekholm U, Grondahl K, Branemark PI, Lindstrom J, Jacobsson M. Reconstruction of severely resorbed edentulous maxillae using osseointegrated fixtures in immediate autogenous bone grafts. Int J Oral Maxillofac Implants 1990;5:233–246.
15. Kahnberg KE, Nystrom E, Bartholdsson L. Combined use of bone grafts and Branemark fixtures in the treatment of severely resorbed maxillae. Int J Oral Maxillofac Implants 1989; 4:297–304.
16. Nystrom E, Kahnberg KE, Gunne J. Bone grafts and Branemark implants in the treatment of the severely resorbed maxilla: A 2-year longitudinal study. Int J Oral Maxillofac Implants 1993;8:45–53.
17. Wood RM, Moore DL. Grafting of the maxillary sinus with intraorally harvested autogenous bone prior to implant placement. Int J Oral Maxillofac Implants 1988;3:209–214.
18. Jensen J, Sindet-Pedersen S. Autogenous mandibular bone grafts and osseointegrated implants for reconstruction of the severely atrophied maxilla: A preliminary report. J Oral Maxillofac Surg 1991;49:1277–1287.
19. Keller EE, van Roekel NB, Desjardins RP, Tolman DE. Prosthetic-surgical reconstruction of the severely resorbed maxilla with iliac bone grafting and tissue-integrated prostheses. Int J Oral Maxillofac Implants 1987;2: 155–165.
20. Loukota RA, Isaksson SG, Linner EL, Blomqvist JE. A technique for inserting endosseous implants in the atrophic maxilla in a single stage procedure. Br J Oral Maxillofac Surg 1992;30:46–49.
21. Small SA, Zinner ID, Panno FV, Shapiro HJ, Stein JI. Augmenting the maxillary sinus for implants: Report of 27 patients. Int J Oral Maxillofac Implants 1993;8:523–528.
22. Jensen OT, Perkins S, Van de Water FW. Nasal fossa and maxillary sinus grafting of implants from a palatal approach: Report of a case. J Oral Maxillofac Surg 1992;50:415–418.
23. Tidwell JK, Blijdorp PA, Stoelinga PJW, Brouns JB, Hinderks F. Composite grafting of the maxillary sinus for placement of endosteal implants. A preliminary report of 48 patients. Int J Oral Maxillofac Surg 1992;21:204–209.
24. Triplett RG, Schow SR. Autologous bone grafts and endosseous implants: complementary techniques. J Oral Maxillofac Surg 1996; 54:486–494.

25. Zinner ID, Small SA. Sinus-lift graft: Using the maxillary sinuses to support implants. J Am Dent Assoc 1996;127:51–57.
26. Peleg M, Mazor Z, Chaushu G, Garg AK. Sinus floor augmentation with simultaneous implant placement in severely atrophic maxilla. J Periodontol 1998;69:1397–1403.
27. Peleg M, Mazor Z, Garg AK. Augmentation grafting of the maxillary sinus and simultaneous implant placement in patients with 3 to 5 mm of residual alveolar bone height. Int J Oral Maxillofac Implants 1999;14:549–556.
28. Boyne PJ. The Use of Bone Graft Systems in Maxillary Implant Surgery. [Proceedings of the 50th Annual Meeting of the American Institute of Oral Biology, 29 Oct–3 Nov 1993, Palm Springs, CA.] 1994:107–114.
29. Daelemans P, Hermans M, Godet F, Malevez C. Autologous bone graft to augment the maxillary sinus in conjunction with immediate endosseous implants: A retrospective study up to 5 years. Int J Periodontics Restorative Dent 1997:17;27–39.
30. Razavi R, Zena RB, Khan Z, Gould AR. Anatomic site evaluation of edentulous maxillae for dental implant placement. J Prosthodont 1995;4:90–94.
31. Chanavaz M. Maxillary sinus: Anatomy, physiology, surgery, and bone grafting related to implantology—Eleven years of surgical experience (1979–1990). J Oral Implantol 1990; 16:199–209.
32. Cuenin MF, Pollard BK, Elrod CW. Maxillary sinus morphology in differential dental diagnosis. Gen Dent 1996;44:328–331.
33. Ulm CW, Solar P, Gsellman B, Matejka M, Watzek G. The edentulous maxillary alveolar process in the region of the maxillary sinus—A study of physical dimension. Int J Oral Maxillofac Surg 1995;24:279–282.
34. Marx RE, Garg AK. Bone structure, metabolism, and physiology: Its impact on dental implantology. Implant Dent 1998;7:267–276.
35. Lane JM. Bone graft substitutes. West J Med 1995;163:565–566.
36. Frame JW. Hydroxyapatite as a biomaterial for alveolar ridge augmentation. Int J Oral Maxillofac Surg 1987;16:642–655.
37. Pinholt EM, Bang G, Haanaes HR. Alveolar ridge augmentation in rats by combined hydroxylapatite and osteoinductive material. Scand J Dent Res 1991;99:64–74.
38. Misch CE, Dietsh F. Bone-grafting materials in implant dentistry. Implant Dent 1993;2: 158–167.
39. Second-hand bones? [editorial]. Lancet 1992; 340:1443.
40. Rummelhart JM, Mellonig JT, Gray JL, Towle HJ. A comparison of freeze-dried bone allograft and demineralized freeze-dried bone allograft in human periodontal osseous defects. J Periodontal 1989;60:655–663.
41. Mellonig JT. Decalcified freeze-dried bone allograft as an implant material in human periodontal defects. Int J Periodontics Restorative Dent 1984;4:40–55.
42. Tatum OH Jr, Lebowitz MS, Tatum CA, Borgner RA. Sinus augmentation: Rationale, development, long-term results. N Y State Dent J 1993;59:43–48.
43. Tatum OH Jr. Osseous grafts in intra-oral sites. J Oral Implantol 1996;22:51–52.
44. Fetner AE, Hartigan MS, Low SB. Periodontal repair using PerioGlas in nonhuman primates: Clinical and histologic observations. Compendium 1994;15:932, 935–938.
45. Schepers E, de Clercq M, Ducheyne P, Kempeneers R. Bioactive glass particulate materials as a filler for bone lesions. J Oral Rehabil 1991; 18:439–452.
46. Schepers EJ, Ducheyne P, Barbier L, Schepers S. Bioactive glass particles of narrow size range: A new material for the repair of bone defects. Implant Dent 1993;2:151–156.
47. McAllister BS, Margolin MD, Cogan AG, Buck D, Hollinger JO, Lynch SE. Eighteen-month radiographic and histologic evaluation of sinus grafting with anorganic bovine bone in the chimpanzee. Int J Oral Maxillofac Implants 1999;14:361–368.
48. Wagner J. Clinical and histological case study using resorbable hydroxylapatite for the repair of osseous defects prior to endosseous implant surgery. J Oral Implantol 1989;15: 186–192.
49. Moy PK, Lundgren S, Holmes RE. Maxillary sinus augmentation: Histomorphometric analysis of graft materials for maxillary sinus floor augmentation. J Oral Maxillofac Surg 1993; 51:857–862.

50. Jensen OT, Greer R. Immediate placement of osseointegrating implants into the maxillary sinus augmented with mineralized cancellous allograft and Gore-Tex: Second stage surgical and histological findings. In: Laney WR, Tolman DE (eds). Tissue Integration in Oral, Orthopedic and Maxillofacial Reconstruction. [Proceedings of the Second International Congress on Tissue Integration in Oral, Orthopedic, and Maxillofacial Reconstruction, 23–27 Sept 1990, Rochester, MN.] Chicago: Quintessence, 1992:321–333.
51. Nishibori M, Betts NJ, Salama H, Listgarten MA. Short-term healing of autogenous and allogeneic bone grafts after sinus augmentation: A report of 2 cases. J Periodontol 1994;65:958–966.
52. Wheeler SL, Holmes RE, Calhoun CJ. Six-year clinical and histologic study of sinus-lift grafts. Int J Oral Maxillofac Implants 1996;11:26–34.
53. Lorenzetti M, Mozzati M, Campanino PP, Valente G. Bone augmentation of the inferior floor of the maxillary sinus with autogenous bone or composite bone grafts: A histologic-histomorphometric preliminary report. Int J Oral Maxillofac Implants 1998;13:69–76.
54. Lazzara RJ. The sinus elevation procedure in endosseous implant therapy. Curr Opin Periodontol 1996;3:178–183.
55. Koole R, Bosker H, van der Dussen FN. Late secondary autogenous bone grafting in cleft patients comparing mandibular (ectomesenchymal) and iliac crest (mesenchymal) grafts. J Craniomaxillofac Surg 1989;17(suppl 1):28–30.
56. Shirota T, Ohno K, Motohashi M, Michi K. Histologic and microradiologic comparison of block and particulate cancellous bone and marrow grafts in reconstructed mandibles being considered for dental implant placement. J Oral Maxillofac Surg 1996;54:15–20.
57. Block MS, Kent JN, Kallukaran FU, Thunthy K, Weinberg R. Bone maintenance 5 to 10 years after sinus grafting. J Oral Maxillofac Surg 1998;56:706–714.
58. Urist MR, Dowell TA, Hay PH, Strates BS. Inductive substrates for bone formation. Clin Orthop 1968;59:59–96.
59. Becker W, Urist MR, Tucker LM, Becker BE, Ochsenbein C. Human demineralized freeze-dried bone: Inadequate induced bone formation in athymic mice. A preliminary report. J Periodontol 1995;66:822–828.
60. Becker W, Lynch S, Lekholm U, et al. A comparison of ePTFE membranes alone or in combination with platelet-derived growth factors and insulin-like growth factor-I or demineralized freeze-dried bone in promoting bone formation around immediate extraction socket implants. J Periodontol 1992;63:929–940.
61. Pinholt EM, Haanaes HR, Donath K, Bang G. Titanium implant insertion into dog alveolar ridges augmented by allogenic material. Clin Oral Implants Res 1994;5:213–219.
62. Becker W, Becker BE, Caffesse R. A comparison of demineralized freeze-dried bone and autologous bone to induce bone formation in human extraction sockets. J Periodontol 1994;65:1128–1133 [erratum 1995;66:309].
63. Smiler D, Holmes RE. Sinus lift procedure using porous hydroxyapatite: A preliminary clinical report. J Oral Implantol 1987;13:239–253.
64. Jensen OT. Allogeneic bone or hydroxylapatite for the sinus lift procedure? J Oral Maxillofac Surg 1990;48:771.
65. Boyne PJ, Marx RE, Nevins M, et al. A feasibility study evaluating rhBMP-2/absorbable collagen sponge for maxillary sinus floor augmentation. Int J Periodontics Restorative Dent 1997;17:11–25.
66. Boyne PJ, Nath R, Nakamura A. Human recombinant BMP-2 in osseous reconstruction of simulated cleft palate defects. Br J Oral Maxillofac Surg 1998;36:84–90.
67. Boyne PJ. Animal studies of the application of rhBMP-2 in maxillofacial reconstruction. Bone 1996;19(suppl 1):83S–92S.
68. Nevins M, Kirker-Head C, Nevins M, Wozney JA, Palmer R, Graham D. Bone formation in the goat maxillary sinus induced by absorbable collagen sponge implants impregnated with recombinant human bone morphogenetic protein-2. Int J Periodontics Restorative Dent 1996;16:8–19.
69. Hollinger JO, Schmitt JM, Hwang K, Soleymani P, Buck D. Impact of nicotine on bone healing. J Biomed Mater Res 1999;45:294–301 [erratum 1999;46:438–439].

70. Borris TJ, Weber CR. Intraoperative nasal transillumination for maxillary sinus augmentation procedures: A technical note. Int J Oral Maxillofac Implants 1998;13:569–570.
71. Abrahams JJ, Glassberg RM. Dental disease: A frequently unrecognized cause of maxillary sinus abnormalities? AJR Am J Roentgenol 1996;166:1219–1223.
72. Misch CM. The pharmacologic management of maxillary sinus elevation surgery. J Oral Implantol 1992;18:15–23.
73. Peterson LJ. Antibiotic prophylaxis against wound infections in oral and maxillofacial surgery. J Oral Maxillofac Surg 1990;48:617–620.
74. Betts NJ, Miloro M. Modification of the sinus lift procedure for septa in the maxillary antrum. J Oral Maxillofac Surg 1994;52:332–333.
75. Ulm CW, Solar P, Krennmair G, Matejka M, Watzek G. Incidence and suggested surgical management of septa in sinus-lift procedures. Int J Oral Maxillofac Implants 1995;10:462–465.
76. Regev E, Smith RA, Perrott DH, Pogrel MA. Maxillary sinus complications related to endosseous implants. Int J Oral Maxillofac Implants 1995;10:451–461.

CHAPTER

9 Augmentation and Grafting for the Maxillary Anterior Alveolar Ridges

The anterior maxilla is the most challenging region of the dentition to restore (Fig 9-1).[1–4] Bone grafting to support esthetics is key in this prominent area because the underlying ridge must support both the implant restoration and the soft tissue to achieve a long-lasting, esthetic result. These factors are particularly important in cases involving two or more teeth. Osseointegration of dental implants, particularly in the anterior maxilla, depends on adequate trabecular bone density, ridge height and width,[5] and systemic bone health. The clinician must evaluate all of these factors to ensure that implants can maintain osseointegration during function.[6–11] Furthermore, the clinician must take advantage of all available clinical, laboratory, and communication technologies to meet the patient's functional and esthetic needs.[12]

Bone augmentation is required when anterior tooth loss leads to the loss of bone volume needed for proper implant positioning.[13,14] The diameter of the implant, compared with that of natural teeth, can create challenges associated with the cervical esthetics of the crown. Other unique problems that may limit ideal placement of implants in the anterior maxilla include *(1)* a resorbed (from periodontal disease) or fractured (from extraction) facial cortical plate over the maxillary roots of the teeth; *(2)* close proximity of the nasal and maxillary sinus cavities; *(3)* lateral extension of the incisive canal; *(4)* facial concavities; and *(5)* reduced turnover and health of bone caused by aging or metabolic disease (which may not be revealed until after implant placement) (Fig 9-2). Attention must also be paid to developing a healthy and esthetic soft tissue result and a natural emergence profile,[15–22] with soft tissue grafting undertaken as needed.[23–28] Thus, the clinician must develop a comprehensive treatment plan that allows the surgeon, the laboratory technician, and the restorative clinician to visualize the anticipated result before treatment begins.

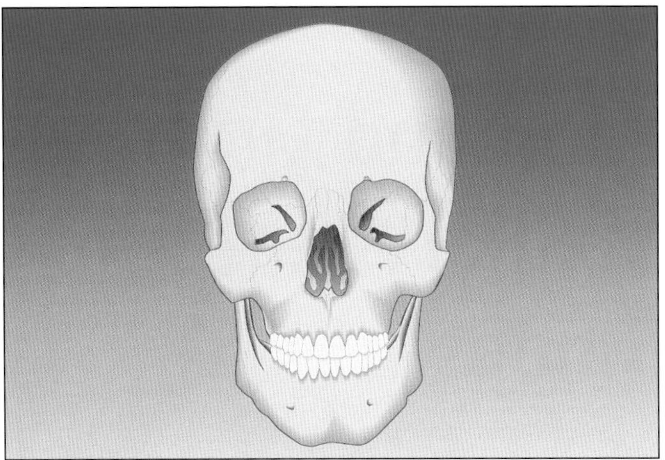

Fig 9-1
From simple restorations to complex reconstruction, the prominence and visibility of the anterior maxilla always presents challenges.

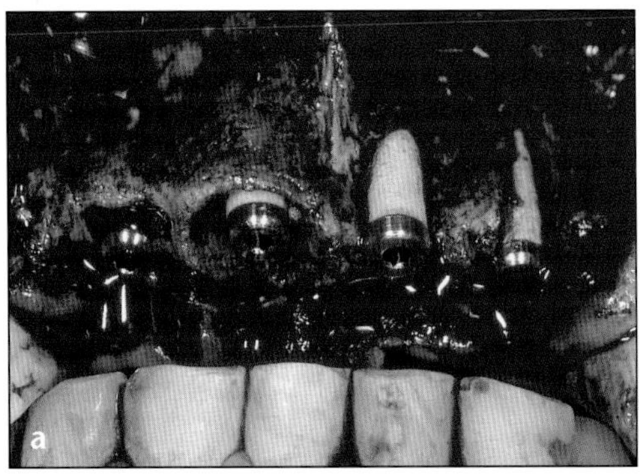

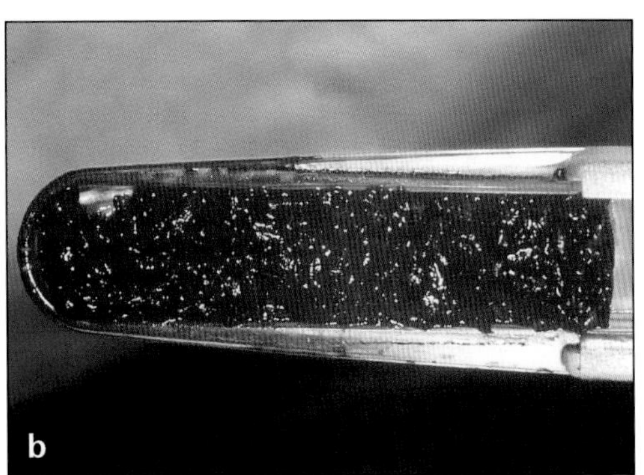

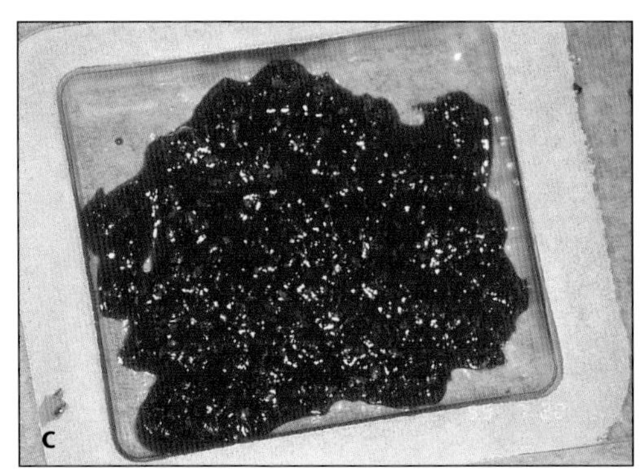

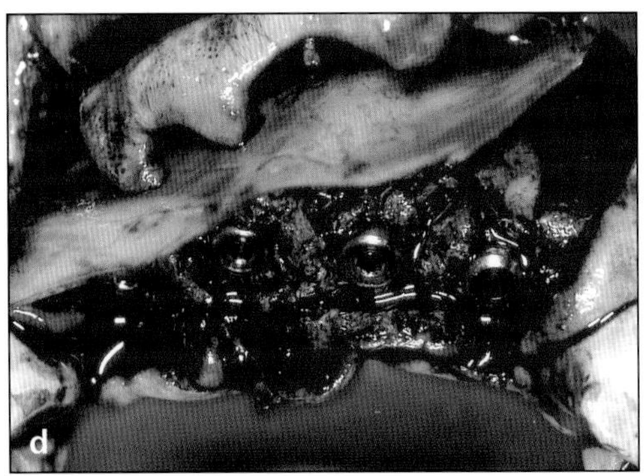

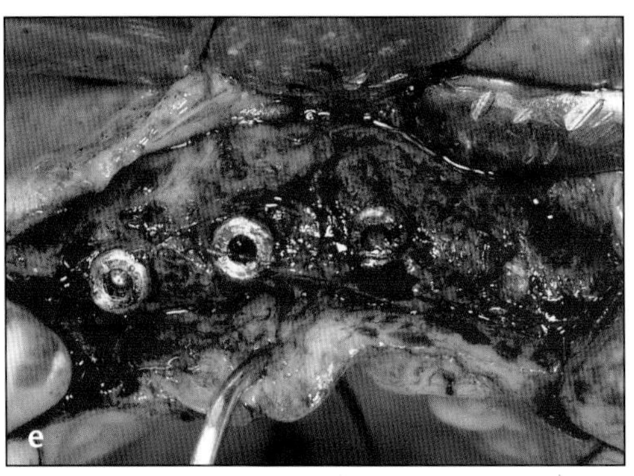

Fig 9-2 Bone volume must be adequate not only for proper face contour and lip support but also for exact positioning and angulation and correct intermaxillary relationship of subsequent implants.

(a) This partially resorbed maxilla required grafting and implants.

(b) A bone shaver can provide particulate bone, even from the implant area, while the ridge is simultaneously smoothed.

(c) As little as 2 mL of particulate bone can adequately cover the buccal surface of two exposed implants.

(d) A thin piece of lamellar allogeneic bone can be placed over the implants to help keep the particulate bone in place and keep soft tissue cells from invading the area where bone growth alone is desired.

(e) After 6 months, the implants show perfect coverage; extra bone can be removed from the head of the fourth implant at this stage 2 procedure.

Evaluating Tissues to Determine Grafting Needs

During treatment planning for implant placement in the anterior maxilla, the clinician must analyze the topography of the edentulous ridge, particularly from the incisogingival and faciolingual positions. Adequate bone must be available to accommodate the number and length of implants needed to support the planned restoration and the soft tissue architecture.[29] The examination is done clinically and radiographically. If even more information is needed, a computerized tomography (CT) or spiral tomography scan[30] may be used to obtain a three-dimensional view. This implant placement technology is complemented by the three-dimensional placement of abutments via computer-aided design/computer-assisted manufacture (CAD/CAM) technology to help provide functional and esthetic satisfaction for the patient.[31] Additionally, a waxup of the ridge as well as the missing tooth or teeth can be requested from the laboratory.

The approach to implant restoration will depend on whether a single tooth or multiple teeth are being restored[32–41] and whether implant placement is immediate or delayed.[42–46] If more than two teeth are missing, reducing the number of implants can improve the esthetic outcome by enhancing the peri-implant soft tissue architecture at the pontic area.[47] The clinician can then take steps to develop the inter-implant papillae. If there are the same number of implants as there are missing teeth, creating the illusion of papillae can be difficult.[48–50]

Anterior Ridge Augmentation Methods

To determine whether and how to augment the anterior alveolar ridge of the maxilla, the clinician must consider the crown-to-implant ratio and the incisal edge position in relation to the implant body. The morphology of the defect must also be considered because it will determine which techniques or graft materials will be used. Ridge augmentation techniques (separately or in combination) to accommodate implant placement in the anterior maxilla include nasal floor elevation with grafting (see chapter 10), ridge spreading using osteotomes, corticocancellous autogenous block bone grafting (see chapter 5), and guided tissue regeneration (see chapter 3). Table 9-1 lists the classifications of ridge augmentation techniques according to the severity of the ridge deficiencies. Generally, if 4 to 10 mm of ridge thickness is available, a variety of office-based procedures can be considered. More severely resorbed or otherwise grossly deficient ridges require more extensive treatment.

Mucogingival reconstruction may also be required in anterior maxillary restoration cases. If horizontal and vertical dimensions of the ridge deficiency are within 3 mm of their original contour, good results can be achieved using soft tissue augmentation procedures, such as pedicle connective tissue grafts and free onlay or inlay connective tissue grafts harvested from the palatal mucosa. These grafting procedures can be performed prior to implant placement or during the submerged healing phase.[51–53]

Table 9-1 Classification of ridge augmentation techniques

Ridge thickness	Procedure
8 to 10 mm	Barrier membranes alone
7 to 8 mm	Particulate graft and barrier membrane with pin fixation
6 to 7 mm	Osteotomes for ridge expansion
5 to 6 mm	Allogeneic block of bone
4 to 5 mm	Autogenous block of bone
1 to 4 mm	Downfracture of the maxilla or titanium mesh crib (both with autogenous bone) or distraction osteogenesis

Barrier Membranes

If the ridge is at least 8 to 10 mm in buccopalatal width and the interarch ridge relationship is appropriate, then an implant can usually be placed adequately in bone. On occasion, some grafting may be required for esthetics or to cover a few exposed threads of the implant. In this scenario, a barrier membrane with titanium reinforcement struts can be considered.[8] Clinical experience and the published literature have shown that bone defects in a ridge of this width can be treated effectively without bone graft materials and using only guided bone regeneration (GBR). In fact, the results are so predictable that soft tissue management often becomes the most serious obstacle to successful use of implant-supported prosthetics in the anterior region.[51]

Use of barrier membranes for GBR in the maxilla, such as the Gore-Tex titanium-reinforced submerged membrane (W. L. Gore, Flagstaff, AZ), can follow a one- or two-stage approach. Embedded titanium struts allow the membrane to safely envelop the bone defect while effectively keeping the membrane off the bone (provided the titanium struts are bent appropriately and the membrane is tacked into position). If sufficient bone is available for placing the implant and primary stability is not a concern, then the membrane and implant can be placed simultaneously in a one-stage approach to treat any minor dehiscences or fenestrations. The membrane can be removed approximately 6 months later, and prosthetic treatment can commence. When local maxillary bone is insufficient for the placement of the implant because of the patient's esthetic and functional needs, barrier membranes can be placed first to help regenerate the bone in the area of the defect. The membrane can then be removed approximately 9 months later, and the implant can be placed at a second-stage surgery. Prosthetic treatment can commence approximately 3 months after implant placement.

Particulate Graft and Membranes with Pin Fixation

If the ridge is at least 7 to 8 mm buccopalatally, a membrane with some particulated graft material should be considered. The graft material can consist of autogenous bone, an allograft (such as demineralized or mineralized freeze-dried bone [FDBA]), or an alloplast/xenograft. Autogenous grafts regenerate bone, while alloplasts and xenografts create an osteoconductive

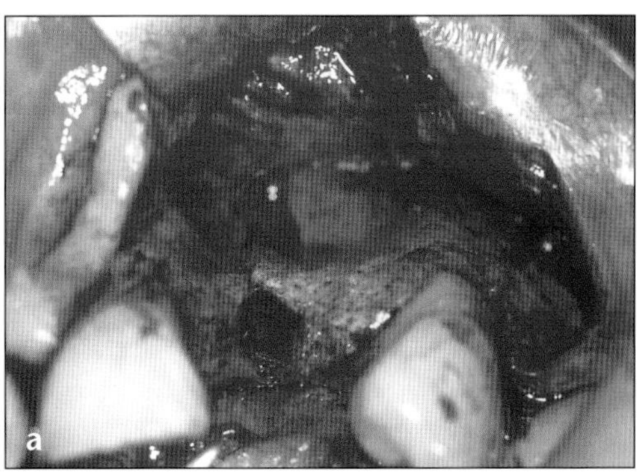
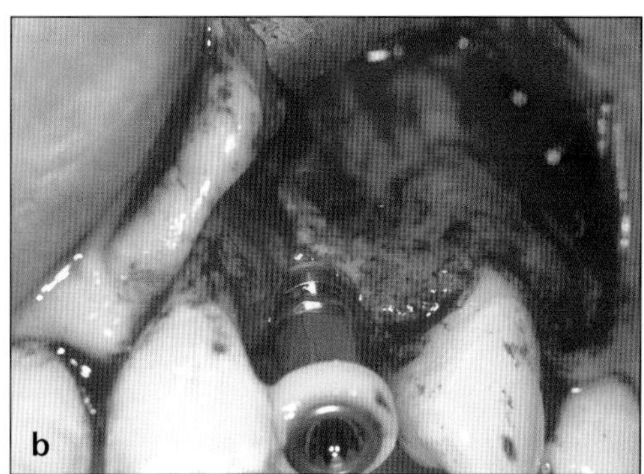
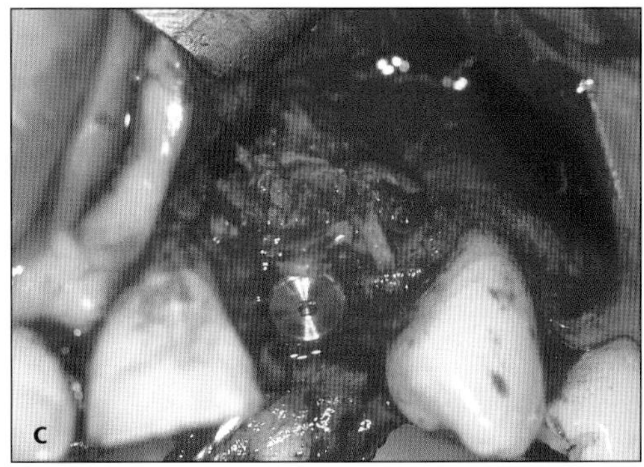
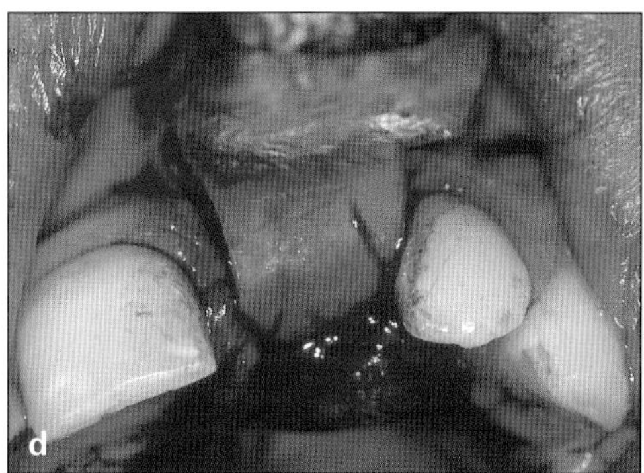
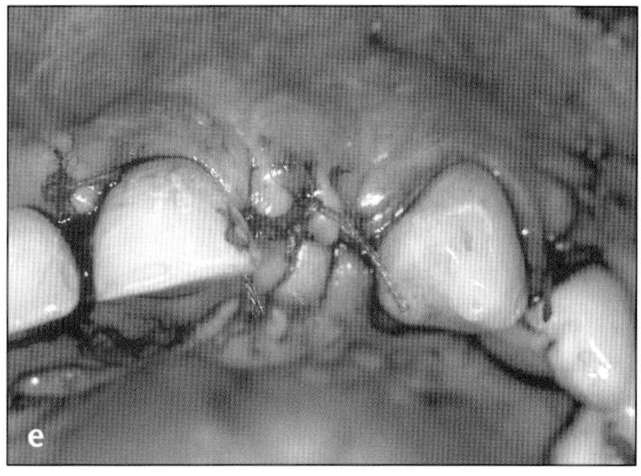

Fig 9-3 Use of barrier membranes in the maxilla following a one-stage approach.

(a) Bone dehiscence has occurred at the time of implant placement.

(b) Good stability is achieved despite implant exposure.

(c) Autogenous bone is obtained from the newly formed socket during careful drilling and is sufficient to provide good coverage in this patient.

(d) A resorbable collagen membrane is cut to fit the area and placed at the site.

(e) The flap should be placed exactly in its original position with passive closure and sutured to achieve primary closure.

scaffolding to facilitate bone regeneration. Allografts with collagen[54,55] or other types of resorbable membranes (eg, AlloDerm [LifeCell, Branchburg, NJ]),[56,57] including fixed bioabsorbable membranes,[58] can be used for ridge augmentation (Fig 9-3). However, the literature generally reports more predictable results with nonresorbable membranes, even when placed simultaneously with implants (Fig 9-4).[59] The best results have been obtained when implant placement is delayed for several weeks and when only a single implant is placed.[60]

Several researchers have demonstrated the effective use of GBR even in cases of more severe bone loss. In one study, human DFDBA was used with submembranous space creation to augment bone prior to implant placement.[61]

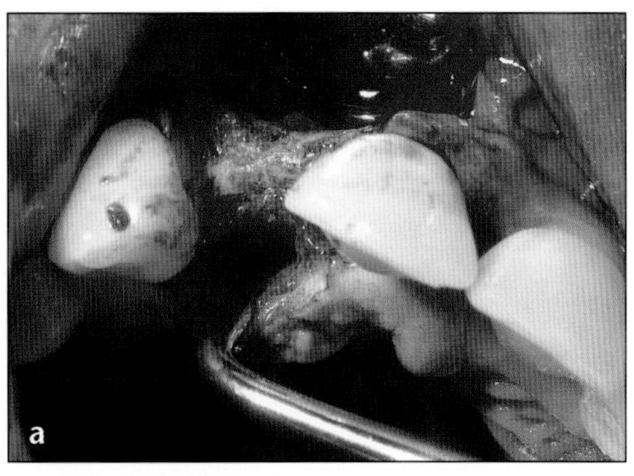

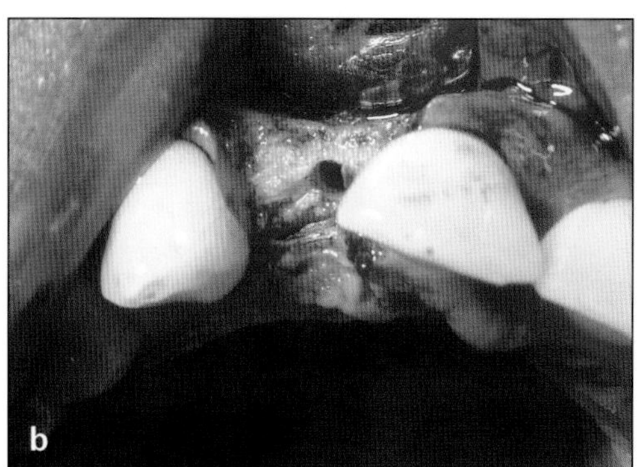

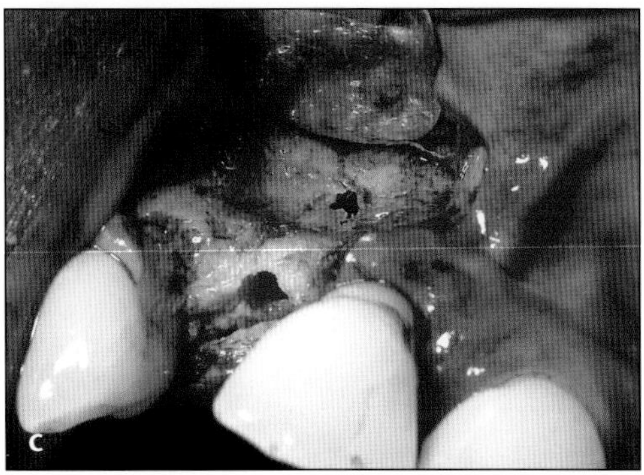

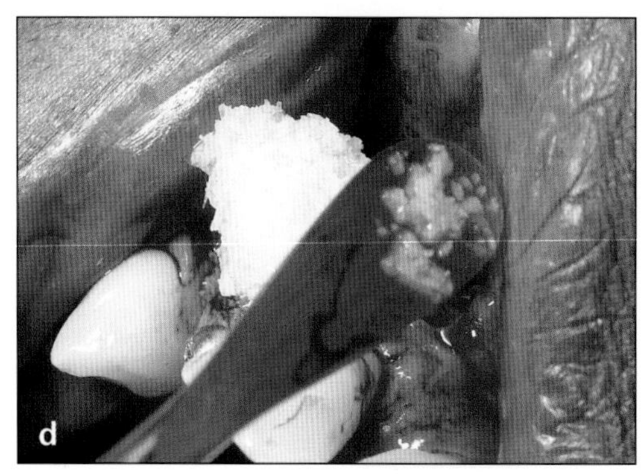

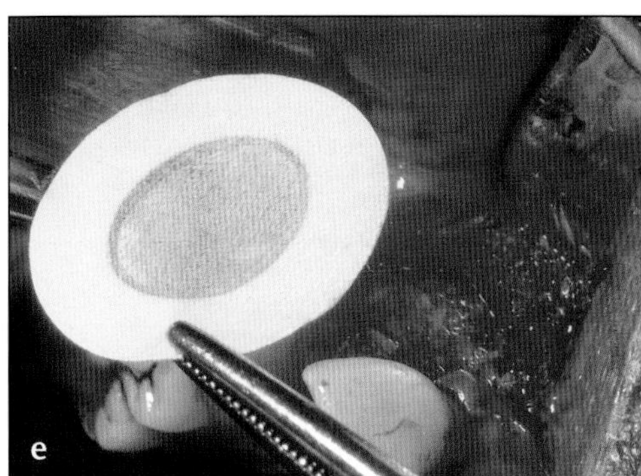

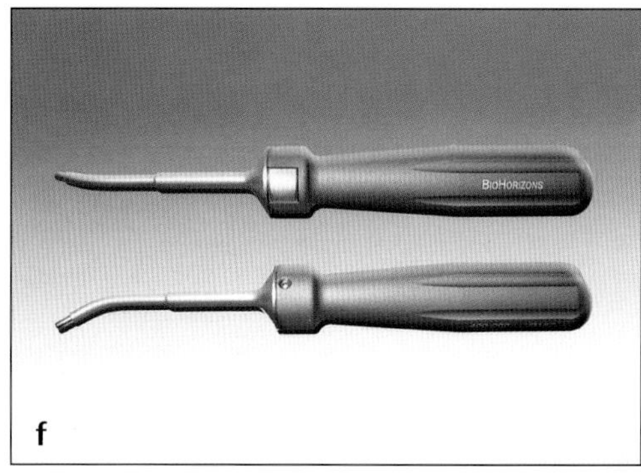

Fig 9-4 If the ridge is at least 8 to 12 mm in buccopalatal width, dehiscences can be corrected with the use of GBR membranes with or without bone graft materials.

(a) A single-tooth site in the anterior maxilla also poses a challenge in terms of bone height and width and the need to provide symmetry with the contralateral site.

(b) A single-tooth edentulous site can present the illusion of containing good bone width and height; concavities filled with connective tissue can give the appearance of having a good thickness of bone, even when palpated.

(c) Although it had the appearance of adequate bone, flap reflection reveals a deep concavity that gives way to bone dehiscence during drilling.

(d) In this patient, the placement of allogeneic particulate bone with the membrane was preferred.

(e) A Gore-Tex membrane was chosen for this patient because it provides good adaptation and coverage to the area. This nonresorbable membrane will be removed during the stage 2 procedure.

(f) The use of the Auto-Tac system (BioHorizons, Birmingham, AL) with resorbable or nonresorbable tacks is ideal to help keep the membrane immobilized.

Osteotomes for Ridge Expansion

If the ridge is at least 6 to 7 mm, then osteotomes can be used to expand and augment the ridge to provide appropriate amounts of bone for function, and the ridge can generally be modified to provide good esthetics as well.

Using osteotomes to expand a narrow anterior alveolar ridge prior to implant placement offers a particularly versatile approach for the clinician. Key advantages of the osteotome technique include minimal or no drilling, conservation of osseous tissue, improvement of bone density, and implant-to-bone interface with a denser bone. The osteotomy for an endosseous

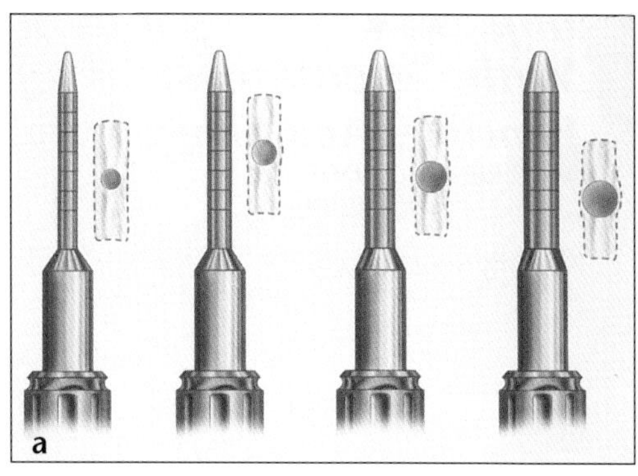
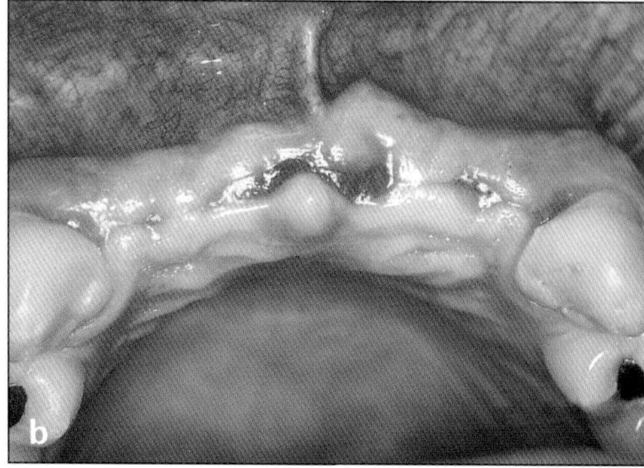
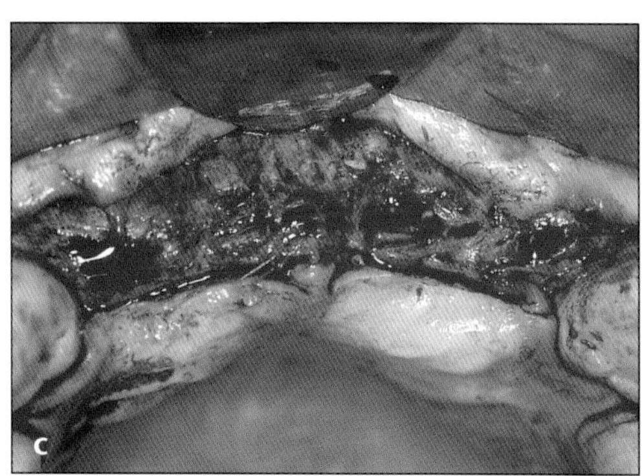
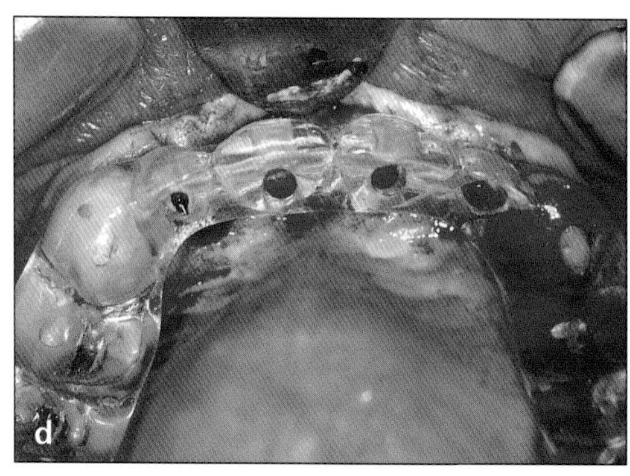
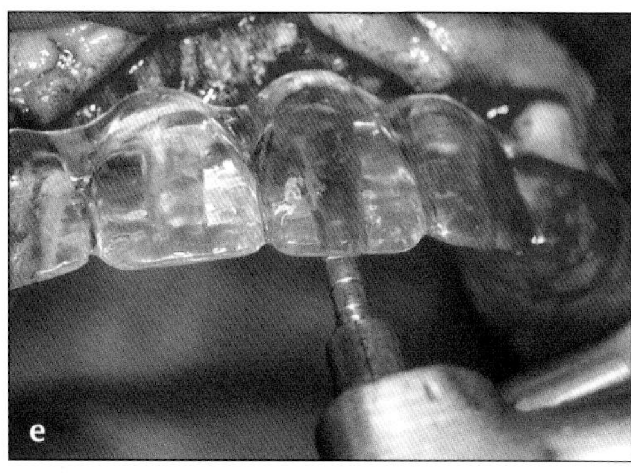
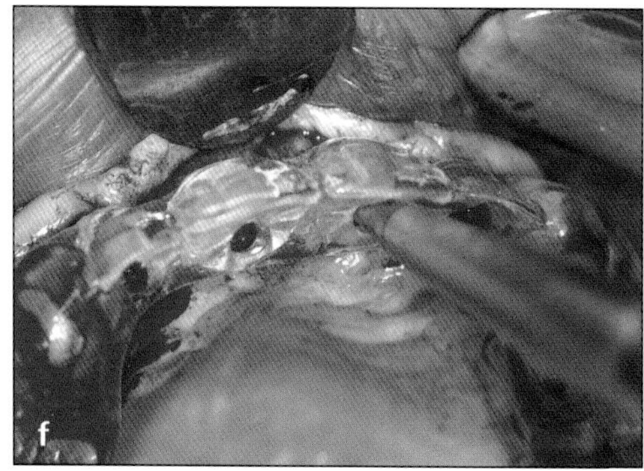

Fig 9-5 Osteotomes can be used to expand and augment the ridge to provide appropriate bone for function. The bone is compacted and relocated rather than removed, increasing the chances of implant survival.

(a) Osteotomes of increasing diameter (0.03 to 0.06 mm) are used to create an osteotomy to accommodate a specific implant system. (From Saadoun AP, Le Gall MG. Implant site preparation with osteotomes: Principles and clinical application. Pract Periodontics Aesthet Dent 1996;8:453–463. Used with permission.)

(b) Preoperative view showing a thin ridge in the anterior maxilla missing four incisors. A flap is reflected in order to gain access and visibility.

(c) The flap is reflected and retracted to expose the ridge.

(d) A surgical template is positioned to determine the appropriate osteotomy sites.

(e) The smallest diameter drill for the particular implant system is used first to reach the correct depth for the implant, which is then selected.

(f) An osteotome of the same diameter as the drilled osteotomy (or slightly larger, eg, 0.03 mm or less) is introduced into the site. Osteotomes of larger diameter are used to reach the appropriate depth based on the size of implant to be placed. The osteotomes are either slowly rotated in by hand or by gentle tapping with a mallet. The final osteotome should approximate the implant shape and diameter.

(continued)

implant is created by removing bone from the site using drills of progressively larger diameter, the last of which is approximately the same diameter and length as the implant. Where dense bone predominates, this traditional drilling approach is generally appropriate. However, when poor-density bone predominates at the proposed implant site—which is most often the case in the maxilla—a more conservative approach should be used. Using osteotomes of progressively larger diameter that can be pushed or malleted into the alveolar ridge actually compacts the bone. The poor-density bone at the implant site is effectively relocated rather than removed, as it is through drilling, thus increasing the chances of an implant's survival once it is in place (Fig 9-5). Other indications for ridge expansion include the need to improve esthetics, reduce maxillary undercuts, alter emergence angles, and match opposing landmarks.

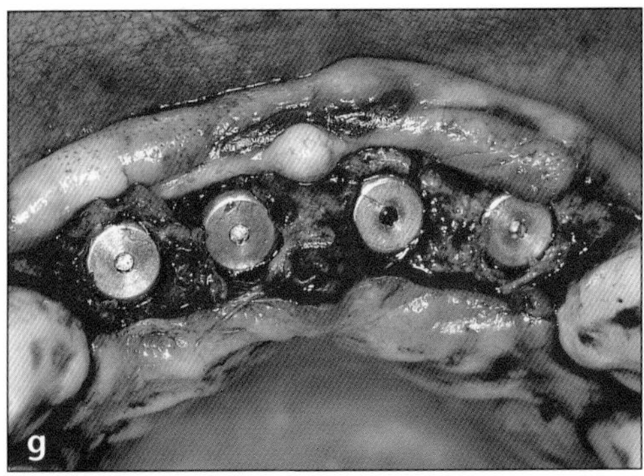

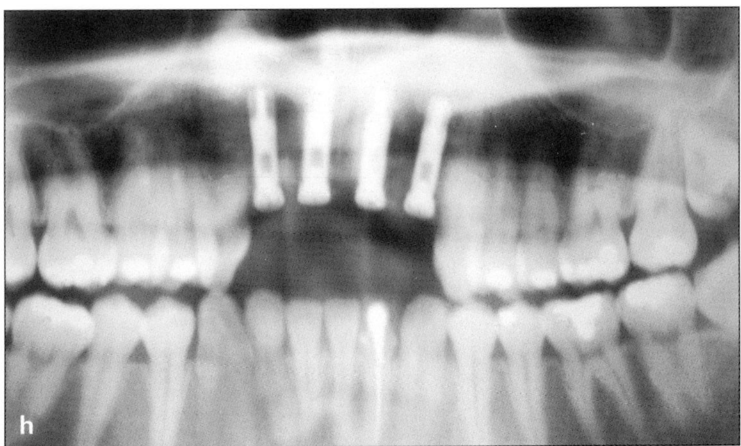

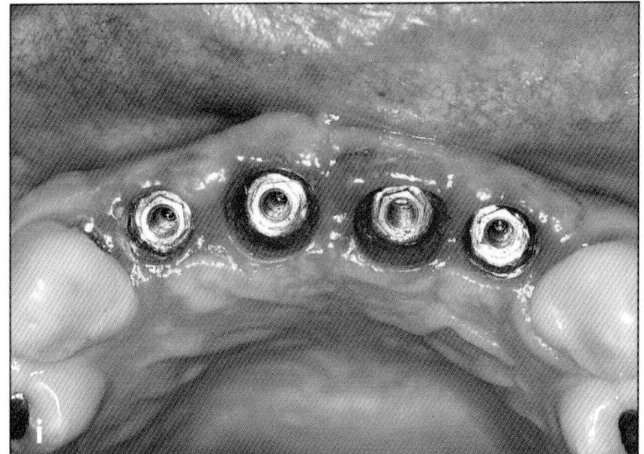

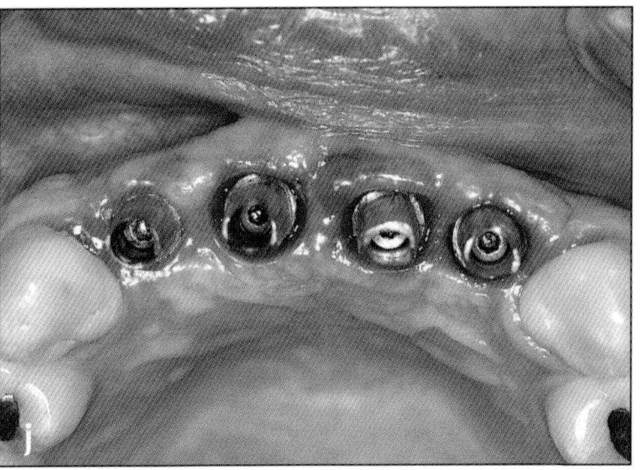

Fig 9-5 *(cont)*
(g) The implant should have a self-tapping design. Implants of 3.75 × 15 mm are shown.

(h) Postoperative radiograph showing implants in place.

(i) Occlusal view of the ridge shows the increased buccopalatal dimension created with osteotomes.

(j) Fixed abutments are shown on the dental implant in preparation for fixed prosthetics.

Allogeneic Block Bone Grafts

If the ridge is at least 5 to 6 mm buccopalatally, then an allogeneic/FDBA should be considered. Allografts have been used for years as viable alternatives to autogenous bone grafts. They eliminate many of the disadvantages associated with autogenous grafts, including morbidity, limited volume and dimension of bone, and harvesting time. In cases requiring good structural support, such as ridge augmentation, blocks of allogeneic bone can be used predictably to serve as a scaffolding that will eventually resorb and be replaced with host bone (Fig 9-6).

Allogeneic bone materials should contain both the collagen and mineral components of bone. For example, the Puros J-block (Zimmer Dental, Carlsbad, CA) is harvested and processed to eliminate the cells, moisture, fats, and lipids but to maintain the collagen and mineral components. In general, the criteria for using allogeneic block grafts are the same as the criteria for using autogenous block grafts described later in this chapter, with the following exceptions:

1. When an allogeneic bone block is used, both the recipient site and the block graft should be decorticated.
2. Barrier membranes are required with autogenous blocks of bone only if more than 50% of the surface is particulated. However, with the allogeneic block, barrier membranes are recommended in all cases.
3. The autogenous block does not require rehydration; however, the J-block is rehydrated prior to use, preferably in nonactivated platelet-rich plasma (PRP).

Corticocancellous Block Grafts

If the ridge is at least 4 to 5 mm wide, then an autogenous bone block should be used.[9,62–66] Ridges with a crestal width of less than 6 mm typically require bone grafting prior to implant therapy. On the facial and lingual areas, at least 2 mm of bone must surround the implant. Thus, for the clinician to place a 4-mm-diameter implant, an 8- to 10-mm bone bed is required buccolingually. While alloplastic grafting materials can be used to augment the ridge in the posterior maxilla and in the mandible,[67] autogenous bone from the anterior mandible or the ramus is highly recommended for augmentation of the anterior maxilla requiring more than 4 to 5 mm of additional ridge width. Corticocancellous block grafts harvested from the chin (see chapter 6) or ramus (see chapter 5) typically will provide adequate bone to overcome width deficiencies in the anterior maxilla extending up to four teeth or to increase both height and width in the areas of one to two teeth.[68–71]

For example, a 2003 study concluded that mandibular block onlay grafts offer extremely reliable results for increasing the width of the anterior maxilla before implant placement.[72] Autogenous block grafts from the chin or ramus revascularize quickly and demonstrate a relatively low rate of resorption.[73] A barrier membrane may also be useful if more than 50% of the grafted area is particulate graft material. In another 2003 study reporting the use of symphyseal bone cores for vertical augmentation of the alveolar ridge, sites were additionally grafted with DFDBA in conjunction with a titanium-reinforced expanded polytetrafluoroethylene (e-PTFE) membrane.[74] Results of this study also indicated an increased ridge width.

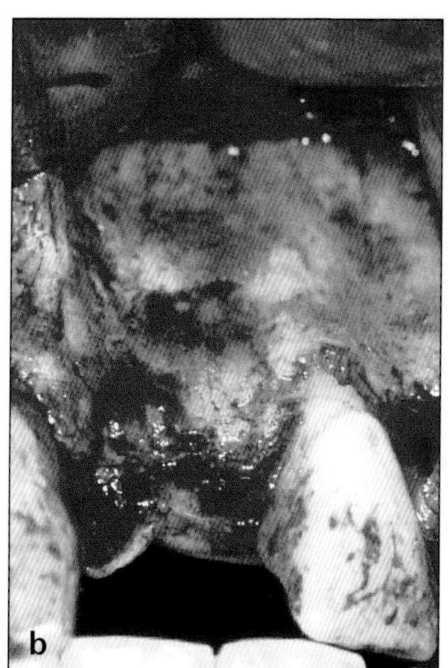

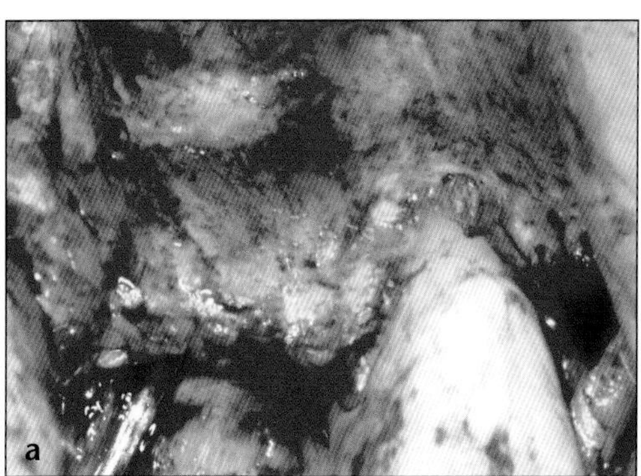

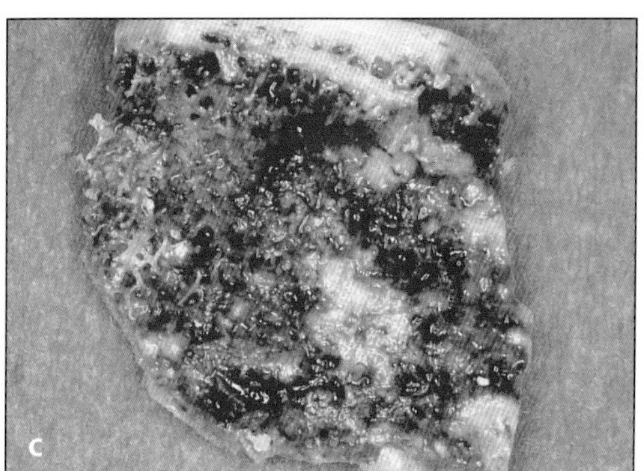

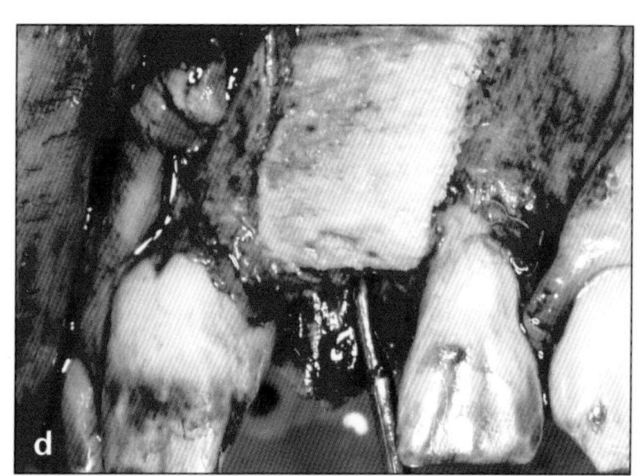

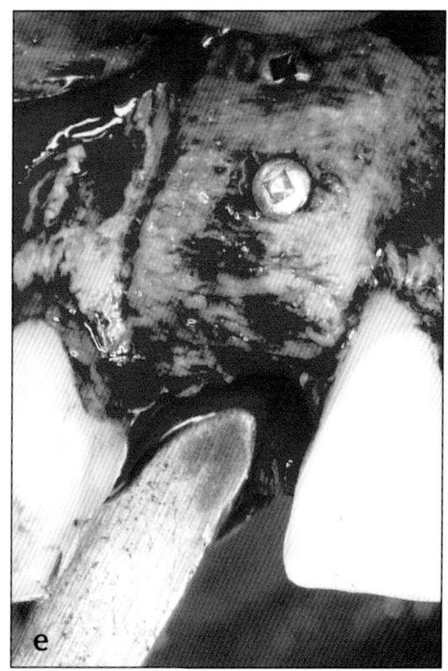

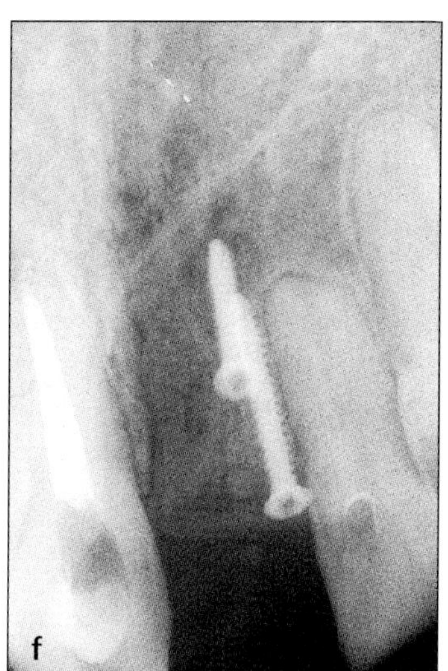

Fig 9-6 Particulate autografts, particulate allografts or alloplasts, and autogenous or allogeneic blocks are all valid options in the preplanning stage. Analyzing and evaluating the patient's healing potential within the boundaries of the bone defect will determine the best option.

(a) Elevating a full-thickness flap with adequate release enables visualization and grafting of the defect area.

(b) The side with the ridge defect and the contralateral side need to match with respect to bony volume and anatomy.

(c) The block is sculpted for the best possible fit in the deficient area.

(d) The block is placed in the defect to check for adaptation and contoured as necessary for good fit and initial stability.

(e) Block grafts of any kind should be stabilized and screwed in place, preferably with more than one screw, to provide as much adaptation as possible to the host bone and to minimize rotation or micromovement.

(f) The retaining screws (shown radiographically) will be removed at the time of implant placement.

Fig 9-6 *(cont)*
(g) Soft tissue dissection can provide a tension-free flap to reduce soft tissue dehiscence from adjacent muscle pull.

(h) The buccal flap is repositioned after careful dissection to permit it to be tension free. It was designed, replaced, and sutured so that both papillae remain intact.

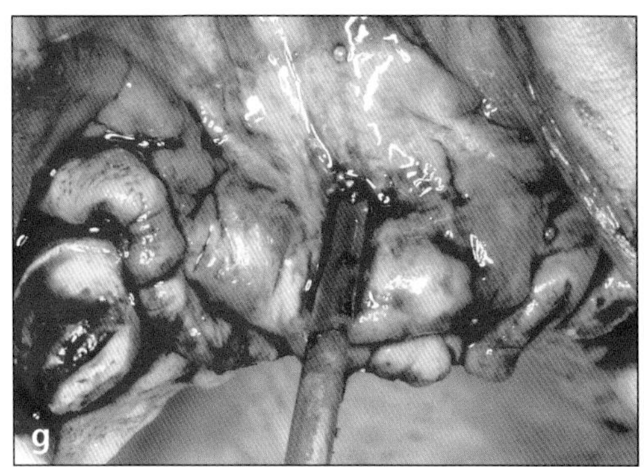

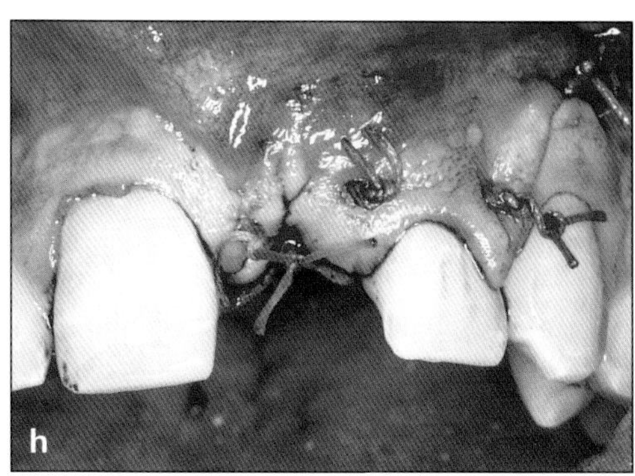

Autogenous Bone Block

Clinicians should use their own discretion in prescribing antibiotics and anti-inflammatory medications before and after surgery. Some clinicians have suggested using ibuprofen 1 hour prior to surgery and for 3 to 7 days afterward. Amoxicillin can also be prescribed for use before and after surgery. In the area of the maxillary alveolar defect, 2% lidocaine with 1:100,000 epinephrine may be used as a local anesthetic; articaine is also an alternative.

An incision is made on the palatal aspect of the maxillary ridge to elevate a split-thickness mucosal flap. The periosteum is then incised over the crest. Divergent releasing incisions are made adjacent to the bordering teeth, and a full-thickness flap is elevated to expose the defect. Proper flap reflection and careful incision are crucial. By exposing the recipient area, the clinician can verify the need for the graft as well as the optimal amount of bone required.

Before any intraoral donor bone is harvested, the recipient site should be debrided and irrigated to remove any potentially inflammatory tissue or scar tissue. Osteoinduction and osteoconduction will be delayed by the presence of fibrous (scar) tissue or complicated if epithelial tissue remains. This can lead to fibrous healing instead of bone formation.[75,76] A piece of bone wax can be placed into the defect area and modeled to approximate the dimensions of the bone graft. The bone wax can then be removed and used as a template for harvesting an appropriate-sized block graft. Alternatively, other sterile materials can be cut to shape and used as a template. The host bone should be perforated with a small round bur to increase the availability of osteogenic cells, which can accelerate revascularization and improve union of the graft to the host bone.

The graft, which should be placed as soon as possible after harvesting, is contoured to eliminate sharp edges and to ensure maximal contact with the bone in the defect. Typically, 1.0- to 1.6-mm-diameter titanium alloy screws are used to affix the graft to the host bone. Small discrepancies should also be filled with particulate cancellous bone from the harvest site.

A tension-free closure over these grafts is important. Prior to suturing, the buccal periosteum of the mucosal flap should be scored with a scalpel and undermined to allow a greater advancement of the soft tissue. The incisions are then closed using 3–0 chromic interrupted mattress sutures. This approach minimizes tension and maintains coverage. The provisional removable partial denture should be adjusted to avoid contact with the grafted area (Fig 9-7).

Antibiotics and Adjunctive Techniques

Amoxicillin or clindamycin can be administered 1 hour before the operation and continued for up to 1 week afterward. Dexamethasone can be prescribed the day of surgery and continued for several days postoperatively. Complications such as membrane exposure, infection, and plaque accumulation can be addressed in subsequent appointments. Serious exposure of the membrane may require regrafting or membrane removal, whereas minor exposure may require simply applying a topical antimicrobial (eg, chlorhexidine) as necessary.

The final reconstructed recipient ridge should be at least 8 to 10 mm in width to allow for possible graft resorption and remodeling and yet still result in an adequate width for placement of standard-diameter implants.

The recipient site should be allowed to heal for 4 to 8 months following grafting before the implant is placed. Graft fracture, wound dehiscence (with implant and graft exposure), and a higher rate of implant failure are more likely when implants are placed simultaneously with the graft[77] or GBR[78] instead of in a two-stage approach. Performing the surgery in stages enhances prosthetic alignment, obviating the need for remodeling or additional securing of the graft. A two-stage approach also allows the clinician to deal with any resorption that takes place so that the implant has a more secure base. While some research shows positive results for immediate loading of single-tooth implants in the anterior maxilla, conditions involving augmentation require more study.[79] Some clinical studies report that graft failures are often related to infection at the recipient site, premature loading of the grafts with transitional prostheses, and mucosal flap dehiscence with subsequent graft exposure to the oral cavity.[80]

Use of a Titanium Mesh Crib for Onlay Bone Graft or Le Fort I Downfracture of the Maxilla

For severely resorbed ridges and/or ridge-relation discrepancies, use of a titanium mesh crib or a Le Fort I downfracture of the maxilla and an interpositional bone graft can be considered.[81] Additionally, if a residual bone stock is available, distraction osteogenesis can provide a viable alternative to these two approaches.

Titanium mesh crib with autogenous bone

Vertical defects often require a technique-sensitive procedure using an onlay autogenous graft supported by a nonresorbable titanium mesh crib (Fig 9-8).[82,83] These defects occur in patients who have had tooth extractions because of significant bone loss from periodontal disease, fractured roots, or pulpal pathology.[84]

Le Fort I downfracture of the maxilla

Research and clinical experience support the reconstruction of the severely atrophic maxilla via a Le Fort I downfracture with interpositional bone grafting along with dental implants, either immediate or de-

Fig 9-7 Ridge augmentation of the anterior maxilla with an autogenous bone block.

(a) Loss of teeth due to trauma often leads to very narrow ridges because socket grafting is not possible.

(b) Extremely thin anterior ridges with huge concavities left by the loss of the two central incisors due to trauma.

(c) The area is slightly recontoured with a surgical oval-shaped bur to obtain a more favorable surface in which to place the grafts.

(d) The residual midline crest, which is nothing more than the nasal spine, is eliminated to favor block placement in an optimal position and minimize the necessary recontouring of the block.

(e) Perforations are made in the cortical bone with a no. 1701 cylindrical bur (Brasseler, Savannah, GA) while avoiding getting too close to the adjacent teeth.

(f) Perforations facilitate the vascular formation and cell migration through the openings, enabling integration of harvested and host bone. Trauma reduces the amount of cancellous bone, so the harvested block should have some cancellous quality to provide viable cells to the remaining buccal, cortical, and palatal bone.

(continued)

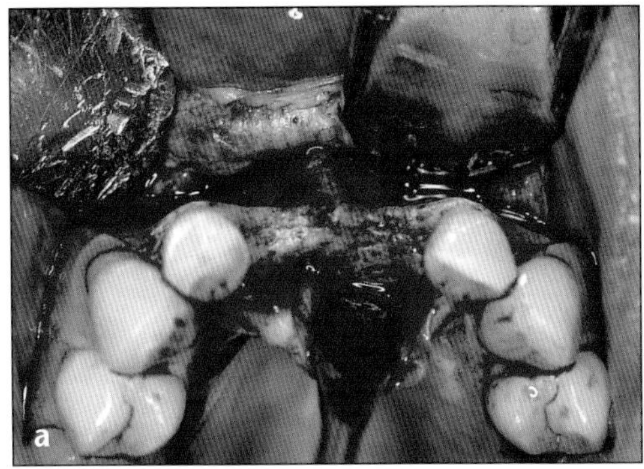

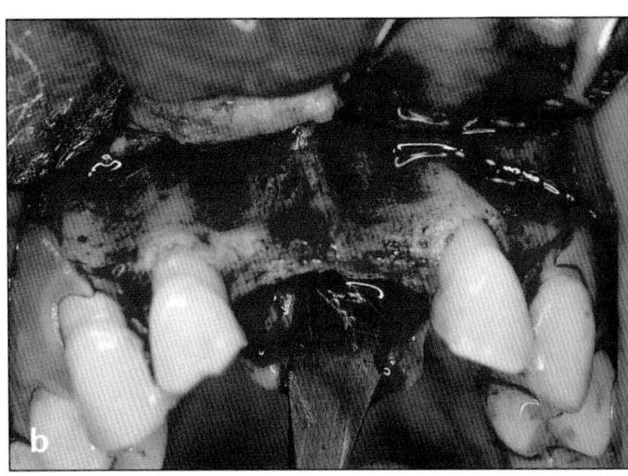

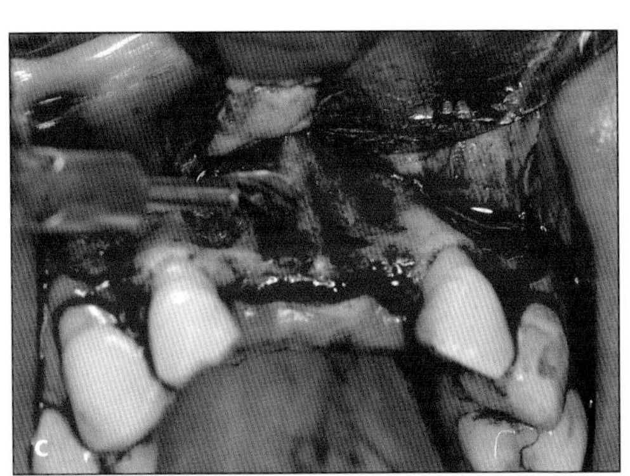

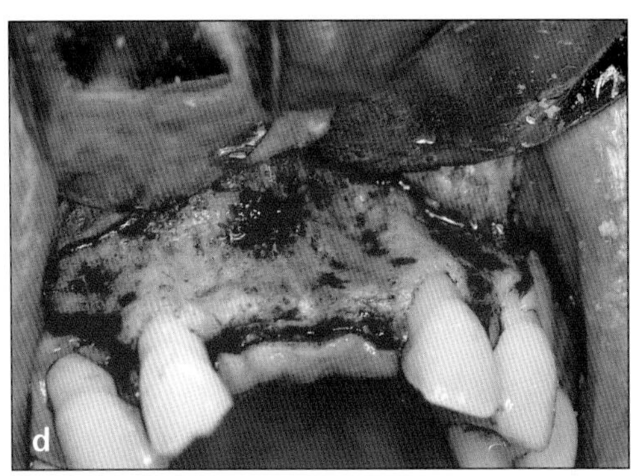

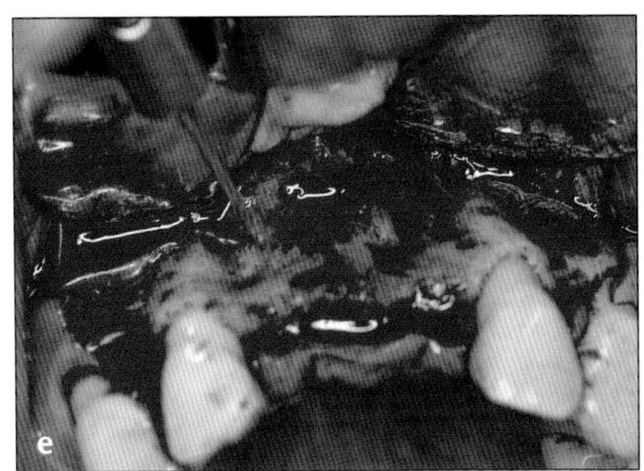

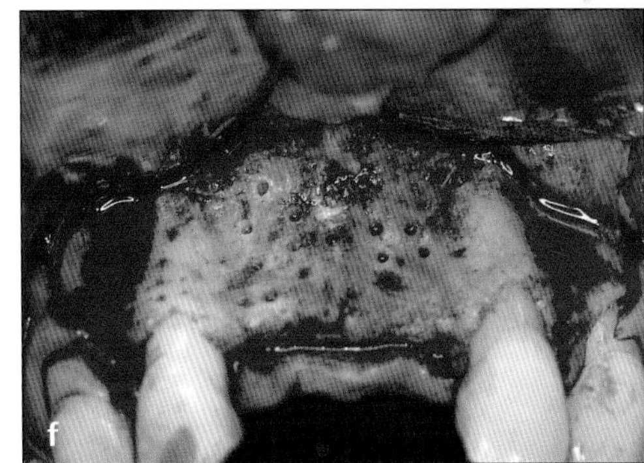

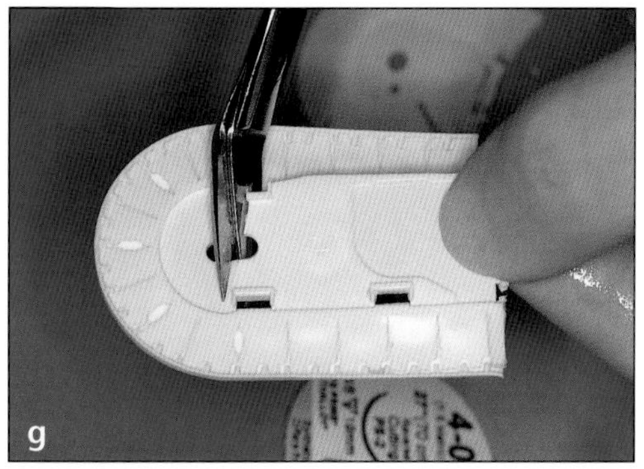

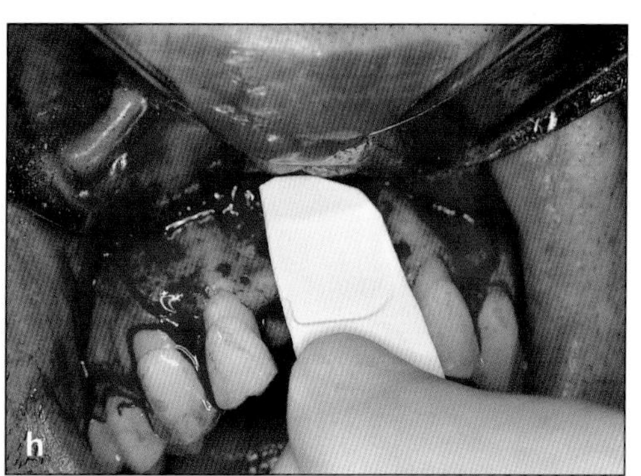

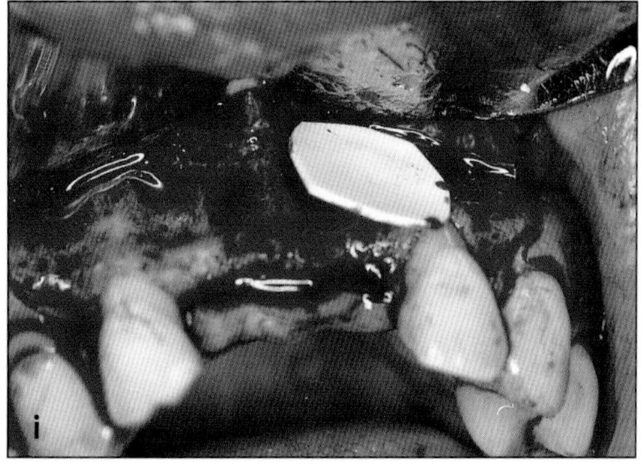

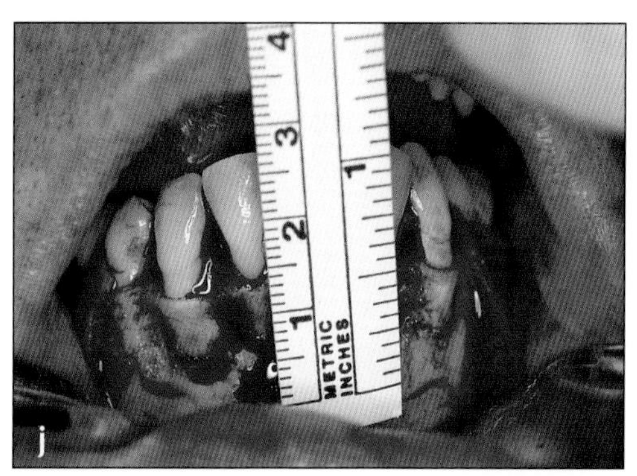

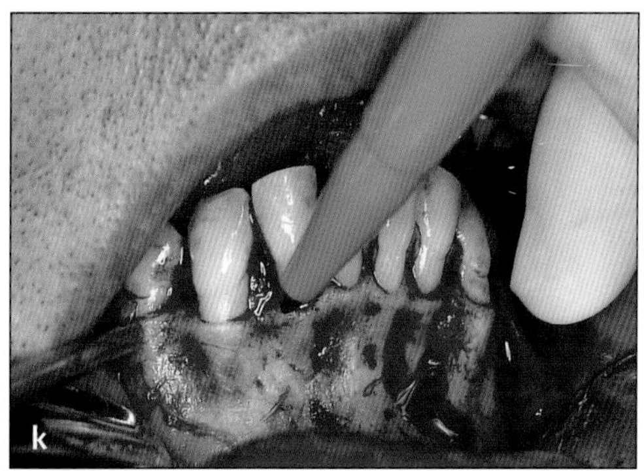

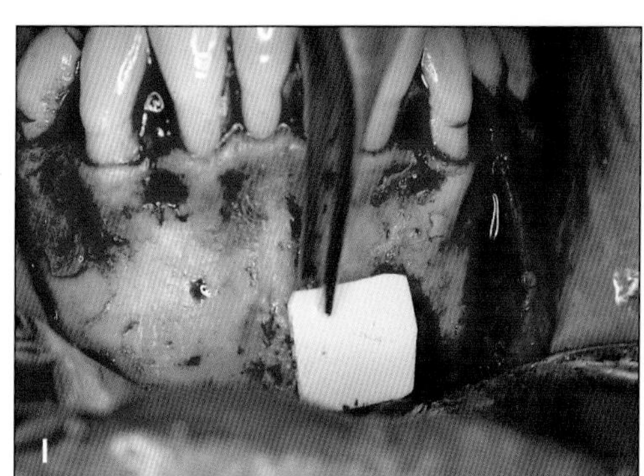

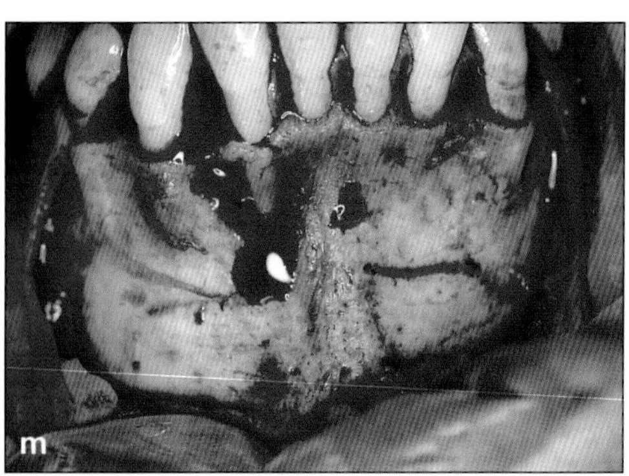

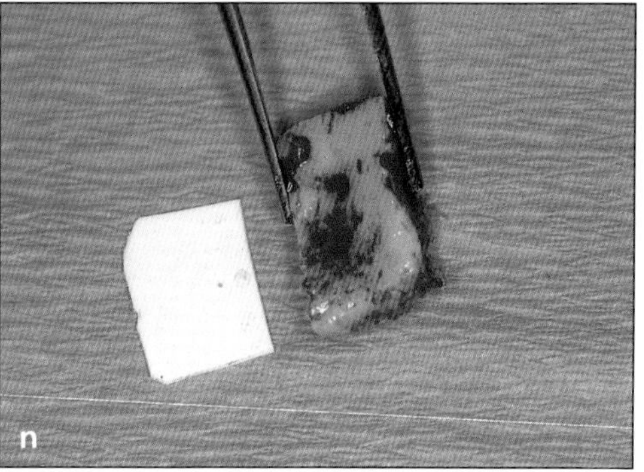

Fig 9-7 *(cont)*
(g) A mold of the defect will help the clinician obtain blocks that fit as accurately as possible. Something as simple and readily available as the piece of plastic that carries the suture can be used.

(h) The flat piece of sterile plastic is held against the defect to help visualize the desired size and shape of the block.

(i) The mold is cut and shaped appropriately. This reduces the amount of cutting and shaping of the bone block and also minimizes both the risk for damage and the chance of harvesting blocks that are too small or too large for the recipient site.

(j) A ruler is used to help determine the length of the anterior incisors. Radiographs are also useful for this purpose; however, magnification must be taken into consideration.

(k) A sterile surgical marker can be used to indicate where the apices of the incisors are situated and the area from which the bone can be safely harvested.

(l) The previously cut mold is transported to the anterior mandible.

(m) Markings are made where a no. 1701 bur will be used to cut the blocks down to the medullary bone.

(n) If the steps are followed carefully and the block is cut fully and deeply enough, it should be easy to retrieve in one piece with the help of a chisel. The anteriormost cut should be made at a 45-degree bevel to allow the chisel to slide in easily. It is better to obtain a slightly larger block of bone than what is needed, provided it does not increase morbidity and the adjacent anatomy permits it.

Fig 9-7 *(cont)*
(o) A hemostatic collagen material such as Avitene (MedChem Products, Woburn, MA) can be used to fill the donor sites so as to stop the bleeding.

(p) This resorbable hemostatic material can be lifted with tissue pliers and easily packed into the donor sites.

(q) In addition to its hemostatic effects, this material helps create a scaffold that will add volume to the sites. If desired, particulate or putty graft material can be placed into the donor site at this time.

(r) The blocks of bone are placed in their correct position and affixed with two screws apiece to prevent rotation and micromovement.

(s) An occlusal view shows overcontouring that will compensate for the expected resorption. If the blocks do not resorb enough and remain too bulky, they can be shaved down as needed with a large oval surgical bur.

(t) Good dissection of the flap to divide stretchable mucosa from nonstretchable periosteum is very important in this patient, in whom contour volume was augmented and primary closure of the flap is necessary.

(u) Occlusal view showing that the contour of the anterior maxillary ridge has already been restored to its original form. The provisional crowns placed according to the resorbed maxilla are positioned further back. Implants will be placed in the correct three-dimensional position and later restored with central incisor crowns in an optimal intermaxillary relationship.

(continued)

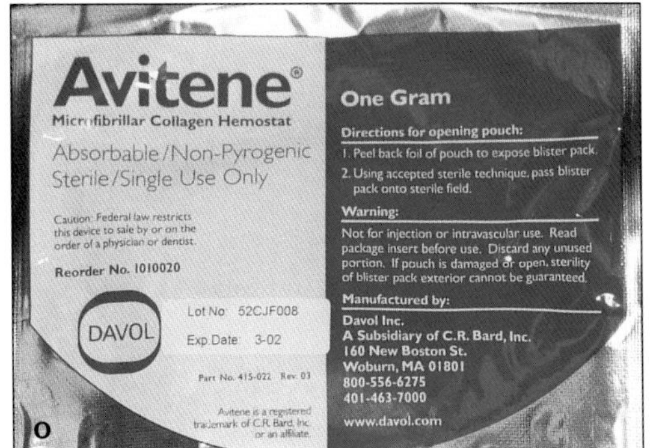

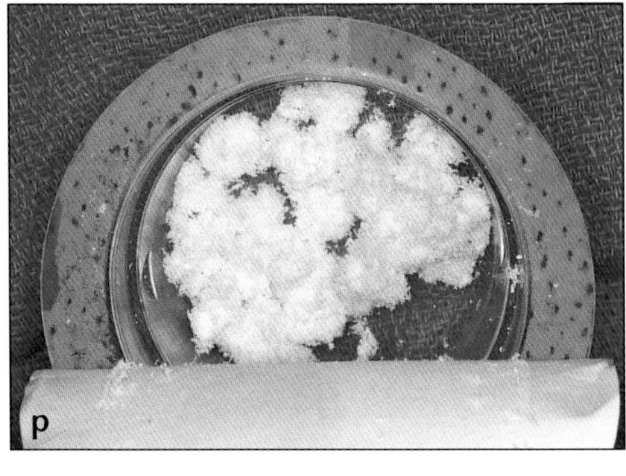

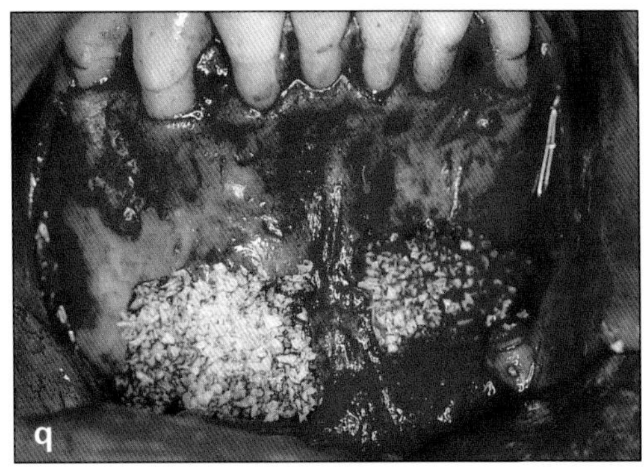

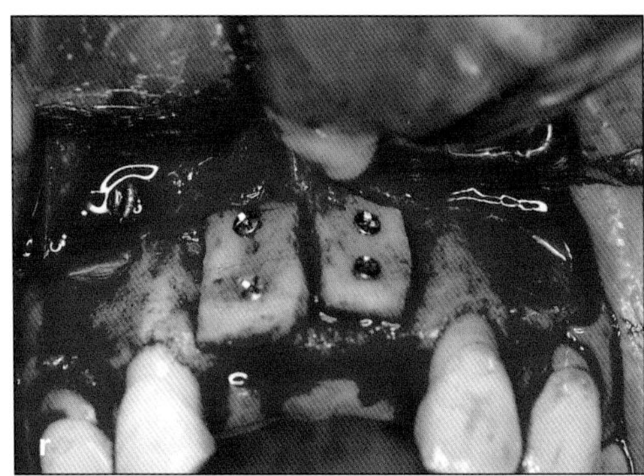

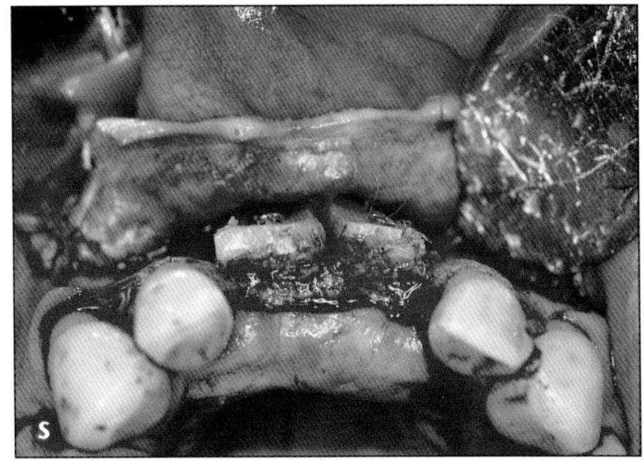

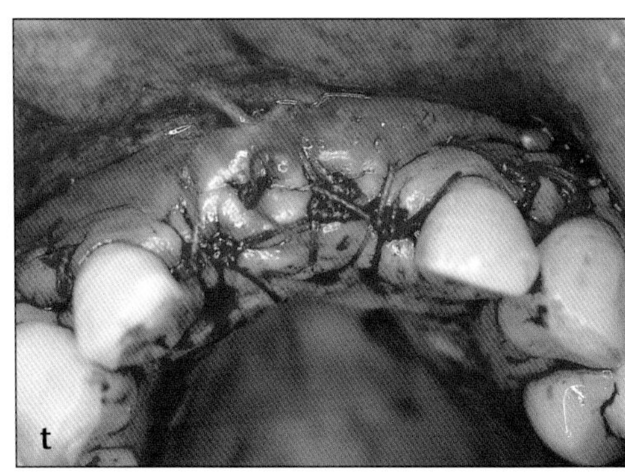

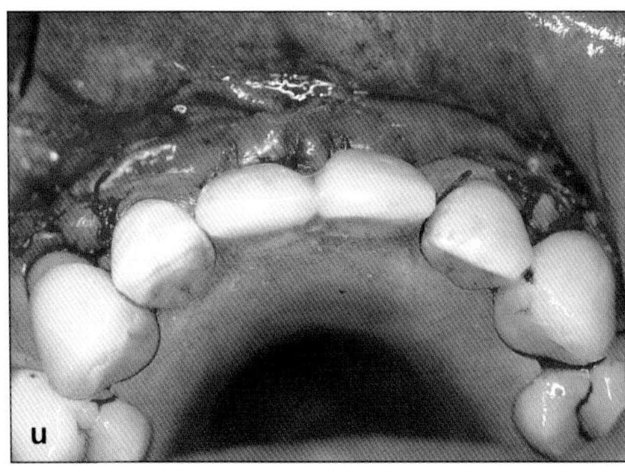

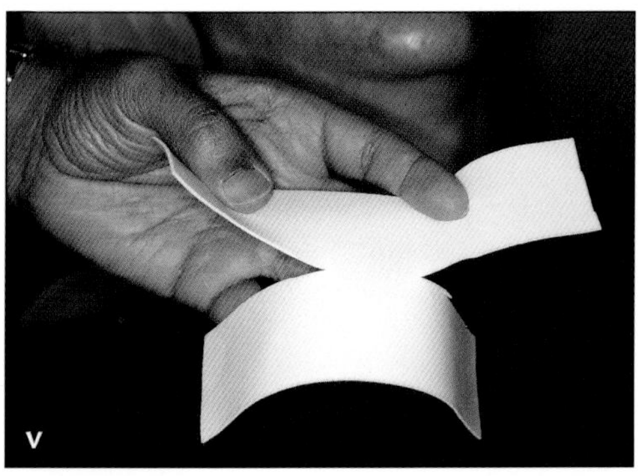

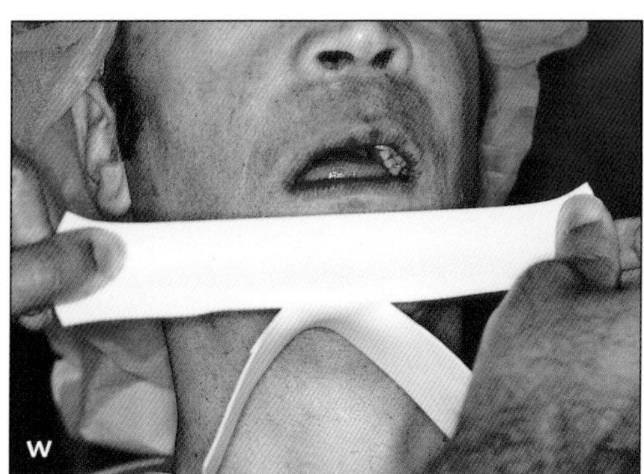

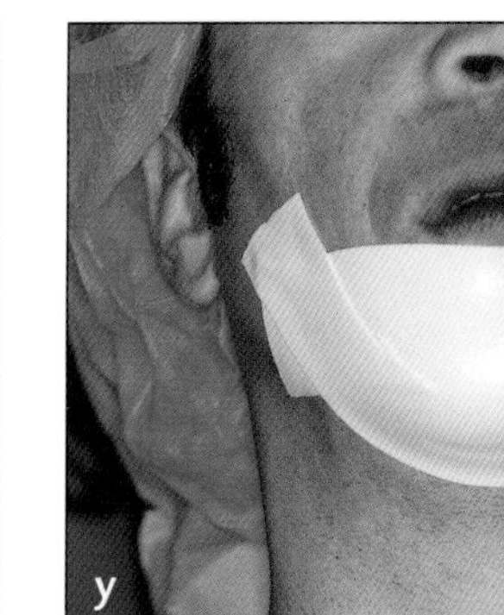

Fig 9-7 *(cont)*
(v) A band of stretchable foam tape approximately 20 × 5 cm wide is cut lengthwise, sparing 4 to 5 cm in the middle.

(w) The superior portion of the band is stretched underneath the lower lip and taped back.

(x) The inferior portion of the band is stretched under the chin and taped upward.

(y) This dressing gives the patient protection and comfort and supports the mentalis muscle (which was partially detached from the anterior mandible) and the soft tissues.

layed. In such cases, the maxillary reconstruction involves a Le Fort I osteotomy and downfracture followed by the harvesting of cancellous marrow from the posterior iliac crest, which is grafted to the maxilla between the stable and downfractured maxillary components.[85] Subsequently, implants are placed in the reconstructed maxilla, followed by the placement of implant-retained overdentures. The long-term stability of Le Fort I maxillary downfractures with interpositional bone grafting has been well documented[86,87] and should always be a consideration of the dental team.[88,89]

Stage 1 Surgery for Implant Placement

Once the clinician has obtained the ideal amount of bone in the anterior maxilla, a surgical template is fabricated to identify the incisal edge of the final prosthesis and to ensure proper implant positioning in relation to neighboring teeth. A soft tissue incision may be made on the crest of the ridge to permit ideal reflection. As mentioned, the implant site should be more than 5 mm wide at this point. The greater the implant diameter, the more esthetically pleasing the cervical portion of the crown will be.

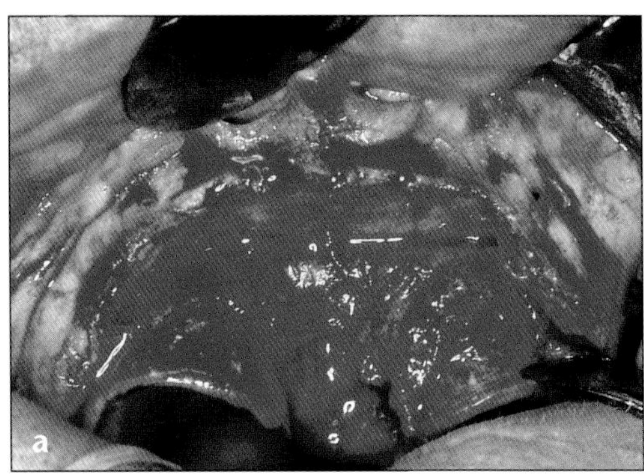

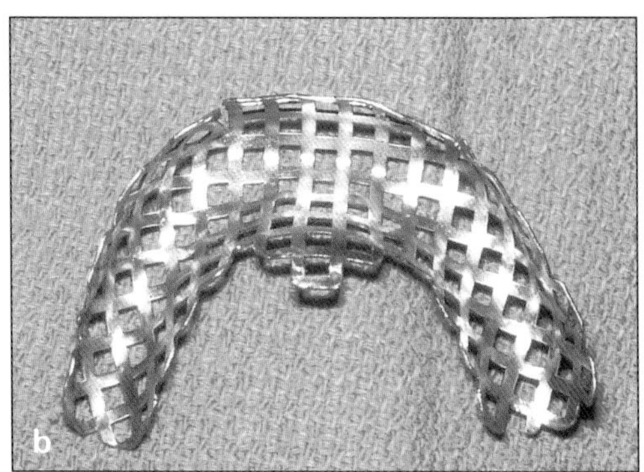

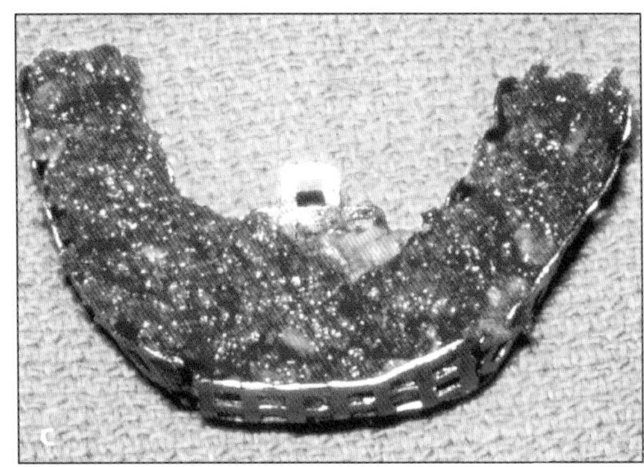

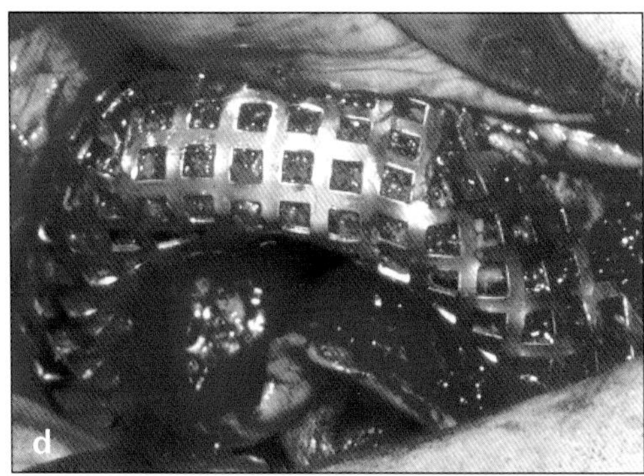

Fig 9-8 Vertical defects often require a technique-sensitive procedure using an onlay autogenous graft supported by a nonresorbable titanium mesh crib.

(a) The highly resorbed maxilla requires extensive bone-harvesting procedures.

(b) An impression of the patient's maxilla is taken and the cast is waxed to the ideal volume according to the desired intermaxillary relationship. Titanium mesh is then shaped over the idealized waxup of the maxillary cast.

(c) The titanium mesh is filled with particulated bone that was harvested from the posterior hip.

(d) This bone-filled titanium mesh is affixed to the recipient area with screws. Extensive flap release is necessary, and a vestibuloplasty is usually performed at a later stage.

The vertical position of the implant should balance the marginal level of bone around the implant (remembering that 1 mm of bone is typically lost around the implant neck during the first year of function) and the biologic height of soft tissues (generally 3 to 4 mm). Thus, the implant neck should be placed 2.0 to 2.5 mm apical of the anticipated buccogingival margin of the restoration.[6] This approach allows for a proper implant emergence profile while the biologic width and height are maintained over long-term function.

On the mesiodistal aspect, a minimum space of 1.5 to 2.0 mm should remain between tooth and implant. Between two adjacent implants, the distance should be at least 3 to 4 mm. Additional interimplant bone support is also helpful because it helps to ensure a full gingival papilla. In the buccolingual dimension, the implant should be placed as far to the buccal as possible while still allowing for use of restorative materials of an adequate thickness and for an appropriate screw-access hole. Care should be taken to maintain or create a minimum of 2 to 3 mm of bone thickness buccal to the dental implant.[6]

To allow for a proper emergence profile, the clinician should maintain 2 to 3 mm of bone labial to the implant.[90] Placing the implant further in a palatal direction results in an undercontoured restoration with a modified ridge flap design for the final restoration. Such conditions can hinder hygiene and compromise esthetics. Placing the implant too far to the labial also jeopardizes esthetics by creating a bulky, overcontoured crown that cannot be corrected with angulated abutments. If a case calls for placing an implant in a palatal direction because of anatomic or clinical limitations, the implant should be placed 1 mm apically for every 1 mm it is placed palatally.[91]

If cemented abutments are used, the implant should be located exactly in the center of the long axis of the future implant-supported crown. For screw-retained abutments, the implant should be placed slightly palatal to the long axis of the crown to allow the clinician to access the connecting screw palatally.[92] Generally, internal connection implants are recommended for the esthetic zone.

Stage 1 indexing technique

Stage 1 indexing is a relatively simple procedure that is recommended for implant placement in the esthetic zone. When the implant is placed, the clinician takes an impression of the head of the implant using sterile methods and materials, recording its relation to adjacent teeth by means of a "pick-up" impression coping attached to the implant. Once this index is removed, the clinician completes the surgery. This index, study casts of the mandible and maxilla, bite registration, and a shade selection are then shipped to the laboratory. An anatomically correct abutment and provisional crown can now be fabricated by the laboratory using as a guide an implant analog attached to the impression coping and retrofitted into the study casts using what is essentially the altered cast technique. When the implant is uncovered at stage 2 surgery, the clinician can attach the custom abutment and the provisional crown to the implant. Helping to form gingival contours as early as possible, this method bypasses the use of a healing abutment and may obviate the need for a subsequent soft tissue surgery for papilla regeneration procedures since the gingival topography surrounding the restoration conforms to the tooth fabricated for this particular patient. The indexing impression taken at stage 1 surgery thus provides orientation for the guided tooth form that facilitates early soft tissue healing and contouring as soon as stage 2 surgery is completed. At the placement of the provisional restoration at stage 2 surgery, the clinician can fashion the soft tissue for optimal esthetic results. Another benefit of the stage 1 impression technique is superior soft tissue contour and esthetics when stage 2 surgery begins because the provisional crown has been fabricated by the laboratory based on the specific patient's oral needs and dimensions. As the soft tissue heals, it also adapts to the provisional crown's surface, predetermined by the indexing and impression information given to the laboratory. Thus, when the last impression is made, soft tissue contours and crown stability are optimized. The distance between the bone crest and the contact point between the teeth or crowns should not exceed 5 mm. This distance allows the bone to support the gingival margin and the interproximal papillae needed for optimal esthetics.[93–97]

Implants ideally should be placed at the same angulation as the lingual two thirds of the natural tooth. The implant should be angled through the incisal edge of the surgical guide for cement-retained prostheses and through the cingulum in screw-retained prostheses.[98-102] Provisional restorations are used to further guide the healing soft tissues and develop the crown emergence profile. Any transmucosal loading from the provisional restoration during the healing period must be avoided. Otherwise, bone regeneration may be limited and membrane exposure more likely. Fixed provisional prostheses are a good choice to deter movement. If the provisional restoration is removable, it should be aggressively recontoured to eliminate implant contact during healing.

Stage 2 Surgery for Abutment Connection

To ensure an esthetically pleasing restoration, the clinician should use an appropriate gingivoplasty procedure to uncover the implant body. A horizontal incision may be made on the palatal aspect of the ridge, extending from the line angles of the two adjacent teeth. The tissue is then reflected toward the labial crest and the implant head is exposed.

The prefabricated and custom-designed abutments, along with the prefabricated provisional restorations, are placed at this time to allow for optimal maturation of the soft tissues at the site. All periodontal plastic surgery procedures should be performed at this time to allow for optimal soft tissue esthetics. The tissues are placed slightly coronal to the gingival margin on the adjacent teeth, and interdental sutures are placed. Sutures are removed after 1 week; the soft tissue usually requires 6 to 8 weeks to mature before final abutment selection or final impressions.[103-106]

Note that following abutment connection, the maturing peri-implant soft tissues tend to recede slightly. The clinician must consider this tendency to ensure that the tissue changes do not compromise the planned emergence profile of the restoration. Thus, following abutment-connection surgery and keratinized soft tissue esthetic procedures around the implant site, a 6- to 8-week provisional phase is recommended before final impressions are taken (Fig 9-9).[6]

The clinician should consider implant positioning in the anterior maxilla based primarily on the prosthesis needed to satisfy the patient's functional and esthetic needs, not on the availability of local bone. This goal has been described in the literature as *restoration-driven* rather than *bone-driven* implant placement.[107-109] Bone and soft tissue augmentation are often required to achieve these results. When single teeth are to be replaced, three-dimensional placement of the implant is essential. The restoration-driven dental team has been described as facilitators of esthetics who adhere to the following criteria[110]:

1. Reverse planning (designing the placement of the implant and the amount of grafting required based on the ultimate function and esthetics of the final prosthetic plan), surgical templates, and ideal implant positioning
2. Esthetically oriented surgical procedures
3. Bone augmentation procedures
4. Soft tissue management for esthetics

Augmentation and implant placement in the anterior maxilla, the most challenging region of the dentition to restore, require criteria no less demanding than these.

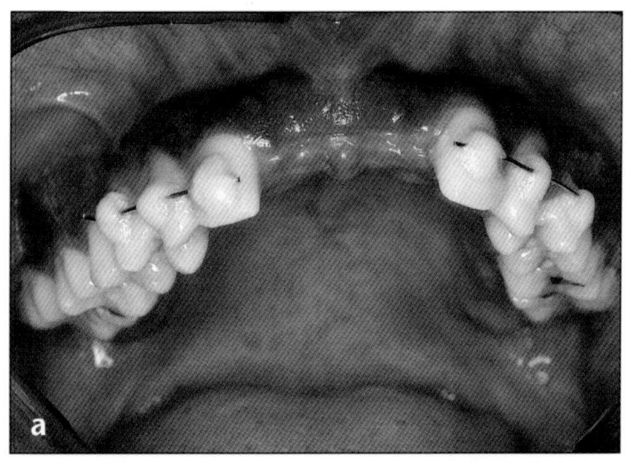

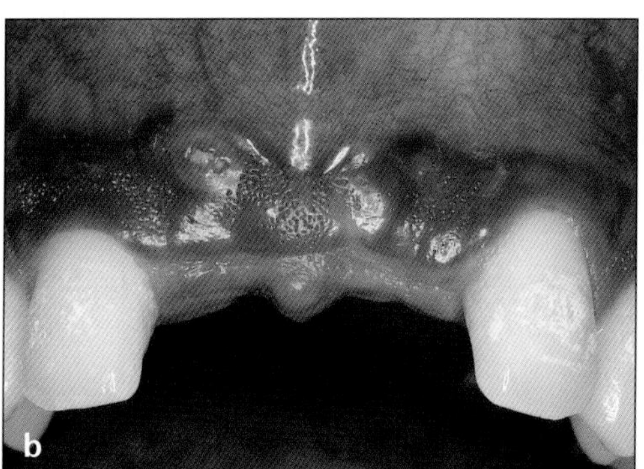

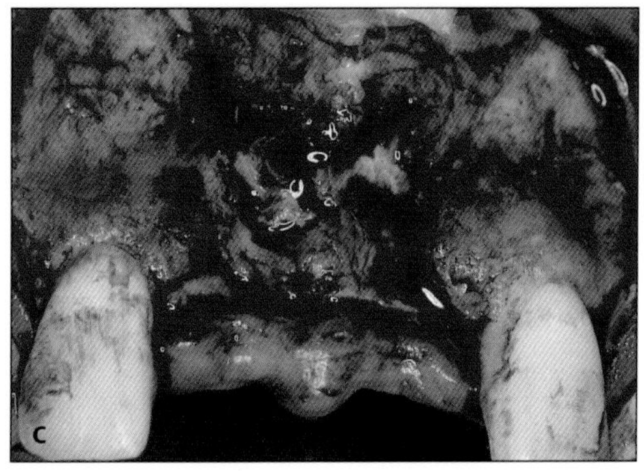

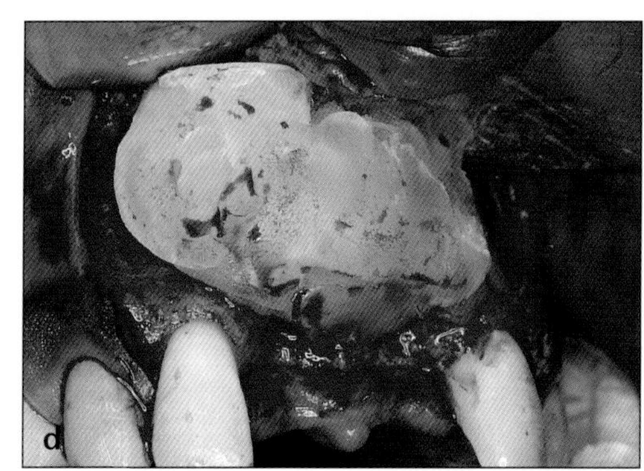

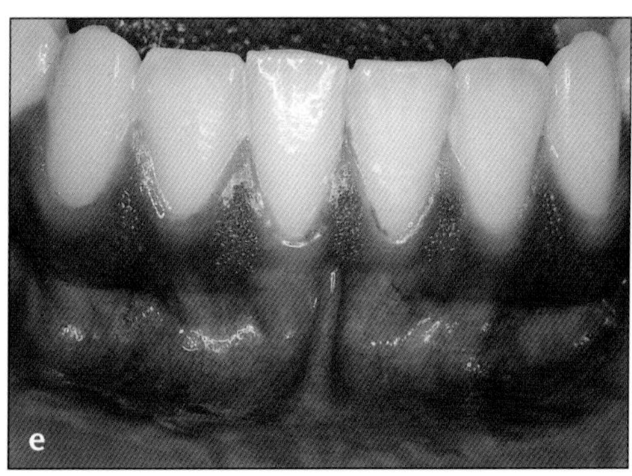

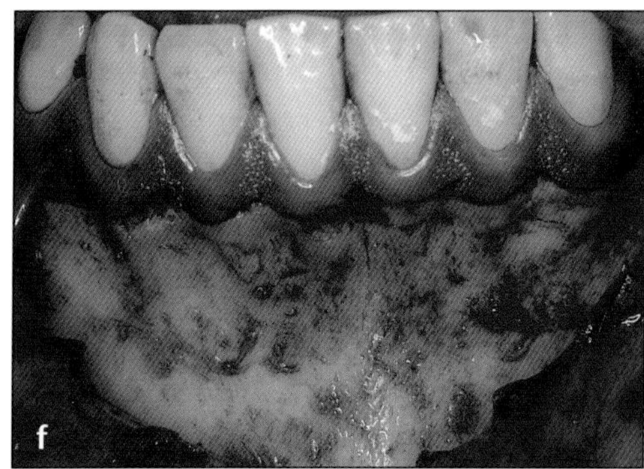

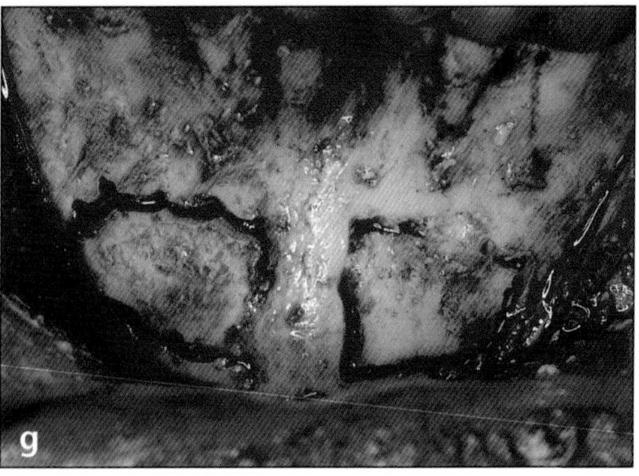

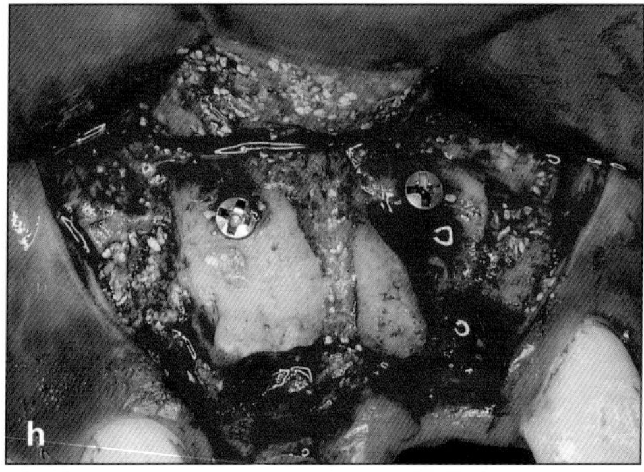

Fig 9-9 Two-stage ridge augmentation and implant placement procedure.

(a) Maxillary condition following alveolar ridge fracture and the loss of the two maxillary central incisors due to trauma.

(b) A closer look helps determine what has been lost: two central incisors and their buccal plates. Part of the defect area has been filled in by granulation tissues that will require removal.

(c) An extended flap is designed with incisions distal to the lateral teeth to provide ample working space; an extensive, easy-to-dissect flap; and incision lines far from the grafted area.

(d) A bone-wax mold of the area serves as a surgical template and helps the clinician remove a bone block of the correct size and shape from the chin.

(e) The donor site is evaluated to determine which of the three different incision designs used for the anterior mandibular bone block harvest is most appropriate: intrasulcular, attached gingival, or vestibular.

(f) The attached gingival incision was chosen for this patient to minimize the chance of blunting the thin, scalloped papillae with an intersulcular incision or damaging the high frenum or labial frenum or causing a scar band in the vestibule with a vestibular incision.

(g) Two bone blocks are harvested according to the mold taken of the defect area. The bone block is cut down to cancellous bone with a no. 1701 bur and retrieved using a chisel.

(h) The bone blocks are placed on the anterior maxilla and affixed with titanium screws. In this case, only one screw was used per block because the blocks fit perfectly in each space after careful molding.

Fig 9-9 *(cont)*
(i) A mouth-guard type of removable denture with maxillary central incisors was given to the patient postsurgery. Alternatively, an Essix appliance (Raintree Essix, Metairie, LA) may be used. A common tissue-borne partial denture would not guarantee separation of pressure from the prosthesis and the surgical site as this one does.

(j) Note the excellent condition of the tissues 1 week after the surgery, at the time of suture removal.

(k) After 6 months, implants are placed in the areas of the central incisors. Implant indexing at the time of placement allows the clinician to provide the patient with provisional crowns when the implants are uncovered. Atlantis System impression posts (Atlantis Components, Cambridge, MA) are easily screwed into the implants before the flap is replaced.

(l) Bite registration material is injected around the impression posts and several adjacent teeth. The impression posts are then unscrewed and sent, along with preliminary casts and shade selection, to the laboratory for custom abutment and provisional crown fabrication.

(m) Four months later, the characteristics of the gingiva are carefully evaluated to determine which uncovering technique will provide the best function and esthetics in the area.

(n) The good height, shape, and condition of the three papillae (right, middle, and left) called for a papilla-sparing incision placed slightly palatally to allow for apical repositioning of the soft tissue and to provide an adequate band of attached gingiva.

(o) This Atlantis abutment, created using CAD/CAM technology, shows the exact transverse anatomy of a maxillary central incisor and provides an excellent periodontal environment and esthetics for the final restoration.

(continued)

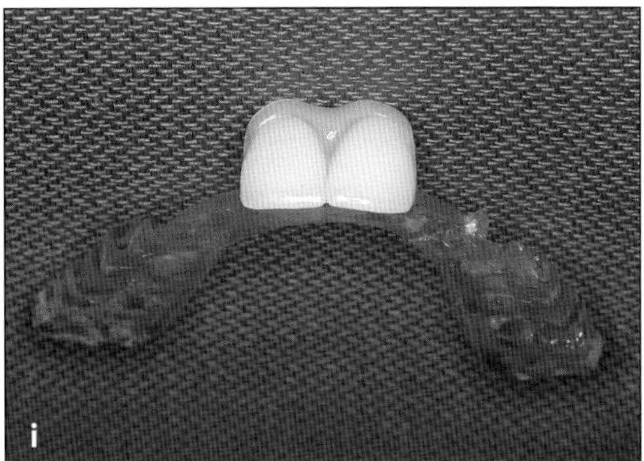
i

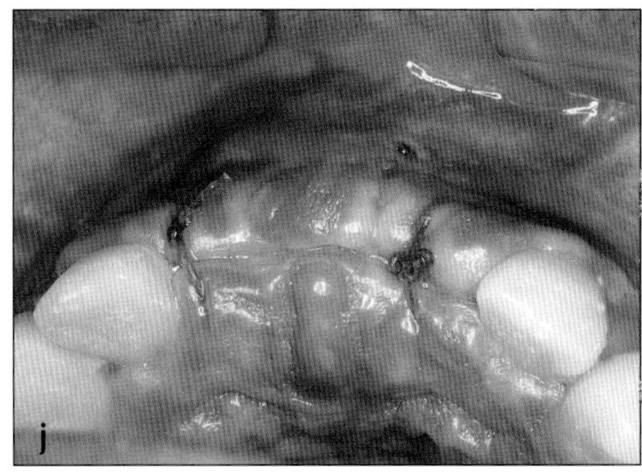
j

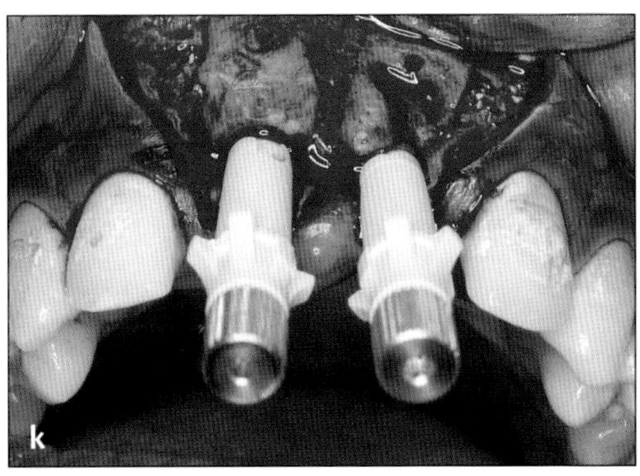
k

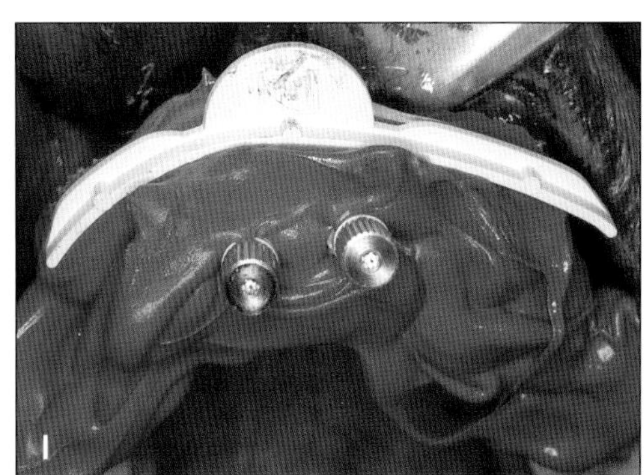
l

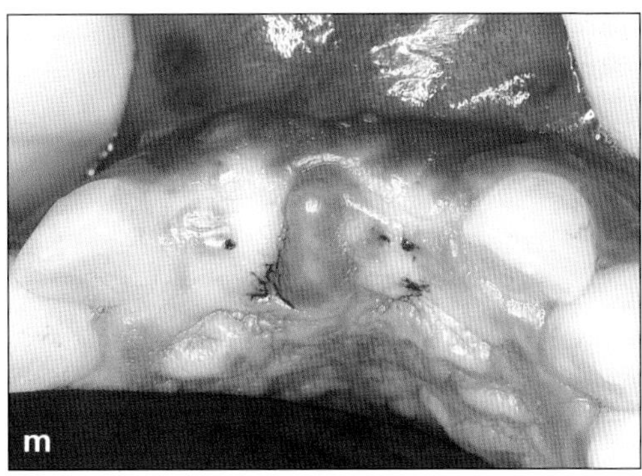
m

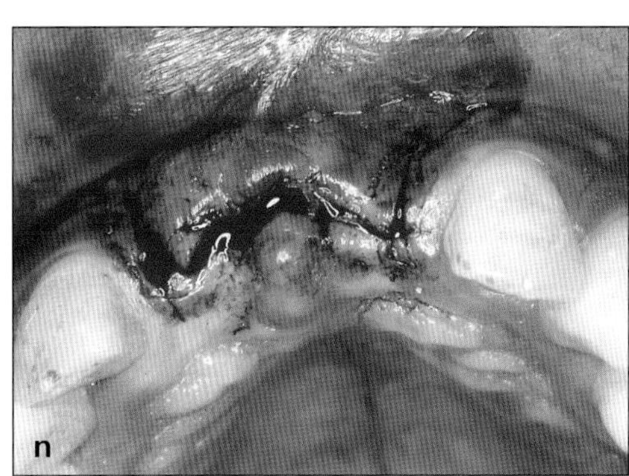
n

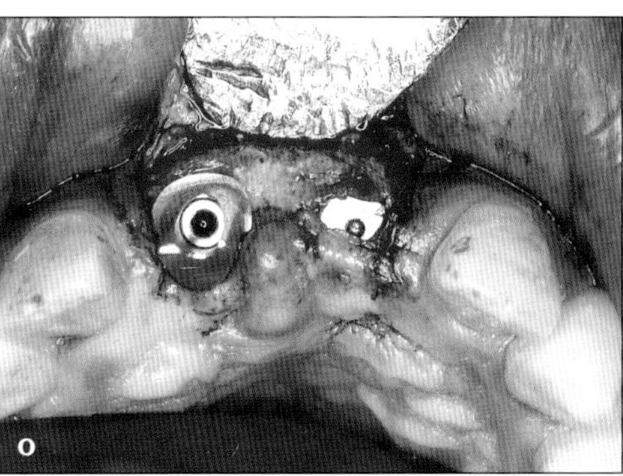
o

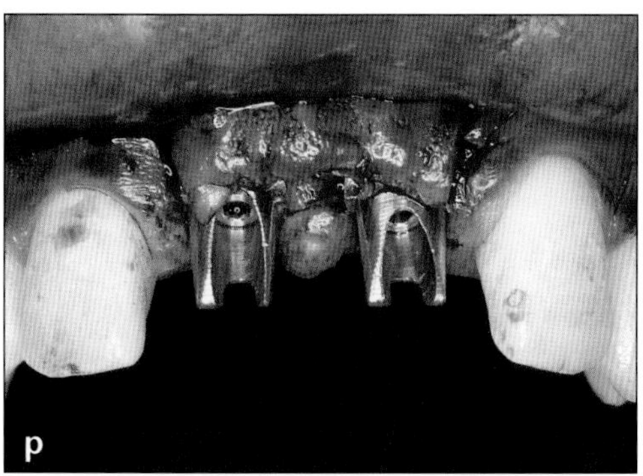

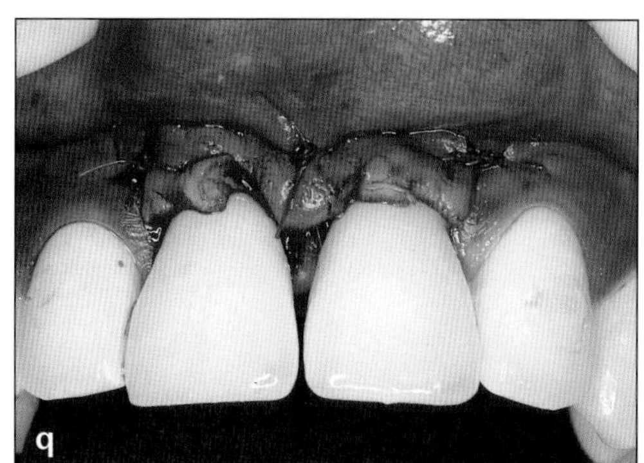

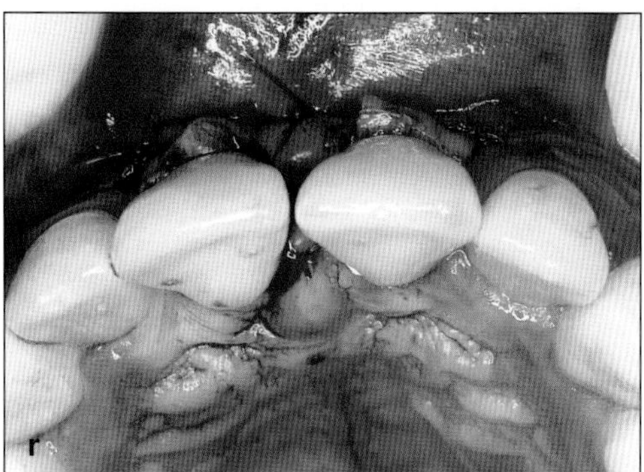

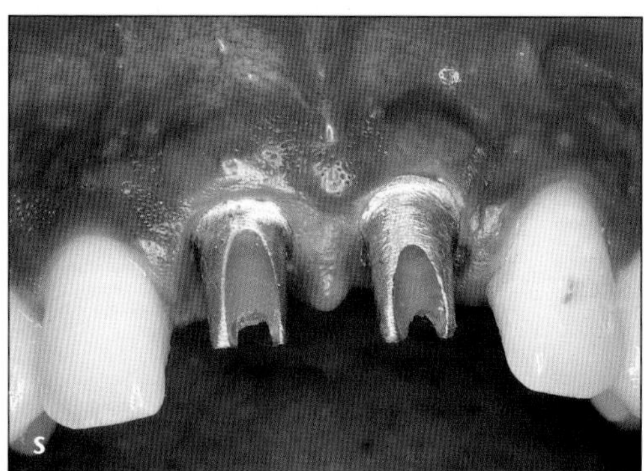

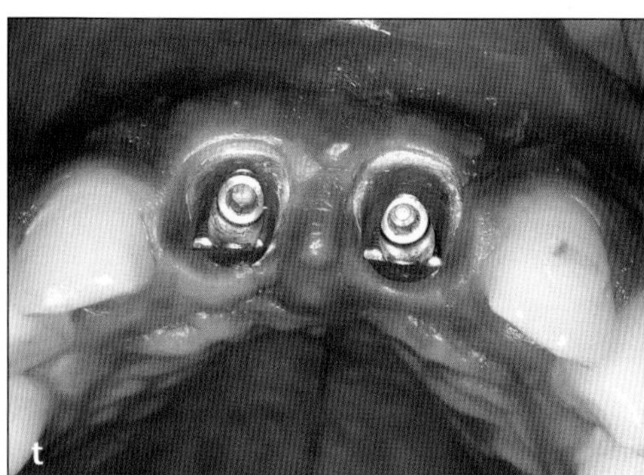

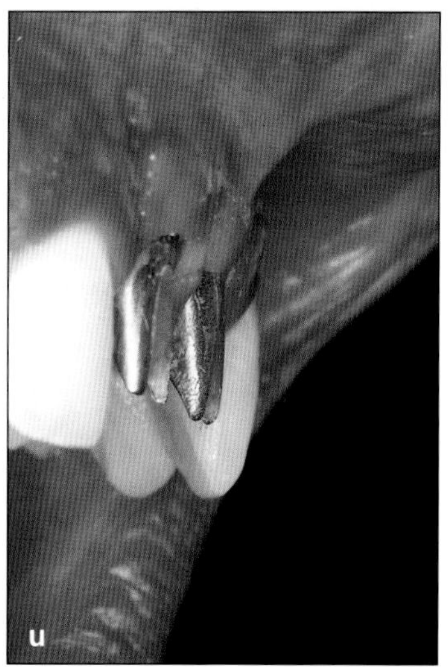

Fig 9-9 *(cont)*
(p) Both Atlantis abutments are screwed into the implants and the flap is replaced. The papillae were preserved as planned.

(q) The Atlantis provisional crowns are cemented before suturing. Their contour and smooth finish will help the soft tissues around them heal toward the correct anatomy. All excess temporary cement should be carefully eliminated to avoid interference with the healing process.

(r) An occlusal view shows how anatomically correct abutments yield anatomically correct provisional crowns, stimulating anatomically correct healing.

(s) Results that satisfy both patient and clinician can be obtained when every step of a treatment plan targeted toward retaining the natural anatomy of the hard and soft tissue is carefully followed. The gingiva around the abutments is of the correct height and width and is ready for impressions for definitive porcelain crowns.

(t) An occlusal view permits appreciation of the natural buccal contour of the two central incisor abutments.

(u) The optimal angulation favors the intermaxillary relationship that is essential in the anterior maxilla.

Table 9-2 Potential complications of augmentation and grafting for the maxillary anterior alveolar ridges

Complication	Cause	Preventive measures
Damage to adjacent teeth	Placement of fixation screws into tooth roots or periodontal ligament space	Use caution when drilling holes for the placement of fixation screws and while placing the screws.
Inadequate ridge size after grafting	Grafting with inadequate amount of graft material; resorption of graft	Take accurate preoperative measurements, use a waxup of the ridge to determine the ideal ridge size and shape, and minimize resorption by using intraoral bone and membrane barriers.
Incision dehiscence in recipient area	Inadequate release of flap; poor closure of donor site; postoperative edema; hematoma	Be sure to release the flap adequately by incising the periosteum and blunt dissection and then suturing the flap carefully. Use ice packs and anti-inflammatory drugs and consider corticosteroids postoperatively to minimize edema.
Graft not attaching to recipient site	Imprecise adaptation of graft to host bone; interpositional soft tissue between graft and host bone; inadequate decortication of host bone; inadequate time for graft maturation	Be sure to reflect the soft tissue flap carefully and completely, curette any soft tissue left on the host bone, decorticate the host bone, modify both the host bone and the graft to allow precise adaptation of the graft to the recipient site, and allow at least 5 months for graft maturation.
Fracture of buccal bone while using osteotomes	Using osteotomes on a narrow ridge; not using a proper sequence of osteotomes	Use osteotomes only if the ridge width is at least 6 mm; use a set of gradually larger diameter osteotomes after starting with a very small diameter; make sure that there is cancellous bone to expand and that the ridge is not all cortical bone.

Potential Complications

Preventing early complications involves using pressure dressings, topical ice packs, and anti-inflammatory drugs to reduce swelling; prescribing analgesics for pain control; and instructing the patient about the importance of meticulous oral hygiene. Edema is very common following surgery, although its intensity may vary. In most cases, swelling decreases rapidly during the first 2 days postsurgery and complete dissipation occurs within 1 week. Table 9-2 lists other potential complications, along with common reasons for their occurrence and techniques with which to minimize them.

References

1. Gregory-Head BL, McDonald A, Labarre E. Treatment planning for success: Wise choices for maxillary single-tooth implants. J Calif Dent Assoc 2001;29:766–771.
2. Derbabian K, Chee WW. Simple tools to facilitate communication in esthetic dentistry. J Calif Dent Assoc 2003;31:537–542.
3. Jivraj SA, Chee WW. An interdisciplinary approach to treatment planning in the esthetic zone. J Calif Dent Assoc 2003;31:544–549.
4. Chee WW. Treatment planning and soft-tissue management for optimal implant esthetics: A prosthodontic perspective. J Calif Dent Assoc 2003;31:559–563.
5. Eufinger H, Konig S, Eufinger A, Machtens E. Significance of the height and width of the alveolar ridge in implantology in the edentulous maxilla. Analysis of 95 cadaver jaws and 24 consecutive patients [in German]. Mund Kiefer Gesichtschir 1999;3(suppl 1):S14–S18.
6. Jovanovic SA, Paul SJ, Nishimura RD. Anterior implant-supported reconstructions: A surgical challenge. Pract Periodontics Aesthet Dent 1999;11:551–558.
7. Paul SJ, Jovanovic SA. Anterior implant-supported reconstructions: A prosthetic challenge. Pract Periodontics Aesthet Dent 1999; 11:585–590.
8. John V, Gossweiler M. Implant treatment planning and rehabilitation of the anterior maxilla: Part 1. J Indiana Dent Assoc 2001;80: 20–24.
9. John V, Gossweiler M. Implant treatment planning and rehabilitation of the anterior maxilla, Part 2: The role of autogenous grafts. J Indiana Dent Assoc 2002;81:33–38.
10. Conte GJ, Rhodes P, Richards D, Kao RT. Considerations for anterior implant esthetics. J Calif Dent Assoc 2002;30:528–534.
11. Levine RA, Katz D. Developing a team approach to complex aesthetics: Treatment considerations. Pract Proced Aesthet Dent 2003; 15:301–306.
12. Amet EM, Milana JP. Restoring soft and hard dental tissues using a removable implant prosthesis with digital imaging for optimum dental esthetics: A clinical report. Int J Periodontics Restorative Dent 2003;23:269–275.
13. Andersson B, Odman P, Lindvall AM, Lithner B. Single-tooth restorations supported by osseointegrated implants: Results and experiences from a prospective study after 2 to 3 years. Int J Oral Maxillofac Implants 1995;10: 702–711.
14. Jemt T. Regeneration of gingival papillae after single-implant treatment. Int J Periodontics Restorative Dent 1997;17:326–333.
15. Touati B, Guez G, Saadoun A. Aesthetic soft tissue integration and optimized emergence profile: Provisionalization and customized impression coping. Pract Periodontics Aesthet Dent 1999;11:305–314.
16. Cobb GW, Reeves GW, Duncan JD. Guided tissue healing for single-tooth implants. Compend Contin Educ Dent 1999;20:571–578, 580–581.
17. Sullivan RM. Perspectives on esthetics in implant dentistry. Compend Contin Educ Dent 2001;22:685–692.
18. Davarpanah M, Martinez H, Celletti R, Tecucianu JF. Three-stage approach to aesthetic implant restoration: Emergence profile concept. Pract Proced Aesthet Dent 2001;13: 761–767.
19. Velvart P. Papilla base incision: A new approach to recession-free healing of the interdental papilla after endodontic surgery. Int Endod J 2002;35:453–460.
20. Flanagan D. An incision design to promote a gingival base for the creation of interdental implant papillae. J Oral Implantol 2002;28: 25–28.
21. Reddy MS. Achieving gingival esthetics. J Am Dent Assoc 2003;134:295–304.
22. Kan JY, Rungcharassaeng K. Interimplant papilla preservation in the esthetic zone: A report of six consecutive cases. Int J Periodontics Restorative Dent 2003;23:249–259.
23. Azzi R, Etienne D, Takei H, Fenech P. Surgical thickening of the existing gingiva and reconstruction of interdental papillae around implant-supported restorations. Int J Periodontics Restorative Dent 2002;22:71–77.
24. Mathews DP. The pediculated connective tissue graft: A technique for improving unaesthetic implant restorations. Pract Proced Aesthet Dent 2002;14:719–724.
25. Cranin AN. Implant surgery: The management of soft tissues. J Oral Implantol 2002;28: 230–237.
26. Harris RJ. Soft tissue ridge augmentation with an acellular dermal matrix. Int J Periodontics Restorative Dent 2003;23:87–92.

27. Evian CI, al-Maseeh J, Symeonides E. Soft tissue augmentation for implant dentistry. Compend Contin Educ Dent 2003; 24:195–198, 200–202, 204–206.
28. Mahn DH. Esthetic soft tissue ridge augmentation using an acellular dermal connective tissue allograft. J Esthet Restorative Dent 2003;15:72–78.
29. Eufinger H, Konig S, Eufinger A. The role of alveolar ridge width in dental implantology. Clin Oral Investig 1997;1:169–177.
30. Dixon DR, Morgan R, Hollender LG, Roberts FA, O'Neal RB. Clinical application of spiral tomography in anterior implant placement: Case report. J Periodontol 2002;73:1202–1209.
31. Boudrias P, Shoghikian E, Morin E, Hutnik P. Esthetic option for the implant-supported single-tooth restoration—Treatment sequence with a ceramic abutment. J Can Dent Assoc 2001;67:508–514.
32. Kan JY, Rungcharassaeng K. Site development for anterior single implant esthetics: The dentulous site. Compend Contin Educ Dent 2001; 22:221–226, 228, 230–231.
33. Norton MR. Single-tooth implant-supported restorations. Planning for an aesthetic and functional solution. Dent Update 2001;28: 170–175.
34. Haas R, Polak C, Furhauser R, Mailath-Pokorny G, Dortbudak O, Watzek G. A long-term follow-up of 76 Branemark single-tooth implants. Clin Oral Implants Res 2002;13:38–43.
35. Gibbard LL, Zarb G. A 5-year prospective study of implant-supported single-tooth replacements. J Can Dent Assoc 2002;68:110–116.
36. Zarb JP, Zarb GA. Implant prosthodontic management of anterior partial edentulism: Long-term follow-up of a prospective study. J Can Dent Assoc 2002;68:92–96.
37. Romeo E, Chiapasco M, Ghisolfi M, Vogel G. Long-term clinical effectiveness of oral implants in the treatment of partial edentulism. Seven-year life table analysis of a prospective study with ITI dental implants system used for single-tooth restorations. Clin Oral Implants Res 2002;13:133–143.
38. Mayer TM, Hawley CE, Gunsolley JC, Feldman S. The single-tooth implant: A viable alternative for single-tooth replacement. J Periodontol 2002;73:687–693.
39. Attard N, Barzilay I. A modified impression technique for accurate registration of peri-implant soft tissues. J Can Dent Assoc 2003; 69:80–83.
40. Smukler H, Castellucci F, Capri D. The role of the implant housing in obtaining aesthetics: Generation of peri-implant gingivae and papillae—Part 1. Pract Proced Aesthet Dent 2003;15:141–149.
41. Andersson L, Emami-Kristiansen Z, Hogstrom J. Single-tooth implant treatment in the anterior region of the maxilla for treatment of tooth loss after trauma: A retrospective clinical and interview study. Dent Traumatol 2003; 19:126–131.
42. Klokkevold PR, Han TJ, Camargo PM. Aesthetic management of extractions for implant site development: Delayed versus staged implant placement. Pract Periodontics Aesthet Dent 1999;11:603–610.
43. Wheeler SL, Vogel RE, Casellini R. Tissue preservation and maintenance of optimum esthetics: A clinical report. Int J Oral Maxillofac Implants 2000;15:265–271.
44. Raigrodski AJ, Block MS. Clinical considerations for enhancing the success of implant-supported restorations in the aesthetic zone with delayed implant placement. Pract Proced Aesthet Dent 2002;14:21–28.
45. Anson D. Maxillary anterior esthetic extractions with delayed single-stage implant placement. Compend Contin Educ Dent 2002;23: 829–830, 833–836, 838 passim.
46. Schiroli G. Immediate tooth extraction, placement of a Tapered Screw-Vent implant, and provisionalization in the esthetic zone: A case report. Implant Dent 2003;12:123–131.
47. Edelhoff D, Spiekermann H, Yildirim M. A review of esthetic pontic design options. Quintessence Int 2002;33:736–746.
48. el Askary AS. Multifaceted aspects of implant esthetics: The anterior maxilla. Implant Dent 2001;10:182–191.
49. Priest G. Predictability of soft tissue form around single-tooth implant restorations. Int J Periodontics Restorative Dent 2003;23:19–27.
50. Gadhia MH, Holt RL. A new implant design for optimal esthetics and retention of interproximal papillae. Implant Dent 2003;12: 164–169.
51. Yildirim M, Hanisch O, Spiekermann H. Simultaneous hard and soft tissue augmentation for implant-supported single-tooth restorations. Pract Periodontics Aesthet Dent 1997;9: 1023–1031.
52. Weber HP, Fiorellini JP, Buser DA. Hard-tissue augmentation for the placement of anterior dental implants. Compend Contin Educ Dent 1997;18:779–784, 786–788, 790–791.

53. Wang HL, Kimble K, Eber R. Use of bone grafts for the enhancement of a GTR-based root coverage procedure: A pilot case study. Int J Periodontics Restorative Dent 2002;22:119–127.
54. Wang HL, Carroll MJ. Guided bone regeneration using bone grafts and collagen membranes. Quintessence Int 2001;32:504–515.
55. Iasella JM, Greenwell H, Miller RL, et al. Ridge preservation with freeze-dried bone allograft and a collagen membrane compared to extraction alone for implant site development: A clinical and histologic study in humans. J Periodontol 2003;74:990–999.
56. Fowler EB, Breault LG, Rebitski G. Ridge preservation utilizing an acellular dermal allograft and demineralized freeze-dried bone allograft: Part I. A report of 2 cases. J Periodontol 2000:71:1353–1359.
57. Fowler EB, Breault LG, Rebitski G. Ridge preservation utilizing an acellular dermal allograft and demineralized freeze-dried bone allograft: Part II. Immediate endosseous implant placement. J Periodontol 2000;71:1360–1364 [erratum 2000;71:1670].
58. Zubillaga G, Von Hagen S, Simon BI, Deasy MJ. Changes in alveolar bone height and width following post-extraction ridge augmentation using a fixed bioabsorbable membrane and demineralized freeze-dried bone osteoinductive graft. J Periodontol 2003;74:965–975.
59. Cornelini R, Cangini F, Covani U, Andreana S. Simultaneous implant placement and vertical ridge augmentation with a titanium-reinforced membrane: A case report. Int J Oral Maxillofac Implants 2000;15:883–888.
60. Nemcovsky CE, Artzi Z. Comparative study of buccal dehiscence defects in immediate, delayed, and late maxillary implant placement with collagen membranes: Clinical healing between placement and second-stage surgery. J Periodontol 2002;73:754–761.
61. Tal H, Oelgiesser D, Moses O. Preimplant guided bone regeneration in the anterior maxilla. Int J Periodontics Restorative Dent 1997;17:436–447.
62. Raghoebar GM, Batenburg RH, Vissink A, Reintsema H. Augmentation of localized defects of the anterior maxillary ridge with autogenous bone before insertion of implants. J Oral Maxillofac Surg 1996;54:1180–1185.
63. Nystrom E, Ahlqvist J, Kahnberg KE, Rosenquist JB. Autogenous onlay bone grafts fixed with screw implants for the treatment of severely resorbed maxillae. Radiographic evaluation of preoperative bone dimensions, postoperative bone loss, and changes in soft-tissue profile. Int J Oral Maxillofac Surg 1996;25:351–359.
64. Widmark G, Andersson B, Ivanoff CJ. Mandibular bone graft in the anterior maxilla for single-tooth implants. Presentation of surgical method. Int J Oral Maxillofac Surg 1997;26:106–109.
65. Proussaefs P, Lozada J, Kleinman A, Rohrer MD. The use of ramus autogenous block grafts for vertical alveolar ridge augmentation and implant placement: A pilot study. Int J Oral Maxillofac Implants 2002;17:238–248.
66. Balaji SM. Management of deficient anterior maxillary alveolus with mandibular parasymphyseal bone graft for implants. Implant Dent 2002;11:363–369.
67. Sandor GK, Kainulainen VT, Queiroz JO, Carmichael RP, Oikarinen KS. Preservation of ridge dimensions following grafting with coral granules of 48 post-traumatic and post-extraction dento-alveolar defects. Dent Traumatol 2003;19:221–227.
68. Marx RE, Garg AK. Bone structure, metabolism, and physiology: Its impact on dental implantology. Implant Dent 1998;7:267–276.
69. Ramp LC, Jeffcoat RL. Dynamic behavior of implants as a measure of osseointegration. Int J Oral Maxillofac Implants 2001;16:637–645.
70. Buser D, Ingimarsson S, Dula K, Lussi A, Hirt HP, Belser UC. Long-term stability of osseointegrated implants in augmented bone: A 5-year prospective study in partially edentulous patients. Int J Periodontics Restorative Dent 2002;22:109–117.
71. Nystrom E, Ahlqvist J, Legrell PE, Kahnberg KE. Bone graft remodelling and implant success rate in the treatment of the severely resorbed maxilla: A 5-year longitudinal study. Int J Oral Maxillofac Surg 2002;31:158–164.
72. McCarthy C, Patel RR, Wragg PF, Brook IM. Dental implants and onlay bone grafts in the anterior maxilla: Analysis of clinical outcome. Int J Oral Maxillofac Implants 2003;18:238–241.
73. Hunt DR, Jovanovic SA. Autogenous bone harvesting: A chin graft technique for particulate and monocortical bone blocks. Int J Periodontics Restorative Dent 1999;19:165–173.

74. Kaufman E, Wang PD. Localized vertical maxillary ridge augmentation using symphyseal bone cores: A technique and case report. Int J Oral Maxillofac Implants 2003;18: 293–298.
75. Smiler DG. Bone grafting: Materials and modes of action. Pract Periodontics Aesthet Dent 1996;8:413–416.
76. Costantino PD, Hiltzik D, Govindaraj S, Moche J. Bone healing and bone substitutes. Facial Plast Surg 2002;18:13–26.
77. Misch CM, Misch CE. The repair of localized severe ridge defects for implant placement using mandibular bone grafts. Implant Dent 1995;4:261–267.
78. Kohavi D. Simultaneous and staged approaches for guided bone regeneration. Compend Contin Educ Dent 2000;21:495–498, 500, 502 passim.
79. Lorenzoni M, Pertl C, Zhang K, Wimmer G, Wegscheider WA. Immediate loading of single-tooth implants in the anterior maxilla. Preliminary results after one year. Clin Oral Implants Res 2003;14:180–187.
80. Triplett RG, Schow SR. Autologous bone grafts and endosseous implants: Complementary techniques. J Oral Maxillofac Surg 1996;54: 486–494.
81. Thor A. Reconstruction of the anterior maxilla with platelet gel, autogenous bone, and titanium mesh: A case report. Clin Implant Dent Relat Res 2002;4:150–155.
82. Proussaefs P, Lozada J, Kleinman A, Rohrer MD, McMillan PJ. The use of titanium mesh in conjunction with autogenous bone graft and inorganic bovine bone mineral (bio-oss) for localized alveolar ridge augmentation: A human study. Int J Periodontics Restorative Dent 2003;23:185–195.
83. Artzi Z, Dayan D, Alpern Y, Nemcovsky CE. Vertical ridge augmentation using xenogenic material supported by a configured titanium mesh: Clinicohistopathologic and histochemical study. Int J Oral Maxillofac Implants 2003; 18:440–446.
84. Stambaugh R. Aesthetic ridge and extraction site augmentation for anterior implant placement without barrier membrane. Pract Periodontics Aesthet Dent 1997;9:991–998.
85. Cutilli BJ, Smith BM, Bleiler R. Reconstruction of a severely atrophic maxilla using a Le Fort I downgraft and dental implants: Clinical report. Implant Dent 1997;6:105–108.
86. Perez MM, Sameshima GT, Sinclair PM. The long-term stability of LeFort I maxillary downgrafts with rigid fixation to correct vertical maxillary deficiency. Am J Orthod Dentofacial Orthop 1997;112:104–108.
87. Wolford LM, Stevao ELL. Correction of jaw deformities in patients with cleft lip and palate. Baylor University Med Center Proc 2002;15:250–254.
88. Wardrop RW, Wolford LM. Maxillary stability following downgraft and/or advancement procedures with stabilization using rigid fixation and porous block hydroxyapatite implants. J Oral Maxillofac Surg 1989;47:336–342.
89. Macmillan AR, Tideman H. The stability of the downgrafted maxilla in the cleft lip and palate patient. Ann R Australas Coll Dent Surg 1994;12:232–239.
90. Belser UC, Bernard JP, Buser D. Implant-supported restorations in the anterior region: Prosthetic considerations. Pract Periodontics Aesthet Dent 1996;8:875–883.
91. Potashnick SR. Soft tissue modeling for the esthetic single-tooth implant restoration. J Esthet Dent 1998;10:121–131.
92. Davidoff SR. Developing soft tissue contours for implant-supported restorations: A simplified method for enhanced aesthetics. Pract Periodontics Aesthet Dent 1996;8:507–513.
93. Tarnow DP, Magner AW, Fletcher P. The effect of the distance from the contact point to the crest of bone on the presence or absence of the interproximal dental papilla. J Periodontol 1992;63:995–996.
94. Tarnow DP, Cho SC, Wallace SS. The effect of inter-implant distance on the height of inter-implant bone crest. J Periodontol 2000;71: 546–549.
95. Grossberg DE. Interimplant papilla reconstruction: Assessment of soft tissue changes and results of 12 consecutive cases. J Periodontol 2001;72:958–962.
96. Choquet V, Hermans M, Adriaenssens P, Daelemans P, Tarnow DP, Malevez C. Clinical and radiographic evaluation of the papilla level adjacent to single-tooth dental implants. A retrospective study in the maxillary anterior region. J Periodontol 2001;72:1364–1371.
97. Kois JC, Kan JY. Predictable peri-implant gingival aesthetics: Surgical and prosthodontic rationales. Pract Proced Aesthet Dent 2001; 13:691–698.

98. Bosse LP, Taylor TD. Problems associated with implant rehabilitation of the edentulous maxilla. Dent Clin North Am 1998;42: 117–127.
99. Dario LJ, Aschaffenburg PH, English R Jr, Nager MC. Fixed implant rehabilitation of the edentulous maxilla: Clinical guidelines and case reports. Part I. Implant Dent 1999;8: 186–193.
100. Dario LJ, Aschaffenburg PH, English R Jr, Nager MC. Fixed implant rehabilitation of the edentulous maxilla: Clinical guidelines and case reports. Part II. Implant Dent 2000; 9:102–109.
101. Henry PJ. A review of guidelines for implant rehabilitation of the edentulous maxilla. J Prosthet Dent 2002;87:281–288.
102. Glavas P, Moses MS. Stage I indexing to replace a failed implant in an edentulous arch: A clinical report. J Prosthet Dent 2003;89: 533–535.
103. Lazzara RJ. Managing the soft tissue margin: The key to implant aesthetics. Pract Periodontics Aesthet Dent 1993;5:81–88.
104. Tarlow JL. Procedure for obtaining proper contour of an implant-supported crown: A clinical report. J Prosthet Dent 2002;87:416–418.
105. Vogel RC. Enhancing implant esthetics with ideal provisionalization. J Indiana Dent Assoc 2002;81:11–14.
106. Padbury A Jr, Eber R, Wang HL. Interactions between the gingiva and the margin of restorations. J Clin Periodontol 2003;30:379–385.
107. Garber DA. The esthetic dental implant: Letting restoration be the guide. J Am Dent Assoc 1995;126:319–325.
108. Garber DA, Belser UC. Restoration-driven implant placement with restoration-generated site development. Compend Contin Educ Dent 1995;16:796, 798–802, 804.
109. el Askary A el-S. Esthetic considerations in anterior single-tooth replacement. Implant Dent 1999;8:61–67.
110. Francischone CE, Vasconcelos LW, and Brånemark PI. Esthetic optimization of implant supported single tooth restorations. In: Osseointegration and Esthetics in Single Tooth Rehabilitation. São Paulo: Quintessence, 2000:77–91.

CHAPTER

10 Subnasal Elevation and Bone Augmentation

The anterior maxilla commonly lacks sufficient bone height for implant placement. To augment both the quantity and quality of bone in the anterior maxillary residual crest, a subnasal elevation followed by bone grafting may be performed. This useful technique can predictably elevate the nasal mucosa 3 to 5 mm prior to grafting and is indicated when the residual crest is less than 10 mm in height. Prior to implant insertion, the recipient bone bed in the anterior maxilla should ideally be at least 6 mm wide and 13 mm high.[1] This allows for the placement of longer implants (10 to 13 mm), which increase the success of implant restoration in this area.[2–4] The technique also deters penetration of the implant into the nasal cavity, which has been shown to occur frequently when the transverse alveolar dimension of the anterior maxilla has significantly diminished.[5]

For the subnasal elevation, the periosteum of the labial aspect of the anterior maxilla is reflected to expose the inferior and/or lateral piriform rim (Figs 10-1 and 10-2). A nasal undercut region is typically present in the area of the lateral-inferior piriform rim, and in this region, the nasal mucosa can be elevated (Fig 10-3). Particulated graft material is typically used to augment this area. In patients with unilateral or bilateral edentulism, antral-nasal inlay composite grafts can also be used.[6] For the edentulous patient with a compromised anterior maxillary region, a complete-arch onlay graft can be used to reduce the interarch space and to create an arch with a

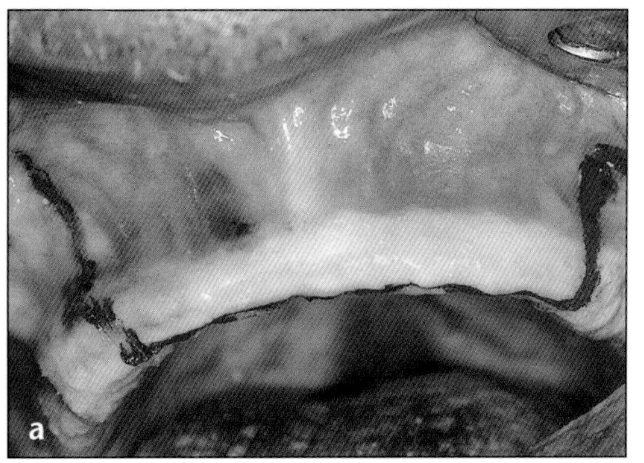

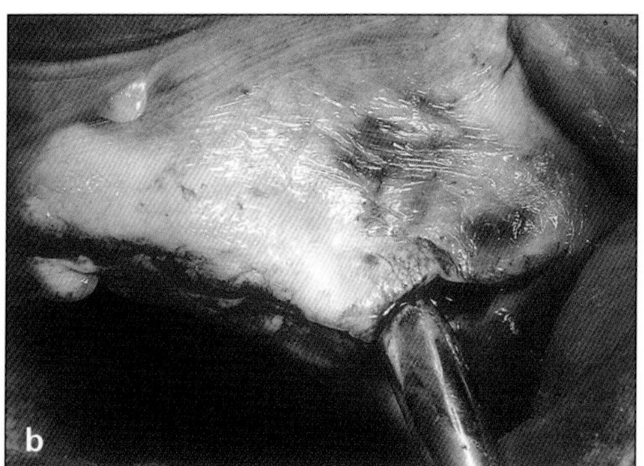

Fig 10-1
A midcrestal incision and two high vertical divergent incisions will provide a flap that can be reflected adequately to provide access and visibility for the nasal spine and piriform rims. Here the initial incision is performed on a cadaver specimen *(a)* and on an actual patient *(b)*.

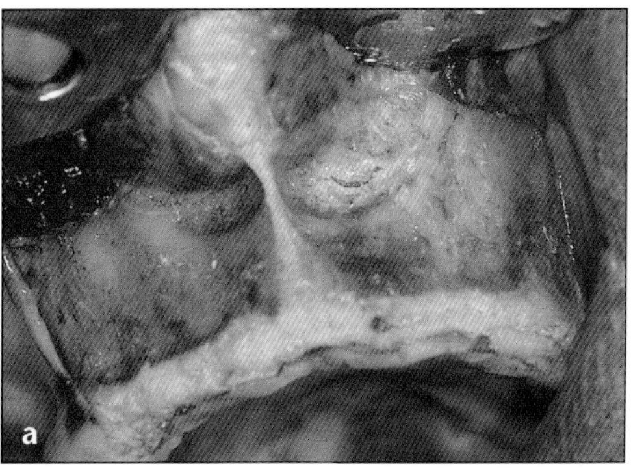

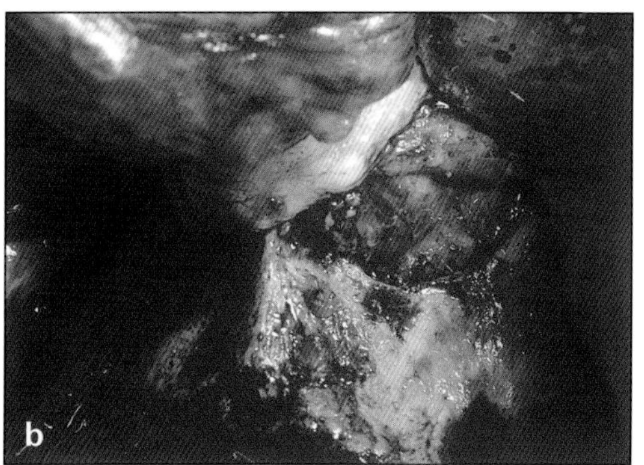

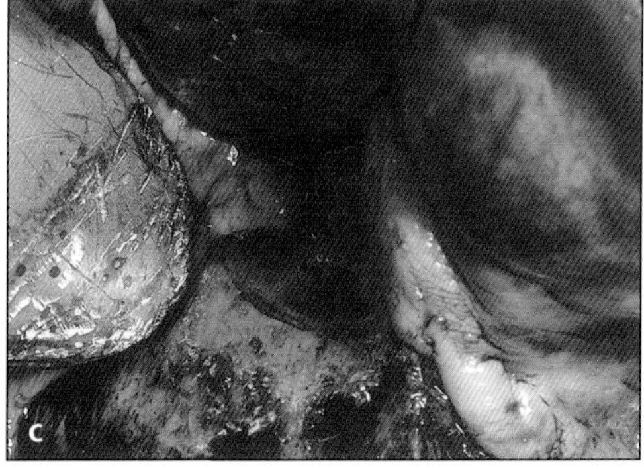

Fig 10-2
The flap reflection, shown here in a cadaver *(a)* and an actual patient *(b and c)*, should be done with a sharp periosteal elevator to prevent tearing the periosteum or mucosa and should also permit a careful separation of the mucosa from the nasal lining.

more ideal size and shape.[7,8] In totally edentulous patients, however, a complete-arch onlay graft may not be possible because of an inadequate arch space or a short upper lip.

A significantly resorbed maxilla, which often presents with reverse architecture in the anterior maxilla where retained or supererupted mandibular incisors have accelerated resorption into the basal bone, may leave only a few millimeters or complete dehiscence of the anterior nasal floor. In these situations, a 5- to 7-mm block graft is placed following nasal mucosal elevation, and an inferior septoplasty is performed. When performed in conjunction with alveolar augmentation, this procedure provides additional stability and vertical dimension for the implants.

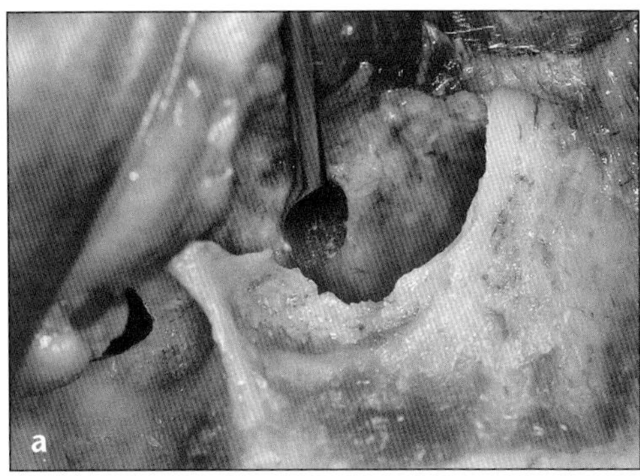

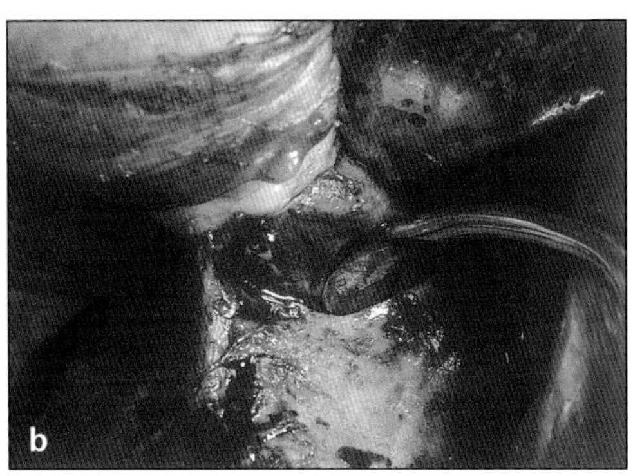

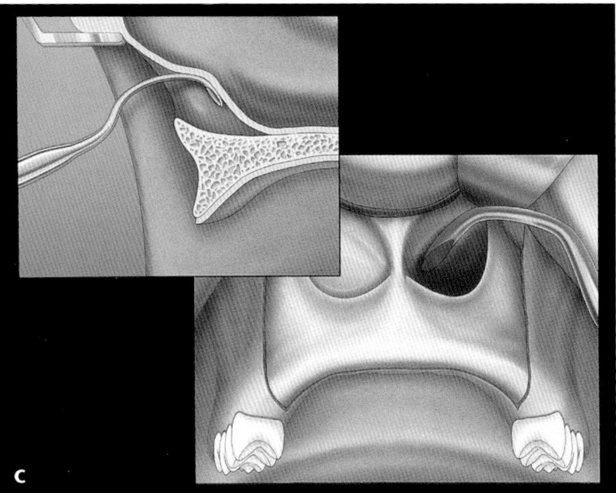

Fig 10-3
(a) The nasal mucosa should be carefully dissected to detach it from the bone starting at the piriform rim and continuing into the nasal floor. Note the separation of mucosa from bone in this cadaver demonstration.

(b) Excessive pressure could give way to a perforation. This mucosa is thicker and more resistant than the sinus membrane, but a tear here calls for a water-tight closure with resorbable sutures or aborting of the procedure because bacterial contamination could enter the grafted site from the nasal cavity.

(c) Lateral and frontal view of the correct way to hold the curette, with the concavity of the curette oriented toward the bone.

Despite these augmentation measures, inlay or onlay grafting procedures do not always adequately restore enough vertical bone to accommodate a fixed prosthesis. In that case, a continuous bar overdenture is a prudent prosthetic choice.[6]

In some respects, the nasal lift is similar to the maxillary sinus lift; both are performed using a soft tissue curette to elevate the mucosa. Because the nasal mucosa is generally much thicker and more tear resistant than the maxillary sinus membrane, there is less chance of perforation during elevation, and it is easier to elevate. An underlying elastic fiber makes it adhere more firmly to the underlying bone; therefore, significant pressure must be applied to elevate the nasal mucosa. The clinician should bear in mind that if a perforation occurs in the mucosa, it is imperative to suture it closed and obtain a water-tight closure to minimize the chance of bacterial flora from the nose migrating into the graft and causing contamination and infection.

This chapter outlines a step-by-step technique for performing a nasal sinus lift and subsequent grafting and also provides an overview of the nasal anatomy and vasculature, of which the surgeon must have a good working understanding before undertaking this procedure.

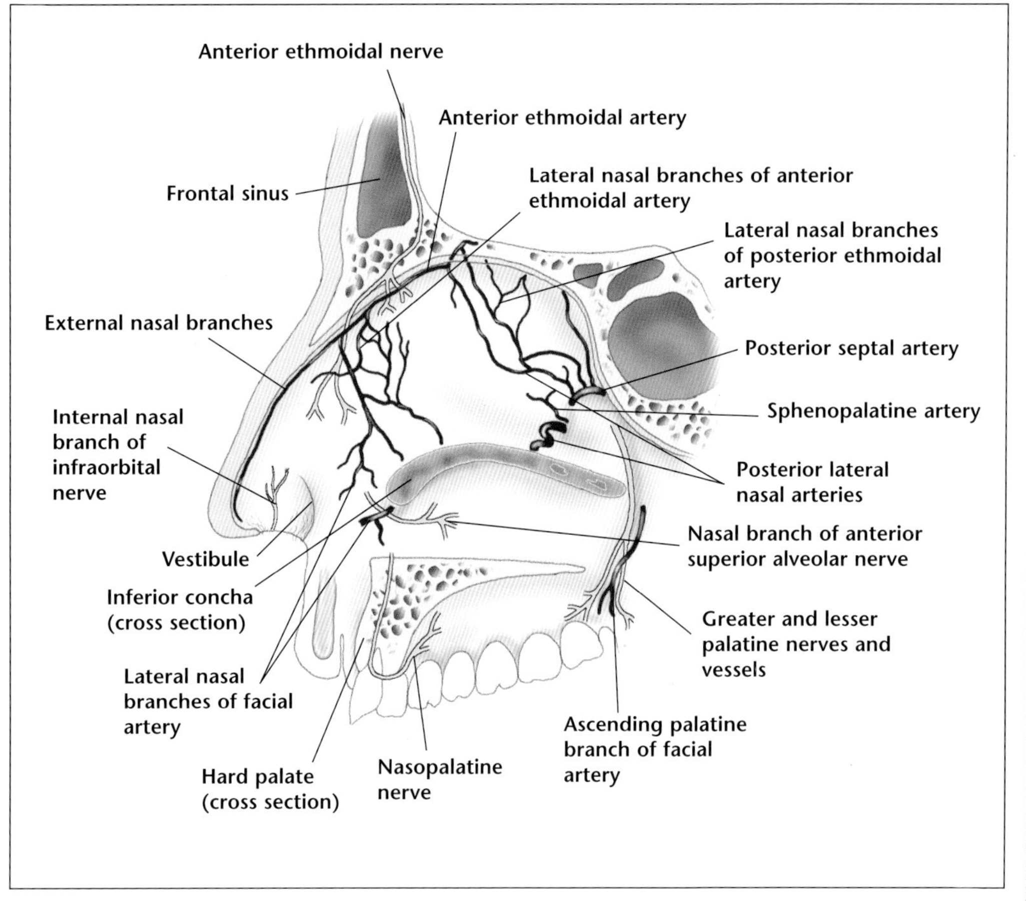

Fig 10-4
The septum—and the nasal cavity in general—is highly vascularized. This may be to warm the air before it reaches the bronchi and lungs. The arterial blood supply to the nose is derived from the terminal branch of the maxillary artery, which supplies the sphenopalatine artery, which in turn supplies the lateral and medial walls of the nasal chamber. The anterior and posterior ethmoidal arteries supply the vestibule and the anterior portion of the septum. A few blood vessels from the greater palatine artery pass through the incisive canal of the palate to reach the anterior part of the nose. Sensory innervation to the nose is also important in that it provides reflexes (such as the sneeze reflex) to keep foreign particles out of the respiratory system. For this surgery, it is critical for the surgeon to be familiar with the orientation of the anterior ethmoidal and nasopalatine nerves.

Nasal Anatomy and Vasculature

To successfully perform a subnasal elevation, the surgeon must consider the nasal structure, vasculature, innervation, and soft tissues in the operative area.

The arterial blood supply to the nose is derived from the external and internal carotid arteries. The terminal branch of the maxillary artery (a branch of the external carotid artery) supplies the sphenopalatine artery, which in turn supplies the lateral and medial walls of the nasal chamber. The anterior and posterior ethmoidal arteries (branches of the ophthalmic artery, which itself is a branch of the internal carotid artery) supply the vestibule and the anterior portion of the septum. A few blood vessels from the greater palatine artery pass through the incisive canal of the palate to reach the anterior part of the nose (Fig 10-4).

Selection of Bone-Grafting Material

Because of its significant osteogenic properties, autogenous bone is recommended for use in grafting the nasal fossa. This material allows for the most rapid bone formation and is the best option where significant bone augmentation or repair is required. Autogenous bone can be harvested from the iliac crest or the tibia; from intraoral sites such as the mandibular symphysis, maxillary tuberosity, ramus, or exostoses; or from debris from an implant osteotomy.[9–11] Local bone defects in the anterior maxilla usually require only small grafts, which can be obtained intraorally,[1] and the procedure can be easily accomplished in an office setting with the patient under parenteral sedation and/or local anesthesia.[11]

The use of morselized and compressed cancellous or corticocancellous bone is preferred, and alloplasts and allografts may be used to expand the autogenous graft.[12] The use of these materials alone is not currently recommended for subnasal grafting because more evidence is needed to establish their effectiveness. Platelet-rich plasma (PRP) can added to the graft mix, if desired, to improve graft handling and enhance the graft maturation rate and bone density.

Procedure

A chlorhexidine antiseptic scrub and rinse can be used to prepare the surgical site. Iodophor or chlorhexidine antiseptics can be used for preoperative extraoral scrubbing of the skin.

Infiltration anesthesia has been successfully used for this procedure; however, a more significant regional anesthesia occurs when the secondary division of the maxillary nerve (V2) is blocked. Block anesthesia produces a longer anesthetic effect in the maxilla than does infiltration anesthesia. With this technique, anesthesia of the hemimaxillary side of the nose, cheek, lip, and sinus area can be achieved, preferably using a long-acting anesthetic (bupivacaine or etidocaine). Proper angulation of the needle prevents penetration into the nasal cavity through the medial wall of the pterygopalatine fossa. Lidocaine 2% with 1:100,000 epinephrine is then infiltrated into the labial mucosa and palatal region to decrease initial hemorrhaging and to allow the surgeon to evaluate the effectiveness of the local anesthesia.

A full-thickness incision is made on the crest of the maxillary ridge, from the distal end of the canine region to the distal end of the contralateral canine region. A vertical lateral releasing incision is then made at its distal extensions. The full-thickness tissue flap is reflected to expose the anterior maxilla to the nasal spine and the inferior and/or lateral piriform rim.

A nasal undercut region is typically formed at the junction of the lateral-inferior piriform rim that often corresponds to the area where implants will be placed (canine area). The nasal mucosa in this region is elevated with a soft tissue curette in a manner similar to that used to elevate the mucoperiosteum in subantral augmentation procedures. Depending on the depth of the impression behind the piriform rim, the nasal mucosa is elevated approximately 3 to 5 mm and then augmented with graft material. In this manner, 3 to 5 mm of additional bone height can be obtained for implant placement. If additional bone height is obtained, the patient's air inspiration may be affected unless the inferior nasal concha is removed.

For subnasal augmentation, approximately 5 mL of cortical and trabecular

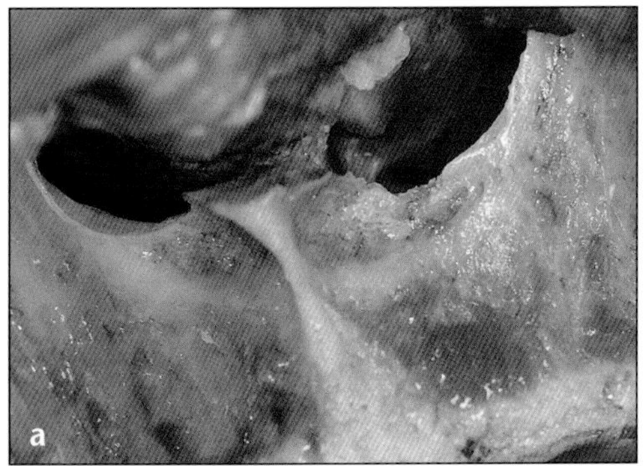

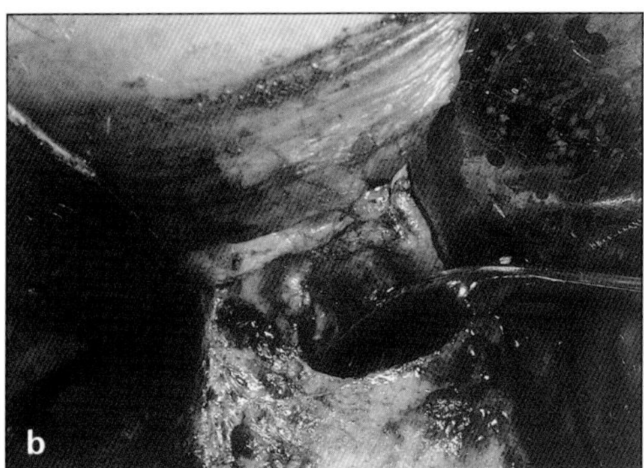

Fig 10-5
Nasal cavity with mucosa reflected in a cadaver *(a)* and patient *(b)*. The amount of nasal mucosa that is reflected in depth should be enough to provide bone surrounding the apex of the implant regardless of the angle at which it is placed.

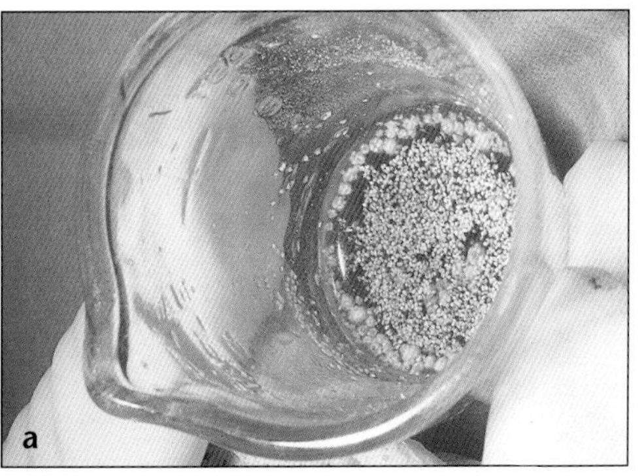

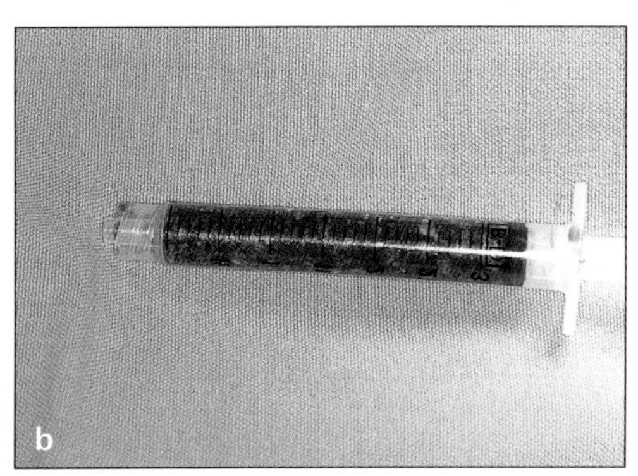

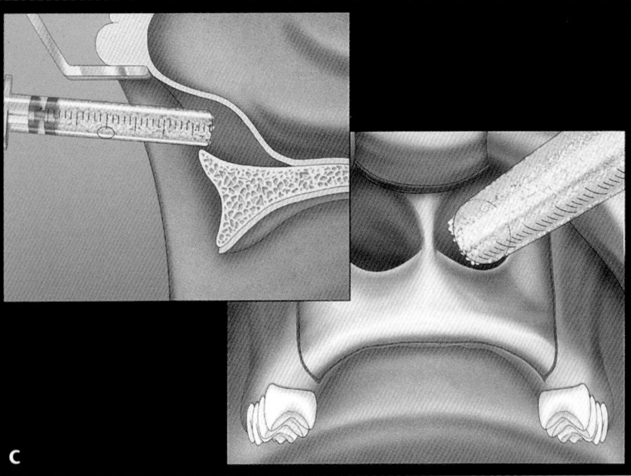

Fig 10-6
The graft material of choice for this nasal elevation case was autogenous bone mixed with allogeneic bone in a 1:1 ratio *(a)*. A sterile plastic syringe with the tip cut off is used as a graft carrier *(b)*, and the material is injected into the recipient site *(c)*.

autogenous bone is harvested from the mandibular symphysis or tibia. If necessary for volume expansion, this bone can then be mixed with freeze-dried bone allograft in a 1:1 ratio (a minimum of 40% autogenous bone is recommended for this procedure) and compressed into a 1- to 3-mL tuberculin syringe. The mixture is applied from the posteriormost regions of the nasal space to the anteriormost labial region of the nasal spine and piriform rim (Figs 10-5 to 10-8).

Fig 10-7
Delivery of graft material in a cadaver *(a)* and a patient *(b)*. A modified amalgam plugger is used to condense the graft particles and pack them into the graft recipient site *(c and d)*.

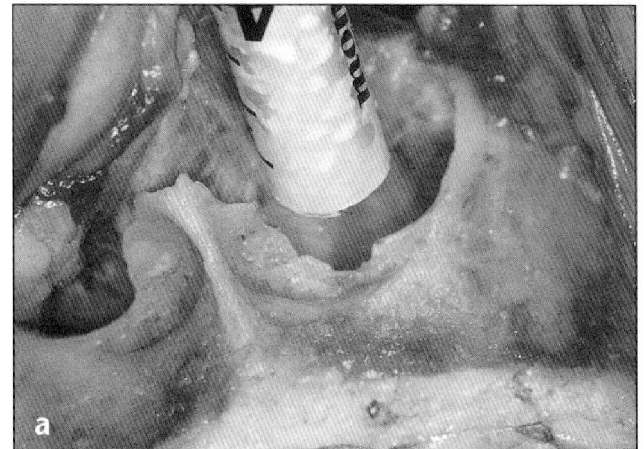

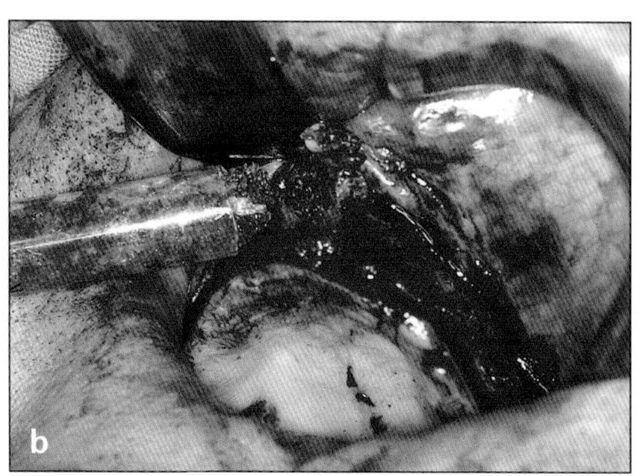

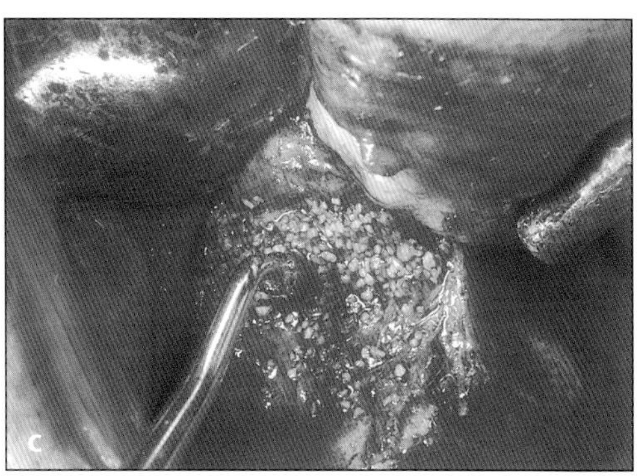

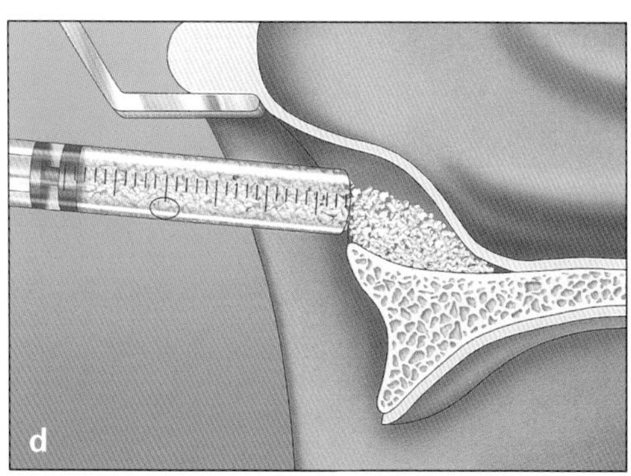

Fig 10-8
Completely filled sinus cavity in a cadaver *(a)* and a patient *(b)*. The clinician should take care not to overfill the area.

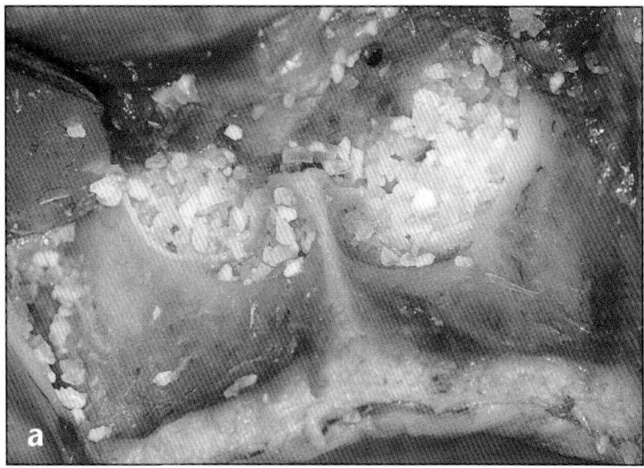

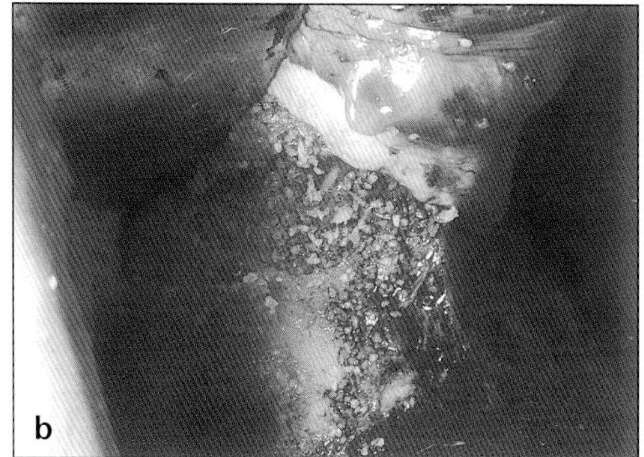

When subnasal augmentation is performed in conjunction with iliac graft reconstruction of the maxilla, a 2- to 5-mm septal reduction is performed on the anterior septum, taking care to avoid tearing the mucosal lining of the basal septum. A 5- to 7-mm-high block graft is fixed with one or two miniscrews placed laterally; the miniscrews can be left permanently if facial augmentation is performed over them. This provides enough stabilization for standard implants. If additional ridge width is needed, block grafts from the anterior mandible or ramus can be affixed to the buccal aspect of the anterior maxilla (Figs 10-9 and 10-10). After maturation of the graft, appropriately sized implants can be placed.

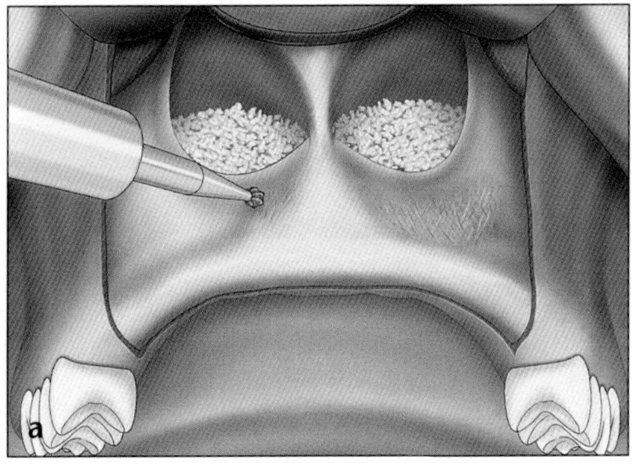

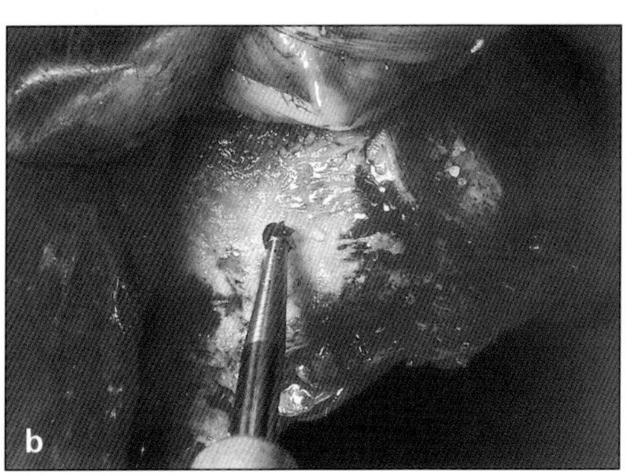

Fig 10-9
A large pineapple-shaped bur is also used to modify the recipient site to allow for good adaptation of a block bone graft. Sites that require a nasal lift procedure for additional bone height typically require a block bone graft for additional bone width as well. The buccal wall of the anterior maxilla is perforated repeatedly with a small round bur to promote bleeding.

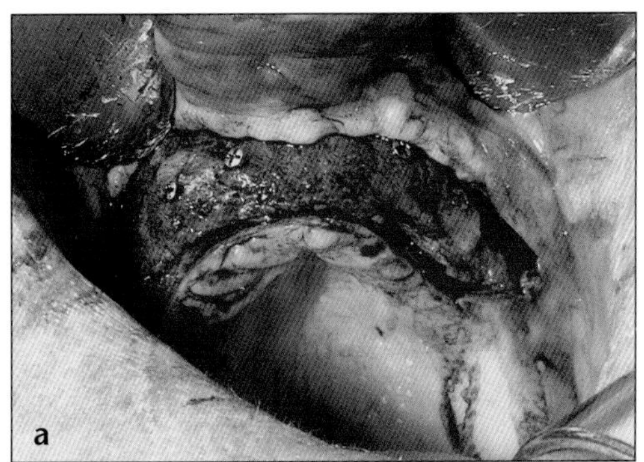

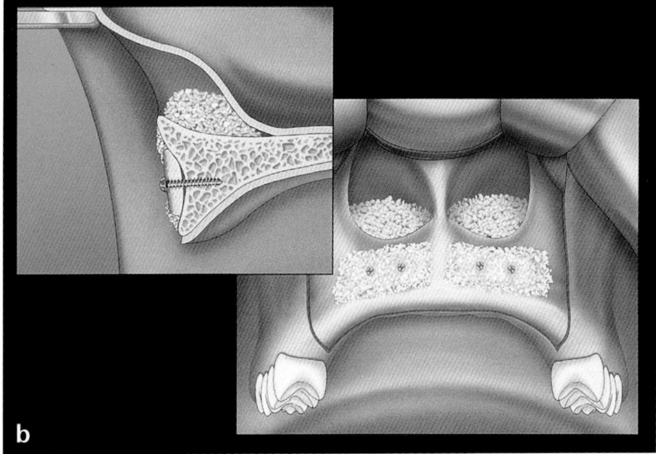

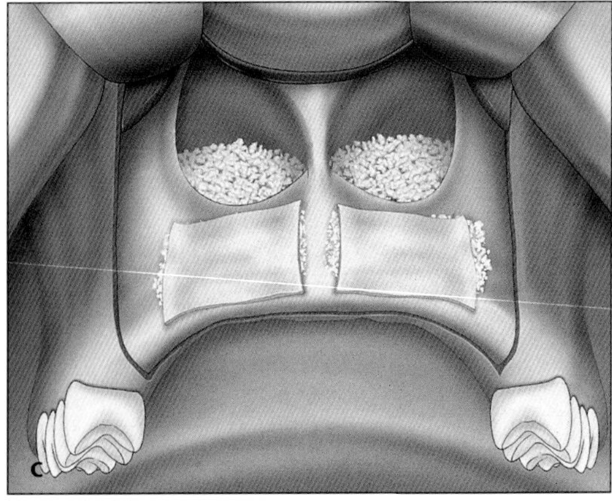

Fig 10-10
The bone blocks are affixed with screws *(a)*. Lateral and anterior views *(b)* illustrate the vertical and horizontal gains. Membranes can be placed over the bone block but should not be placed in the area of the nasal lift procedure *(c)*.

Prior to suturing, the periosteum of the mucosal flap covering the graft is horizontally scored with a scalpel to allow for tension-free flap advancement and wound closure. The primary crestal incision and the vertical releasing incisions are closed with 4-0 chromic sutures in either an interrupted or a continuous mattress fashion. This area should be permitted to heal for 4 to 6 months before implant placement.[3,7] The provisional partial or complete denture should also be adjusted and relined to avoid contact with the grafted area.

The postoperative instructions are similar to those for most oral surgery or sinus manipulation procedures. After 1 week, the patient should begin using a chlorhexidine mouthrinse twice a day for the next 2 weeks to reduce the risk of infection. For at least 1 week following surgery, the patient should avoid blowing his or her nose and creating negative pressure while sucking liquid through a straw and smoking cigarettes (smoking can also compromise healing of the intraoral and subnasal graft regions). The patient also should cough with an open mouth to relieve pressure.

Potential Complications

Bleeding is rarely a concern during the subnasal elevation and bone augmentation procedures. If bleeding does occur, pressure, hemostatic agents, bone wax, or electrocautery can be used to contain the vessels. Postoperative swelling in the region is common, but the pain is less severe than that which follows a sinus grafting procedure or the placement of mandibular implants.

Inadequate soft tissue management causes the most devastating effect during the immediate postoperative phase. Blood supply to the graft can be compromised by improper flap design, and excessive tension on the incision line can cause it to open and expose the graft. Delayed healing, leakage of graft material into the oral cavity, and increased risk of infection may result.

During placement, an implant may penetrate the nasal fossa or even the maxillary sinus because of insufficient grafting of the area. If this occurs, the implant can become accidentally displaced into the sinus or nasal cavity during the healing period. Tight fixation of the implants should always be confirmed at the time of surgery, and any implant that is mobile or inadequately stabilized should be removed.[7]

When the implant is not placed sufficiently in bone, especially when soft tissue may adhere to the implant, downgrowth of the epithelium may compromise osseointegration. However, at least three studies have reported that during healing, no undesirable side effects occurred secondary to incidental penetration of titanium screws into the maxillary sinus or nasal cavity, providing the implant was located sufficiently in bone.[13-15]

If an implant or graft becomes infected, local spread of inflammation from an infected maxillary implant can cause rhinitis or sinusitis. Maxillary sinusitis can also occur when an implant becomes displaced and acts as a foreign body, causing chronic infection.[16]

If septoplasty procedures are performed, care must be taken to avoid septal displacement or deviation. This generally does not occur if only the anterior inferior septal area is resected.[17]

Conclusion

Subnasal elevation is a useful procedure that is extremely predictable when using at least 50% autogenous bone. It provides additional bone height in the anterior maxilla for patients who are otherwise good candidates for dental implants. Procedures to increase the bone width are also frequently required in order to allow for implant placement.

References

1. Raghoebar GM, Batenburg RH, Vissink A, Reintsema H. Augmentation of localized defects of the anterior maxillary ridge with autogenous bone before insertion of implants. J Oral Maxillofac Surg 1996;54:1180–1185.
2. Keller EE, Tolman DE, Eckert SE. Maxillary antral-nasal inlay autogenous bone graft reconstruction of compromised maxilla: A 12-year retrospective study. Int J Oral Maxillofac Implants 1999;14:707–721.
3. Lundgren S, Nystrom E, Nilson H, Gunne J, Lindhagen O. Bone grafting to the maxillary sinuses, nasal floor and anterior maxilla in the atrophic edentulous maxilla: A two-stage technique. Int J Oral Maxillofac Surg 1997; 26:428–434.
4. Lozada JL, Emanuelli S, James RA, Boskovic M, Lindsted K. Root-form implants placed in subantral grafted sites. J Calif Dent Assoc 1993;21:31–35.
5. Tataryn RW, Torabinejad M, Boyne PJ. Healing potential of osteotomies of the nasal sinus of the dog. Oral Surg Oral Med Oral Pathol Oral Radiol Endod 1997;84:196–202.
6. Keller EE, Eckert SE, Tolman DE. Maxillary antral and nasal one-stage inlay composite bone graft: Preliminary report on 30 recipient sites. J Oral Maxillofac Surg 1994;52:438–447.
7. Adell R, Lekholm U, Grondahl K, Branemark PI, Lindstrom J, Jacobsson M. Reconstruction of severely resorbed edentulous maxillae using osseointegrated fixtures in immediate autogenous bone grafts. Int J Oral Maxillofac Implants 1990;5:233–246.
8. Keller EE, Tolman DE, Brånemark PI. Surgical reconstruction of advanced maxillary resorption with composite grafts. In: Worthington P, Brånemark PI (eds). Advanced Osseointegration Surgery: Application in the Maxillary Region. Chicago: Quintessence, 1992;146–161.
9. Misch CE, Dietsh F. Bone-grafting materials in implant dentistry. Implant Dent 1993;2: 158–167.
10. Koole R, Bosker H, van der Dussen FN. Late secondary autogenous bone grafting in cleft patients comparing mandibular (ectomesenchymal) and iliac crest (mesenchymal) grafts. J Craniomaxillofac Surg 1989;17(suppl 1):28–30.
11. Garg AK. Practical Implant Dentistry. Dallas: Taylor, 1996:89–101.
12. Hising P, Bolin A, Branting C. Reconstruction of severely resorbed alveolar ridge crests with dental implants using bovine bone mineral for augmentation. Int J Oral Maxillofac Implants 2001;16:90–97.
13. Brånemark PI, Adell R, Albrektsson T, Lekholm U, Lindstrom J, Rockler B. An experimental and clinical study of osseointegrated implants penetrating the nasal cavity and maxillary sinus. J Oral Maxillofac Surg 1984; 42:497–505.
14. Jensen J, Sindet-Pedersen S, Oliver AJ. Varying treatment strategies for reconstruction of maxillary atrophy with implants: Results in 98 patients. J Oral Maxillofac Surg 1994;52: 210–216.
15. Jensen J, Sindet-Pedersen S. Autogenous mandibular bone grafts and osseointegrated implants for reconstruction of the severely atrophied maxilla: A preliminary report. J Oral Maxillofac Surg 1991;49:1277–1287.
16. Ueda M, Kaneda T. Maxillary sinusitis caused by dental implants: Report of two cases. J Oral Maxillofac Surg 1992;50:285–287.
17. Garg AK. Nasal sinus lift: An innovative technique for implant insertions. Dent Implantol Update 1997;8:49–53.

PART

IV

Future Directions

CHAPTER

11

Biologic Growth Factors and Bone Morphogens in Bone Regeneration Procedures

Perhaps the most promising research currently underway on bone regeneration is the incorporation of biologic growth factors and bone morphogens. In general, these biologic proteins are intimately involved in regulating the cellular events that occur during repair of bone and other tissues in the body. Such processes include cell proliferation, chemotaxis, mitosis, differentiation, and matrix synthesis. Growth factors bind to specific receptors on target cell surfaces, leading to a complex cascade of intracellular events that culminates in bone formation. The basic theory is that by clinically applying an added number of these bone-building "orchestrators" to a wound site, they may in effect jump-start and perhaps even improve the body's normal osteoregenerative potential. Some researchers even speculate that in the not-too-distant future, growth factors and bone morphogens may eventually make the use of other bone graft materials—even autogenous bone—obsolete. The potential also exists for achieving earlier and better osseointegration of dental implants.

Such biologic treatments are just beginning to enter the market for orthopedic applications. InFuse Bone Graft (Medtronic Sofamore Danek, Memphis, TN) received Food and Drug Administration (FDA) approval in early 2002 for use in spinal fusion surgery. This product consists of two collagen sponges that can be soaked in recombinant human bone morphogenetic protein-2 (rhBMP-2) and placed into the defect or inserted into a titanium cage for spinal surgery (Fig 11-1). Another biologic product, Stryker Biotech OP-1 (Stryker Biotech, Natick, MA), received a Humanitarian Device Exemption from the FDA in

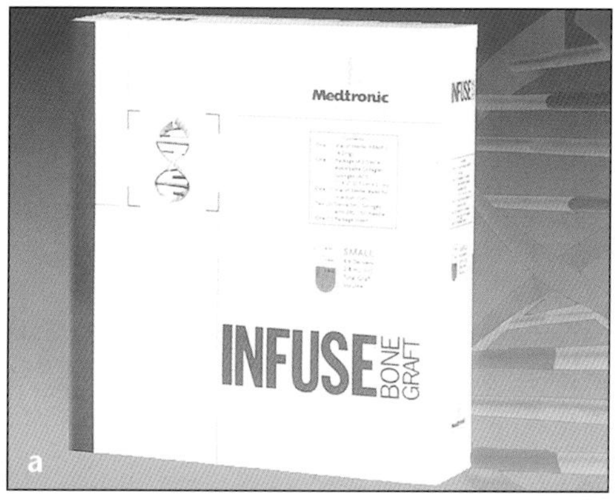

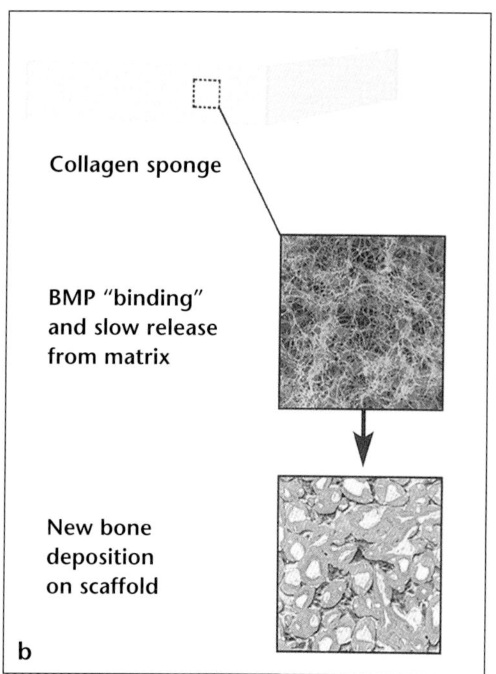

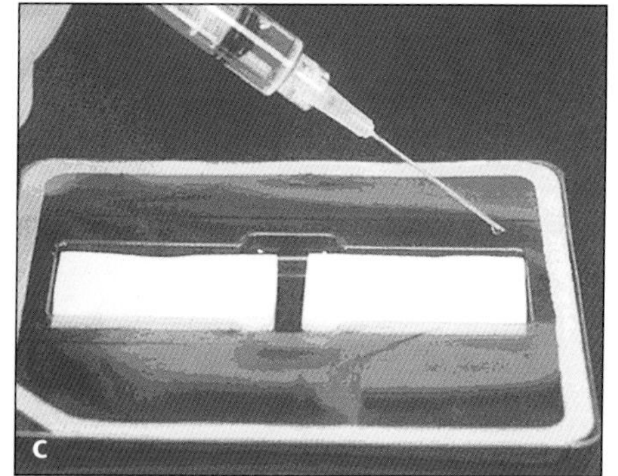

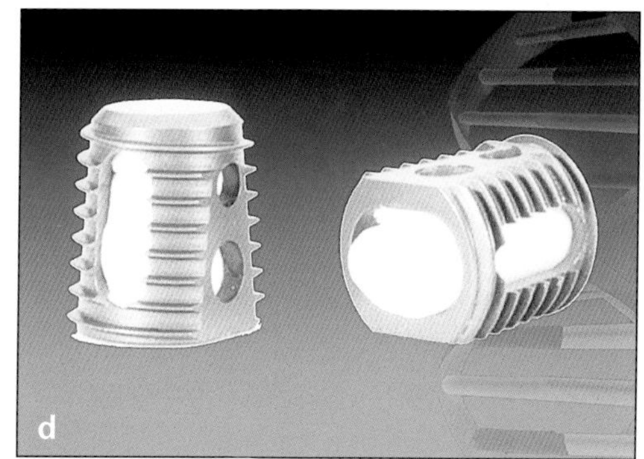

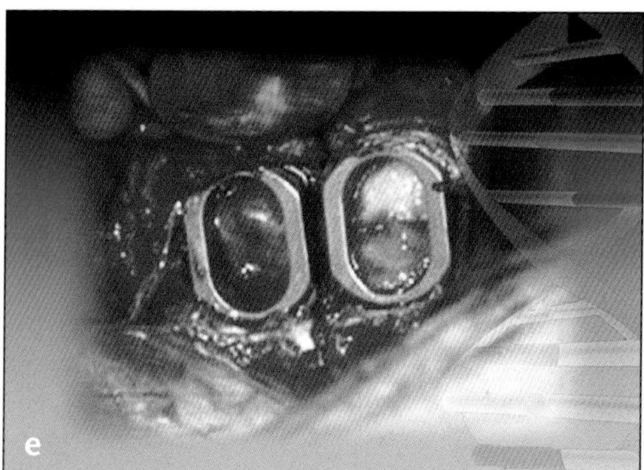

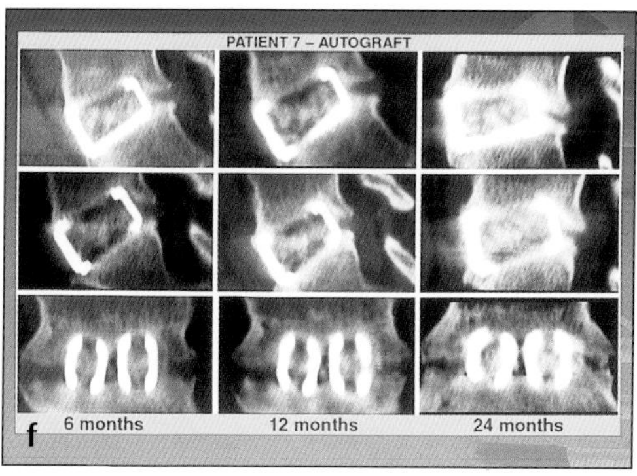

Fig 11-1

(a) Small package of the InFuse material, which contains two collagen sponges and rhBMP-2.

(b) When used as a carrier for rhBMP-2, an absorbable collagen sponge retains the rhBMP-2 at the surgical site and provides a favorable environment for bone formation.

(c) Absorbable collagen sponges act as carriers to deliver rhBMP-2.

(d) Tapered interbody titanium cages filled with autogenous iliac crest bone grafts or with collagen sponges soaked in rhBMP-2 are used for lumbar spine surgery in patients with degenerative lumbar disc disease.

(e) Two titanium cages filled with the rhBMP-2–saturated collagen sponges have been placed at the spinal surgical site. This comparative clinical study randomly divided the subjects into two groups that underwent interbody fusion via two tapered fusion cages: one group of 143 patients with rhBMP-2 on an absorbable collagen sponge and the other of 132 patients with autogenous anterior iliac crest grafts. At 24 months, the fusion rate was 5.8% higher in the BMP group (94.5% fusion rate) than in the control group (88.7% fusion rate).

(f) A serial computerized tomography (CT) image shows the right cage (upper), the left cage (middle), and a coronal view of both (lower) at 6, 12, and 24 months, revealing evidence of bony induction and early incorporation of bone in both groups.

2001 for use in no more than 4,000 adult cases per year requiring treatment for nonunions of tibia secondary to trauma in which autografts have failed or are not feasible. The product was also approved in 2001 by the European Agency for Evaluation of Medicinal Products for the same application, without limitation on number of cases, in all 15 European Union countries plus Iceland and Norway. Thus far no biologic treatments have been approved for maxillofacial reconstruction; however, as of this writing a large, multicenter, phase 3 clinical trial is underway on rhBMP-2, one of the most promising growth factors for use in dental applications.

Several other individual growth factors and their specific functions in bone healing have also been identified and tested for their ability to affect bone growth. These include platelet-derived growth factor (PDGF), insulin-like growth factor (IGF), fibroblastic growth factor (FGF), and transforming growth factor-beta (TGF-β). This chapter describes their function in bone formation and provides information on the current state of research for each factor.

Growth Factors

Platelet-Derived Growth Factor

PDGF is one of the principal wound-healing hormones. It plays several important roles in bone formation and regeneration, including *(1)* increasing the number of healing cells (including osteoblasts) present at the wound site; *(2)* transforming endothelial mitoses into functioning capillaries; *(3)* debriding the wound site; and *(4)* providing a second-phase source of growth factors for continued bone regeneration.[1] Its primary effect is as a potent mitogen, initiating cell division, and as a chemotactic factor for cells of mesenchymal origin, including osteoblasts. Several subtypes of PDGFs exist; they consist of homodimers or heterodimers of the PDGF-A and PDGF-B gene products. Sources of PDGF include platelets as well as activated macrophages and bone matrix.[2] The most intense area of PDGF research involves the use of platelet-rich-plasma (PRP), as described below.

Because growth factors are cell-specific, meaning that particular growth factors work only to stimulate specific cell types, many researchers studying the usefulness of PDGF have also focused on combining it with other growth factors to optimize complete tissue regeneration. Much of the research on such PDGF combinations—particularly with IGF—has addressed their usefulness for periodontal regeneration,[3] including a recent clinical trial (FDA phase 1 and 2) of 38 patients with moderate to severe periodontitis. At 6 to 9 months postsurgery, patients treated with a combination of PDGF-BB and IGF-1 (150 μg/mL of each) experienced a statistically significant 43% mean bone fill (with 2.1 mm vertical bone height), whereas control groups receiving either sham surgery or carrier alone experienced an average 18.5% fill (with 0.8 mm vertical bone height).[4]

Lee et al demonstrated the ability of PDGF to induce bone regeneration earlier than guided bone regeneration alone.[5] His team placed 500 ng of PDGF-BB in molded poly(L-lactide) membranes and inserted them into defects of various sizes in four rabbit calvaria. At 4 weeks, the dome-shaped treated membranes obtained almost complete bone formation (28% new bone) compared with untreated membranes (13% new bone). Controls did not completely refill until 12 to 18 weeks.

In a few canine studies, researchers have demonstrated that the PDGF-IGF combination may also enhance bone growth around implants and accelerate osseointegration. In a study by Lynch et al, 40 implants with apical holes containing either the PDGF-IGF combination or carrier alone were assessed after 1 and 3 weeks in the mandibular premolars of eight beagle dogs.[6] At 1 week, peri-implant bone fill and bone-to-implant contact were significantly higher in the test group. By 3 weeks, bone fill was still significantly greater in the test group, but bone-to-implant contact differences became insignificant. In another study, Stefani et al also noted significantly earlier bone formation and more bone-to-implant contact (22% vs 17%) within the first 3 weeks in patients treated with the PDGF-IGF combination compared with controls in a histometric study involving immediate implant placement in eight dogs.[7] Yet another study evaluated the PDGF-IGF combination with guided bone regeneration in fresh extraction sockets of four dogs with buccal dehiscences and implants.[8] At 18 weeks, Becker et al observed denser bone and twice as much bone-to-implant contact and area of peri-implant bone fill in the defects treated with the growth factors and expanded polytetrafluoroethylene (e-PTFE) membrane compared with controls receiving membranes alone.[8]

The mechanism by which these growth factor combinations improve bone and periodontal regeneration still must be proven in vivo, as must the specific amounts of the growth factors that would be optimally useful.

Insulin-like Growth Factor

There are two types of IGF—IGF-I and IGF-II—that function similarly but are independently regulated. As their name indicates, IGFs are biochemically and functionally similar to insulin.[1] They are primarily produced by the liver and circulate in the vascular system.[2] Although its direct or indirect effects on bone remodeling are not fully understood, IGF-I appears to stimulate bone formation by increasing cellular proliferation and differentiation as well as bone matrix production. Some evidence suggests IGF-I may mediate the ability of parathyroid hormone to stimulate osteoprogenitor cell proliferation within bones.[9]

As mentioned previously, animal studies suggest that IGF-I works synergistically with PDGF; it initiates better tissue regenerative results in combination than it does on its own. Thus, most in vivo studies have incorporated IGF in combination with this and other growth factors.

Fibroblast Growth Factor

FGFs received their name because of their general growth-promoting effects on most fibroblastic cell types. This growth factor—which occurs in both acidic and basic forms and is stored in bone—also stimulates angiogenesis for vascular invasion of bone, wound healing, and cell migration. Both forms of FGF stimulate bone cell replication, but they can also inhibit matrix synthesis by bone cells under some conditions, and they have no stimulatory effect on mature osteoblasts.[3,10]

Lab studies suggest FGFs may stimulate endothelial and periodontal ligament cell migration and proliferation as well, but only a few positive in vivo studies supporting an enhanced bone regenerative benefit for either orthopedic or craniomaxillofacial applications have been reported.[11-14] Appropriate dosage and delivery systems are important unresolved issues regarding FGF.[13-15]

Transforming Growth Factor-Beta

TGF-β is a multifunctional growth factor synthesized by many cell types, and almost every cell type can be stimulated by at least one of the various TGF-β molecules. It is one of the major growth factors present in bone (as well as platelets) and is structurally related to, but functionally different from, the BMPs. Generally, TGF-β is a weak mitogen for osteoblasts. It has been shown to be chemotactic for bone cells and may increase or decrease their proliferation depending on various conditions. It has also been shown to stimulate type-1 collagen synthesis.[2,3] Several in vivo studies have shown that TGF-β can induce new cartilage and bone, but only if it is planted in proximity to a bony site.[3] As with IGF, in vitro evidence suggests that TGF-β may exert more powerful bone-forming effects in combination with PDGF.[16] In vivo studies demonstrate that TGF-β_1 can induce bone closure of calvarial defects in rabbits,[17] enhance fracture healing in rabbit tibiae,[18] and promote osseous wound healing in rats.[19] These studies also suggest that TGF-β_1 has a dose-related effect on bone induction, but that a higher dose does not always generate more bone.

Two recent animal studies suggest that TGF-β_1 may be a useful adjunct to guided tissue regeneration (GTR) in inducing greater early bone formation. Mohammed et al studied TGF-β_1 with GTR in Class II furcation defects in the mandibular premolars of 24 sheep.[20] Defects treated with TGF-β_1 and membrane had significantly greater mean bone volume at 6 weeks (59%) than did those treated with membrane (53%) or carrier alone (43%). Ruskin et al also noted statistically more bone formation at 8 weeks in surgically created alveolar defects in 13 foxhounds when TGF-β_1 and a membrane were used (84%) compared with when TGF-β_1 (61%) or a carrier alone (30%) were used.[21]

Platelet-Rich Plasma

Although the application of growth factors shows great promise for enhancing wound healing and bone regeneration, approved pharmaceutical formulations are still not forthcoming. In addition, procuring growth factors for eventual clinical use is likely to be an expensive proposition. Therefore, as an alternative source of growth factors, PRP has become an increasingly popular clinical tool for several types of surgery, including oral bone-regenerative procedures.

PRP is a concentrated autologous source of several growth factors, particularly PDGF, TGF-β_1, and TGF-β_2, as well as vascular endothelial growth factor (VEGF), IGF, and other growth factors possibly contained within platelets. Once the clinician prepares PRP by extracting a small amount of the patient's own blood and then sequestering and concentrating the platelets—a process that requires 20 to 30 minutes in an outpatient clinical setting—PRP can be used to enhance graft material, to form a growth factor–rich membrane,[22] or to enhance a traditional barrier membrane. PRP's fibrinogen component also makes it an excellent hemostatic tool, tissue sealant, wound stabilizer, and graft condenser through the creation of a gel-like substance that allows for sculpting and excellent adherence in defects.

It has been shown radiographically that adding PRP to graft material significantly accelerates the rate of bone formation and improves trabecular bone density as compared with sites treated only with autogenous graft material.[22,23] Widespread clinical reports and recent published research also suggest that PRP significantly enhances soft tissue healing; reduces bleeding, edema, and scarring; and decreases patients' self-reported pain levels postoperatively.[24–29] Some evidence even suggests that adding PRP to graft material leads to growth of bone that is more dense than native bone,[23,30] a potential benefit that has not been reported in studies where BMPs or growth factors are applied alone. PRP growth factors are particularly attractive for use in patients with conditions that typically reduce the success of bone grafts and osseointegration, including those with an edentulous and severely atrophic maxilla, osteoporosis, and tissues that have been scarred and altered by prior dental disease.[31]

The concentrated levels of PDGF and TGF-β in PRP (in addition to the presence of other growth factors and proteins) appear to provide benefits that lead to more rapid and effective bone regeneration. The beneficial effects of these growth factors can perhaps best be understood through a description of the components and biology of PRP.

PRP components and bone healing

An understanding of how PRP growth factors may enhance bone grafts and implant osseointegration requires a description of the components of PRP and their roles in wound and bone healing (Fig 11-2).

Specific studies of PRP have identified at least three important factors in the alpha granules of the sequestered platelets: PDGF, TGF-β_1, and TGF-β_2.[32–34] In addition, other studies have documented the presence of VEGF and IGF-I in platelets from peripheral human blood tests.[35–39]

PDGF is considered one of the principal healing hormones in any wound, and platelets are the greatest source of this growth factor in the human body.[23] PDGF isolated from human platelets consists of homodimers (AA or BB) or heterodimers (AB) of the two PDGF gene products, with the heterodimers predominating. Two different PDGF homodimers, PDGF-AA and -BB, are 56% autologous, encoded by different genes, and independently regulated. Recent evidence indicates that the PDGF-AB heterodimer and PDGF-BB homodimer have equivalent activity and are equally potent in stimulating DNA synthesis in human fibroblasts.[40,41]

PDGF-AA and PDGF-BB were found to be potent mitogens for human periodontal ligament cells, maximally enhancing the mitogenic response 10- and 12-fold, respectively; furthermore, the mitogenic response for both PDGF isoforms increased, depending on the dosage. A 1989 study identifies two receptor subunit molecules, alpha and beta, for PDGF.[42] The AA isoform binds only alpha-receptor dimers, while the BB isoform binds all combinations of alpha- and beta-receptor dimers. The number of receptor-binding sites for each isoform is thought to determine the mitogenic potency of each isoform in a given cell type. Thus, the strategy behind PRP use is amplification and acceleration of the effects of growth factors contained in platelets, the universal initiators of almost all wound healing (Fig 11-3).

TGF-β_1 and -β_2 are multifunctional cytokines involved in general connective tissue repair and bone regeneration. Their most important role appears to be the chemotaxis and mitogenesis of osteoblast precursors and the stimulation of deposition of collagen matrix for wound healing and bone formation.[23] These growth factors also enhance bone formation by increasing the rate of stem cell proliferation and, to some degree, inhibit osteoclast formation and, thus, bone resorption.[43,44] Bone and platelets contain approximately 100 times more TGF-β than do any other tissues, and osteoblasts contain the greatest number of TGF-β receptors.[45]

PRP also contains fibrin, fibronectin, and vitronectin, cell-adhesion molecules

Fig 11-2
(a) Proper technique preserves cell viability when whole blood is separated into its main components, such as these packed red blood cells from a blood bank.

(b) A bag of concentrated platelets from a blood bank.

(c) A bag of blood plasma from a blood bank.

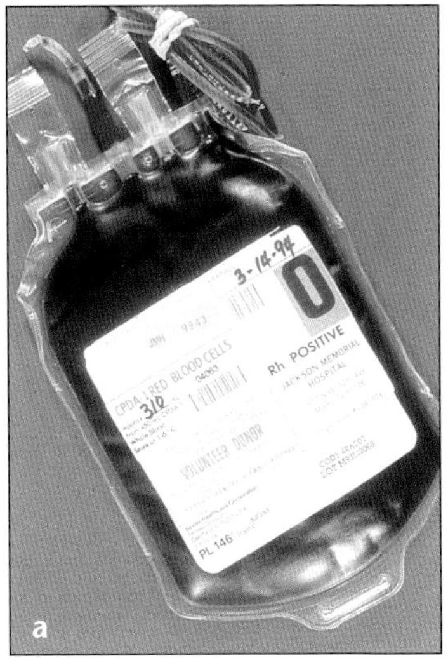

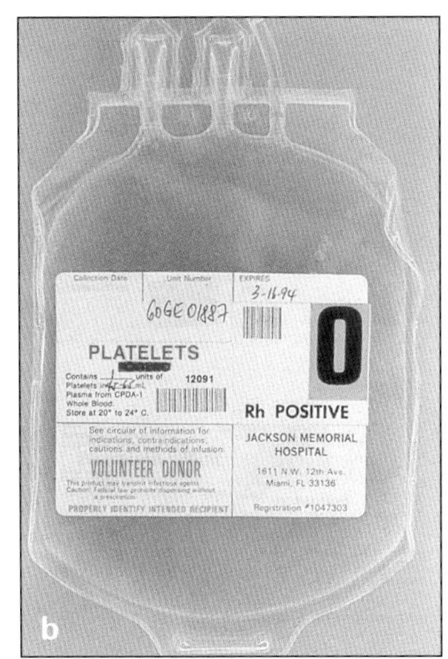

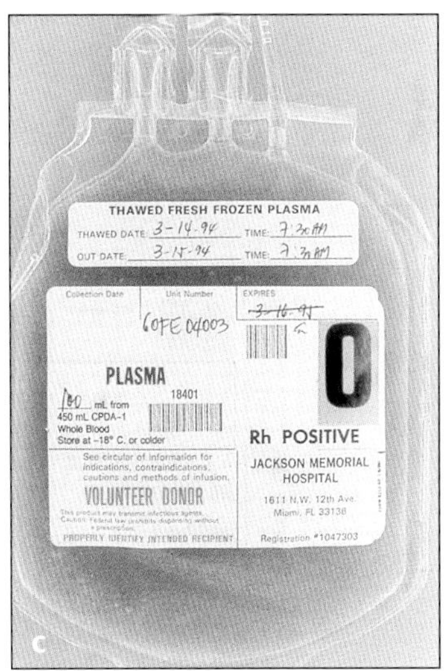

Fig 11-3
A device designed and priced for office use separates 20 to 60 mL of blood drawn from a patient into its components.

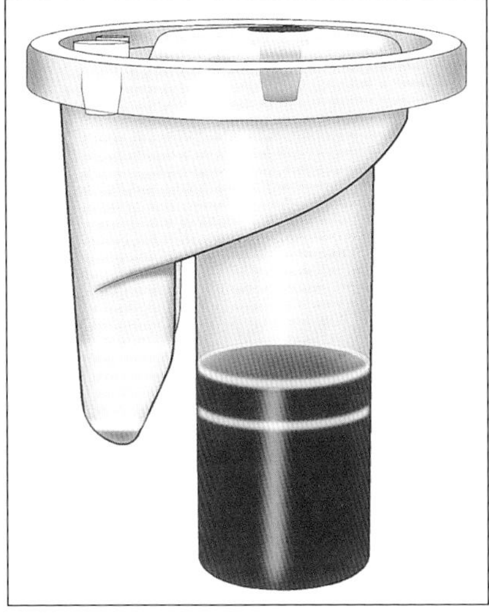

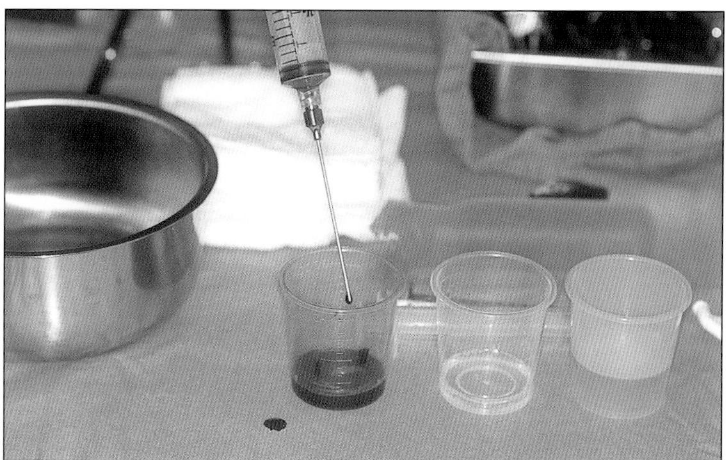

Fig 11-4
PRP is placed on the surgical field. A mixture of thrombin and calcium chloride is used to activate the concentrated platelets to release their growth factors and to initiate gelling for better clinical handling.

that support cell migration (osteoconduction) (Fig 11-4).[46] The dense fibrin net that PRP provides is also hemostatic, and it helps to bind graft material and to stabilize the blood clot in the defect once applied, possibly acting as a barrier membrane to impede the migration of epithelial and connective tissue cells.[46] Its hemostatic and wound-sealing effects have proven useful in cardiovascular, orthopedic, plastic, and other surgeries. PRP also modulates and upregulates one growth factor's function in the presence of the other growth factors. This feature separates PRP growth factors from recombinant growth factors, which focus only on a single regeneration pathway.[22]

Bone Morphogenetic Proteins

Although bone morphogenetic proteins (BMPs) are often referred to as a category of growth factors, they are actually a distinct group of proteins. Bone-related growth factors exist primarily in bone matrix and are released during remodeling or in response to trauma. When this occurs, the growth factors modulate or stimulate the neighboring osteoprogenitor (differentiated) cells that are already present in the area, inducing and aiding bone formation. Because they rely on the presence of local osteoprogenitor cells, however, growth factors cannot induce bone growth in ectopic sites. Their effect is also limited in large bony defects.[47]

The main advantage of BMPs, which are also found in extracellular bone matrix, is that they do not require existing osteoprogenitor cells to form bone. BMPs are osteoinductive factors that can stimulate mesenchymal cells to differentiate into cartilage- and bone-forming cells (Fig 11-5).[48] Unlike true growth factors, however, they are not mitogenic for many cells and cell types.[49] In embryonic development, BMPs affect the direction of cell differentiation and also act as positional signals, providing information needed to form a growth pattern that culminates in the adult form. Whether the ability to form such a pattern also exists in adult bone regeneration is still unclear, but the properties of BMPs essentially allow them to create an unlimited amount of new bone.[47]

The development of bone can occur in two ways. With intramembranous ossification, mesenchymal cells differentiate di-

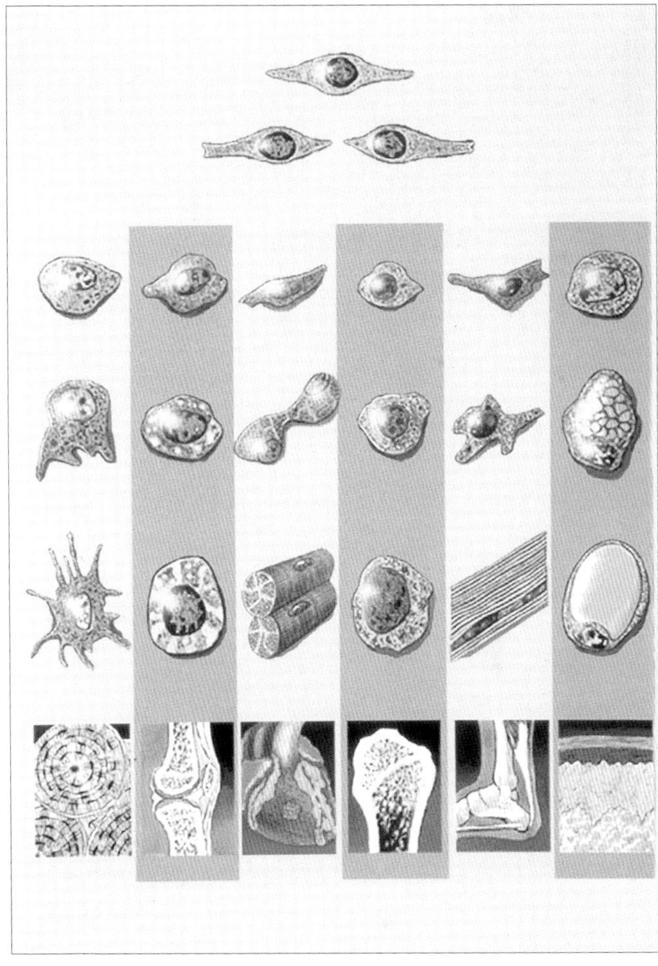

Fig 11-5
Growth factors can stimulate mesenchymal stem cells to differentiate according to the body's needs. For example, a mother cell can change into a chondroblast or epithelial cell. Likewise, BMPs can stimulate mesenchymal cells to differentiate into bone-forming cells (osteoblasts).

rectly to bone. This occurs in the flat bones of the craniofacial skeleton. With endochondral ossification, cartilage provides a blueprint for bone morphogenesis, and this ephemeral blueprint is subsequently replaced by bone. This is how most bones in the human skeleton are formed.[50] BMPs appear to be capable of influencing both types of bone formation.[51,52]

Marshall Urist is credited with the earliest work that isolated BMPs during the 1960s. He discovered that this extractable protein in demineralized bone matrix was responsible for inducing bone formation when implanted ectopically in an animal.[53] Early on, isolating and purifying BMPs was difficult because only trace amounts exist in bone. In 1988, Wang et al made a major advancement by identifying three different BMPs in bovine bone, characterizing their amino acid sequences, and then isolating recombinant clones for each one that were used to screen the corresponding human DNA libraries.[54] This led to the discovery of recombinant human BMP-1, -2a, and -3. Since then, the number of known BMPs has increased to at least 15, each of which has a slightly different amino acid structure.[55] Most of these BMPs are related to one another and are classified as part of the TGF-β superfamily because of their amino acid sequences.

Although it has been decades since BMPs were isolated, progress on their clinical usefulness has proceeded fairly slowly as researchers continue to grapple with

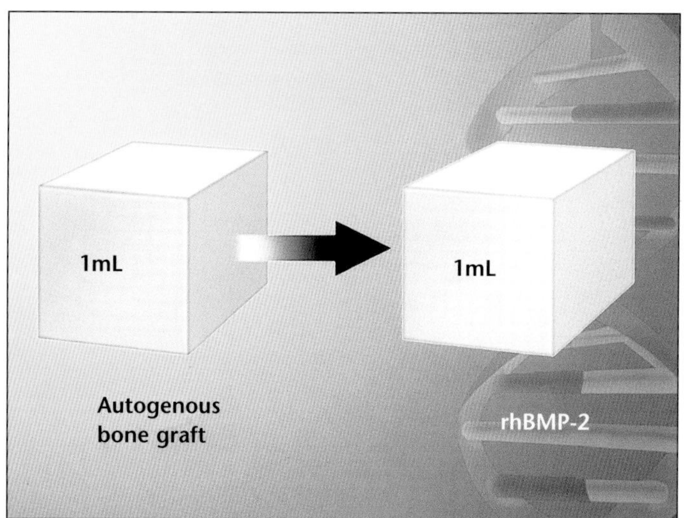

Fig 11-6
The volumetric relationship of InFuse on collagen to autogenous bone when grafting. The relationship between rhBMP-2 and autograft is 1:1—1 mL of InFuse on a collagen sponge will generate the same amount of bone as 1 mL of autogenous bone graft material.

long-standing problems, including identifying adequate carriers to immobilize the BMPs for a sufficient duration (an area of intense research at the present time),[56] determining optimal dosages, and completing reliable studies on BMP use in specific maxillofacial sites.[57]

Nonetheless, recombinant DNA technology has allowed the production of BMP-2 and BMP-7, also known as osteogenic protein-1 (OP-1), in large quantities. They are the most extensively researched BMPs to date, having undergone human clinical trials and received limited approval for use in orthopedics for large segmental bone defects. There is still relatively limited experience with human recombinant BMPs in the craniomaxillofacial area, however. Studies on these bone-inducing proteins are discussed in the following section.

Recombinant Human BMP-2

As stated earlier, the primary activity of rhBMP-2 appears to be differentiating mesenchymal precursor cells into mature osteoblasts and/or chondroblasts. In addition, rhBMP-2 is chemotactic for some osteoblastic-type cells.

RhBMP-2 has been shown to induce the complete sequence of endochondral ossification. Its application results in local induction of cartilage, which is subsequently replaced by bone and marrow. It also appears to play a particularly important role in the early stage of osteoinduction.[58] As increasing amounts of rhBMP-2 are implanted into a site, the time required for bone formation to occur decreases. It has also been shown that large amounts of rhBMP-2 result in concurrent formation of cartilage and bone. These findings indicate that rhBMP-2 may influence both the direct bone formation pathway and the endochondral sequence (Fig 11-6).[51]

Cross-species applications of rhBMP-2 have demonstrated its ability to support healing of critical-sized defects. Results from a study of rhBMP-2 in a canine model showed an extensive amount of bone regeneration after rhBMP-2 was surgically implanted in 5-mm mandibular premolar defects compared with controls receiving no BMPs. The benefits were observed histometrically in terms of height (means of 3.5 vs 0.8 mm in controls) and new bone area (means of 8.4 vs 0.4 mm in controls).[59]

In another canine model, mandibular premolars were extracted and rectangular bone defects measuring 10 × 8 × 7 mm were created and filled with either rhBMP-2 or an untreated carrier.[60] In the control group, there was virtually no bone formation during the 12-week computerized tomography (CT) and histologic observation period. In the rhBMP-2–treated group, however, new bone was found in all defects from 4 weeks onward, with complete fill seen by week 12. Qualitative CT scans also showed that the bone had integrated well with the surrounding cortical host bone and was similarly dense by 12 weeks.

Another study in canine models evaluated the regenerative ability of rhBMP-2 in horizontal circumferential defects along root surfaces with a history of periodontal disease.[61] Results of this study showed a significantly greater amount of new bone formation in the sites treated with rhBMP-2 than in control sites.

In a histomorphometric analysis of extracted maxillary premolars from rats, Matin et al noted significantly faster bone reformation in sockets implanted with rhBMP-2 compared with controls, with greater bone height and total area after 14, 28, and 56 days.[62] Comparable completed healing in both groups was observed at day 84. This may be explained by the greater numbers of proliferating cells and densely populated differentiating mesenchymal cells that were observed on the rhBMP-2 sockets in the early stage.

Studies have also focused on the use of rhBMP-2 rather than graft material for cases requiring maxillary sinus augmentation. In the first clinical study, Boyne et al evaluated 11 of 12 patients who underwent sinus elevation with rhBMP-2 in an absorbable collagen sponge carrier.[63] All patients experienced induced bone formation, averaging 8.5 mm in height. The regenerated maxillary bone in 8 of the 11 patients was judged suitable for accommodating implants following the BMP treatment. Histologic analysis of bone cores removed during implant placement showed a density similar to that of native bone.

In an animal study, Nevins et al histologically showed more rapid bone formation in sinuses augmented with rhBMP-2 compared with untreated controls.[64] More recently, Wada et al used a canine model to show comparable results in bone quality and quantity achieved when either rhBMP-2 or particulate cancellous bone and marrow harvested from the iliac crest were incorporated into maxillary sinus augmentation.[65]

Several recent studies have also focused on the usefulness of rhBMP-2 to encourage bone formation and osseointegration in dental implant cases.[49] In a pilot clinical study, Cochran et al followed 12 patients who received rhBMP-2 in an absorbable collagen sponge in either extraction sites or sites requiring ridge augmentation prior to implant insertion.[66] Most sites were in the anterior maxilla. Implants were placed from 16 to 30 weeks postoperatively. Three of 10 patients receiving implants required additional grafting prior to implant placement. All implants, including those placed in sites treated only with BMP, were stable during all follow-up visits. Once loaded, they remained immobile and functional during the entire observation period (ranging from 66 to 104 weeks postoperatively). Although the lack of controls makes it impossible to determine how much bone formation could be attributed to the rhBMP-2, the lack of adverse side effects and the long-term success of the implants that were placed indicate that rhBMP-2 can be used safely in these defects and that dental implants placed in bony areas treated with rhBMP-2 can be functionally restored without complication[66] (Fig 11-7).

RhBMP-2 also shows some promise for encouraging earlier osseointegration of implants. For instance, Bessho et al compared the reverse torque value of implants placed with either BMP in a collagen carrier or with an untreated carrier.[67] Six edentulous dogs received 36 total screw implants dispersed among each quadrant. A reverse test at 3 weeks showed that the average for BMP-stimulated implants was more than twice that of the controls, suggesting rapid early bone formation with BMP. Histologic assessment also showed a statistically higher bone contact length at this point compared with controls. However, this difference in contact diminished histologically by week 12, when there was no statistical difference between the test and control groups. Interestingly, the mean reverse torque value for the controls at 12 weeks was not statistically different from that for the BMP implants at 3 weeks.

In a canine model by Sykaras et al, 104 hollow cylinder implants were placed in the extracted mandibular premolar area of 14 foxhound dogs.[68] Half served as controls and half had their implant chambers filled with rhBMP-2 in a collagen sponge. Although there was no difference in bone growth at 2 weeks, the rhBMP-2 group regained statistically more bone than did controls by week 4 (23.48% vs 5.98%) and week 8 (20.94% vs 7.75%). By week 12, there was no significant difference in bone growth, but bone-to-implant contact remained significantly higher for the BMP-treated group (43.78% vs 21.05%). However, complete bone fill of the extraction sites was not achieved.[68]

In a primate study, Hanisch et al demonstrated the capacity of implanted rhBMP-2 to induce dental implant reosseointegration.[69] After creating advanced peri-implantitis defects in four rhesus monkeys treated with implants, they observed three times more bone reformation in the defects treated with rhBMP-2 than in untreated controls (2.6 vs 0.8 mm). Bone-to-implant contact was also statistically better in the treated defect areas compared with the controls (29% vs 4%).

Other researchers using canine models have noted similar improvements in the rate and extent of bone formation compared with controls when rhBMP-2 was used with dental implants.[70–72] However, osseointegration results have tended to be variable, perhaps because of varying dosages, carrier materials, or implant and defect characteristics.[68,73,74]

Recombinant BMP-7/ Osteogenic Protein-1

The use of recombinant DNA techniques to produce BMP-7 (also known as OP-1) has allowed extensive research on its clinical usefulness thus far, primarily in orthopedic cases. As mentioned earlier, an orthopedic OP-1 product was approved in the European Union to treat very large segmental bone defects; the FDA also granted a limited-use approval for this orthopedic indication. Research on the use of OP-1 for human maxillofacial applications is relatively limited, but animal and some human studies have been published.

Like rhBMP-2 and other BMPs, OP-1 has been shown in animal models to be capable of initiating endochondral bone formation.[75] OP-1 has been shown in vivo to form new bone and to promote osteoblast growth as well as in vitro to maintain the osteoblast phenotype, indicating that it may be centrally involved in overall bone homeostasis.[76] It has also been shown to induce cementogenesis in furcation de-

Fig 11-7 The usefulness of rhBMP-2 to encourage bone formation for augmentation grafting for the maxillary sinus has been documented.

(a) Lyophilized rhBMP-2 prior to reconstitution for use in maxillary sinus elevation trials.

(b) Strips of collagen sponges soaked with lyophilized rhBMP-2.

(c) A window in the lateral wall of the maxilla provides access to the maxillary sinus cavity and reveals an intact schneiderian membrane, which has been carefully elevated to avoid tears and to contain the rhBMP-2.

(d) After careful elevation of the sinus membrane, the collagen strip saturated with rhBMP-2 is introduced into the sinus cavity.

(e) The clinician introduces the collagen membrane strips one by one into the cavity, making sure that no air pockets (empty spaces) are created.

(f) A modified amalgam plugger (3- to 5-mm-diameter tip) is ideal for packing the rhBMP-2–laden collagen sponge strips into the cavity.

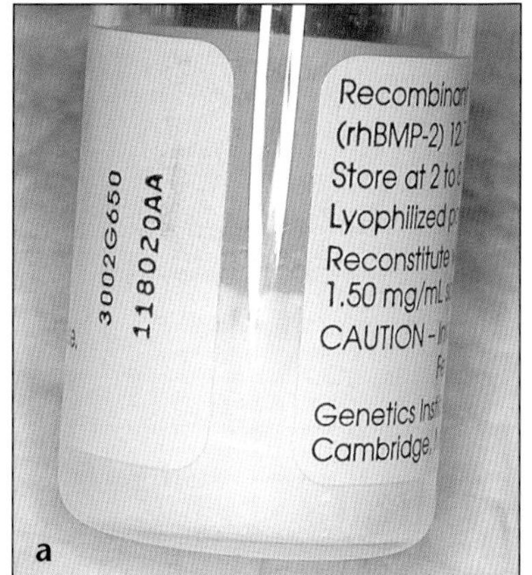

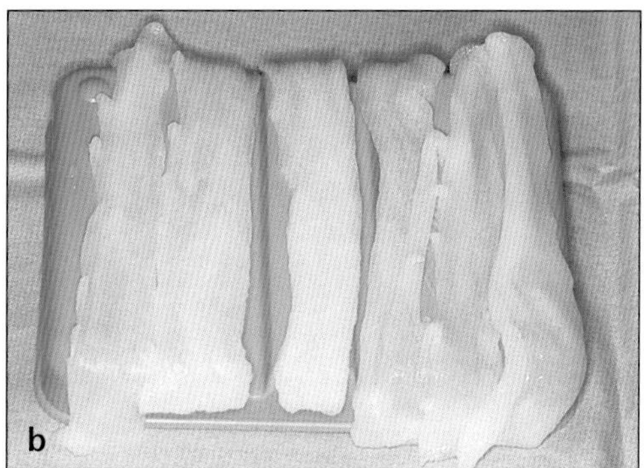

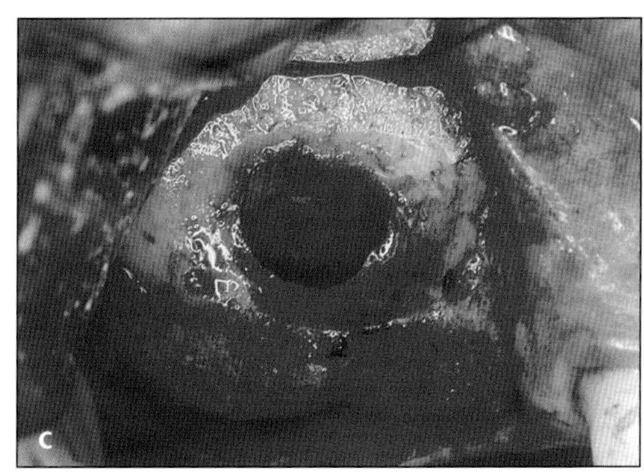

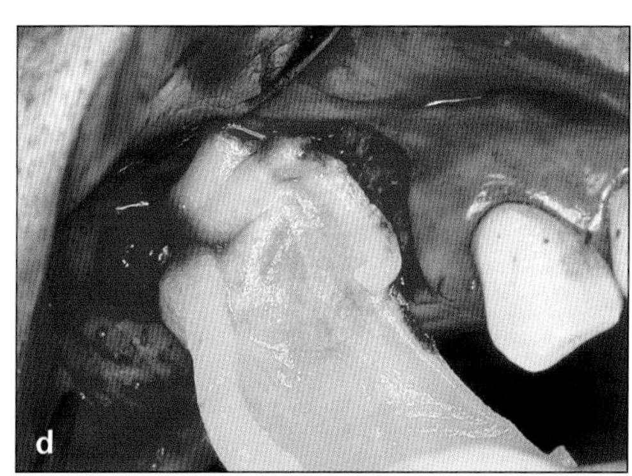

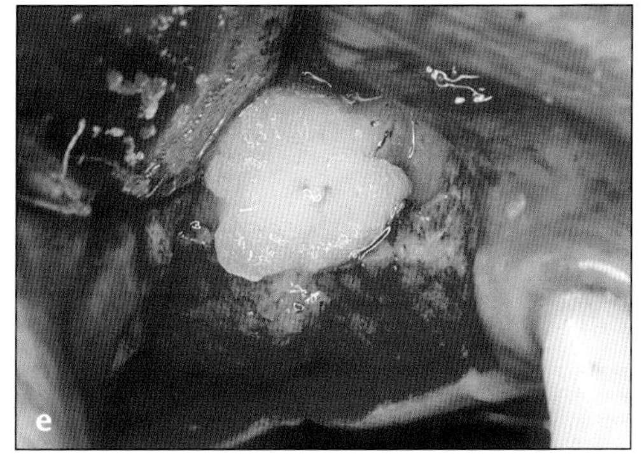

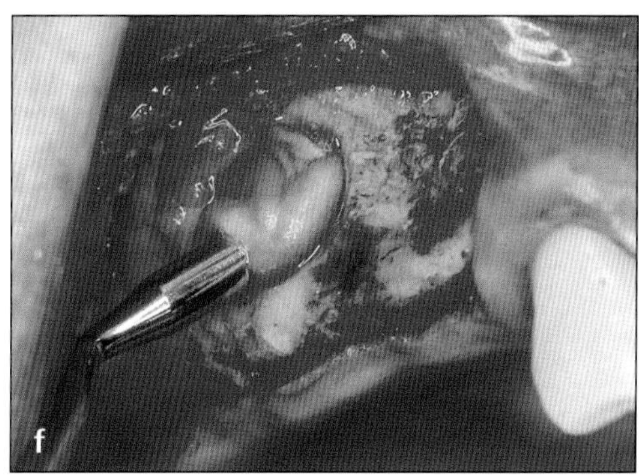

fects of the baboon[77-79] and the dog,[80] indicating that OP-1 may play a specific role in regenerating periodontal tissues.

In the most recent baboon study by Ripamonti et al, 12 furcation defects in the mandibular premolar area of three baboons were treated with OP-1, rhBMP-2, or a combination of both.[79] A histologic analysis 60 days postoperatively revealed that OP-1–treated sites showed substantial cementogenesis but relatively limited bone formation. Sites treated only with rhBMP-2 showed little cementogenesis but significantly more bone formation than either the OP-1 sites or those treated with the combination of rhBMP-2 and OP-1. The combination treatment led to the least amount of bone and attachment formation, although this may be because of dosages or other variables in the normal bone healing sequence.

In a study by Giannobile et al using higher dosages of OP-1, a substantial amount of bone regeneration—as well as cementogenesis and attachment formation—were noted in Class III mandibular furcation defects created in 18 beagle dogs.[80] A histomorphometric analysis at 8 weeks showed that bone formation was significant compared with defects receiving only surgery or the collagen carrier alone.

In two other animal studies, OP-1 was also shown to induce good-quality bone formation in extraction sites treated with immediately placed implants as well as close bone apposition to the implants compared with untreated controls.[81,82] However, Rutherford et al noted that significantly less bone was seen closely apposed to the threaded surface when the distance from implant to socket wall exceeded 3 mm.[83] Evidence of better bone quantity and quality compared with untreated controls was also seen in as few as 3 weeks in extraction sockets treated with OP-1 but not implants.[83]

Some studies have focused on the use of OP-1 in maxillary sinus augmentation, but its usefulness in encouraging bone formation in these challenging cases has been unpredictable. In a study by Margolin et al, two sinus lifts were performed in each of 15 chimpanzees.[84] The sites were then treated with natural bone mineral and one of three different dosages of OP-1 (0.25, 0.6, or 2.5 mg OP-1 per gram); with a collagen matrix and one of the three OP-1 dosages; or with a collagen matrix alone. Radiographic and histologic evidence showed that the best quantity and quality of bone formed with the 2.5 mg/1 g collagen matrix OP-1 graft by 7.5 months. The bone was deemed suitable for dental implantation.

In a study by van den Bergh et al,[57] three human sinus lift patients received the same 2.5-mg dosage of OP-1 in a collagen carrier, while another three received autogenous bone grafts. A clinical and histologic assessment after 6 months, however, showed that only one patient in the OP-1–treated group had well-vascularized, good-quality bone that could accommodate implant placement. Among the other test patients, one experienced no bone formation, and the other showed some bone-like formation but with substantial flexible tissue. However, all of the autogenous grafted sites showed new bone growth similar to normal maxillary bone. In a follow-up study, Groenveld et al followed the patient who experienced no bone growth for an additional 6 months.[81] However, no additional bone formed in the OP-1–treated site; in fact, most of the new bone was lost. The authors suggested this may have been caused by a lack of mechanical loading.

Terheyden et al[82] attempted to improve these outcomes by combining OP-1 and Bio-Oss in a study involving five miniature pigs who underwent bilateral maxillary sinus augmentation. One side received the combination treatment and the other was treated with Bio-Oss alone. Dental implants were placed simultaneously in each site. At 6 months, acceptable bone regeneration levels had occurred in both treatment groups; however, significantly better bone-to-implant contact percentages were noted in the sites receiving the combination treatment compared with the sites treated with Bio-Oss alone (80% vs 36%). The test sites also underwent earlier bone apposition—beginning as early as week 2—compared with controls, in which bone apposition was not seen until week 8.

Terheyden's group also investigated a novel approach to using OP-1 in mandibular reconstruction by implanting it in the latissimus dorsi muscle of miniature pigs and thereby prefabricating a vascularized bone graft. When this graft was transplanted into the mandibular defects and affixed with miniature plates, the reconstructive result was deemed significantly superior in terms of volume, shape, and contour compared to control sites treated with a combination of OP-1 and Bio-Oss.[85,86]

Future Directions

While further promising preclinical and clinical research continues to refine the usefulness of BMPs as an alternative to available bone graft materials, novel gene therapy approaches aimed at harnessing the power of these biologic mediators are also being investigated.[87] For instance, researchers at the University of Michigan and elsewhere have used ex vivo cellular reengineering methods to transfer genes encoding BMPs.[88,89] The actual gene transfer is accomplished in a tissue culture environment; the transduced cells, carrying the foreign genes, are then placed back into the host. In animal models, these researchers showed that several cell types, including osteoblasts, can express the BMP-7 gene after being infected with an adenoviral vector.[88] Researchers at the University of Virginia showed that it is possible to directly deliver the BMP-2 gene in vivo to tissue via an adenoviral vector (as opposed to ex vivo cellular reengineering) and thus achieve healing of mandibular defects.[90]

References

1. Marx RE, Carlson ER, Eichstaedt RM, Schimmele SR, Strauss JE, Georgeff KR. Platelet-rich plasma: Growth factor enhancement for bone grafts. Oral Surg Oral Med Oral Pathol Oral Radiol Endod 1998;85:638–646.
2. Rose LF, Rosenberg E. Bone grafts and growth and differentiation factors for regenerative therapy: A review. Pract Proced Aesthet Dent 2001;13:725–734.
3. Cochran DL, Wozney JM. Biological mediators for periodontal regeneration. Periodontol 2000 1999;19:40–58.
4. Howell TH, Fiorellini JP, Paquette DW, Offenbacher S, Giannobile WV, Lynch SE. A phase I/II clinical trial to evaluate a combination of recombinant human platelet-derived growth factor-BB and recombinant human insulin-like growth factor-I in patients with periodontal disease. J Periodontol 1997;68:1186–1193.
5. Lee SJ, Park YJ, Park SN, et al. Molded porous poly (L-lactide) membranes for guided bone regeneration with enhanced effects by controlled growth factor release. J Biomed Mater Res 2001;55:295–303.
6. Lynch SE, Buser D, Hernandez RA, et al. Effects on the platelet-derived growth factor/insulin-like growth factor-I combination on bone regeneration around titanium dental implants. Results of a pilot study in beagle dogs. J Periodontol 1991;62:710–716.
7. Stefani CM, Machado MA, Sallum EA, Sallum AW, Toledo S, Nociti FH Jr. Platelet-derived growth factor/insulin-like growth factor-1 combination and bone regeneration around implants placed into extraction sockets: A histometric study in dogs. Implant Dent 2000;9:126–131.
8. Becker W, Lynch SE, Lekholm U, et al. A comparison of ePTFE membranes alone or in combination with platelet-derived growth factors and insulin-like growth factor-I or demineralized freeze-dried bone in promoting bone formation around immediate extraction socket implants. J Periodontol 1992;63:929–940.

9. Tokimasa C, Kawata T, Fujita T, et al. Effects of insulin-like growth factor-I on nasopremaxillary growth under different masticatory loadings in growing mice. Arch Oral Biol 2000;45:871–878.
10. The potential role of growth and differentiation factors in periodontal regeneration. J Periodontol 1996;67:545–553.
11. Inui K, Maeda M, Sano A, et al. Local application of basic fibroblast growth factor minipellet induces the healing of segmental bony defects in rabbits. Calcif Tissue Int 1998;63: 490–495.
12. Hosokawa R, Kikuzaki K, Kimoto T, et al. Controlled local application of basic fibroblast factor (FGF-2) accelerates the healing of GBR. An experimental study in beagle dogs. Clin Oral Implants Res 2000;11:345–353.
13. Rossa C Jr, Marcantonio E Jr, Cirelli JA, Marcantonio RA, Spolidorio LC, Fogo JC. Regeneration of Class III furcation defects with basic fibroblast growth factor (b-FGF) associated with GTR. A descriptive and histometric study in dogs. J Periodontol 2000;71:775–784.
14. Aspenberg P, Thorngren KG, Lohmander LS. Dose-dependent stimulation of bone induction by basic fibroblast growth factor in rats. Acta Orthop Scand 1991;62:481–484.
15. Schliephake H, Jamil MU, Knebel JW. Experimental reconstruction of the mandible using polylactic acid tubes and basic fibroblast growth factor in alloplastic scaffolds. J Oral Maxillofac Surg 1998;56:616–626.
16. Mott DA, Mailhot J, Cuenin MF, Sharawy M, Borke J. Enhancement of osteoblast proliferation in vitro by selective enrichment of demineralized freeze-dried bone allograft with specific growth factors. J Oral Implantol 2002; 28:57–66.
17. Beck LS, Deguzman L, Lee WP, et al. Rapid publication. TGF-beta 1 induces bone closure of skull defects. J Bone Miner Res 1991;6: 1257–1265.
18. Lind M, Schumacker B, Soballe K, Keller J, Melsen F, Bunger C. Transforming growth factor-beta enhances fracture healing in rabbit tibiae. Acta Orthop Scand 1993;64: 553–556.
19. Joyce ME, Roberts AB, Sporn MB, Bolander ME. Transforming growth factor-beta and the initiation of chondrogenesis and osteogenesis in the rat femur. J Cell Biol 1990;110: 2195–2207.
20. Mohammed S, Pack AR, Kardos TB. The effect of transforming growth factor beta one (TGF-beta 1) on wound healing, with or without barrier membranes, in a Class II furcation defect in sheep. J Periodontal Res 1998;33: 335–344.
21. Ruskin JD, Hardwick R, Buser D, Dahlin C, Schenk RK. Alveolar ridge repair in a canine model using rhTGF-beta 1 with barrier membranes. Clin Oral Implants Res 2000;11: 107–115.
22. Garg AK, Gargenease D, Peace I. Using a platelet-rich plasma to develop an autologous membrane for growth factor delivery in dental implant therapy. Dent Implantol Update 2000;11:41–44.
23. Marx RE, Carlson ER, Eichstaedt RM, Schimmele SR, Strauss JE, Georgeff KR. Platelet-rich plasma: Growth factor enhancement for bone grafts. Oral Surg Oral Med Oral Pathol Oral Radiol Endod 1998;85:638–646.
24. Marx RE. Platelet-rich plasma: A source of multiple autologous growth factors for bone grafts. In: Lynch SE, Genco RJ, Marx RE (eds). Tissue Engineering: Application in Maxillofacial Surgery and Periodontics. Chicago: Quintessence, 1999:71–82.
25. Tischler M. Platelet-rich plasma. The use of autologous growth factors to enhance bone and soft tissue grafts. N Y State Dent J 2002; 68:22–24.
26. Petrungaro PS. Using platelet-rich plasma to accelerate soft tissue maturation in esthetic periodontal surgery. Compend Contin Educ Dent 2001;22:729–732, 734, 736 passim.
27. Marx RE. Clinical effects of platelet-rich plasma on soft-tissue healing. Presented at the First Symposium on Platelet-Rich Plasma and Its Growth Factors, Lake Buena Vista, FL, 28 Feb–2 Mar 2002.
28. Krauser JT. PRP and PepGen P-15: Case report on a bilateral sinus graft. Presented at the First Symposium on Platelet-Rich Plasma and Its Growth Factors, Lake Buena Vista, FL, 28 Feb–2 Mar 2002.
29. Misch DM. The use of platelet-rich plasma in oral reconstruction with dental implants. Presented at the First Symposium on Platelet-Rich Plasma and Its Growth Factors, Lake Buena Vista, FL, 28 Feb–2 Mar 2002.
30. Marx RE. Biology of platelet-rich plasma and growth factors. Presented at the First Symposium on Platelet-Rich Plasma and Its Growth Factors, Lake Buena Vista, FL, 28 Feb–2 Mar 2002.

31. Marx RE, Garg AK. Bone graft physiology with use of platelet-rich plasma and hyperbaric oxygen. In: Jensen OT (ed). The Sinus Bone Graft. Chicago: Quintessence, 1999: 183–189.
32. Bowen-Pope DF, Malpass TW, Foster DM, Ross R. Platelet-derived growth factor in vivo: Levels, activity, and rate of clearance. Blood 1984;64:458–469.
33. Wickenhauser C, Hillienhof A, Jungheim K, et al. Detection and quantification of transforming growth factor beta (TGF-beta) and platelet-derived growth factor (PDGF) release by normal human megakaryocytes. Leukemia 1995;9:310–15.
34. Ledent E, Wasteson A, Berlin G. Growth factor release during preparation and storage of platelet concentrates. Vox Sang 1995;68:205–209.
35. Hartmann K, Baier TG, Loibl R, Schmitt A, Schonberg D. Demonstration of type I insulin-like growth factor receptors on human platelets. J Recept Res 1989;9:181–198.
36. Stuart CA, Meehan RT, Neale LS, Cintron NM, Furlanetto RW. Insulin-like growth factor-I binds selectively to human peripheral blood monocytes and B-lymphocytes. J Clin Endocrinol Metab 1991;72:1117–1122.
37. Kooijman R, Willems M, De Haas CJ, et al. Expression of type I insulin-like growth factor receptors on human peripheral blood mononuclear cells. Endocrinology 1992;131:2244–2250.
38. Taylor VL, Spencer EM. Characterisation of insulin-like growth factor-binding protein-3 binding to a novel receptor on human platelet membranes. J Endocrinol 2001;168:307–315.
39. Auernhammer CJ, Fottner C, Engelhardt D, Bidlingmaier M, Strasburger CJ, Weber MM. Differential regulation of insulin-like growth factor-(IGF) I and IGF-binding protein (IGFBP) secretion by human peripheral blood mononuclear cells. Horm Res 2002;57:15–21.
40. Gope R. The effect of epidermal growth factor & platelet-derived growth factors on wound healing process. Indian J Med Res 2002;116: 201–206.
41. Muller C, Richter S, Rinas U. Kinetics control preferential heterodimer formation of platelet-derived growth factor from unfolded A- and B-chains. J Biol Chem 2003;278:18330–18335.
42. Seifert RA, Hart CE, Phillips PE, et al. Two different subunits associate to create isoform-specific platelet-derived growth factor receptors. J Biol Chem 1989;264:8771–8778.
43. Centrella M, Massague J, Canalis E. Human platelet-derived transforming growth factor-beta stimulates parameters of bone growth in fetal rat calvariae. Endocrinology 1986;119; 2306–2312.
44. Mohan S, Baylink DJ. Bone growth factors. Clin Orthop 1991;(263):30–48.
45. Lind M. Growth factors: Possible new clinical tools. A review. Acta Orthop Scand 1996;67: 407–417.
46. Lekovic V, Camargo PM, Weinlaender M, Vaslic N, Kenney EB, Madzarevic M. Comparison of platelet-rich plasma, bovine porous bone mineral, and guided tissue regeneration versus platelet-rich plasma and bovine porous bone mineral in the treatment of intrabony defects: A reentry study. J Periodontol 2002; 73:198–205.
47. Lee MB. Bone morphogenetic proteins: Background and implications for oral reconstruction. A review. J Clin Periodontol 1997;24: 255–265.
48. Reddi A, Cunningham NS. Initiation and promotion of bone differentiation by bone morphogenetic proteins. J Bone Miner Res 1993; 8(suppl 2):S499–S502.
49. Salata LA, Franke-Stenport V, Rasmusson L. Recent outcomes and perspectives of the application of bone morphogenetic proteins in implant dentistry. Clin Implant Dent Relat Res 2002;4:27–32.
50. Reddi AH. Bone morphogenesis and modeling: Soluble signals sculpt osteosomes in the solid state. Cell 1997;89:159–161.
51. Wozney JM. The potential role of bone morphogenetic proteins in periodontal reconstruction. J Periodontol 1995;66:506–510.
52. Wang EA, Rosen V, D'Alessandro JS, et al. Recombinant human bone morphogenetic protein induces bone formation. Proc Natl Acad Sci U S A 1990;87:2220–2224.
53. Urist MR. Bone: Formation by autoinduction. Science 1965;150:893–899.
54. Wang EA, Rosen V, Cordes P, et al. Purification and characterization of other distinct bone-inducing factors. Proc Natl Acad Sci U S A 1988;85:9484–9488.
55. Vehof JW, Haus MT, de Ruijter AE, Spauwen PH, Jansen JA. Bone formation in transforming growth factor beta-I-loaded titanium fiber mesh implants. Clin Oral Implants Res 2002;13:94–102.

56. Murphy WL, Mooney DJ. Controlled delivery of inductive proteins, plasmid DNA and cells from tissue engineering matrices. J Periodontal Res 1999;34:413–419.
57. van den Bergh JP, ten Bruggenkate CM, Groeneveld HH, Burger EH, Tuinzing DB. Recombinant human bone morphogenetic protein-7 in maxillary sinus floor elevation surgery in 3 patients compared to autogenous bone grafts. A clinical pilot study. J Clin Periodontol 2000;27:627–636.
58. Okubo Y, Bessho K, Fujimura K, Kusumoto K, Ogawa Y, Iizuka T. Expression of bone morphogenetic protein in the course of osteoinduction by recombinant human bone morphogenetic protein-2. Clin Oral Implants Res 2002;13:80–85.
59. Sigurdsson TJ, Lee MB, Kubota K, Turek TJ, Wozney JM, Wikesjo UM. Periodontal repair in dogs: Recombinant human bone morphogenetic protein-2 significantly enhances periodontal regeneration. J Periodontol 1995;66:131–138.
60. Nagao H, Tachikawa N, Miki T, et al. Effect of recombinant human bone morphogenetic protein-2 on bone formation in alveolar ridge defects in dogs. J Oral Maxillofac Surg 2002;31:66–72.
61. Kinoshita A, Oda S, Takahashi K, Yokota S, Ishikawa I. Periodontal regeneration by application of recombinant human bone morphogenetic protein-2 to horizontal circumferential defects created by experimental periodontitis in beagle dogs. J Periodontol 1997;68:103–109.
62. Matin K, Nakamura H, Irie K, Ozawa H, Ejiri S. Impact of recombinant human bone morphogenetic protein-2 on residual ridge resorption after tooth extraction: An experimental study in the rat. Int J Oral Maxillofac Implants 2001;16:400–411.
63. Boyne PJ, Marx RE, Nevins M, et al. A feasibility study evaluating rhBMP-2/absorbable collagen sponge for maxillary sinus augmentation. Int J Periodontics Restorative Dent 1997;17:25.
64. Nevins M, Kirker-Head C, Nevins M, Wozney JA, Palmer R, Graham D. Bone formation in the goat maxillary sinus induced by absorbable collagen sponge implants impregnated with recombinant human bone morphogenetic protein-2. Int J Periodontics Restorative Dent 1996;16:8–19.
65. Wada K, Niimi A, Watanabe K, Sawai T, Ueda M. Maxillary sinus floor augmentation in rabbits: A comparative histologic-histomorphometric study between rhBMP-2 and autogenous bone. Int J Periodontics Restorative Dent 2001;21:252–263.
66. Cochran DL, Jones AA, Lilly LC, Fiorellini JP, Howell H. Evaluation of recombinant human bone morphogenetic protein-2 in oral applications including the use of endosseous implants: 3-year results of a pilot study in humans. J Periodontol 2000;71:1241–1257.
67. Bessho K, Carnes DL, Cavin R, Chen HY, Ong JL. BMP stimulation of bone response adjacent to titanium implants in vivo. Clin Oral Implants Res 1999;10:212–218.
68. Sykaras N, Triplett RG, Nunn ME, Iacopino AM, Opperman LA. Effect of recombinant human bone morphogenetic protein-2 on bone regeneration and osseointegration of dental implants. Clin Oral Implants Res 2001;12:339–349.
69. Hanisch O, Tatakis DN, Rohrer MD, Wohrle PS, Wozney JM, Wikesjo UM. Bone formation and osseointegration stimulated by rhBMP-2 following subantral augmentation procedures in nonhuman primates. Int J Oral Maxillofac Implants 1997;12:785–792.
70. Fiorellini JP, Buser D, Riley E, Howell TH. Effect on bone healing of bone morphogenetic protein placed in combination with endosseous implants: A pilot study in beagle dogs. Int J Periodontics Restorative Dent 2001;21:41–47.
71. Sigurdsson TJ, Fu E, Tatakis DN, Rohrer MD, Wikesjo UM. Bone morphogenetic protein-2 for peri-implant bone regeneration and osseointegration. Clin Oral Implants Res 1997;8:367–374.
72. Cochran DL, Nummikoski PV, Jones AA, Makins SR, Turek TJ, Buser D. Radiographic analysis of regenerated bone around endosseous implants in the canine using recombinant human bone morphogenetic protein-2. Int J Oral Maxillofac Implants 1997;12:739–748.
73. Sigurdsson TJ, Nguyen S, Wikesjo UM. Alveolar ridge augmentation with rhBMP-2 and bone-to-implant contact in induced bone. Int J Periodontics Restorative Dent 2001;21:461–473.

74. Cochran DL, Schenk R, Buser D, Wozney JM, Jones AA. Recombinant human bone morphogenetic protein-2 stimulation of bone formation around endosseous dental implants. J Periodontol 1999;70:139–150.
75. Rutherford RB, Wahle J, Tucker M, Rueger D, Charette M. Induction of reparative dentine formation in monkeys by recombinant human osteogenic protein-1. Arch Oral Biol 1993;38:571–576.
76. Cook SD, Rueger DC. Osteogenic protein-1. Biology and applications. Clin Orthop 1996;(324):29–38.
77. Ripamonti U, Reddi AH. Growth and morphogenetic factors in bone induction: Role of osteogenin and related bone morphogenetic proteins in craniofacial and periodontal bone repair. Crit Rev Oral Biol Med 1992;3:1–14.
78. Ripamonti U, Heliotis M, Ruger DC, Sampath TK. Induction of cementogenesis by recombinant human osteogenic protein-1 (hop-1/bmp-7) in the baboon (*Papio ursinus*). Arch Oral Biol 1996;41:121–126.
79. Ripamonti U, Crooks J, Petit JC, Rueger D. Periodontal tissue regeneration by combined applications of recombinant human osteogenic protein-1 and bone morphogenetic protein-2: A pilot study in Chacma baboons (*Papio ursinus*). Eur J Oral Sci 2001;109:241–248.
80. Giannobile WV, Ryan S, Shih MS, Su DL, Kaplan PL, Chan TC. Recombinant human osteogenic protein-1 (OP-1) stimulated periodontal wound healing in class III furcation defects. J Periodontol 1998;69:129–137.
81. Groenveld HH, van den Bergh JP, Holzmann CM, ten Bruggenkate CM, Tuinzing DB, Burger EH. Histological observations of a bilateral maxillary sinus floor elevation 6 and 12 months after grafting with osteogenic protein-1 device. J Clin Periodontol 1999;26:841–846.
82. Terheyden H, Jepsen S, Moller B, Tucker MM, Rueger DC. Sinus floor augmentation with simultaneous placement of dental implants using a combination of deproteinized bone xenografts and recombinant human osteogenic protein-1. A histometric study in miniature pigs. Clin Oral Implants Res 1999;10:510–521.
83. Rutherford RB, Sampath TK, Rueger DC, Taylor TD. Use of bovine osteogenic protein to promote rapid osseointegration of endosseous dental implants. Int J Oral Maxillofac Implants 1992;7:297–301.
84. Margolin MD, Cogan AG, Taylor M, et al. Maxillary sinus augmentation in the nonhuman primate: A comparative radiographic and histologic study between recombinant human osteogenic protein-1 and natural bone mineral. J Periodontol 1998;69:911–919.
85. Terheyden H, Jepsen S, Rueger DR. Mandibular reconstruction in miniature pigs with prefabricated vascularized bone grafts using recombinant human osteogenic protein-1: A preliminary study. Int J Oral Maxillofac Surg 1999;28:461–463.
86. Terheyden H, Warnke P, Dunsche A, et al. Mandibular reconstruction with prefabricated vascularized bone grafts using recombinant human osteogenic protein-1: An experimental study in miniature pigs. Part II: Transplantation. Int J Oral Maxillofac Surg 2001;30:469–478.
87. Baum BJ, Kok M, Tran SD, Yamano S. The impact of gene therapy on dentistry: A revisiting after six years. J Am Dent Assoc 2002;133:35–44.
88. Krebsbach PH, Gu K, Franceschi RT, Rutherford RB. Gene therapy-directed osteogenesis: BMP-7–transduced human fibroblasts form bone in vivo. Hum Gene Ther 2000;11:1201–1210.
89. Oakes DA, Lieberman JR. Osteoinductive applications of regional gene therapy: Ex vivo gene transfer. Clin Orthop 2000;(379 suppl):S101–S112.
90. Alden TD, Beres EJ, Laurent JS, et al. The use of bone morphogenetic protein gene therapy in craniofacial bone repair. J Craniofac Surg 2000;11:24–30.

Index

Page numbers followed by "t" denote tables; those followed by "f" denote figures

B

C

O

P

R

S

T

U

V

W

X